Parasites in Human Tissues

We dedicate this book to the memory of our mentor,

the late Professor Paul Chester Beaver.

His vision, dedication, and direction still serve as an inspiration to those of us who studied under him.

Parasites in Human Tissues

Thomas C. Orihel, PhD
William Vincent Professor of Tropical Diseases
Department of Tropical Medicine
School of Public Health and Tropical Medicine
Tulane University
New Orleans, LA

Lawrence R. Ash, PhD
Professor of Infectious and Tropical Diseases
Department of Epidemiology
School of Public Health
University of California, Los Angeles
Los Angeles, CA

ASCP PRESS

American Society of Clinical Pathologists
Chicago, IL

Publishing Team
Jennifer Schima (editorial)
Renee Kastar (marketing)
Michael Methe (design/production)
Joshua Weikersheimer (publishing direction)

Plate 8:1 was reproduced from the *American Journal of Veterinary Research* (1981;42:1400).
Plate 8:2 was reproduced from *Microbiological Reviews* (1983;47:84).
Plate 20:1 was reproduced from *Acta Cytologica* (1989;33:557).
Plate 20:3 was reproduced from the *Journal of Histotechnology* (1991;14:1799).
4 **was reproduced from *Acta Cytologica* (1987;32:491).**
12 **was reproduced from *The Laboratory Diagnosis of Infectious Diseases, Vol. I.* 1988: 929.**
18 **was reproduced from the *Annals of Internal Medicine* (1987:106:396).**

Notice
Trade names and equipment and supplies described herein are included as suggestions only. In no way does their inclusion constitute an endorsement or preference by the American Society of Clinical Pathologists. The ASCP did not test the equipment, supplies, or procedures and, therefore, urges all readers to read and follow all manufacturers' instructions and package insert warnings concerning the proper and safe use of products.

Library of Congress Cataloging in Publication Data
Orihel, Thomas C.
Parasites in Human Tissues/Thomas C. Orihel, Lawrence R. Ash.
p. cm.
Includes bibliographical references and index.
ISBN 0-89189-379-2
1. Parasitic diseases—Diagnosis. 2. Parasites—Identification.
I. Ash, Lawrence R. II. Title.
[DNLM: 1. Parasites—atlases. 2. Parasitic Diseases—diagnosis—atlases. QZ 17 069p 1994]
RC119.075 1994
616.9'6—dc20
DNLM/DLC 94-22474
for Library of Congress CIP

Printed in Hong Kong

99 98 97 96 95 5 4 3 2 1

"What I wish here to emphasize is that
a correct knowledge of the diseases of man caused
by worms, and all that is connected with them,
is the more difficult to attain the more
the parasites of animals are ignored."

Arthur Looss, 1911

Table of Contents

Preface

Our goal in the preparation of this book is to provide pathologists, research scientists, and others working in clinical and diagnostic settings with a comprehensive guide to the identification of parasites encountered in human tissues.

The number of parasites found in human tissues is much greater than one might realize. Several common parasites, as adults or larvae, are sequestered in the tissues and consequently are rarely encountered, poorly described, and not easily identified. There are other species, ordinarily rare parasites of humans, that have become opportunistic pathogens in immunocompromised or immunodeficient hosts and about which we know very little. Additionally, people who have exotic food preferences or who travel to tropical regions where parasitic diseases are endemic frequently acquire parasitic infections that are rarely seen or recognized in temperate climates.

Zoonotic parasites contribute substantially to the list of parasites found in human tissues, and the number of new ones increases each year. Medical parasitologists and pathologists are less familiar with these new species, and although they are readily found in the tissues, specific identification is usually a problem. Again, published descriptions of the microanatomy of these parasites are rare. Although in some instances their morphological features in host tissues have been described, details are meager and descriptions are often buried in the zoological literature.

Just as objects that mimic parasite stages are found in feces and in blood, there are also nonparasitic elements in tissues that must be differentiated from parasites. We have made an effort to introduce the microscopist to some of these nonparasitic elements, but it is impossible to describe the full range of possibilities.

The number of investigators who devote their time to this aspect of parasitology are few, and there are few repositories for slide collections of parasites in tissues. Fortunately, we had access to institutional collections as well as our own personal collections. Colleagues from around the world provided additional materials, enabling us to obtain a fairly complete assemblage of tissue parasites. As a consequence, we feel that our guide to parasites that have been encountered in human tissues is reasonably comprehensive. This book includes approximately 700 color photomicrographs of organisms in histologic sections; the accompanying text summarizes the biology and life histories of these organisms as well as their clinical presentations and pathology. Our goal is to assist the reader in making a diagnosis and to provide some insight as to how infections might be acquired.

Our account of each parasite or group of parasites is not exhaustive. In many cases the reader may wish to look at original case reports or review articles for additional information. We provide references at the end of each presentation, but they are limited to those sources that offer the most useful and current information on the morphology and identification of each parasite. Because some of the opportunistic protozoan parasites have become very important clinically in recent years, we provide more references pertaining to them, especially very current sources that deal with morphology and diagnosis.

We believe that this work will complement our earlier ***Atlas of Human Parasitology,*** which offered a comprehensive guide to the identification of parasites found in feces, blood, and urine. Hopefully, the information presented in the two texts will enhance the capacity of pathologists, clinicians, technologists, and researchers to identify parasites that invade the human body.

Thomas C. Orihel
Lawrence R. Ash
1995

Many of the clinical images that appear in this book were obtained from colleagues from around the world. The names of these individuals are listed below. References to clinical images consist of a symbol (➡) and a number.

➡ **3** courtesy of L.M. Sloan.
➡ **11** courtesy of D. LePay.
➡ **13** courtesy of W.A. Krotoski.
➡ **15** courtesy of F. Martinez, Cali, Colombia.
➡ **22** courtesy of Y. Yazaki, Asahikawa, Japan.
➡ **27** courtesy of A.M. Polderman, Leiden, Holland.
➡ **28** courtesy of P. Morera, San Jose, Costa Rica.
➡ **31** courtesy of M.D. Little.
➡ **36** courtesy of R.C. Lowrie, Jr.
➡ **42** courtesy of R. Javier Vasquez, Panama.
➡ **46** courtesy of M.L. Eberhard.
➡ **48** courtesy of AFIP.
➡ **55** courtesy of L. Measures, Mont-Joli, Canada.
➡ **64** courtesy of J.H. Smith.
➡ **68** courtesy of J.H. Smith.
➡ **70** courtesy of K. Yamashita, Ube, Japan.
➡ **77** courtesy of M.L. Eberhard.
➡ **78** courtesy of G. Baskin.
➡ **79** courtesy of P.E. Newman.
➡ **82 & 83** courtesy of A. Lopez-Villegas and A. D'Alessandro, Cali, Colombia.
➡ **85** courtesy of A.D.M. Bryceson, London, England.

Acknowledgements

Many colleagues have contributed to the preparation of this book. In addition to the personal collections of the authors, a substantial portion of the slide materials used in the preparation of the images are housed in the laboratories of the Department of Tropical Medicine at Tulane University School of Public Health and Tropical Medicine. They were drawn from the collection of the late Paul C. Beaver, who accumulated slide materials over a period of almost 35 years. Slides were sent to Professor Beaver by scores of investigators who sought his expertise in the identification of parasites found in tissues submitted for diagnosis. Unfortunately, it is not possible to name each of these contributors.

In addition, significant amounts of parasite material were contributed to the collection by the faculty of the departments of Tropical Medicine and Parasitology, including A. D'Alessandro, J. Esslinger, R. Jung, M.D. Little, and R. Yaeger, and the departments of pathology in the Medical Center and the Tulane Regional Primate Research Center. Parasitology graduate students also made important contributions to the collection over the years.

In several instances, we obtained specimens from the parasite collections housed in the United States National Museum Parasite Collection (ARS/USDA) in Beltsville, Maryland, and the Armed Forces Institute of Pathology in Washington, D.C. We are indebted to the curators of these collections for their generous assistance.

The remainder of contributions came from colleagues all over the world who, upon request, generously provided us with the specific parasite materials from which we have generated the images published here. Although it is always difficult to try to list every person who has provided help, we shall attempt to be as complete as possible. If any contributor's name has been inadvertently omitted, our gratitude is no less sincere and we are certainly most appreciative of their assistance. We are extremely grateful to each of the following: H. Akahane, J. Alroy, E.M. Andersen, K. Ando, A.P. Anzil, F. Ardoin, M.J. Arrowood, K. Baird, A.R. Barr, M. Bartlett, C.M. Bedrossian, D. Bowman, R. Bryan, A. Bryceson, E.U. Canning, J.Y. Chai, A. Cheever, T.M. Chesney, S.Y. Cho, F. Cogswell, K. Cove, J.H. Cross, A. Curry, D. Despommier, O. Ditrich, J.P. Dubey, G. Dutton, M.L. Eberhard, W.J. Foreyt, J.K. Frenkel, B. Furner, C.A. Garcia, C.H. Gardiner, B.G. Gazzard, M. Grady, I. Greene, J.R. Greenwood, M. Grossman, Y. Gutierrez, C. Harbut, E.L. Howes, W. H. Hutchinson, H. Isaacs, M. Kearney, H. Kim, H. Kutsumi, D. LePay, J.R. Lichtenfels, S.B. Lucas, W. Margaretten, A.J. Martinez, A. Marty, W. Mason, J. Mead, L. Measures, H. Mehlhorn, E. Mendoza, I. Miyazaki, P. Morera, R. Neafie, R. Orozco-Florian, T. Oshima, R. Pamphlett, S. Pampiglione, C. Panosian, J.C. Petithory, P. Pfitzer, A. Polderman, A.K. Purohit, J. Remington, B. Rodriguez, L. Rosen, F. Roussel, M. Scaglia, D.A. Schwartz, S. Siegel, J.H. Smith, J.W. Smith, M. Sohn, T. Sun, I. Tada, W. Travis, C.H. Tse, J. Turner, M. Valkounova, G. Visvesvara, M. Voge (deceased), R. Weber, L.H. Weiland, M. Wittner, K. Yamashita, Y. Yazaki, C. Yii, Y. Yoshida, and M. Zeuthen.

In addition to the individuals listed above who contributed microscopic slide material for our use, we are pleased to acknowledge other colleagues who have most generously provided us with 2 x 2 transparencies that we use directly in the text. Many of these illustrations are unique and are of clinical material that otherwise would have been unavailable to us. For these photographs we acknowledge the individual and the publication source if the material has been previously published.

Sincere appreciation is extended to the staff of the UCLA Louise Darling Biomedical Library, in particular Mrs. Marie Saito, for their help in providing access to the scientific literature.

The authors also wish to thank Dr. Jackeline Alger, who assisted in the preparation of the manuscript, and Nora Comiskey, who generously gave her time to proofreading the manuscript.

A special note of thanks goes to Dr. Mark Eberhard, who painstakingly reviewed the manuscript and offered many valuable criticisms that were much appreciated.

Finally, we would like to acknowledge the staff of the ASCP Press and the excellent support they gave us. In particular, we wish to thank Joshua Weikersheimer, director of the ASCP Press, for his advice on the preparation of the manuscript and for the enormous amount of effort he put into preparing the color separations for this book. He and his editing team also handled the large volume of text and legend material in an excellent fashion.

Introduction

Parasites take an enormous toll on human health and the quality of life in societies throughout the world. The list of the major parasitic diseases of medical importance is modest in size and includes, most prominently, malaria, amebiasis, soil-transmitted nematodiases (ascariasis, trichuriasis, and hookworm disease), schistosomiases, filariases, leishmaniases, and trypanosomiases. Additionally, with the emergence of the acquired immunodeficiency syndrome (AIDS), a number of parasitic diseases previously thought to be of minor health importance or not known at all are now recognized as the cause of significant human disease (eg, cryptosporidiosis, microsporidiosis).

The perception that only a limited number of parasite species infect people, particularly in the more advanced and developed regions of the world, is an illusion. Coombs and Crompton (1991) compiled a listing of well over 300 species of helminths alone that have been recorded from humans. Even though many of these are rare, there is the need to recognize and accurately identify these parasites regardless of the frequency with which they are found. As stated so frequently, the world is a much smaller place because of the efficiency of modern transportation. People can be exposed to a myriad of parasitic infections in far-off places and are not diagnosed until they return home. "Exotic" parasites also enter this country in their immigrant hosts and often become a medical problem only after their arrival.

The parasitologist or pathologist has ready access to most of the parasites that inhabit the digestive tract and the organs that communicate with it (eg, the liver, lung). Consequently, these parasites are well described and easily identified without the need to examine them in tissue sections. However, there are numerous helminth species that are tissue parasites and are rarely encountered in their adult stages (eg, filarial worms in lymphatics, schistosomes in blood vessels). In other words, the adult parasites may be fairly well described, but because of their limited geographical distribution they are rarely found in histopathological specimens outside endemic areas and may pose diagnostic problems for all except the most experienced parasitologists or pathologists.

There is a much larger group of parasite species, the majority of which are nematode parasites of animals, that accidentally infect humans worldwide. Unfortunately, this group of parasites, with the possible exception of the etiologic agents of cutaneous and visceral larva migrans, is rarely addressed in parasitology or infectious disease textbooks. These zoonotic infections result from transmisssion by a vector, ingestion of infective stages in improperly cooked foods, or exposure to other contaminated or infected substances. Most of these infections tend to be cryptic (ie, nonpatent) and sometimes are asymptomatic. The parasites may undergo considerable growth and development over periods of weeks or months and then die in the tissues, often without provoking a significant host inflammatory response. On the other hand, a few cause symptoms almost immediately (*Anisakis, Eustrongylides*), while others manifest chronic symptoms of cutaneous or visceral larva migrans (*Ancylostoma braziliense, Gnathostoma* species). More often than not, the parasites die in the tissues and degenerate, resulting in the loss of important morphological features, which seriously hinders identification.

The protozoa often pose difficult diagnostic problems even among the species that are well known to us. In addition, there are other species that invade human tissues that are relatively new to us and have been described only in recent years (eg, *Naegleria fowleri, Acanthamoeba* species, *Balamuthia mandrillaris*). The tissue stages of several coccidian parasites (*Cryptosporidium* species, *Toxoplasma gondii, Neospora caninum, Sarcocystis* species) also have been described only recently or, in some cases, they are still unknown. Other organisms, such as the microsporidia, are of such small size that standard histological preparations are inadequate for diagnosis and one must resort to electron microscopy or the use of specialized staining techniques.

One also must not overlook the invasion of human tissues by a wide variety of arthropods. Only a very few species (eg, *Sarcoptes, Demodex*) are obligate parasites, but many others infest the human tissues as part of their life cycle and may cause typically transitory but sometimes very serious disease (eg, cutaneous- and ophthalmo-myiasis). Although under ordinary circumstances most of these can be identified from the recovery of the intact organisms, many others are subjected to histopathologic examination. Our coverage would have been incomplete without a discussion of the arthropods that may invade human tissues.

Unfortunately, in addition to the wide range of parasites that one might expect to encounter in the tissues, there are also nonparasite objects that, because of their structural form and vague similarity to parasites, are often confused with parasites. We have provided a sampling of these, which we discuss under artifacts.

The gross morphologic features of virtually all parasites are sufficiently described to establish their taxonomic status. However, their microscopic morphological structure is less well known. There is an ongoing series of publications, **Microscopic Anatomy of Invertebrates** (Harrison, 1991-1993), that provides very useful information on the microscopic anatomy of groups that include parasites and other invertebrate organisms. Volumes of particular relevance to our presentations are cited where appropriate.

The protozoa, because of their size and their unicellular nature, are among the best-characterized parasite species.

Among the helminths, the nematodes have received the most attention with respect to anatomical studies at the microscopic level. The early work of the Chitwoods (1950) and the recent work of the Birds (1992) have provided considerable knowledge and insight into the organization and structure of the nematodes per se.

To date, there has not been a comprehensive effort to focus on the identification of parasites found in sections of human tissues or to provide key morphological criteria for their recognition. Parasites in human tissues have been reviewed in the literature largely in terms of the pathological processes associated with their presence. Two publications, Binford and Connor's **Pathology of Tropical and Extraordinary Diseases**, published in 1976, and Gutierrez's **Diagnostic Pathology of Parasitic Infections with Clinical Correlation**, published in 1990, provide substantial details on parasite morphology, but their primary emphasis is on a description of the pathology produced by the organisms. Chitwood and Lichtenfels (1972) made the initial effort to provide morphologic criteria for the identification of metazoan parasites found in the tissues of vertebrate hosts. Their extensively illustrated account concentrated on parasites of animals and excluded the protozoa.

Professor Paul C. Beaver at Tulane University has been the acknowledged leader in the study of natural and zoonotic parasites encountered in human tissues. Over a period of four decades (the 1950s to the 1990s), he and his colleagues published numerous individual studies of the morphology of various zoonotic parasites, stressing their diagnostic features.

This present work is limited in its scope to parasite species that have been recovered from human tissues. It focuses on the identification of the parasites based on morphologic features evident in histopathological materials that often may provide only limited material of varying quality for study. We have provided brief accounts of each parasite's life history, because such information may be relevant in establishing how particular infections are acquired. Geographic distribution is mentioned because many parasites have well-defined geographical ranges, and unless an individual has traveled to or resided within an endemic or enzootic zone, infection with the parasite is unlikely. We felt it was important to provide an overview of the clinical manifestations and pathology that each parasite might produce so that the reader can relate them to previously described symptomatology for the same or similar parasites. Finally, details of both the gross and microscopic morphology of the parasites are presented, along with differential features that might be useful in separating organisms that have similar morphologic features.

The illustrations provided have been made from human cases on file in the Tulane University collection, from the authors' personal collections, and from materials provided by colleagues in the United States and abroad. Some illustrations were prepared from parasites collected from their natural hosts rather than from humans, but they represent species that infect humans. Because the slide material available to us was prepared in many different laboratories, variation in the types and qualities of the stain used, especially Hematoxylin and Eosin, will be evident; but we feel that the important structures are clear nonetheless.

We have attempted to provide the best illustrations possible. Many may seem idealized, but they do illustrate structural features better than what one might see in badly degenerating parasites or parasites cut in awkward planes that would be far more difficult to interpret. We have included some illustrations that are less than ideal in order to give the reader some idea of the types of materials that may be offered for diagnosis and the difficulties that may arise in interpreting such materials. Virtually all of our photomicrographs were taken using ordinary brightfield microscopy. We have included some electron photomicrographs (kindly provided by colleagues) when light microscopy did not provide sufficient magnification to readily visualize the parasites, as was true of the microsporidia.

The space that could be devoted to individual parasites was limited, and in some instances our treatment may seem uneven. In some cases the limited information available on a particular organism or its overall importance as a human infection were considerations. However, parasites such as the filarial worms received extensive coverage because not only do they turn up with great frequency, but a wide variety of both human and zoonotic species are found in the tissues of people throughout the world. We have attempted to be judicious in our selection of photomicrographs so as to give a range of the essential morphologic features of the parasites presented. We often had a large number of images from which to select, but size limitations precluded the possibility of showing "everything" about each parasite.

Binford CH, Connor DH. *Pathology of Tropical and Extraordinary Diseases: An Atlas, Vols. I and II.* Washington, DC: Armed Forces Institute of Pathology, 1976.

Bird AF, Bird J. *The Structure of Nematodes.* 2nd ed. San Diego, Calif: Academic Press Inc, 1991.

Chitwood BG, Chitwood MB. *An Introduction to Nematology.* Baltimore, Md: Monumental Printing Co, 1950.

Chitwood MB, Lichtenfels JR. Identification of parasitic metazoa in tissue sections. *Exp Parasitol.* 1972;32:407-519.

Coombs I, Crompton DWT. *A Guide to Human Helminths.* London: Taylor and Francis, 1990.

Gutierrez, Y. *Diagnostic Pathology of Parasitic Infections with Clinical Correlations.* Philadelphia, Pa: Lea and Febiger, 1990.

Parasite Identification

The identification of parasites in human tissues is not an easy task due to the wide variety of organisms encountered, including protozoans, a large and diverse array of helminths (nematodes, trematodes, cestodes), pentastomes, acanthocephalans, and arthropods. Additionally, some free-living species of protozoa and nematodes assume the role of opportunistic parasites and invade human tissues. Their identification can be further complicated by artifacts that resemble parasites in tissue.

Often a diagnostician is provided with only a single slide, with no prospect for additional ones and minimal clinical information regarding the circumstances that prompted medical intervention. A parasite's orientation and poor condition can make identification even more difficult.

Before attempting an identification, it is important to gather as much information as possible about the patient—recent health problems, symptomatology, place of residence, travel history, typical or unusual food preferences, outdoor activities, and unusual environmental exposures. The tissue site from which the lesion was removed is crucial as well.

The general microscopic anatomic features of each of the major groups of parasites are sufficiently different that it is possible, with the aid of a few key morphologic features, to place most of the parasites encountered into one of the following groups:

Protozoa: Protozoans are unicellular organisms with one or more nuclei and various organelles. Trophozoite and cyst stages may be present.

Nematoda: Nematodes have a body cavity (pseudocoelom); a well-developed body wall consisting of a cuticle that may bear striations, annulations, or other surface modifications; and a thin hypodermis that typically has dorsal, ventral, and lateral chords and well-developed, longitudinally oriented, smooth muscles. The body cavity contains the digestive tube and tubular gonads. The sexes are separate.

Trematoda: These organisms lack a body cavity. The body surface (tegument) may be smooth or spinous. Longitudinal, circular, and diagonal smooth muscle fibers are embedded in the parenchymatous matrix of the body. The digestive system consists of a pharynx and tubular intestinal ceca. These organisms are typically hermaphroditic, except for the schistosomes. Trematodes usually have two suckers. Gonads are sacculate.

Cestoda: The tapeworms lack a body cavity and a digestive system. The tegument is smooth. Longitudinal and circular smooth muscle fibers are embedded in the parenchymatous matrix. These organisms are hermaphroditic. The presence of calcareous corpuscles in the epidermis is diagnostic for this group.

Acanthocephala: Acanthocephalans have a body cavity (pseudocoelom), a thick, multilayered tegument that contains the lacunar system, and both circular and longitudinal muscles. Typically, an eversible, spinous proboscis is present. These organisms lack a digestive system. Sexes are separate, and eggs are often free in the pseudocoelom.

Pentastoma: Pentastome organisms have an elongate, cylindrical, or flattened body with many pseudosegments. The body cavity is present but may be reduced. The cuticle may or may not have spines; a pitlike sclerotized opening is present. The organism does not separate into head, thorax, and abdomen. The anterior extremity has a median subterminal mouth and two pairs of hollow, retractile hooks. Distinctive acidophilic glands are present. Larval stages typically parasitize humans, but adults do not.

Arthropoda: Arthropods have a body cavity, a chitinized or sclerotized body wall, and jointed appendages. Striated muscles, a well-developed digestive tract, malpighian tubules, and respiratory tracheae are present. Sexes are separate. Dipteran larvae (maggots) have sclerotized hooks on the anterior end, with respiratory tracheae and paired, platelike spiracles on the posterior end.

In the introduction to each of the major groups of parasites, we discuss and illustrate the group's characteristic morphologic features and the range of variation that exists among its members. This additional information should enable the reader to confirm an impression or preliminary diagnosis, a process that may be difficult if the organism is dead and has undergone some degree of degeneration. The identification process can be made easier, however, if the parasite's tissue preference, clinical presentation, and symptomatology are considered in addition to morphology.

A series of quick reference guides (Tables 1–4) indicate the usual tissue sites in which each parasite is characteristically found, occasionally found, and rarely encountered. These reference guides are more general than specific and are not the "last word." Almost any of these parasites may at some time be found in sites other than those indicated.

Key references, the most current ones available to us, dealing with the morphology and/or biology of particular parasites are listed at the end of each presentation. At the end of the book, there is a list of texts, books, and monographs dealing with groups of parasites. Again, we have chosen those publications that focus on parasite morphology rather than on diseases that the parasites cause.

Finally, you may want to look at other parasites from human or animal tissues for comparative purposes. You can contact investigators who have worked with particular parasite groups or curators of helminth collections (eg, Biosystematic Parasitology Laboratory, USDA, Beltsville, Maryland, and the Harold W. Manter Laboratory, University of Nebraska, Lincoln, Nebraska). Human tissues that contain organisms posing diagnostic problems can be sent to the Armed Forces Institute of Pathology, Washington, DC; the Parasitic Diseases Branch, Centers for Disease Control and Prevention, Atlanta, Georgia; or laboratories such as ours at Tulane University and the University of California, Los Angeles.

Table 1. Quick reference to locations of protozoan parasites in human tissues.

Parasite	Stage	Skin, Subcutaneous	Muscle	Brain, Meninges, Spinal Chord	Lungs, Pulmonary Vessels	Heart	Liver, Gall Bladder	Kidneys, Pancreas	Stomach	Small Intestine, Appendix
Amebae										
Entamoeba histolytica	T	Secondary site		Rare localization	Secondary site	Rare localization	Secondary site	Secondary site		Secondary site
Acanthamoeba species	T/C	Usual site		Usual site	Rare localization					
Balamuthia mandrillus	T/C			Usual site						
Naegleria fowleri	T			Usual site						
Flagellates										
Giardia lamblia	T									Usual site
Leishmania species	A	Usual site					Usual site			
Trypanosoma cruzi	A		Secondary site	Secondary site		Usual site			Rare localization	Rare localization
Ciliates										
Balantidium coli	T									Usual site
Apicomplexans										
Cryptosporidium species	O				Secondary site		Secondary site		Usual site	Usual site
Isospora belli	O				Rare localization					Usual site
Sarcocystis species	CO		Usual site			Usual site				Usual site
Toxoplasma gondii	CO	Secondary site		Usual site	Usual site	Usual site	Secondary site	Secondary site		Secondary site
Neospora species	CO			Usual site						
Plasmodium species	M						Secondary site			
Microspora										
Enterocytozoon bienusi	S				Secondary site		Secondary site	Secondary site		Usual site
Encephalitozoon species	S				Secondary site		Secondary site	Secondary site		Usual site
Septata intestinalis	S				Secondary site		Secondary site	Secondary site		Usual site
Pleistophora species	S		Usual site							
Nosema species	S		Usual site							
Protozoa/Fungus										
Pneumocystis carinii	T/C	Secondary site			Usual site		Secondary site	Secondary site		Secondary site

A = Amastigote
C = Cyst
CO = Coccidian stages
S = Spores and associated microsporidial stages
M = Malarial parasites
T = Trophozoite

(light shading) = Usual site (dark shading) = Secondary site (medium shading) = Rare localization

Colon	Lymph Nodes, Lymphatics	Peritoneal Cavity, Mesenteries	Female Reproductive System	Male Reproductive System	Bladder, Ureters	Eye, Orbit	Bloodstream, Vessels	Buccal Cavity	Spleen, R.E. System	Bone, Bone Marrow	Reference (page)

Table 2. Quick reference to locations of nematode parasites in human tissues.

Parasite	Stage	Skin, Subcutaneous	Muscle	Brain, Meninges, Spinal Chord	Lungs, Pulmonary Vessels	Heart	Liver, Gall Bladder	Kidneys, Pancreas	Stomach	Small Intestine, Appendix
Ascaris lumbricoides	A/L									
Toxocara canis	L									
Toxocara cati	L									
Baylisascaris procyonis	L									
Lagochilascaris species	A/L									
Anisakis species	L									
Pseudoterranova decipiens	L									
Enterobius vermicularis	A									
Ancylostoma duodenale	A/L									
Ancylostoma species	L									
Necator americanus	A/L									
Oesophagostomum species	A/L									
Mammomonogamus species	A									
Angiostrongylus cantonensis	A									
Angiostrongylus costaricensis	A									
Gnathostoma species	L									
Gongylonema species	A									
Rictularia species	A									
Physaloptera species	A									
Thelazia species	A									
Spirocerca species	A									

A = Adult
L = Larva

= Usual site   = Secondary site   = Rare localization

Colon	Lymph Nodes, Lymphatics	Peritoneal Cavity, Mesenteries	Female Reproductive System	Male Reproductive System	Bladder, Ureters	Eye, Orbit	Bloodstream, Vessels	Buccal Cavity	Spleen, R.E. System	Bone, Bone Marrow	Reference (Page)

Table 3. Quick reference to locations of nematode parasites and acanthocephalans in human tissues.

Parasite	Stage	Skin, Subcutaneous	Muscle	Brain, Meninges, Spinal Chord	Lungs, Pulmonary Vessels	Heart	Liver, Gall Bladder	Kidneys, Pancreas	Stomach	Small Intestine, Appendix
Wuchereria bancrofti	A*				Rare localization					
Brugia malayi	A				Rare localization					
Brugia species (zoonotic)	A				Rare localization					
Onchocerca volvulus	A	Usual site								
Onchocerca species (zoonotic)	A	Usual site								
Loa loa	A	Usual site								
Mansonella perstans	A									
Mansonella streptocerca	A	Usual site								
Mansonella ozzardi	A	Usual site								
Dirofilaria immitis	A	Rare localization			Usual site	Secondary site				
Dirofilaria repens	A	Usual site			Rare localization					
Dirofilaria species	A	Usual site								
Meningonema peruzzii	A			Usual site						
Loaina species	A									
Dracunculus medinensis	A	Usual site		Rare localization						
Strongyloides stercoralis	A / L	L: Rare localization			L: Secondary site		L: Rare localization	L: Rare localization		Usual site
Pelodera strongyloides	L	Usual site								
Halicephalobus deletrix	A / L			Usual site		Rare localization				
Trichuris trichiura	A									Secondary site
Trichinella spiralis	A / L		L: Usual site	L: Rare localization						A: Usual site
Capillaria philippinensis	A									Usual site
Capillaria aerophila	A				Usual site					
Capillaria hepatica	A						Usual site			
Anatrichosoma species	A	Usual site								
Dioctophyme renale	A / L	L: Usual site						A: Usual site		
Eustrongylides species	L								Usual site	Usual site
Acanthocephala	A									Usual site

*Includes immature adults of filariae.
Microfilariae not considered.

A = Adult
L = Larva

Light grey = Usual site; Dark grey = Secondary site; Dark grey = Rare localization

Colon	Lymph Nodes, Lymphatics	Peritoneal Cavity, Mesenteries	Female Reproductive System	Male Reproductive System	Bladder, Ureters	Eye, Orbit	Bloodstream, Vessels	Buccal Cavity	Spleen, R.E. System	Bone, Bone Marrow	Reference (Page)

Table 4. Quick reference to locations of cestode and trematode parasites in human tissues.

Parasite	Stage	Skin, Subcutaneous	Muscle	Brain, Meninges, Spinal Chord	Lungs, Pulmonary Vessels	Heart	Liver, Gall Bladder	Kidneys, Pancreas	Stomach	Small Intestine, Appendix
Cestodes										
Coenurus/*Taenia* species	L	Usual	Usual	Usual						
Cysticercus/*Taenia solium*	L	Usual	Usual	Usual		Secondary				
Hydatid/Alveolar	L			Secondary	Secondary		Usual			
Hydatid/Unilocular	L		Rare	Secondary	Usual	Rare	Usual	Rare		
Sparganum	L	Usual	Usual	Secondary	Rare	Rare				
Mesocestoides species	L									
Trematodes										
Heterophyids	A/E					Rare (partial)				Usual
Clonorchis/Opisthorchis	A/E						Usual			
Fasciola/Fascioloides	A/E	Rare					Usual			
Paragonimus species	A/E	Rare	Rare (partial)	Rare	Usual					
Schistosoma mansoni	A/E			Rare (partial)			Secondary			
Schistosoma haematobium	A/E									
Schistosoma japonicum	A/E			Rare (partial)	Rare		Secondary			Rare (partial)
Alaria species	L	Usual								
Philophthalmus species	A									
Arthropods										
Demodex species	A/L	Usual								
Sarcoptes scabiei	A/L	Usual								
Cordylobia species	L	Usual	Usual							
Gasterophilus species	L	Usual					Rare			Secondary
Dermatobia species	L	Usual								
Oestrus ovis	L	Usual								
Hypoderma species	L	Usual								
Cuterebra species	L	Usual								
Tunga penetrans	A	Usual								
Pentastoma	L				Usual		Usual			

A = Adult
L = Larva
E = Eggs

[light grey] = Usual site [dark grey] = Secondary site [medium grey] = Rare localization

Colon	Lymph Nodes, Lymphatics	Peritoneal Cavity, Mesenteries	Female Reproductive System	Male Reproductive System	Bladder, Ureters	Eye, Orbit	Bloodstream, Vessels	Buccal Cavity	Spleen, R.E. System	Bone, Bone Marrow	Reference (Page)

Parasites in Human Tissues

Diagnostic Text and Images

Protozoa

Protozoans are single-celled organisms. Approximately 45,000 species of protozoans have been described, most of which are free living in the soil, water, and other moist environments. We focus on those species that are obligate or opportunistic parasites and cause human disease.

Protozoan Relationships

From a taxonomic perspective, the protozoa are a large and extremely diverse group of organisms. They are classified into six separate phyla (Lee et al, 1985), four of which are of medical importance. Considerable controversy still exists about protozoa classification, which will probably continue to change as new information comes to light.

Phylum Sarcomastigophora

This large group includes the amebae and flagellates. They have one or more nuclei and may have flagella, pseudopodia, or, in some instances, both.

Subphylum Sarcodina

This group includes both commensal and parasitic amebae of humans that are characterized by having pseudopodia. Flagella, if present, usually occur only temporarily. Asexual reproduction is by binary fission. We discuss *Entamoeba histolytica, Acanthamoeba* species, *Balamuthia mandrillaris,* and *Naegleria fowleri.*

Subphylum Mastigophora

The intestinal, blood, and tissue flagellates are members of this group. Typically, they have one or more flagella in the trophozoite stage. Asexual reproduction is by binary fission. Important human parasites of this group include *Giardia lamblia, Leishmania* species, and *Trypanosoma* species.

Phylum Ciliophora

Although this phylum comprises a large number of organisms, only one species parasitizes humans. These organisms have cilia, micronuclei, and macronuclei. They reproduce asexually by binary fission. *Balantidium coli* is the only ciliate we discuss.

Phylum Apicomplexa

These organisms have an apical complex consisting of a series of organelles (micronemes, rhoptries, conoid, and others). Medically important organisms all belong to the Class Sporozoea.

Class Sporozoea

These organisms generally reproduce by both sexual and asexual processes. Oocysts contain infective sporozoites produced by sporogony. Within the Subclass Coccidia are two suborders of medical importance.

1. Eimeriina: In this group, sporozoites typically are enclosed in a sporocyst within an oocyst. These coccidians may have direct or indirect life cycles. The species considered here include *Cryptosporidium parvum, Isospora belli, Sarcocystis* species, *Toxoplasma gondii,* and *Neospora caninum.*

2. Haemosporina: Members of this group have naked sporozoites and motile zygotes (ookinetes). They reproduce by merogony in vertebrate hosts and sporogony in invertebrate hosts. They are transmitted by blood-sucking arthropods. The human malarial parasites, *Plasmodium* species, are the only members of this group that we discuss.

Phylum Microspora

The intracellular parasites of this phylum characteristically have unicellular spores that contain uninucleate or binucleate sporoplasm and have a simple or complex extrusion apparatus with a polar tube. Species that infect humans include *Enterocytozoon bieneusi, Encephalitozoon* species, *Septata intestinalis, Pleistophora* species, and *Nosema* species.

Species of Uncertain Classification

The taxonomic position of *Pneumocystis carinii* remains unsettled. It has features of both fungi and protozoa, but agreement has yet to be attained on its precise classification.

Protozoan Morphology

The protozoa exhibit great diversity morphologically as well as taxonomically. In general, however, all protozoans possess organelles that are similar to those found in metazoan cells. Protozoans are typical eukaryotic organisms. The cell is bounded by a limiting membrane, which is also referred to as a plasma membrane or a pellicle. The cytoplasm is characteristically composed of an ectoplasm and endoplasm, the latter containing the nucleus. Vesicular nuclei are most commonly seen in the parasitic protozoa. In the amebae, these nuclei often contain a small to large karyosome (sometimes inaccurately referred to as a nucleolus or an endosome), which consists of densely packed, DNA-containing chromatin material that is Feulgen positive. Organelles of locomotion include flagella (found in intestinal and blood flagellates), cilia (occurring in *Balantidium coli*), and pseudopodia (temporary extrusions of cytoplasm in the amebae that aid in both locomotion and the feeding process). Reproduction in the amebae, flagellates, and ciliates is an asexual process, usually by binary fission. Most of the intestinal amebae, the flagellates, and the sole ciliate parasite have trophozoite and cyst stages. The cyst stage is the resistant stage that can survive in the external environment and the infective stage for the next host.

The largest group of organisms of medical importance fall within the Phylum Apicomplexa. All of these forms have a complicated set of organelles that form an apical complex used to invade metazoan cells. These organelles are not visible with light microscopy, but good descriptions have been obtained using electron microscopy. Many of these organisms are intracellular parasites and develop within a parasitophorous vacuole. Reproduction in the various groups of apicomplexans varies somewhat but in general involves both sexual and asexual processes. In some, oocysts are produced and excreted in feces; these oocysts contain infective sporozoites resulting from sporogony (eg, *Cryptosporidium*). In the intestinal coccidians (eg, *Cryptosporidium, Isospora, Toxoplasma,* and *Sarcocystis*), oocysts are a resistant thick-walled stage excreted in feces. In these species the sporoblast in the oocyst divides and forms two sporocysts within which the infective sporozoites develop. In the malaria life cycle, (eg, in *Plasmodium falciparum*), infective sporozoites are produced in oocysts within the anopheline mosquito vector and are inoculated into the human host when the female mosquito takes a blood meal.

The microsporidians produce unicellular spores that contain uninucleate or binucleate sporoplasm and an extrusion apparatus, which is referred to as a polar tubule or polar filament. Characteristically, these spores are all small, 1 to 5 µm. Our knowledge of their morphology is largely derived from ultrastructural studies. These spores are probably excreted in feces and urine primarily, but they may also be present in other bodily secretions or excretions.

Although controversy surrounds the classification of *Pneumocystis carinii* as either a protozoan or a fungus, many researchers in recent years consider this organism a fungal parasite. However, we have included this parasite in our discussion because of its importance as an opportunistic infection associated with the acquired immune deficiency syndrome and its prior affinities to the protozoa.

References

Cox FEG. Systematics of parasitic protozoa. In: Kreier JP, Baker JR, eds. *Parasitic Protozoa, Vol I.* 2nd ed. San Diego, Calif: Academic Press Inc; 1991.

Lee JJ, Hunter SH, Bovee EC, eds. *An Illustrated Guide to the Protozoa.* Lawrence, Kan: Society of Protozoologists; 1985.

Perkins, FO. "Sporozoa": Apicomplexa, Microsporidia, Haplosporidia, Paramyxea, Myxosporidia, and Actinosporidia. In: Harrison FW, Corliss JO, eds. *Microscopic Anatomy of Invertebrates, Vol I: Protozoa.* NY: Wiley-Liss Inc; 1991.

Sleigh MA. The nature of protozoa. In: Kreier JP, Baker JR, eds. *Parasitic Protozoa, Vol I.* 2nd ed. San Diego, Calif: Academic Press Inc; 1991.

Vickerman K, Brugerolle G, Mignot JP. Mastigophora. In: Harrison FW, Corliss JO, eds. *Microscopic Anatomy of Invertebrates, Vol I: Protozoa.* NY: Wiley-Liss Inc; 1991.

Entamoeba histolytica

Amebiasis

Approximately half a billion people acquire *Entamoeba histolytica* infection each year. Disease occurs in approximately 10% to 15% of those infected, resulting in 50,000 to 100,000 deaths. Because of its high morbidity and mortality rates, among the protozoa *E. histolytica* ranks second only to malaria in disease importance. Although more than a century has passed since *E. histolytica* was discovered, many aspects of its biology and pathogenicity remain unresolved.

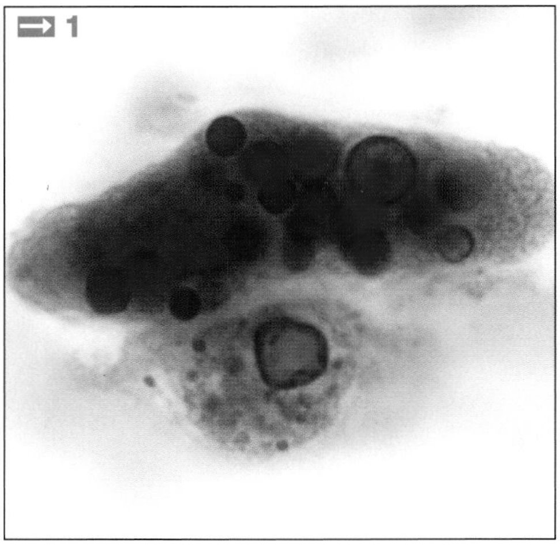

1

Biology and Life Cycle

Trophozoites of *E. histolytica* live and multiply by binary fission in the cecum and colon of the intestine. Trophozoites undergo encystation in the lumen and mature into infective quadrinucleate cysts, which are excreted in feces. Human infection most commonly results from ingestion of infective cysts in food and water contaminated by feces. Pathogenic and nonpathogenic strains of *E. histolytica* are morphologically indistinguishable from one another. Virulent strains of the parasite have the ability to invade tissue, whereas nonpathogenic forms apparently do not. The two forms of the organism can be differentiated by molecular technology, including isoenzyme analysis, typing by monoclonal antibodies to pathogen-specific surface antigens, and analysis of restriction fragment length polymorphism and ribosomal RNA sequences.

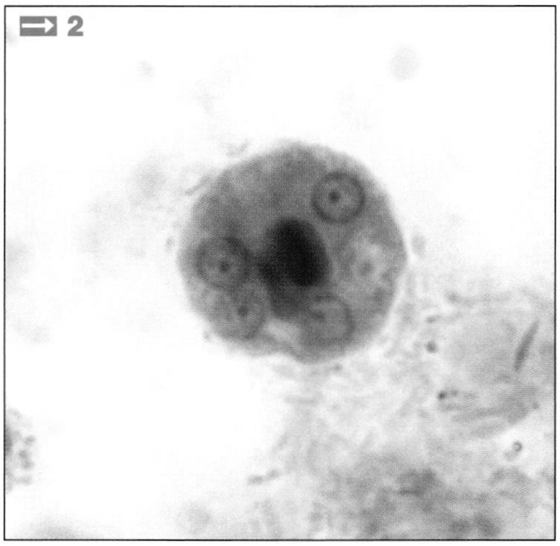

2

The differences between virulent and avirulent strains have led some investigators to propose that a separate species be established for what is now collectively referred to as *E. histolytica*. In 1993, it was proposed that the virulent species be referred to as *E. histolytica* and the nonpathogenic form as *E. dispar*. Tissue-invasive forms initially penetrate and colonize in the wall of the colon. Invasion of intestinal tissue may be limited to this location, but dissemination from this site to virtually every organ and tissue of the body is possible. Although nonhuman primates as well as dogs and cats can be infected by *E. histolytica,* none of these animals constitutes a significant reservoir for human infection.

Pathology and Clinical Manifestations

Luminal amebiasis is usually associated with nonpathogenic strains of *E. histolytica*. Clinical manifestations are absent. Cysts may be excreted for a considerable time (the carrier state), and infections often terminate spontaneously. Trophozoites of invasive strains initiate lysis of the mucosal epithelium in areas where the mucus layer is depleted, which results in the formation of minute, superficial ulcerations. Most frequently, these lesions occur initially in the cecum, appendix, or the ascending portion of the colon. Continued erosion of tissue results in invasion of the lamina propria and submucosa. As trophozoites spread laterally in these layers, the typical flask-shaped ulcers associated with amebiasis are produced (Plate 1:1). Multiple ulcers may develop, and when they coalesce, large areas of ulceration are produced. Although organisms are not seen in the necrotic material of the ulcer, they are readily found in the bordering healthy tissue.

The clinical manifestations of amebic colitis are highly variable and depend on the site and extent of tissue damage. The incubation period before symptomatology develops may vary from less than a week to several months. General malaise, anorexia, weight loss, and abdominal discomfort often precede bouts of acute colitis. Moderate or profuse bloody diarrhea occurs, and a fulminating dysentery may develop. Acute attacks are often followed by symptomless periods with formed stools. This chronic form of amebiasis is more prevalent than acute or subacute amebic colitis. Trophozoite dissemination to other organs and tissues is always secondary to intestinal infection. Extraintestinal amebiasis can develop in the absence of symptomatology associated with colitis; the individual may even be unaware that he was previously infected with *E. histolytica*. Hepatic amebiasis resulting in one or more small to large abscesses is the most common form of extraintestinal disease, but dissemination via the bloodstream to other organs and tissues can occur. Organs and tissues that may be affected include the diaphragm, lung, abdominal wall, and skin via direct extension of lesions from the liver or intestinal tract. Once infection disseminates to the brain, the prognosis is poor. However, lesions that develop in other organs and tissues often resolve without scarring through the use of appropriate chemotherapy.

Parasite Morphology

Entamoeba histolytica has both trophozoite and cyst stages. Trophozoites are found in tissues as well as in feces, whereas cysts occur only in feces. Trophozoites range from 10 to 60 µm, with noninvasive forms usually measuring from 10 to 20 µm and invasive forms measuring 20 µm or more. Living trophozoites have progressive, often explosive motility and extrude fingerlike pseudopodia. It is difficult to see the single nucleus in living trophozoites, but in permanently stained smears the nucleus typically has a small, compact central karyosome and finely granular peripheral chromatin on the inner surface of the nuclear membrane. In virulent strains, trophozoites often contain ingested erythrocytes, which can be seen in both stained and unstained organisms ➡ 1. The mature cyst contains four nuclei ➡ 2, but uninucleate and binucleate cysts are often found in feces. Immature cysts and, more rarely, mature cysts often contain elongated chromatoid bodies with rounded ends. Mature cysts typically measure 10 to 20 µm in diameter.

In sections of tissue containing trophozoites, the characteristic *E. histolytica* nucleus is approximately 3 to 4 µm in diameter, and the punctate central karyosome is usually visible (Plate 1:2, 3, & 6; Plate 2:1, 4–6). If a cluster of trophozoites is present, the nucleus will usually be apparent in only a few. The cytoplasm of trophozoites in section is typically vacuolated, and ingested red blood cells may be recognized. When a Giemsa stain is used, the ingested erythrocytes are pink. Amebae in tissue stain readily with hematoxylin and eosin (H&E) stain and periodic acid–Schiff (PAS) stain. With PAS stain, the organisms become a prominent red color, but the nucleus is not as clearly visible as it is with H&E stain. However, amebae in tissue stained by PAS stand out when seen under lower magnification because of their color (Plate 2:2 & 3).

Organisms with which *E. histolytica* trophozoites might be confused in tissue section are the trophozoites of free-living, pathogenic amebae. For example, free-living, pathogenic amebic trophozoites of the genera *Naegleria* and *Acanthamoeba* are most frequently found in the brain, but they are readily distinguished from *E. histolytica* because their nuclei contain large, prominent karyosomes. Species of *Acanthamoeba* and other leptomyxid amebae (but not *Naegleria*) encyst in human tissues, whereas *E. histolytica* does not. Although inexperienced diagnosticians may have difficulty differentiating between *E. histolytica* trophozoites and histiocytes, differences in staining characteristics of the amebae and histiocytes are apparent. With H&E stains, in trophozoites the nucleus is small and acidophilic, while the cytoplasm is slightly basophilic; in histiocytes the nucleus is larger and basophilic, and the cytoplasm is acidophilic. With PAS, not only do trophozoites of *E. histolytica* stain red but so do histiocytes. Nuclear details must then be studied for proper identification.

References

Chun D, Chandrasoma P, Kiyabu M. Fulminant amebic colitis: a morphologic study of four cases. *Dis Colon Rectum*. 1994;37:535-539.

Clark CG, Cunnick CC, Diamond LS. *Entamoeba histolytica*: is conversion of "nonpathogenic" amebae to the "pathogenic" form a real phenomenon? *Exp Parasitol*. 1992;74:307-314.

Diamond LS, Clark CG. A redescription of *Entamoeba histolytica* (Schaudinn, 1903; emended Walker, 1911) separating it from *Entamoeba dispar* (Brumpt, 1925). *J Euk Microbiol*. 1993;40:340-344.

Kretschmer RR, ed. *Amebiasis: Infection and Disease by Entamoeba histolytica*. Boca Raton, FL: CRC Press; 1990.

Martinez-Palomo A. Amebiasis. In: Ruitenberg EJ, MacInnis AJ, eds. *Human Parasitic Diseases, Vol II*. New York, NY: Elsevier Science Publishing; 1986.

Martinez-Palomo A. Parasitic amebas of the intestinal tract. In: *Parasitic Protozoa, Vol III*. 2nd ed. San Diego, Calif: Academic Press Inc; 1993.

Plate 1

Entamoeba histolytica

Image 1

Amebic ulcer in human colon. In this typical lesion, erosion of the mucosal epithelium extends to the muscularis (H&E, 250x).

Image 2

Several amebae can be seen in this section through an amebic ulcer of the colon. One contains three red-staining erythrocytes, but the nucleus is not visible. Another shows a classic nucleus (dart) containing a central karyosome and fine peripheral chromatin. The cytoplasm contains a single red blood cell. Other amebae (arrows) in this section show neither nuclei nor ingested erythrocytes, but the vacuolated cytoplasm is typical of amebic trophozoites (Giemsa, 1250x).

Image 3

Numerous trophozoites and inflammatory cells are seen in this section through an ulcer of the colon. At moderate magnification, the nuclei of many trophozoites can be seen as small, darker-staining circles within the cytoplasm of the amebae (darts) (H&E, 250x).

Image 4

At high magnification, the nuclei within two of the trophozoites can be seen. The clear space around the trophozoites represents shrinkage of the amebae during the fixation process (H&E, 500x).

Image 5

A large number of amebic trophozoites in a section through the serosa of the colon (H&E, 250x).

Image 6

Nuclei with typical central karyosomes are visible in several of the trophozoites. No erythrocytes are present in any of them (Movat, 750x).

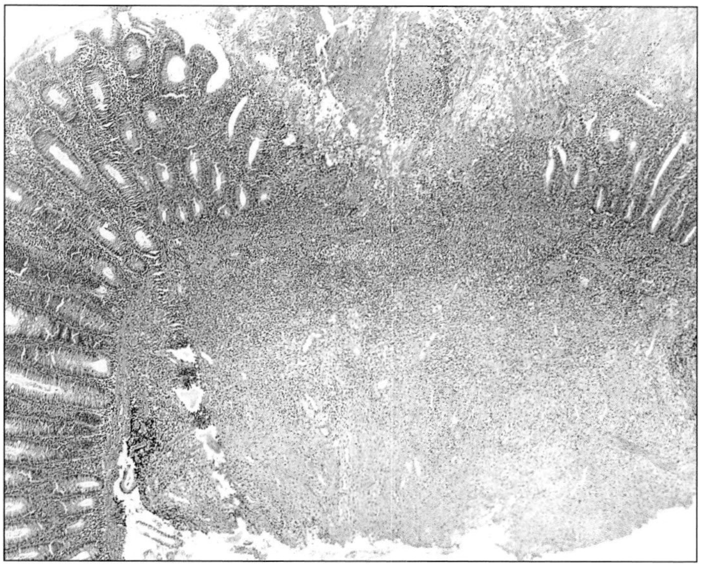

1

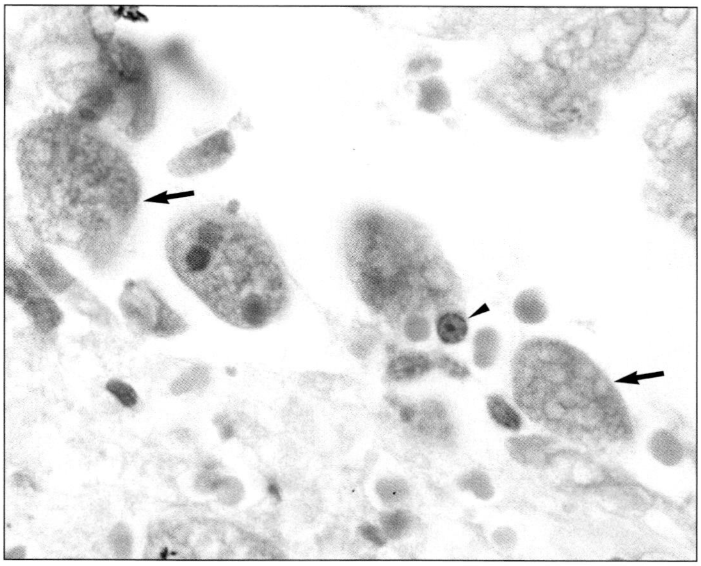

2

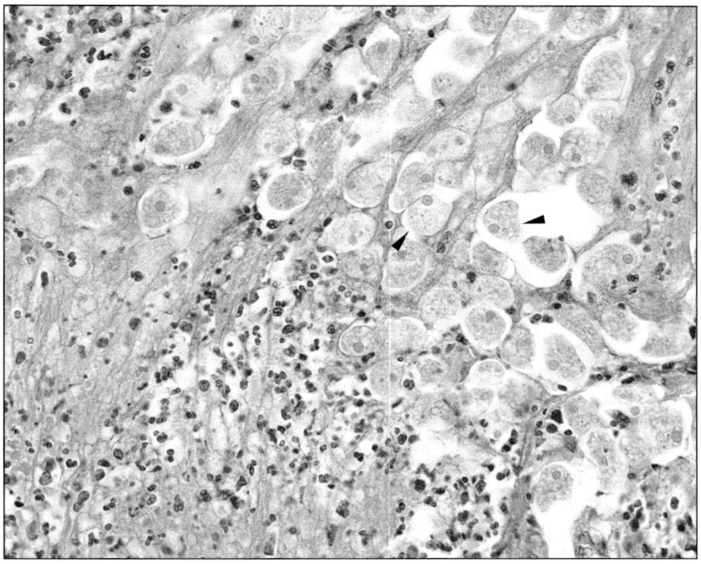

3

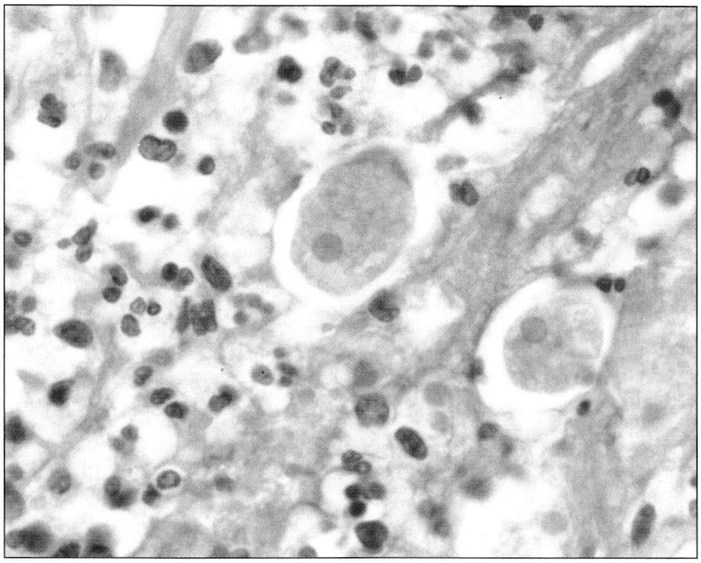

4

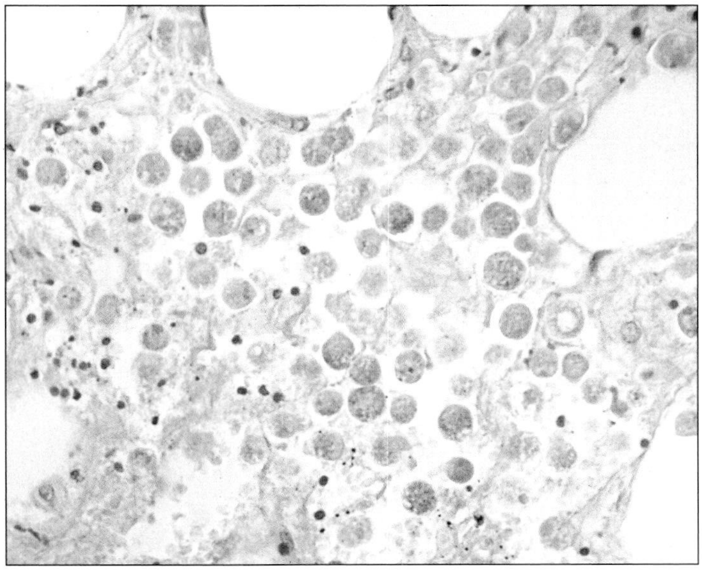

5

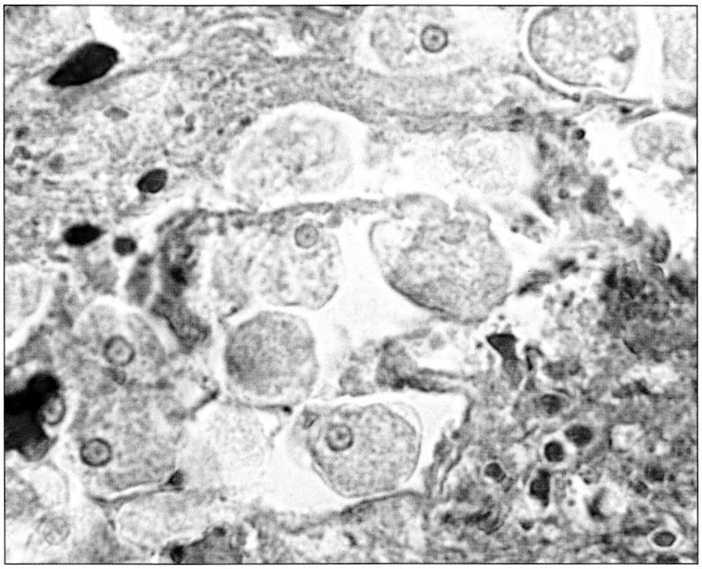

6

Plate 2

Entamoeba histolytica

Image 1

At low magnification, bright-red–staining trophozoites of *E. histolytica* are seen in this section of an amebic liver abscess (PAS, 125x).

Image 2

In this section of a human amebic liver abscess, three trophozoites are visible. Normal hepatic liver cells are seen at one edge of the field. At this moderate magnification, it is possible to see circular nuclei within the cytoplasm of two of the amebae (darts) (H&E, 250x).

Image 3

At higher magnification, several trophozoites are clearly seen. Nuclei are not visible within the cytoplasm (PAS, 525x).

Image 4

Two trophozoites are seen within this section of human diaphragm. The normal architecture of the diaphragm is disrupted considerably. In one of the two amebae, the nucleus is clearly evident (dart), including the karyosome. Only the cytoplasm is visible in the other (H&E, 750x).

Image 5

Section of lung in a case of pulmonary amebiasis. Although several amebae are present, a nucleus is clearly seen in only one of the organisms (dart). At this magnification, one can see the karyosome in the center of the nucleus (H&E, 500x).

Image 6

A cluster of amebic trophozoites is seen in this section through a perianal skin ulcer. Faint outlines of nuclei can be seen in a few organisms, and a few trophozoites have pink-staining red blood cells (darts) in their cytoplasm (H&E, 500x).

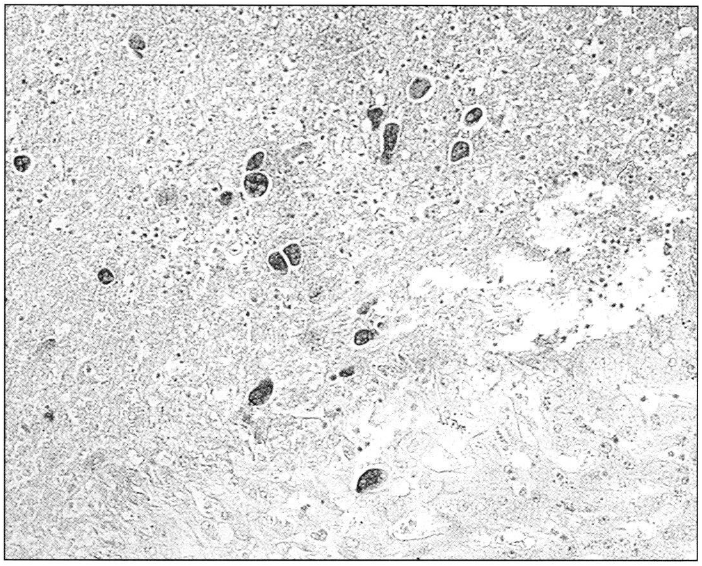

1

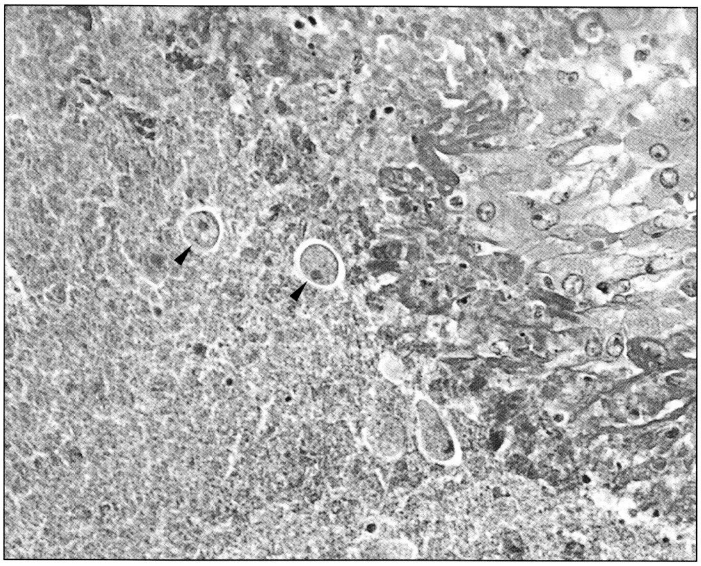

2

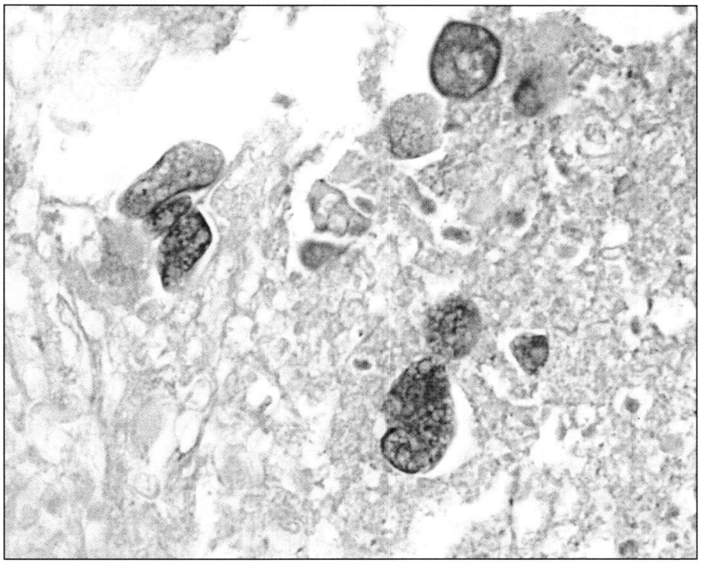

3

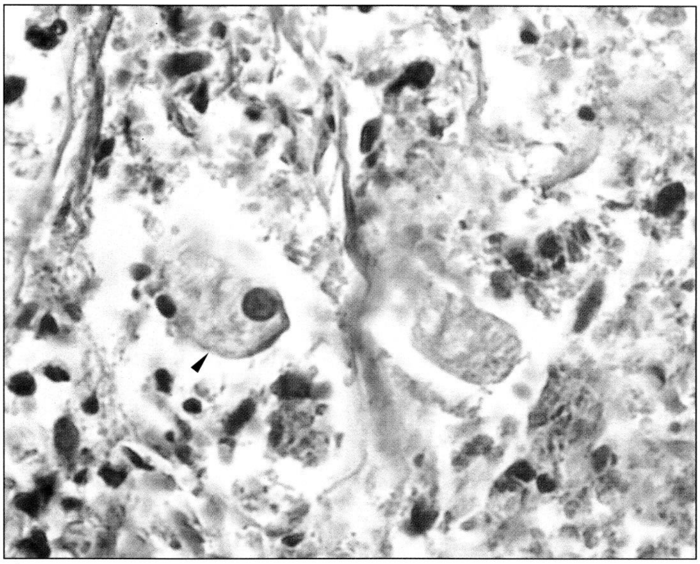

4

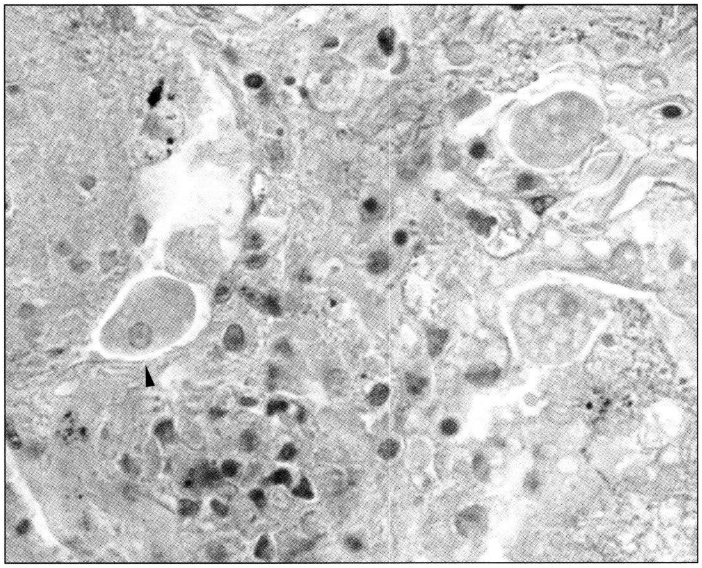

5

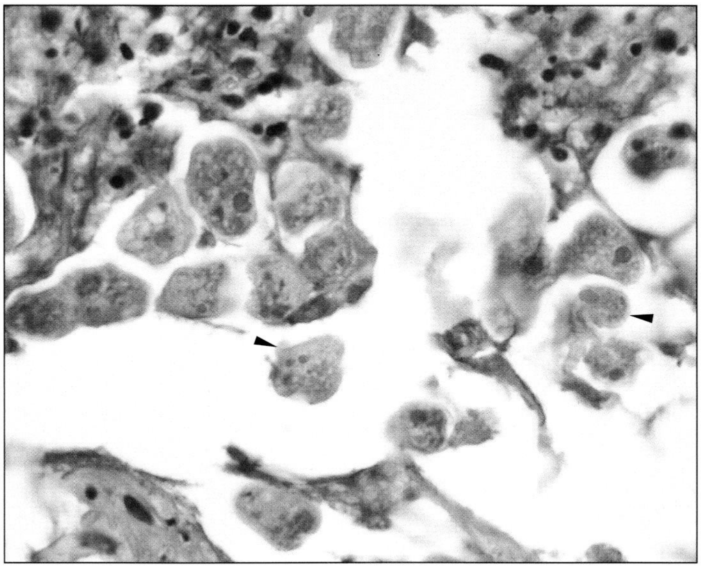

6

Acanthamoeba species and *Balamuthia mandrillaris*

Granulomatous Amebic Encephalitis

Several species of small, free-living amebae found in soil and water and belonging to the genus *Acanthamoeba* cause human infections. Numerous species (*A. astronyxis, A. castellanii, A. hatchetti, A. palestinensis, A. polyphaga,* and *A. rhysodes*) cause disease in the central nervous system and the eye. *Naegleria fowleri*, which is found in soil and water, is another free-living ameba described in humans and is the etiologic agent for primary amebic meningoencephalitis. Specific identification of the free-living amebae involved in human infections on purely morphologic grounds is difficult and is usually accomplished by culture methods, immunodiagnostic procedures, and isoenzyme analysis. *Acanthamoeba* usually produces either a chronic granulomatous amebic encephalitis or amebic keratitis; however, cerebral abscesses caused by these amebae also have been reported in individuals with AIDS. *Balamuthia mandrillaris*, a related free-living ameba of the Order Leptomyxida, has recently been reported to produce amebic granulomas in the brain, which are difficult to distinguish from those caused by *Acanthamoeba* species. Although *Balamuthia* was originally found in a primate (a mandrill), immunofluorescence tests have shown that more than 35 human cases originally attributed to species of *Acanthamoeba* should have been attributed to *Balamuthia*.

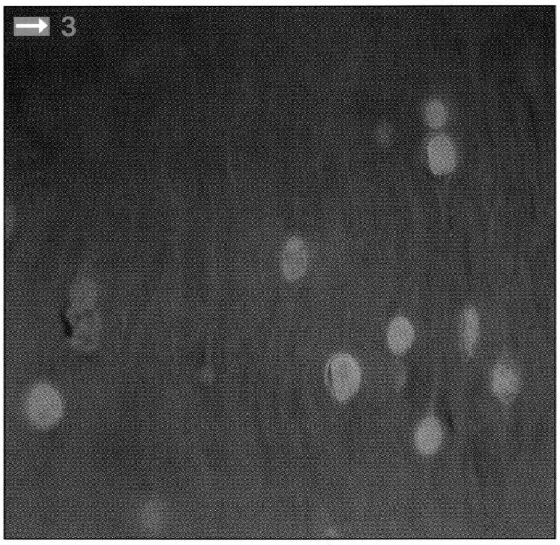

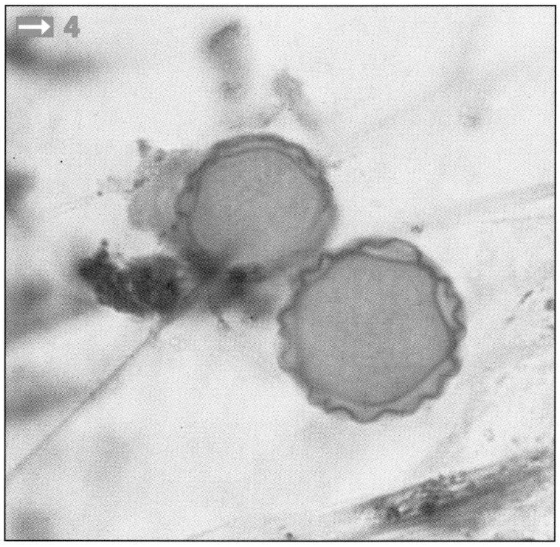

Biology and Life Cycle

Acanthamoeba species reside principally in soil and water, but they have been isolated from cooling towers, air conditioner filters, dust, eye wash stations, contact lenses, and various tissues and organs of human and animal hosts. Trophozoite and cyst stages occur in nature, with cyst stages developing as a result of adverse environmental conditions. Multiplication occurs only in the trophozoite stage with division by binary fission. It appears that species tolerating temperatures of 37°C or higher are those associated with human disease. Human infections seem to result from exposure to contaminated water, soil, or contact lenses. Leptomyxid amebae are also found in soil, but less is known about them. Unlike other soil amebae, however, *Balamuthia* will not grow on bacteria-coated nonnutrient agar plates, though it does well when grown on various mammalian tissue culture monolayers. In axenic liquid media, *Acanthamoeba* grows well but *Balamuthia* does not.

Pathology and Clinical Manifestations

Unlike the primary amebic meningoencephalitis that *Naegleria fowleri* produces, *Acanthamoeba* infection of the brain results from secondary dissemination of organisms: infection spreads through the bloodstream from primary lesions in the lung or the skin. Infection of the respiratory tract probably occurs through cyst inhalation; contamination of skin lesions by water or soil results in primary skin infection. The exact incubation period for infection is not known, but it seems that a considerable amount of time elapses before clinical symptoms begin to appear. In human infections *Acanthamoeba* appears to grow at a slower rate than *Naegleria*, resulting in a more prolonged course of infection. *Acanthamoeba* infection often causes sleepiness, mood swings, and seizures; other symptoms include low-grade fever, stiff neck, nausea, and vomiting.

Grossly, brain lesions on computed tomographic (CT) scans appear as tumorlike masses. In *Acanthamoeba* infections, the CT scan reveals a chronic granulomatous lesion and the presence of multinucleated giant cells. A distinctive feature of *Acanthamoeba* is that both trophozoites and cysts occur in the tissues. Organisms occur throughout brain tissue, but they are often found surrounding the blood vessels. Immunocompromised hosts appear to have a heightened risk of acquiring *Acanthamoeba* infection. Lesions in these hosts typically do not contain multinucleated giant cells.

Acanthamoeba keratitis is a clinical entity distinct from the disease produced in the skin and central nervous system. Chronic infection of the cornea by various species of *Acanthamoeba* was initially associated with penetrating corneal trauma or exposure to contaminated water. However, it now is detected with increasing frequency in contact lens wearers who do not adequately disinfect their contact lenses with heat or who utilize homemade, nonsterile saline solutions for cleaning. Clinical features include severe pain and photophobia, corneal ring infiltrates, a recurrent epithelial breakdown with ulcer formation, and sclerokeratitis. Eradicating the infection, particularly an older established one, is difficult. Corneal transplants frequently become reinfected, apparently from persisting organisms. Fluorescence of organisms after calcofluor white staining aids in their diagnosis ➡ 3

Human infections with the leptomyxid ameba, *Balamuthia*, are less common and are mostly associated with immunocompromised patients or the very young or very old. These infections have clinical features typical of granulomatous amebic encephalitis. A focal necrotizing encephalitis with nonpurulent inflammation of the overlying meninges is present. Amebae also are found in other organs and tissues, including the kidney and adrenal glands.

Parasite Morphology

When seen in culture media, the trophozoites of *Acanthamoeba* species range from 15 to 35 µm in size, have a single nucleus with a large karyosome, and produce thin, spinelike or filamentous pseudopods referred to as acanthopodia. They have a large contractile vacuole that is continuously filling and emptying. Cysts have a double wall and range in diameter from 13 to 20 µm ➡ 4. Their morphology varies depending on the species. The outer wall (the ectocyst) may be rounded, wrinkled, or triangular; the inner wall (the endocyst) may also vary in morphology from smooth to irregular (Plate 4:4). Cysts contain varying numbers of pores (ostioles) that occur at irregular intervals along the cyst wall where the ectocyst is in contact with the endocyst.

In culture, *Balamuthia* species may be highly branched and large, reaching lengths of 15 to 60 µm (mean, 30 µm). They produce broad pseudopodia and usually are uninucleate. Trophozoites may be binucleate but are never multinucleate. The nucleus is approximately 5 µm in diameter, is vesicular, and contains a central karyosome. Cysts are irregularly rounded, are 6 to 30 µm in diameter (mean, 15 µm), and have a thick, wavy, and irregular ectocyst wall and a thinner, spherical endocyst wall. Cysts are primarily uninucleate but may be binucleate.

The size of *Acanthamoeba* trophozoites in tissue is highly variable and depends on their plane of section. Most organisms measure between 8 and 12 µm, but some may reach 20 µm. The cytoplasm is highly vacuolated, and the nucleus has a large karyosome with a halo around it (Plate 3:5). Cysts usually measure between 10 and 15 µm. Although many cysts clearly demonstrate their double-walled structure, many do not (Plate 3:2 & 3). The cyst nucleus is often difficult to see, and the karyosome is much smaller than that in the trophozoite (Plate 3:2).

In tissue section trophozoites of *Balamuthia* usually measure between 15 and 25 µm, but some reach up to 35 µm (Plate 4:2–5). The cytoplasm is highly vacuolated, and the karyosome within the nucleus is not as large or as prominent as the karyosome in *Naegleria* or *Acanthamoeba* (Plate 4:5). Macrophagelike cells are often seen surrounding the amebae. In some instances it is difficult to distinguish organisms from host cells, particularly if the nucleus is not in the plane of section. Cysts of this leptomyxid ameba are also large: they typically measure between 15 and 20 µm but may measure up to 30 µm (Plate 4:6). In an optimal plane of section, the cyst demonstrates a thin outer wall and a much thicker endocyst wall. It is difficult to see the nucleus in the cysts, but refractile granules are often noted within the cytoplasm.

Distinguishing *Acanthamoeba* or leptomyxid amebae from *E. histolytica* and *Naegleria* in tissue section is not difficult. *Acanthamoeba* trophozoites may be found in the central nervous system, eye, skin, and possibly other tissues, whereas the trophozoites of *Naegleria* are usually found only in the central nervous system. The main distinction between *Acanthamoeba* and *Naegleria* in section is that the former encysts in tissue and the latter does not. A considerable size overlap is apparent in trophozoites of *Acanthamoeba* and *Naegleria* in tissue, eliminating this factor as a differential criterion. The trophozoites of *Balamuthia* are usually larger than those of *Acanthamoeba* or *Naegleria*, and their nuclei demonstrate smaller, less clearly defined karyosomes. Cysts of *Balamuthia* have a much thicker wall, are usually spherical, and the internal contents are more globular and refractile than the cysts of *Acanthamoeba*.

References

Anzil AP, Rao C, Wrzolek MA, et al. Amebic meningoencephalitis in a patient with AIDS caused by a newly recognized opportunistic pathogen. *Arch Pathol Lab Med.* 1991;115:21-25.

Garner A. Pathogenesis of acanthamoebic keratitis: hypothesis based an a histological analysis of 30 cases. *Brit J Ophthamol.* 1993;77:366-370.

John DT . Opportunistically pathogenic free-living amebae. In: Kreier JP, Baker JR, eds. *Parasitic Protozoa, Vol III.* 2nd ed. San Diego, Calif: Academic Press Inc; 1993 .

Ma P, Visvesvara GS, Martinez AJ, et al. *Naegleria* and *Acanthamoeba* infections: a review. *Rev Infect Dis.* 1990;12:490-513.

Martinez AJ. Free-living amebas: infection of the central nervous system. *Mt Sinai J Med.* 1993;60:271-278.

Martinez AJ, Guerra AE, Garcia-Tamayo J, et al. Granulomatous amebic encephalitis: a review and report of a spontaneous case from Venezuela. *Acta Neuropathol.* 1994;87:430-434.

Tan B, Weldon-Linne CM, Rhone DP, et al. *Acanthamoeba* infection presenting as skin lesions in patients with the acquired immunodeficiency syndrome. *Arch Pathol Lab Med.* 1993;117:1043-1046.

Visvesvara GS, Martinez AJ, Schuster FL, et al. Leptomyxid ameba: a new agent of amebic meningoencephalitis in humans and animals. *J Clin Microbiol.* 1990;28:2750-2756.

Visvesvara GS, Schuster FL, Martinez AJ. *Balamuthia mandrillaris*, N.G., N. Sp., agent of amebic meningoencephalitis in humans and animals. *J Euk Microbiol.* 1993;40:504-514.

Plate 3

Acanthamoeba

Image 1

Section from the right occipital cortex and overlying meninges from an immunosuppressed patient with *Acanthamoeba* species infection. The cortex demonstrates necrosis, inflammation, and hemorrhage. Cellular infiltration, fibrin, and blood are present in the subarachnoid space (H&E, 50x). (Case courtesy of A. Martinez)

Image 2

Many trophozoites of *Acanthamoeba* species (keyline) are seen encircling a large artery in the brain (fatal case) (H&E, 100x).

Image 3

Several trophozoites of *Acanthamoeba* species are seen in this section of human brain. In two of them (darts), the distinctive large, dark, red-staining karyosomes of the nuclei are clearly visible; in the other organisms, the vacuolated cytoplasm is visible, but the karyosomes are out of the plane of focus (H&E, 1250x).

Image 4

A trophozoite (arrow) and cyst (dart) of *Acanthamoeba* are seen. The large karyosome in the nucleus of the trophozoite is evident. The cyst wall is thick and stains an intense red. *Acanthamoeba* cysts often have this appearance (H&E, 1250x).

Image 5

In this section, the polyhedral appearance of the endocyst is clearly visible. The cyst itself has a diameter of approximately 12 μm. Other trophozoites in the same field are identifiable by their vacuolated cytoplasm, but their karyosomes are not clearly seen (H&E, 1250x).

Image 6

Acanthamoeba trophozoites are present in a granulomatous lesion in a section of human skin. A single trophozoite (dart) is seen. Its nucleus is visible (H&E, 750x).

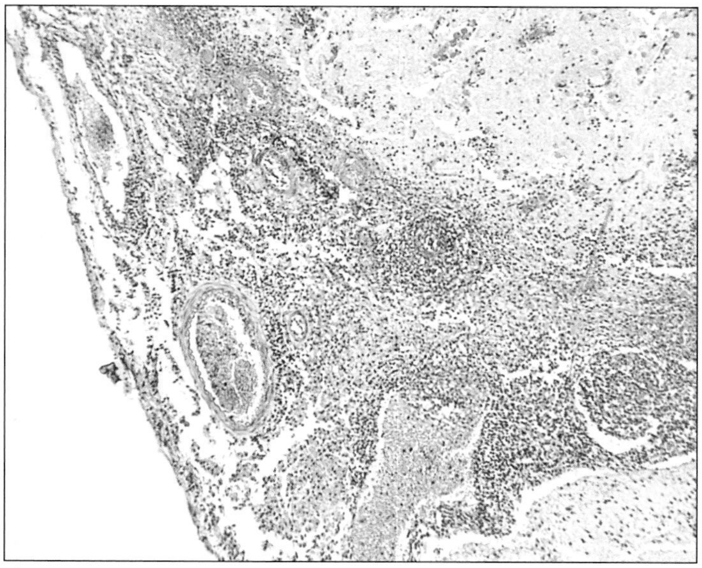

1

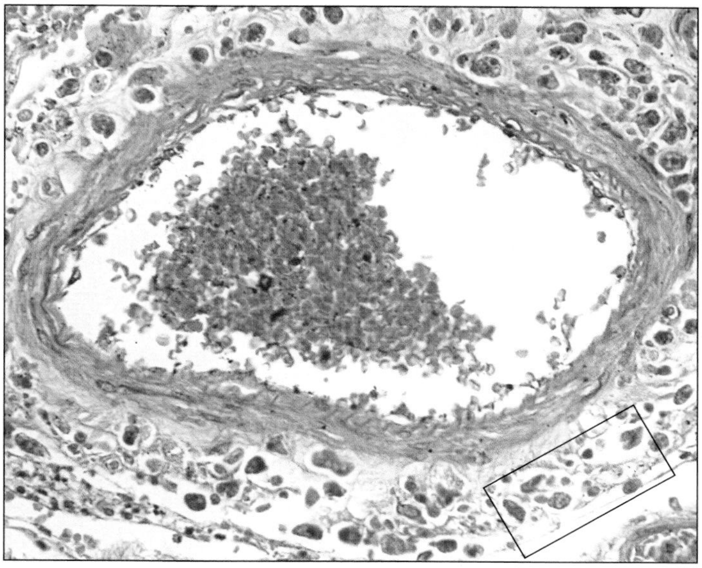

2

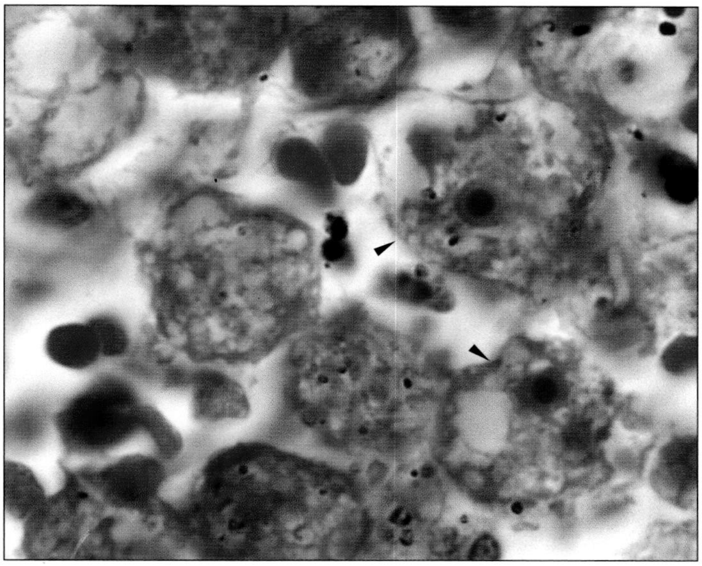

3

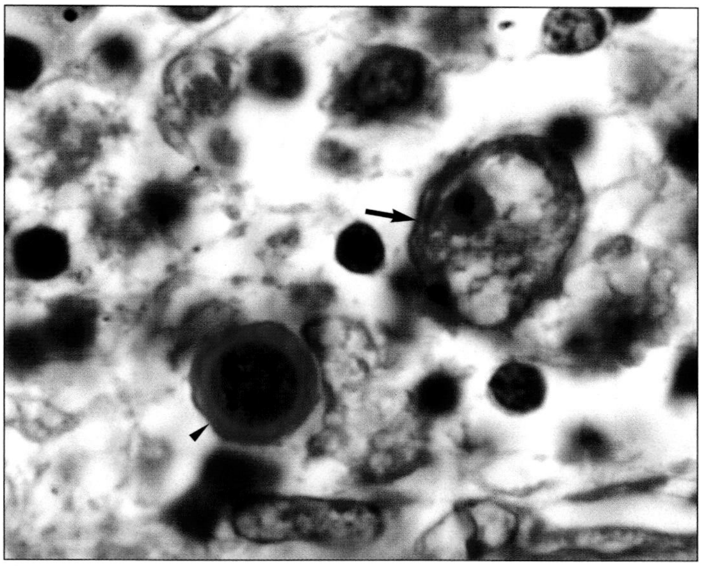

4

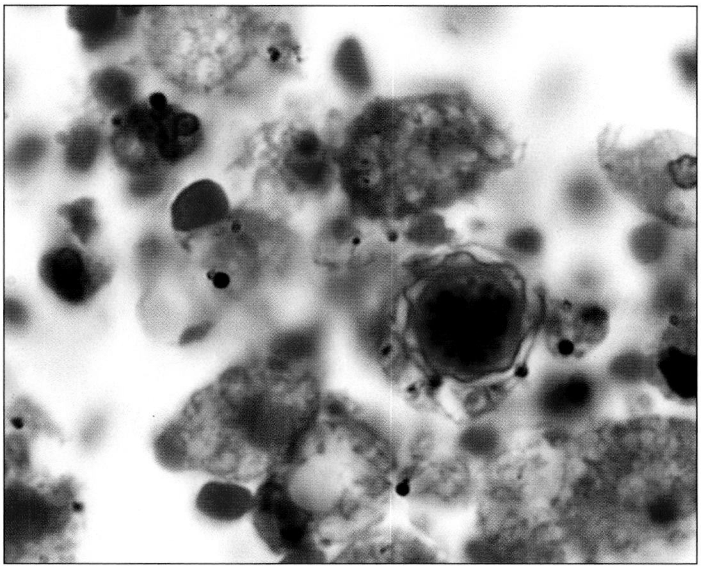

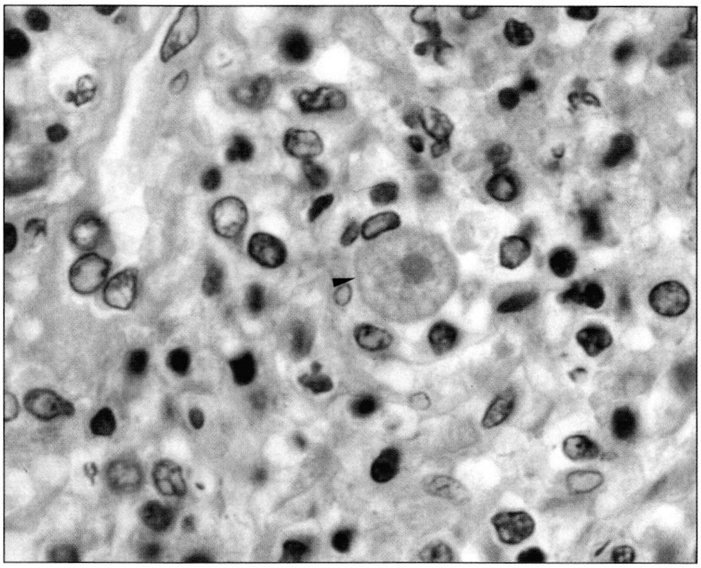

Plate 4

Balamuthia mandrillaris

Image 1

Two rounded cysts (darts) of *Balamuthia* are evident in the wall of a blood vessel in a human brain. Although trophozoites are also present, they are difficult to discern. Organisms are typically found in and around blood vessels (H&E, 250x). (Case courtesy of G. Visvesvara.)

Image 2

At high magnification, a rounded, thick-walled cyst is evident (arrow). A nucleus is visible in the cyst. Two vacuolated trophozoites are also present, but in only one (dart) is a nucleus clearly visible (H&E, 500x). (Case courtesy of G. Visvesvara.)

Image 3

Several trophozoites (darts) of *Balamuthia* in a section of brain. Nuclei are visible within the vacuolated cytoplasm in a number of leptomyxid amebae (H&E, 500x). (Case courtesy of G. Visvesvara.)

Image 4

An elongated *Balamuthia* trophozoite in a section of brain contains a characteristic nucleus with a dark central karyosome that appears to be somewhat more dense at the periphery. The cytoplasm of the organism is vacuolated (H&E, 1000x). (Case courtesy of G. Visvesvara.)

Image 5

A cluster of *Balamuthia* trophozoites partially encircling a blood vessel of the brain. In two trophozoites (darts), nuclei that contain karyosomes are visible; in two others (arrows), vacuolated cytoplasm is evident but nuclei are not in the plane of section (H&E, 500x). (Case courtesy of G. Visvesvara.)

Image 6

A single leptomyxid cyst. The rounded, thick wall surrounds granular cytoplasm with a few prominent globules (H&E, 1250x). (Case courtesy of G. Visvesvara.)

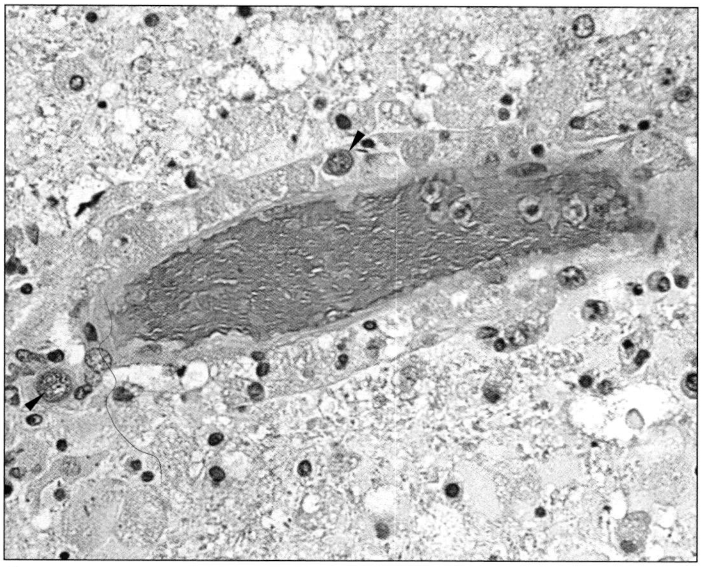

1

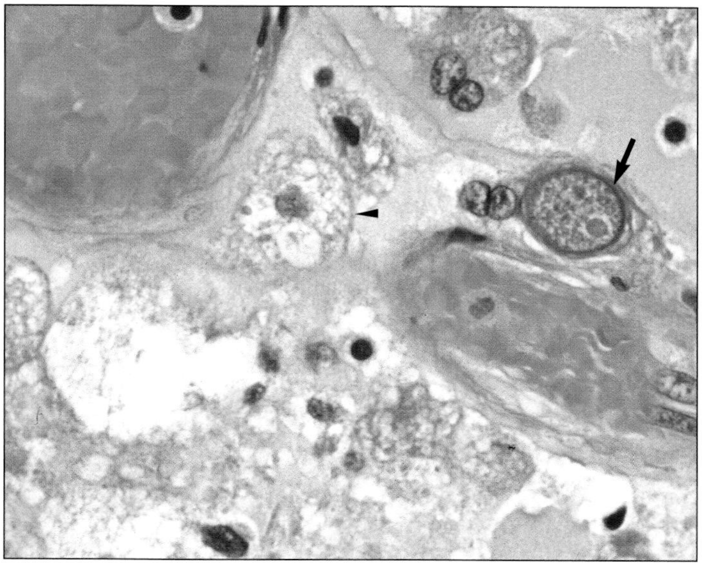

2

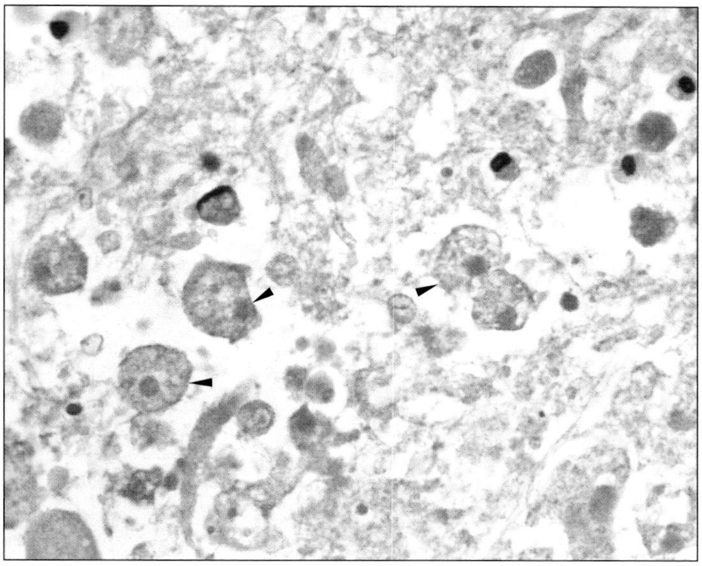

3

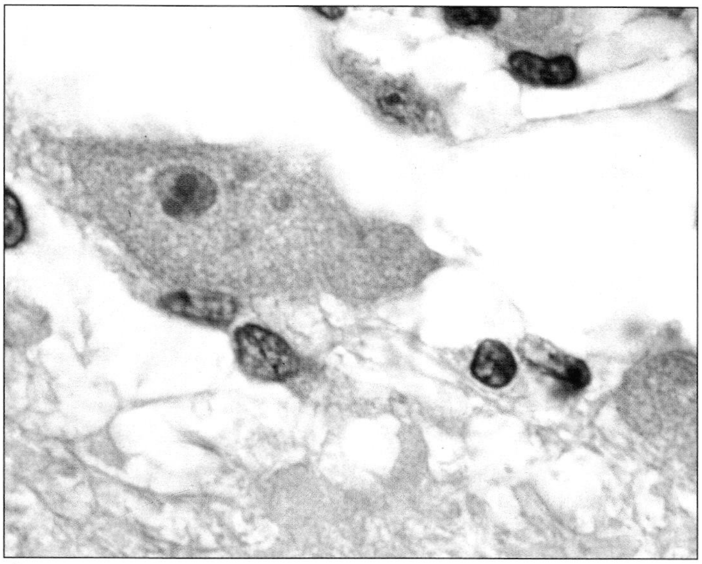

4

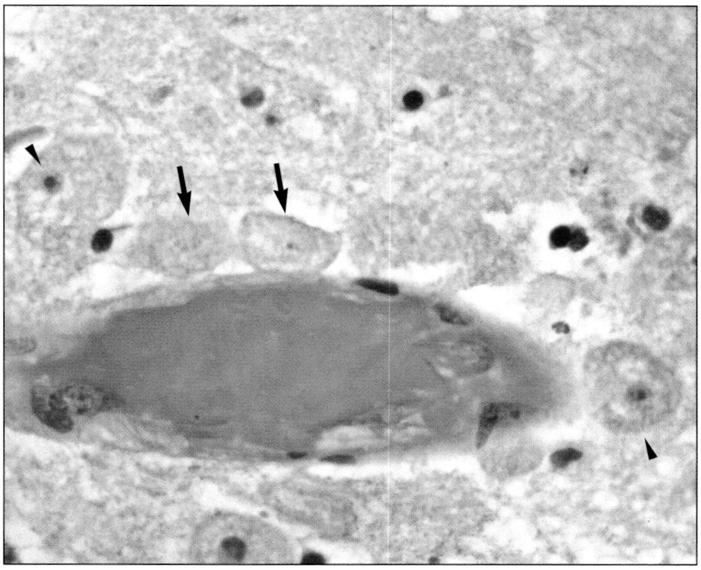

5

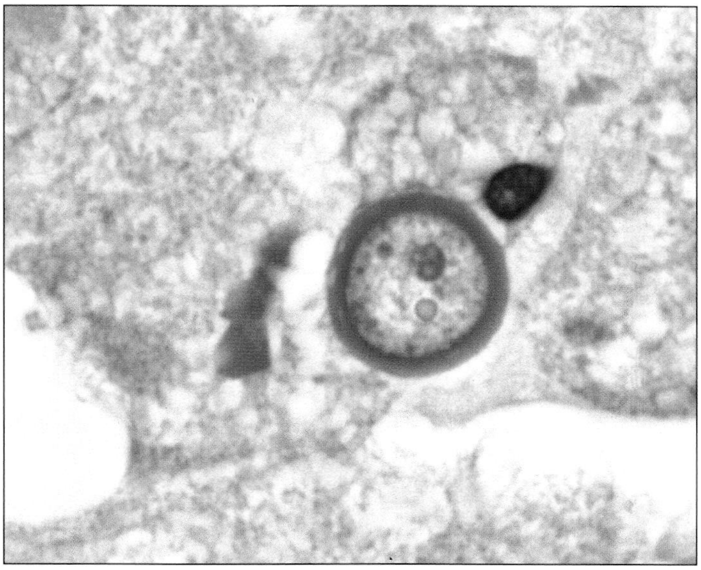

6

Naegleria fowleri

Primary Amebic Meningoencephalitis

The recognition that small, free-living amebae of soil and water cause human disease essentially had its beginnings in the mid-1960s, when what is now identified as *Naegleria fowleri* was found to cause an acute fulminating meningoencephalitis. This infection most frequently involves children or healthy, active young adults who have a history of swimming in extremely warm waters during the summer months. It was only after the discovery of *Naegleria* as the cause of primary amebic meningoencephalitis that species of *Acanthamoeba* and *Balamuthia* were found to also produce an encephalitis in humans but with distinctly different disease characteristics.

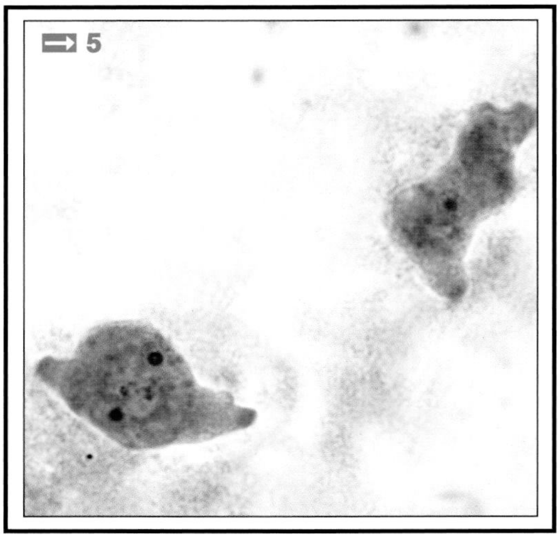

Biology and Life Cycle

Of the *Naegleria* species, only *N. fowleri* has been recognized as a human pathogen. The organism usually lives in water and moist soil. It has three stages in its life cycle: trophozoite, cyst, and a transient flagellated stage, which gives rise to the designation of this species as an ameboflagellate. *Naegleria fowleri* is thermophilic and lives and multiplies at water temperatures of 40 to 45°C. Division is by binary fission of the trophozoite stage. The organism multiplies rapidly in culture media and brain tissue of human or animal hosts. When ameboid trophozoites removed from infected tissues or culture media are placed into distilled water, they transform into the ameboflagellate stage. The ameboflagellates have between one and four terminal flagella; the usual number is two. Multiplication does not occur in the ameboflagellate stage; instead, the organisms revert to the ameboid form. Encystment in nature is probably a response to adverse environmental conditions.

Pathology and Clinical Manifestations

Human infections are most frequently acquired by children and young adults who have been swimming and diving in extremely warm pools of water. Other sources of infection include nasal aspiration of muddy or polluted waters or inhalation of dust that contains cysts. Trophozoites invade the nasal mucosal epithelium and move along unmyelinated olfactory nerves to reach the highly vascular subarachnoid space, where further dissemination to other parts of the central nervous system occurs. After an incubation period of several days to a week or slightly longer, the clinical course of primary amebic meningoencephalitis is rapid. The infection has an abrupt onset characterized by severe headaches, fever, nausea and vomiting, and early signs of an encephalitis. These initial signs and symptoms are suggestive of and difficult to distinguish from acute purulent bacterial meningitis. Coma, seizures, and cardiorespiratory failure ensue rapidly, and death usually occurs within a week of the onset of symptoms. At autopsy, cerebral edema and congestion of leptomeningeal vessels are marked. Histologically, organisms may be seen within inflamed nasal mucosal epithelium. Within the brain, primary involvement of the cortical gray matter is noted, with a purulent leptomeningeal exudate within which amebae are difficult to find (Plate 5:1). Trophozoites but not cysts are frequently seen as clusters of organisms within necrotic tissue (Plate 5:2) or in perivascular spaces associated with small and medium-sized arteries and arterioles.

Parasite Morphology

Living, actively motile trophozoites range from 15 to 30 µm in length by 6 to 9 µm in width, whereas rounded trophozoites measure only 9 to 15 µm. Ameboid trophozoites are occasionally found in cerebrospinal fluid from infected patients. These forms extrude broadly rounded pseudopods (lobopodia) and in their cytoplasm contain one or more contractile vacuoles, which fill and empty continuously. Trophozoites in culture multiply by binary fission and can be large, containing up to eight nuclei before division (➡ 5). In stained trophozoites, the nucleus is 2 to 3 µm in diameter, has a fine nuclear membrane lacking in peripheral chromatin, and contains a large karyosome. The transient ameboflagellate stage is pear shaped and measures approximately 15 by 8 µm. Cysts are 7 to 10 µm in diameter, spherical, and have a smooth wall. In stained specimens, the nucleus is smaller than that in trophozoites and the karyosome is minute.

Trophozoites in tissue usually measure between 7 and 15 µm. Only some demonstrate the characteristic large karyosome; in others it is not within the plane of section (Plate 5:3–6). It is often difficult to see the nuclear membrane; instead, a clear halo is seen around the karyosome. The cytoplasm of the trophozoite appears finely granular and is often vacuolated. Encystation does not occur in tissue.

Other amebae that might be encountered in brain tissue include *Entamoeba histolytica* and other species of free-living amebae of the genera *Acanthamoeba* and *Balamuthia*. In tissue, *E. histolytica* trophozoites are usually larger than *Naegleria*; their nuclei contain minute karyosomes that are readily distinguished from the large karyosomes of *Naegleria* trophozoites, and some contain ingested erythrocytes. Although it is difficult to distinguish the trophozoites of *Naegleria* from those of *Acanthamoeba* in tissue, species of the latter genus, as well as *Balamuthia*, form cysts in tissue. Because cysts of these species in tissue are often as numerous as trophozoites, it is usually not difficult to find them.

References

Carter RF. Description of a *Naegleria* sp. isolated from two cases of primary amebic meningoencephalitis, and of the experimental pathological changes induced by it. *J Pathol.* 1970;100:217-244.

Ma P, Visvesvara GS, Martinez AJ, et al. *Naegleria* and *Acanthamoeba* infections: a review. *Rev Infect Dis.* 1990;12:490-513.

Plate 5

Naegleria fowleri

Image 1

Section of human brain showing necrosis and hemorrhage due to *N. fowleri* infection (H&E, 50x).

Image 2

A large number of trophozoites and a polymorphonuclear leukocyte infiltration (a fatal human case). At this low magnification, one can distinguish the amebae (keyline) from other tissue elements, but it is difficult to discern nuclear detail in the organisms (H&E, 250x).

Image 3

In one of the trophozoites in this field (dart), a typical large karyosome is seen in the nucleus (a fatal case) (H&E, 500x).

Image 4

High magnification demonstrates several trophozoites in which the karyosomes are evident (darts). The cytoplasm of these organisms is irregularly vacuolated (H&E, 1250x). (Case courtesy of W. Earp.)

Image 5

In a hemorrhagic area of brain tissue, a single trophozoite (dart) of *Naegleria* demonstrates a characteristic red-staining karyosome in the nucleus and vacuolated cytoplasm (H&E, 750x).

Image 6

In this cluster of trophozoites, many show the thin nuclear membrane surrounding the typical large karyosomes (H&E, 1250x).

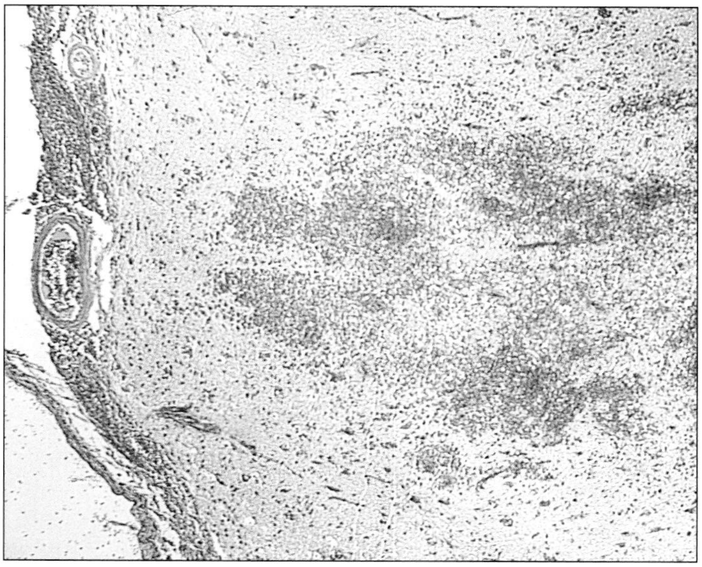

1

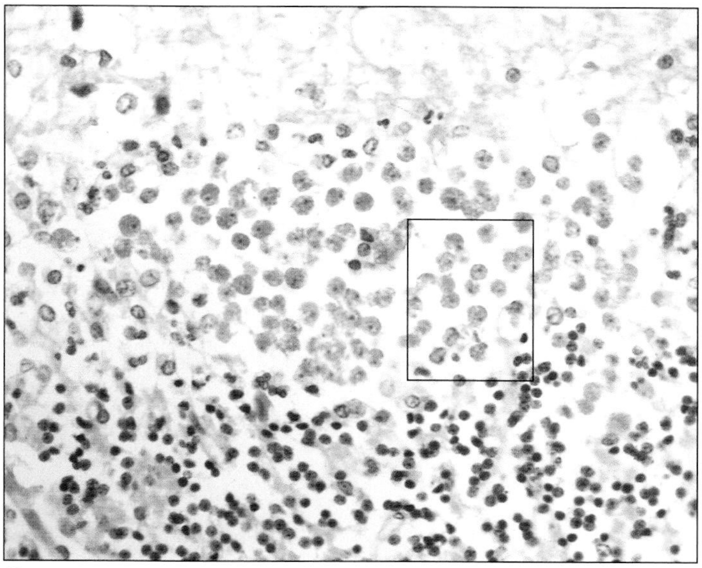

2

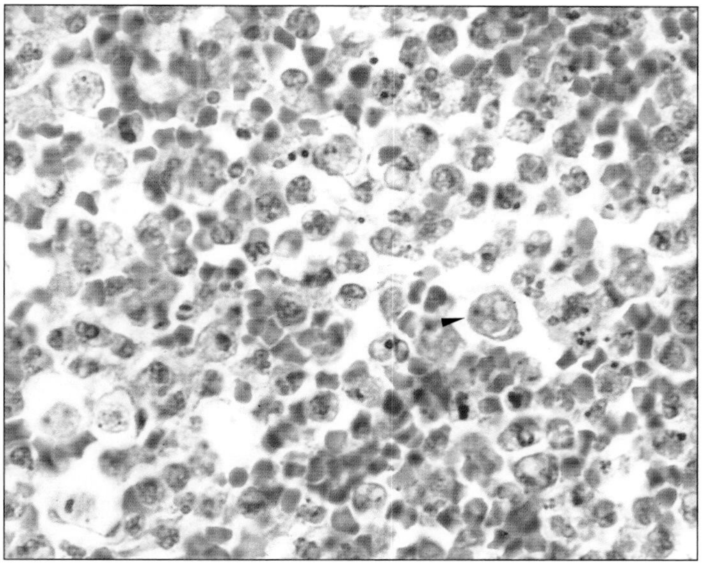

3

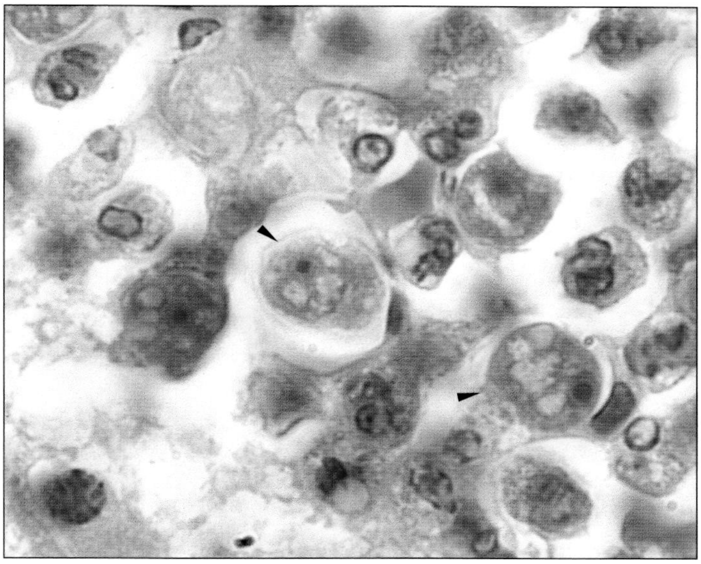

4

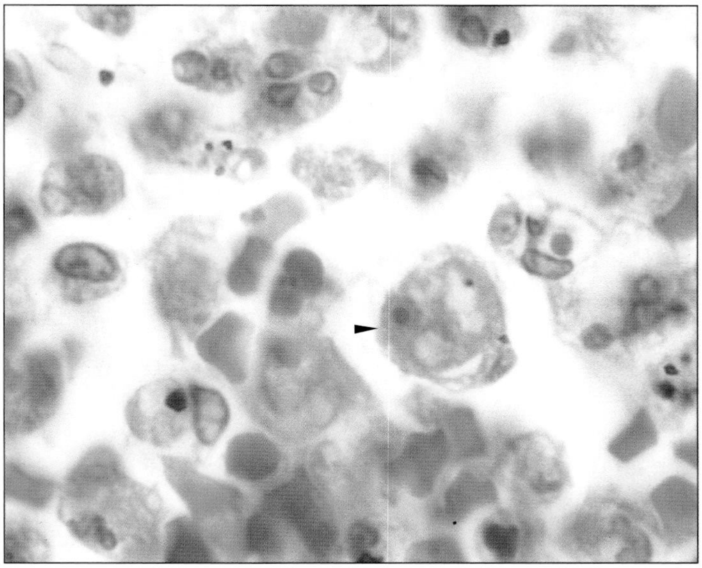

5

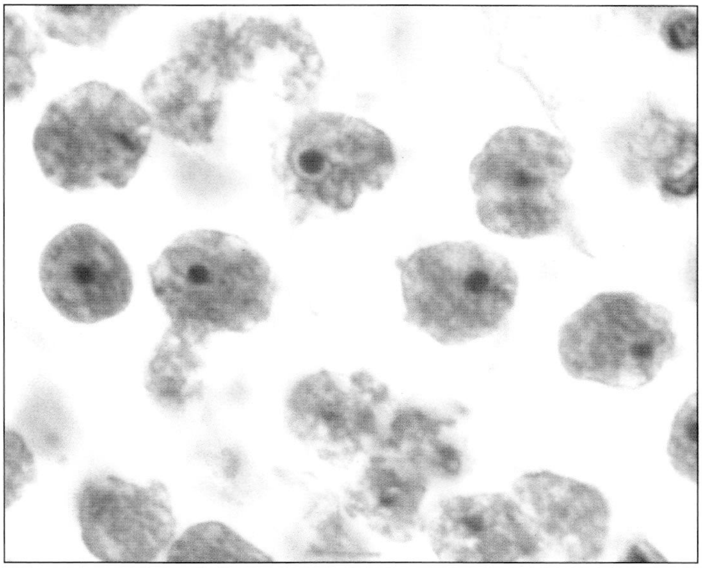

6

Giardia lamblia

Infection with *Giardia lamblia* (also referred to as *Giardia intestinalis* and *Giardia duodenalis*) is now considered the most frequently reported intestinal protozoal parasite causing human diarrhea. This flagellate has a worldwide distribution and is associated with poor hygienic conditions and resultant contamination of water and food. Epidemic outbreaks of this infection have been widely reported in many areas of the United States and other parts of the world. They have usually been associated with waterborne transmission, although in recent years foodborne outbreaks have been reported with more frequency. The increasing utilization of small-bowel biopsies to determine the causes of prolonged diarrhea in patients with AIDS and other conditions has frequently led to the finding of *Giardia* trophozoites in such specimens.

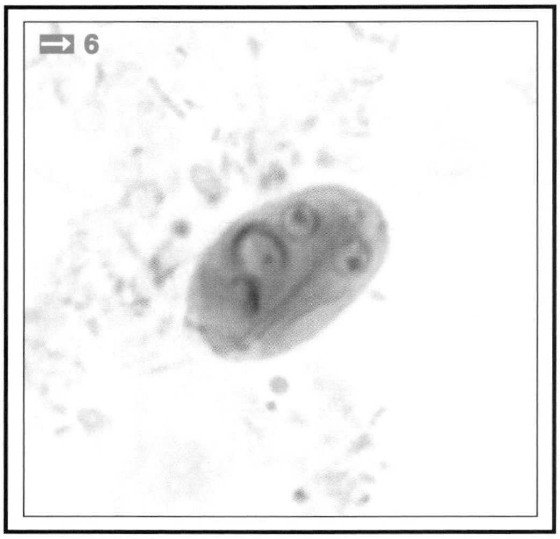

Biology and Life Cycle

Trophozoites of *Giardia* live in the lumen and crypts of the human small intestine. They divide by longitudinal binary fission. Trophozoites are the only stage found in feces in patients with diarrhea, but both trophozoites and cysts can be found in soft fecal specimens. The infective stage of *Giardia* is the mature cyst, which is passed in feces and contains four nuclei. This is the stage usually found in formed stool specimens. Infection is transmitted via the fecal-oral route. Wild animals, particularly the beaver, have been identified as reservoirs for human infection. Domestic pets such as cats and dogs can also be infected with *Giardia*.

Pathology and Clinical Manifestations

For many years *Giardia* was considered to be nonpathogenic, and even today many individuals have no gastrointestinal symptoms when the parasite is present. However, giardiasis can produce a prolonged, foul-smelling, watery diarrhea that lasts for a month or longer in untreated persons. In addition to the diarrhea, individuals report general malaise and fatigue, nausea, anorexia, increased flatulence, cramping, and weight loss. Stool specimens contain large amounts of fat and mucus but no blood. These symptoms of intestinal malabsorption resemble sprue. Pathologic changes include blunting or flattening of villi, loss of the brush border where parasites are attached by their ventral disks, and infiltration of the lamina propria by lymphocytes and granulocytes. Although trophozoites attach to the epithelial cells, the parasites do not actually invade the tissue.

Parasite Morphology

Giardia has both trophozoite and cyst stages. Pear-shaped trophozoites usually measure 12 to 15 µm long, 5 to 9 µm wide, and 2 to 4 µm thick (Plate 6:1). They are rounded anteriorly and tapered posteriorly. On their anterior ventral surface, a shallow, bowl-shaped depression referred to as the ventral disk enables these flagellates to adhere to the mucosal epithelium. Trophozoites have paired nuclei, one on each side of the midline in the anterior portion of the organisms, each of which contains a large central karyosome. Nuclei lack peripheral chromatin. Posterior to the nuclei are one or two curved, transversely oriented median bodies. The positioning of the nuclei and median bodies gives the organism the distinctive "smiling face" appearance associated with stained specimens of *Giardia*. Arising from basal bodies are eight axonemes from which the eight flagella emerge—two anteriorly, four laterally, and two trailing posteriorly. Elliptical mature cysts excreted in feces measure 8 to 19 µm long and 7 to 10 µm wide and contain four nuclei (➡ 6). In cysts, the flagella are retracted into the axonemes, which appear as curved bristlelike structures in the cytoplasm. The cyst wall is a thick membrane, and often the cytoplasm is retracted away from the wall.

Often, only trophozoites are recognized in histologic sections of the small intestine. The trophozoites typically appear as sagittal sections of small crescentic organisms that adhere to the epithelial surface (Plate 6:2–4), or they may appear in ventral views that demonstrate the morphologic characteristics seen in stained smears (Plate 6:5 & 6). Morphologic details of the ventral adhesive disk and other organelles within the trophozoites are generally visible only with electron microscopy.

It is unlikely that *Giardia*, which lives in the lumen, will be confused with other, smaller parasites in histologic sections. Smaller intestinal coccidian parasites occur within the brush border (*Cryptosporidium* species) or within the cytoplasm (*Isospora belli*) of enterocytes. Microsporidian spores are much smaller and also occur in the cytoplasm of epithelial cells.

References

Adam RD. The biology of *Giardia* spp. *Microbiol Rev*. 1991;55:706-732.

Doglioni C, DeBoni M, Cielo R, et al. Gastric giardiasis. *J Clin Pathol*. 1992;45:964-967.

Feely DE, Holberton DV, Erlandsen SL. The biology of *Giardia*. In: Meyer EA, ed. *Giardiasis,* New York, NY: Elsevier Science Publishing; 1990:11-49.

Nemanic PC, Owen RL, Stevens DP, et al. Ultrastructural observations on giardiasis in a mouse model, II: endosymbiosis and organelle distribution in *Giardia muris* and *Giardia lamblia*. *J Infect Dis*. 1979;140:222-228.

Owen RL, Nemanic PC, Stevens DP. Ultrastructural observations on giardiasis in a murine model, I: intestinal distribution, attachment and relationship to the immune system of *Giardia muris*. *Gastroenterology*. 1979;76:757-769.

Plate 6

Giardia lamblia

Image 1

A typical trophozoite in a fecal smear. The paired nuclei are seen on either side of axonemes in the anterior portion of the organism. Two median bodies lie transversely below the nuclei. Flagella are not visible (Trichrome, 1125x).

Image 2

Between two villi one can see at least two sagittal sections of trophozoites adherent to the epithelial surface (arrows) (H&E, 250x).

Image 3

At higher magnification, two organisms can be seen adherent to the epithelial surface (arrows). The crescentic appearance of the trophozoites is evident (H&E, 500x).

Image 4

Under oil immersion magnification, it is difficult to discern any morphologic details of the trophozoites except for the crescentic appearance. Because no other organisms share this unusual appearance, a diagnosis of giardiasis is clear (H&E, 1250x).

Image 5

This section through a crypt provides a ventral view of a trophozoite, which demonstrates the paired nuclei and portions of the central axonemes (H&E, 1250x).

Image 6

In another section through a crypt, portions of two trophozoites are clearly seen in ventral view (arrows). Note the typical paired nuclei. In addition, two trophozoites are seen in their lateral aspect (darts) (H&E, 1250x).

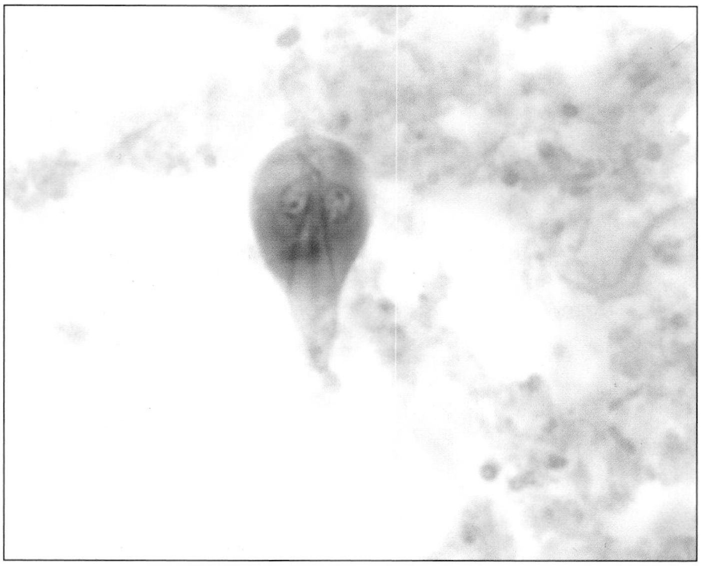

1

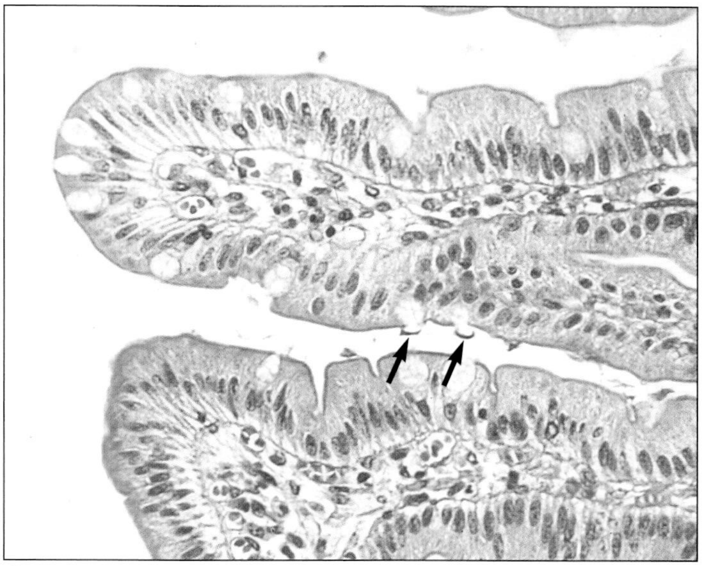

2

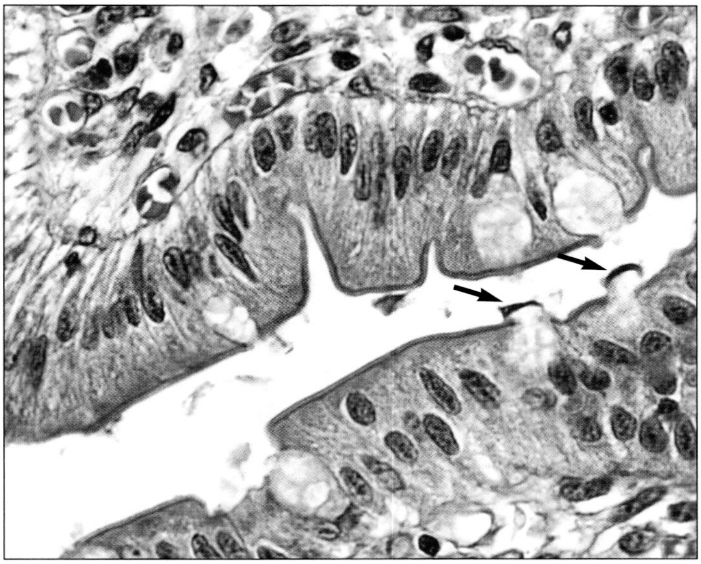

3

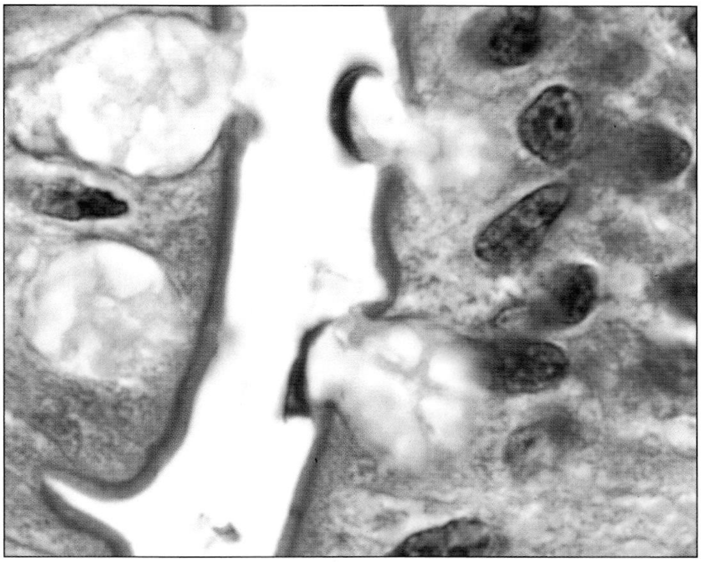

4

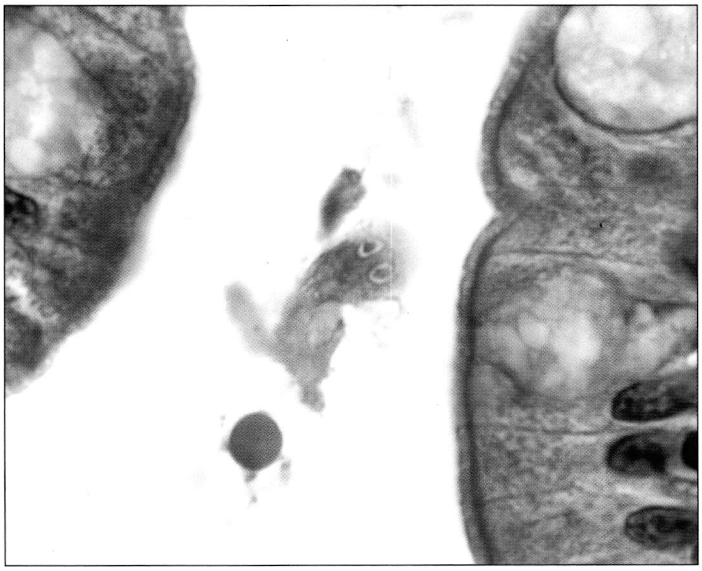

5

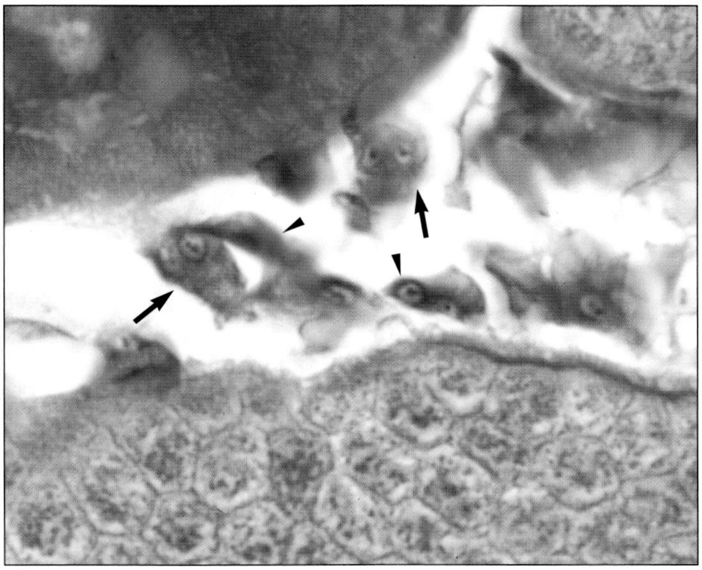

6

Balantidium coli

Balantidium coli is the largest protozoan and the only ciliate parasite of humans. It has worldwide distribution, though it is more common in warmer climates, where it and morphologically similar organisms occur in pigs and monkeys. Although human infections are often seen in people who work with pigs, humans have been shown to be resistant to pig strains of the parasite. In geographic areas where living conditions and personal hygiene are poor, balantidiasis may be transmitted as a human-to-human infection. The colon is the normal site of infection by the large trophozoites, but the parasite rarely disseminates to extraintestinal sites such as the liver, urinary tract, and peritoneal cavity. In tissue sections trophozoites are most likely to be seen in the mucosa and submucosa of the colon and appendix, but deeper involvement of the muscular layers may occur.

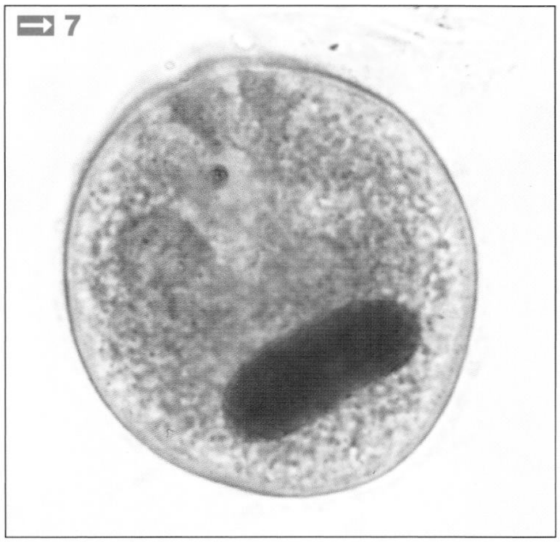

Biology and Life Cycle

Trophozoites colonize the lumen and wall of the colon, where they multiply by longitudinal binary fission and produce cysts. Cysts are the stage encountered in normal fecal specimens, whereas trophozoites are the stage usually found in patients with diarrhea or dysentery. Cysts passed in feces are infective. Infection occurs via the fecal-oral route.

Pathology and Clinical Manifestations

Patients with balantidiasis are either asymptomatic or have symptoms ranging from intermittent diarrhea to severe dysentery, often with blood, mucus, and white blood cells present. Eosinophilia is not a usual feature of the infection. Fever, epigastric distress, and abdominal pain are common. Diarrheal episodes may alternate with periods of constipation. Patients often experience nausea, vomiting, and anorexia, resulting in extreme weakness and weight loss over time. The clinical symptoms are similar to those seen in cases of intestinal amebiasis.

Trophozoites readily invade the wall of the colon and appendix. The ulcers or abscesses that they produce primarily involve the mucosa and submucosa, although invasion of the muscular layers and perforation of the bowel wall may occur. Ulcers are flask shaped, as in intestinal amebiasis, but they are often more shallow and have a wider opening. The adjacent mucosa is not as severely undermined as it is in amebiasis (Plate 7:1). Typical ulcers have ragged edges and necrotic material at the base. Trophozoites are more common in the mucosal and submucosal layers, but they are also found in the muscular layers. On rare occasions, organisms are found in sections of regional lymph nodes, on the peritoneum, and in other organs when extraintestinal dissemination occurs.

Parasite Morphology

Trophozoites measure from 50 to 200 μm in length and from 40 to 70 μm in width. They are ciliated and have two nuclei (a prominent, readily visible, kidney-bean-shaped macronucleus and a smaller, more obscure micronucleus), a characteristic mouth opening called a cytostome, and contractile vacuoles (➡ 7). Cysts are usually spherical, thick walled, and measure between 50 and 70 μm. The macronucleus is visible when the cysts are stained.

Depending on their plane of section, organisms appear as typical trophozoites in sections of tissue: they demonstrate cilia, a large macronucleus, and sometimes the cytostome and contractile vacuoles (Plate 7:2–6). However, in some sections none or only a few of the typical morphologic features may be evident. Because trophozoites are usually present in reasonable numbers, it is not difficult to recognize characteristic features in some of the organisms. Cysts are not found in histologic section; only trophozoites invade tissue.

The features that distinguish *Balantidium* from other protozoa in tissue are its much larger size and the presence of cilia, a large cytostome, and a prominent macronucleus.

References

Arean VM, Koppisch E. Balantidiasis: a review and report of cases. *Am J Pathol.* 1956;32:1089-1115.

Dodd LG. *Balantidium coli* infestation as a cause of acute appendicitis. *J Infect Dis.* 1991;163:1392.

Swartzwelder JC. Balantidiasis. *Am J Dig Dis.* 1950;17:173-179.

Zaman V. *Balantadium coli.* In: Kreier JP, Baker JR, eds. *Parasitic Protozoa, Vol III.* 2nd ed. San Diego, Calif: Academic Press Inc; 1993.

Plate 7

Balantidium coli

Image 1

A section through the edge of an ulcer in human colon. Necrosis extends through the submucosa. The adjacent mucosa appears normal. Ulcers such as this are not unlike what is seen in amebiasis, but in *Balantidium* the opening of the ulcer is wider (H&E, 25x).

Image 2

Three trophozoites of *B. coli* are evident in this section of human colon. In two organisms, the large dark-staining kidney-bean-shaped macronucleus is evident, whereas in the third only a small portion of the macronucleus is in the plane of section (H&E, 125x).

Image 3

Numerous trophozoites are seen in this section of human colon. The characteristic large macronucleus is seen clearly in only a few of the organisms (darts) (H&E, 125x).

Image 4

In this cluster of trophozoites, the macronucleus is evident in three organisms. The cytostome is visible in one trophozoite (dart) (H&E, 250x).

Image 5

A cluster of trophozoites is evident in a crypt. At low magnification, macronuclei are visible in many of the organisms (H&E, 100x).

Image 6

In these trophozoites, macronuclei are seen in different planes of section. In one of these, the cytostome (dart) is also seen (H&E, 250x).

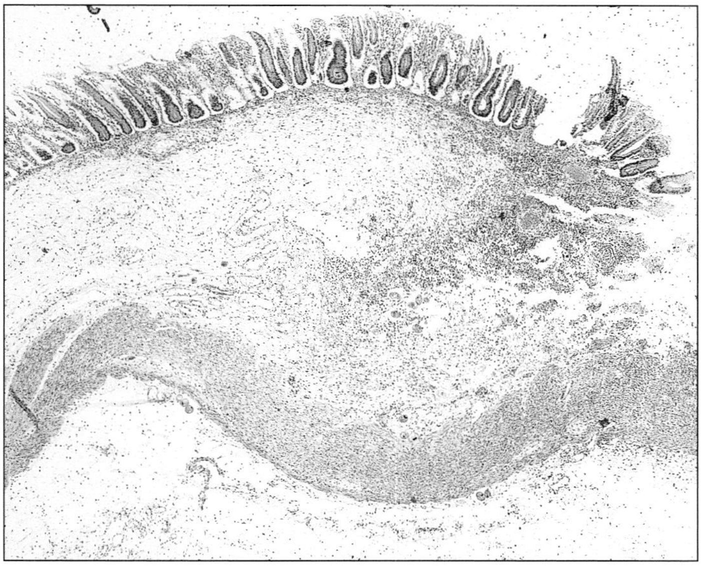
1

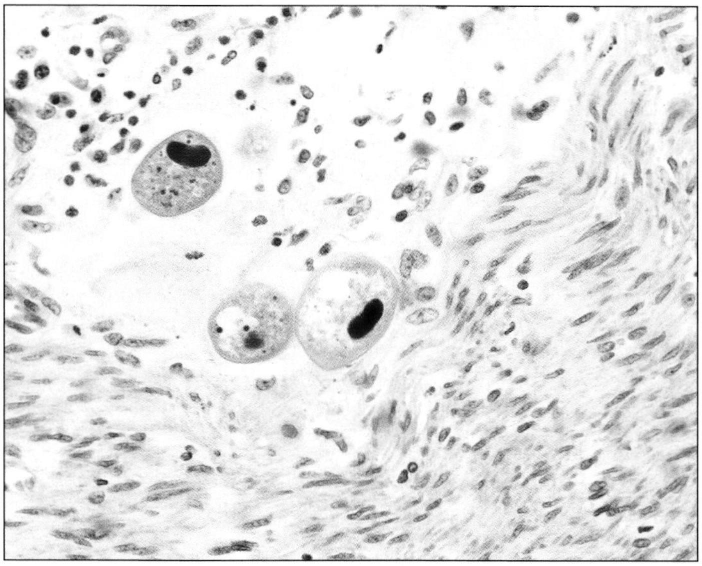
2

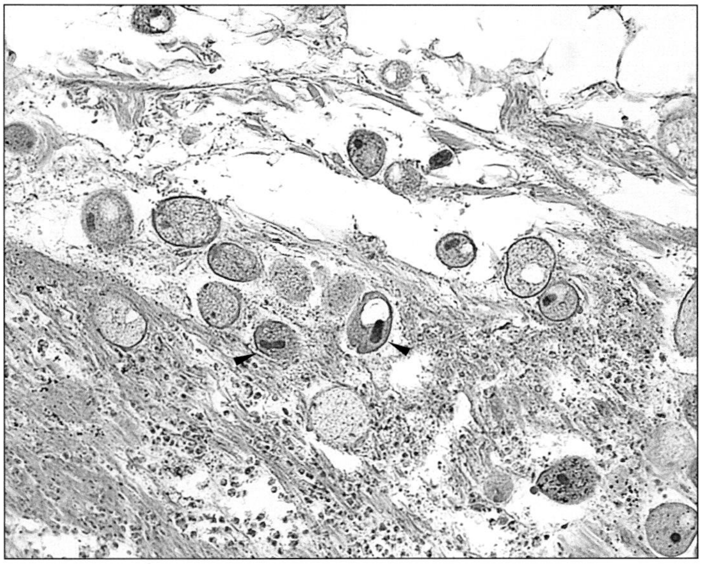
3

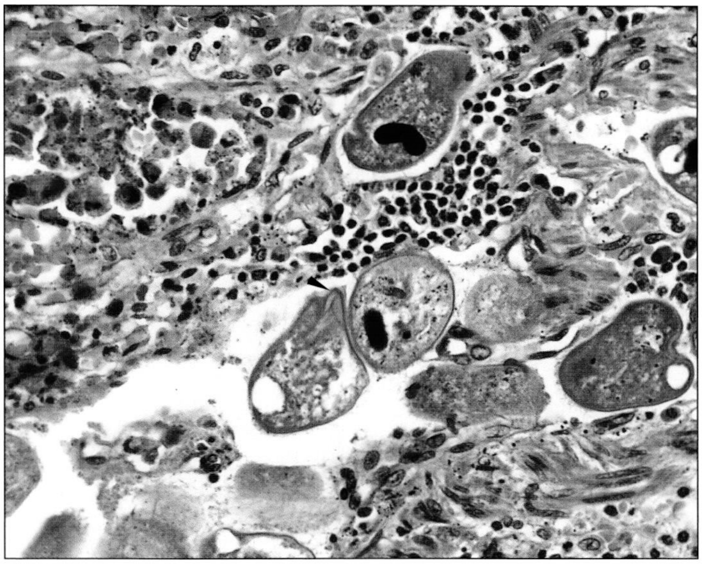
4

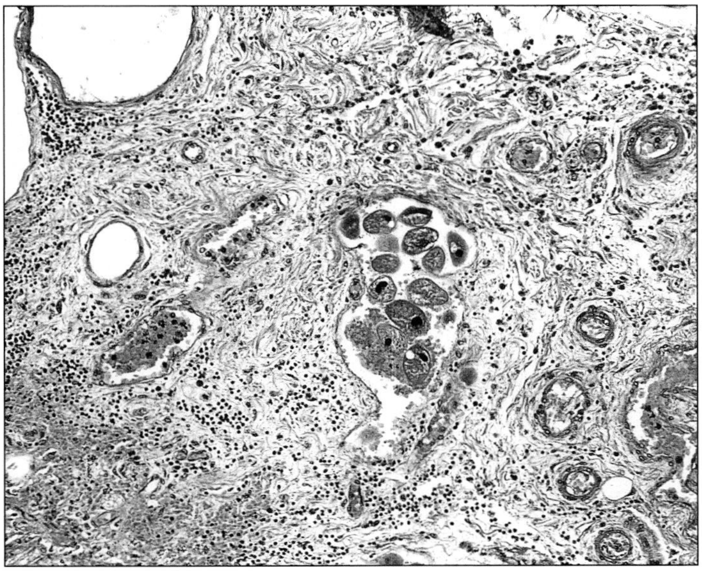
5

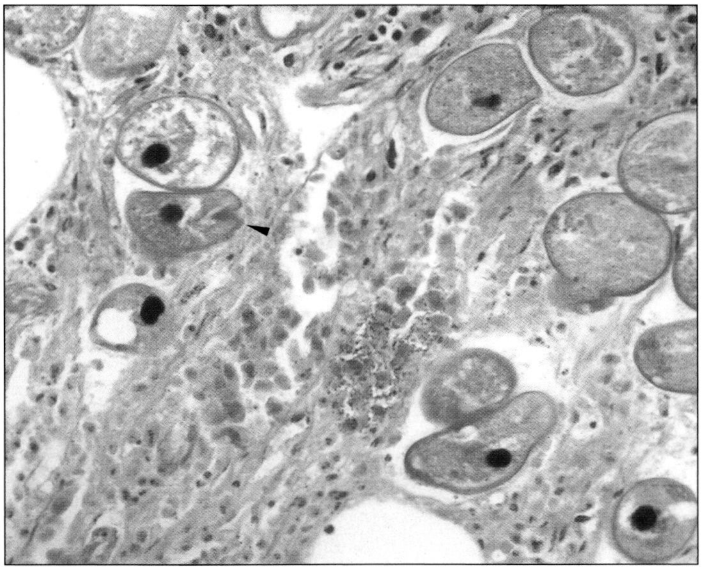
6

Cryptosporidium parvum and *Isospora belli*

Cryptosporidiosis and Isosporiasis

Cryptosporidiosis has only recently emerged as a human disease of significant public health importance. Species of *Cryptosporidium*, an intestinal coccidian, have been known for almost a century and have been described in most vertebrates. Although the parasite has long been known to produce disease in cattle, horses, pigs, and other animals, it was not recognized as a cause of human disease until the early 1980s, when it became known as one of the opportunistic infections associated with AIDS. As studies have progressed, it is now well recognized that *Cryptosporidium* not only causes severe problems in immunocompromised patients, it also causes diarrheal disease in immunocompetent individuals. Surveys of surface water in the United States, many parts of Latin America, and probably worldwide readily demonstrate the presence of the resistant oocyst stage of the organism. Municipal water supplies often become contaminated with fecal wastes, and unless proper filtration methods are used, the result can be diarrheal outbreaks like those in several cities in the United States in recent years. Chlorine levels 30 times higher than those used in water treatment plants are required to kill *Cryptosporidium*; standard chlorination has little effect. *Cryptosporidium parvum*, generally a parasite of cows, is the species considered responsible for most human infections.

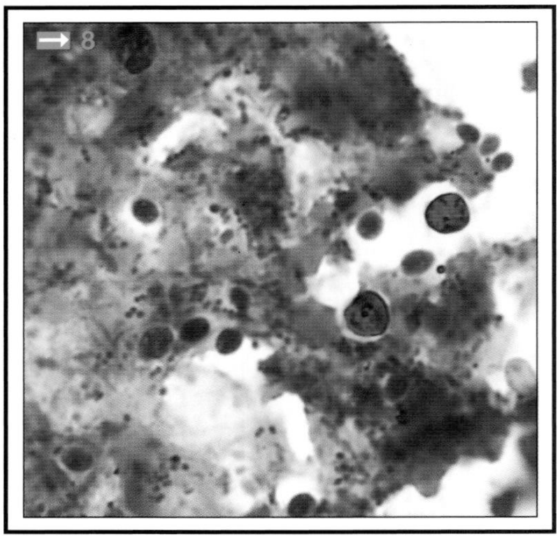

A second intestinal coccidian, *Isospora belli*, has been known for many years to cause human diarrheal disease. This organism also infects both normal and immunocompromised individuals, but the disease is more severe and long lasting in the latter group. Therapy for both isosporiasis and cryptosporidiosis is still inconsistent and often unsuccessful.

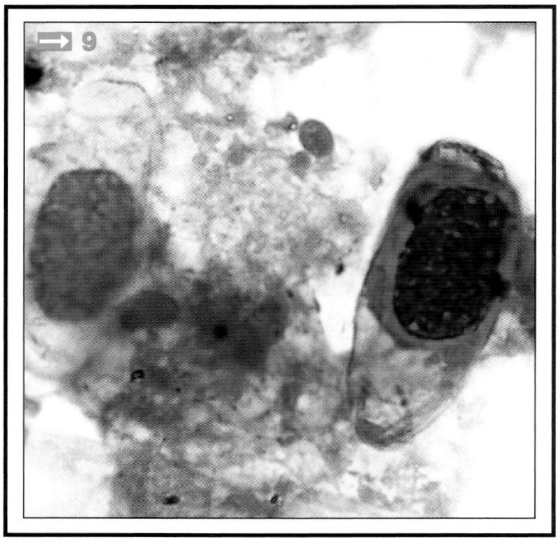

Biology and Life Cycle

The life cycles of both *C. parvum* and *I. belli* involve only a single host. *Cryptosporidium parvum* is an intracellular but extracytoplasmic parasite that colonizes the brush border of enterocytes but does not invade the cytoplasm of the cells. Oocysts containing four sporozoites are the infective stage of the organism. When ingested by a human or animal host, sporozoites emerge and enter the microvillus border, develop into trophozoites, and undergo several cycles of asexual multiplication (schizogony), which results in merozoite formation. When the schizonts rupture, the merozoites invade other cells to continue further schizogony or begin sexual reproduction by forming microgametocytes and macrogametocytes. This continuing schizogony can result in the production of many parasites and is a form of internal autoinfection. Fertilization of macrogametes by microgametes results in the formation of zygotes, which develop a cyst wall and are known as oocysts. The oocysts sporulate while still in the microvillus border and contain four sporozoites. A small percentage of the sporulated oocysts have a thin cyst wall, but the majority have a thicker cyst wall. Only the thick-walled oocysts are excreted in feces; the thin-walled ones rupture in the lumen of the intestine and initiate further intestinal infection. This is another mechanism for building up large numbers of organisms in the intestine. Oocysts are immediately infective when excreted in feces and, in the absence of temperature extremes, they can survive for several months or longer in the external environment. Fecal-oral transmission is the primary route of infection, although infection via inhalation has been documented. The usual incubation period is approximately one week.

Isospora belli differs from *Cryptosporidium* in several important ways. Unsporulated oocysts excreted in feces must develop for a week or slightly less to reach the infective stage. The mature oocyst contains two thin-walled sporocysts, each of which contains four sporozoites. After ingestion of the infective oocyst, the sporozoites emerge and penetrate the cytoplasm of enterocytes, where they undergo both asexual and sexual reproduction. After multiple cycles of schizogony, gametocytes form. A zygote is produced through sexual reproduction and a cyst wall develops around the zygote, forming the oocyst. The oocysts undergo no further development until they pass into the external environment. Because *I. belli* develops only in humans, details of the intracellular development within enterocytes is not as completely known as it is for *Cryptosporidium*.

Pathology and Clinical Manifestations

Acute cryptosporidiosis causes severe watery diarrhea as well as cramping, abdominal pain, nausea, anorexia, and weight loss. In immunocompetent patients, the incubation period ranges from several days to more than a week and is followed by a self-limiting, mild to severe diarrhea that lasts for several days to two weeks or longer. Excretion of moderate to large numbers of oocysts may continue for several days after symptoms cease. In patients with AIDS, the course of infection is initially mild but progresses rapidly to a profuse watery diarrhea, typically with excretion of 10 to 20 L per day. Eating often causes severe abdominal pain and worsens the diarrhea, so that patients refuse to eat and rapidly lose weight, perhaps hastening death.

Histologically, mucosal damage often is extensive and includes villous atrophy and inflammatory cell infiltration throughout the wall extending to the lamina propria. In immunocompromised patients, involvement of the liver, pancreas, and respiratory tract can occur. Developmental stages of the parasite have been found in the epithelium of the gallbladder in patients with cholecystitis, and pathologic conditions may include obstruction and a sclerosing cholangitis (Plate 8:6). Similarly, developmental stages have been found in the pancreatic duct. Respiratory symptomatology includes wheezing, coughing, hoarseness, and shortness of breath. Organisms have been found in the epithelial lining of the trachea, bronchi, and bronchioles (Plate 8:15); however, the parasites have not been reported in alveolar spaces. No consistently satisfactory treatment has been reported for cryptosporidiosis.

As with cryptosporidial infection, the course of *I. belli* infection ranges from no symptoms to a protracted, self-limiting diarrhea in immunocompetent individuals. In immunocompromised patients, the diarrhea is intermittent, prolonged, and more severe, resembling a spruelike syndrome. Pathologically, villi of the small intestinal mucosa are somewhat flattened or exhibit total atrophy. Tissue eosinophilia is not uncommon. Developing stages of the parasite can be found within the cytoplasm of enterocytes. Dissemination of *I. belli* to extraintestinal locations has been reported only rarely. Treatment of this infection is more satisfactory than treatment for cryptosporidiosis, but it usually must be continued for an extended time.

Parasite Morphology

Sporulated *Cryptosporidium* oocysts (4 to 6 µm in diameter) are the resistant stage excreted in feces. They are best seen when the fecal smear is stained with some modification of the acid-fast stain. Oocysts stain pink to bright red and typically contain several prominent black granules (➡ 8). Although trichrome stain, which is frequently used for fecal smears, does not consistently stain these oocysts, it does occasionally stain them well, making it possible to see the four sporozoites inside.

The unsporulated oocysts of *I. belli* are excreted in feces and usually measure 20 to 33 µm long by 10 to 19 µm wide. They taper at the ends, have a double-layered refractile wall, and contain a single sporoblast. Fully developed oocysts in the external environment contain two sporocysts, each of which contains four sporozoites. In acid-fast–stained fecal smears, the oocyst wall is outlined in red and the sporoblast stains positive (➡ 9).

Developmental stages of *Cryptosporidium* can be found at all levels of the alimentary tract, with the jejunum typically the most heavily infected site (Plate 8:1). At the light microscopic level, the parasites are seen as small (3 to 5 µm), spherical structures that are frequently aligned in rows within the brush border of the epithelium (Plate 8:3 & 4). It is difficult if not impossible to visualize or identify the developmental stages unless electron microscopy is utilized. Among the stages identifiable in electron microscopy preparations are trophozoites, schizonts, microgametes and macrogametes, and oocysts containing sporozoites (Plate 8:2). Developmental stages of *I. belli* occur within the cytoplasm of enterocytes, but morphologic details have been incompletely described.

In histologic preparations, the localization of *Cryptosporidium* within the brush border of enterocytes suggests infection with this parasite rather than other coccidian organisms. *Cyclospora cayetanensis*, a recently described intestinal coccidian of humans, produces an unsporulated oocyst that occurs in human feces and resembles *Cryptosporidium*. The oocyst of *Cyclospora* is larger (typically 8 to 10 µm in diameter) and requires approximately five days in the external environment to sporulate. When infective it contains two sporocysts, each with two sporozoites. Electron microscopy of jejunal biopsy specimens has shown that the developmental stages of *Cyclospora* occur within a vacuole at the luminal end of the cytoplasm of enterocytes rather than in the brush border. These developmental stages have been described as measuring 6 to 8 µm long by 1 to 4 µm wide. Thus, *Cyclospora* resembles *I. belli* more closely than it does *Cryptosporidium* with its intracytoplasmic development in enterocytes. With light microscopy of histologic sections, it often is difficult to distinguish *Cyclospora* from *Isospora* on the basis of developmental stages in enterocytes; however, their oocysts in feces are markedly different in size and morphology.

References

Bendall RP, Lucas S, Moody A, et al. Diarrhea associated with cyanobacterium-like bodies: a new coccidian enteritis of man. *Lancet*. 1993;341:590-592.

Connor BA, Shlim DR, Scholes JV, et al. Pathologic changes in the small bowel in nine patients with diarrhea associated with a coccidia-like body. *Ann Intern Med*. 1993;119:377-382.

Current WL, Garcia LS. Cryptosporidiosis. *Clin Microbiol Rev*. 1991;4:325-358.

Giang TT, Pollack G, Kotler DP. Cryptosporidiosis of the nasal mucosa in a patient with AIDS. *AIDS*. 1994;8:555-556.

Godwin TA. Cryptosporidiosis in the acquired immunodeficiency syndrome: a study of 15 autopsy cases. *Hum Pathol*. 1991;22:1215-1224.

Leftkowitch JH, Krumholz S, Feng-Chen KC, et al. Cryptosporidiosis of the human small intestine: a light and electron microscopic study. *Hum Pathol*. 1984;15:746-752.

Ortega YR, Sterling CR, Gilman RH, et al. *Cyclospora* species—a new protozoan pathogen of humans. *N Engl J Med*. 1993;328:1308-1312.

Restrepo C, Macher AM, Radany EH. Disseminated extraintestinal isosporiasis in a patient with acquired immune deficiency syndrome. *Am J Clin Pathol*. 1987;87:536-542.

Ribeiro Jr H daC, Teichborg S, Sun T, et al. Ultrastructure of human cryptosporidial infection: a review. *Prog Clin Parasitol*. 1989;1:143-158.

Sterling CR, Arrowood MJ. Cryptosporidiosis. In: Kreier JP, ed. *Parasitic Protozoa, Vol VI*. 2nd ed. San Diego, Calif: Academic Press Inc; 1993:159-225.

Plate 8

Cryptosporidium parvum

Image 1

Scanning electron micrograph of the heavily infected terminal portion of the ileum of a lamb experimentally infected with *Cryptosporidium parvum*. Many spherical organisms are seen attached to the microvillus brush border (1000x). (Courtesy of S. Tzipori.)

Image 2

Transmission electron micrograph demonstrates various developmental stages of *Cryptosporidium* within the microvillus brush border of an experimentally infected lamb (6000x). (Courtesy of S. Tzipori.)

Image 3

Villus of small intestine demonstrates minute, spherical, basophilic-staining cryptosporidial organisms (darts) within the brush border. At low magnification, one cannot specifically identify *Cryptosporidium,* but the presence of organisms within the brush border strongly suggests this infection (H&E, 500x). (Case courtesy of Y. Gutierrez.)

Image 4

At high magnification, the spherical, basophilic-staining cryptosporidial organisms are clear (darts). Again, it is the location of the organisms rather than their morphology that suggests the infection (H&E, 1250x). (Case courtesy of Y. Gutierrez.)

Image 5

Cryptosporidial organisms (darts) are seen at the luminal aspect of respiratory epithelium of a patient with a history of malignant lymphoma (H&E, 1250x).

Image 6

Cryptosporidial organisms are seen at the surface of bile duct epithelium in an experimentally infected nude mouse. Human bile duct infections with this parasite have been reported (H&E, 750x). (Case courtesy of J. Mead.)

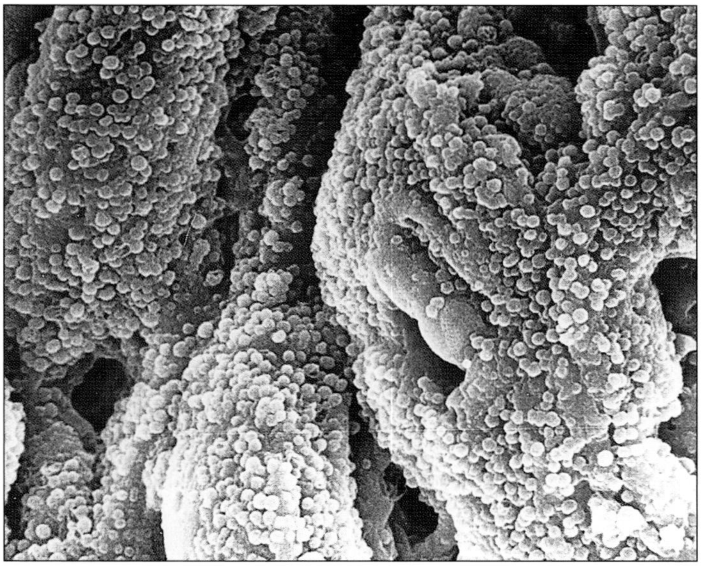

1

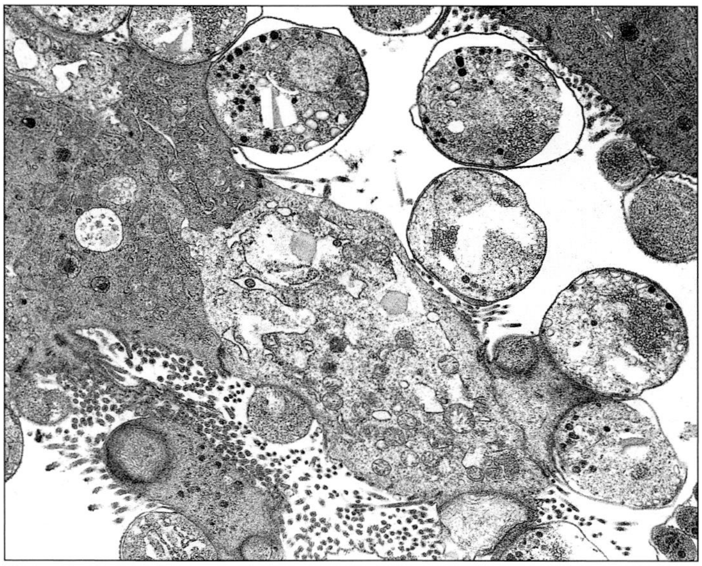

2

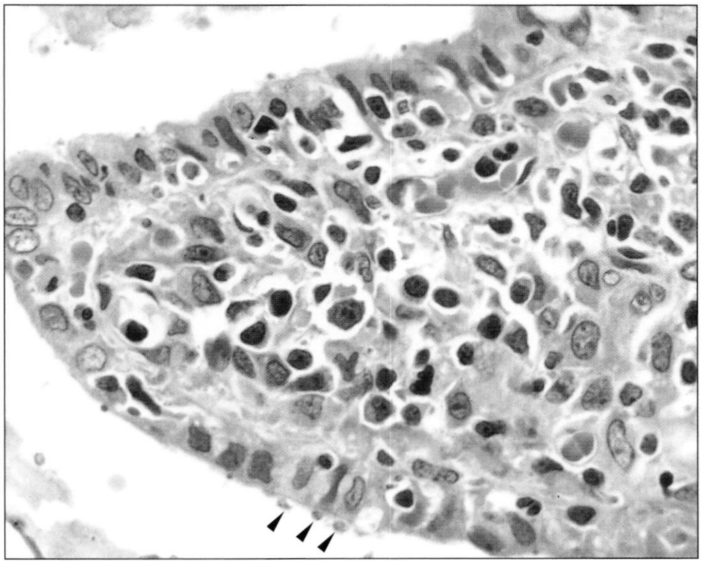

3

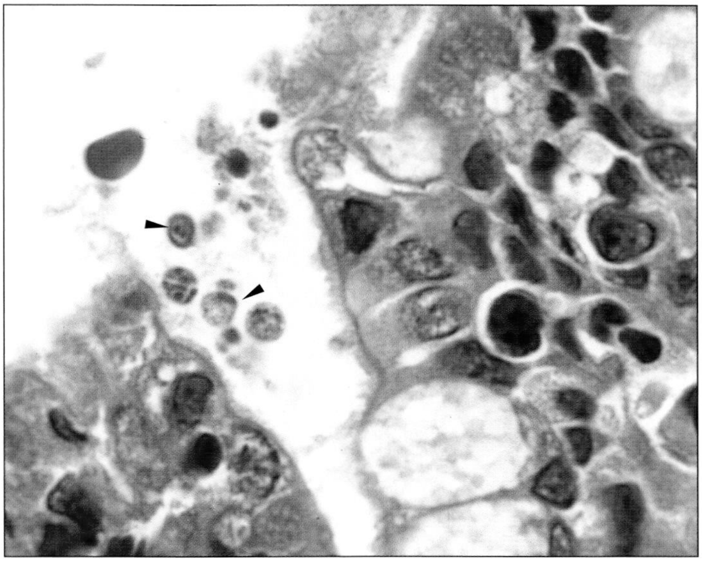

4

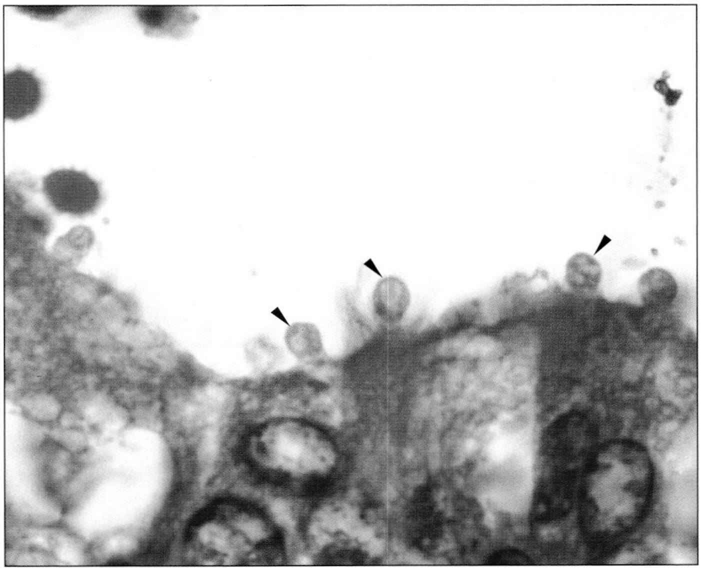

5

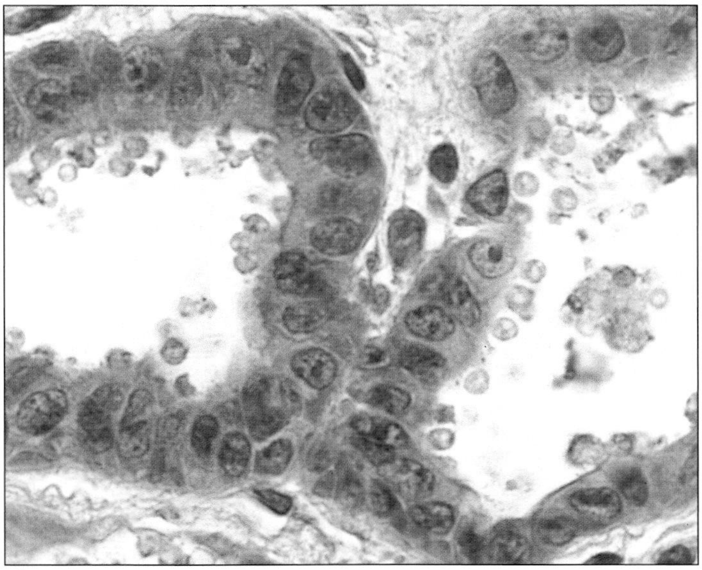

6

Sarcocystis species

Sarcocystosis

Sarcocystosis infection with coccidian parasites of the genus *Sarcocystis* is widely prevalent in livestock and occurs in almost all mammals and birds. Humans may serve as both intermediate and definitive hosts. Two species, *S. hominis* and *S. suihominis*, have a sexual cycle in the human small intestine, resulting in the passage of oocysts and sporocysts in feces. In addition, several morphologic types of tissue cysts (sarcocysts) have been described from muscle tissues of humans. In these instances, it is likely that other animals serve as the true or usual intermediate hosts in the life cycles, and humans are only accidental hosts. Sarcocysts discovered in human tissues, where the infecting organism was unknown, have been referred to as *S. lindemanni*, which represents a number of as yet undescribed species. Because there are many species and they occur in a wide range of definitive and intermediate hosts, the taxonomy and classification of many of these parasites continue to change. Actually, each organism has one or several previous specific names.

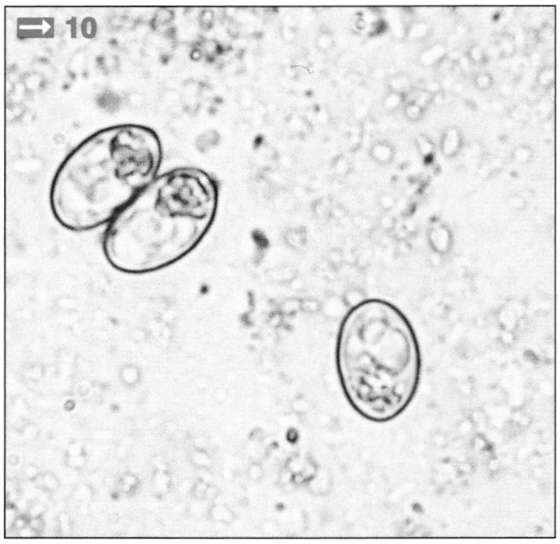

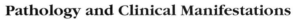

Biology and Life Cycle

Species of *Sarcocystis* have a two-host (predator-prey) life cycle, in which the definitive host (usually a carnivore or omnivore) acquires infection by eating the flesh of the appropriate intermediate host, the prey. In the intestine of the definitive host, bradyzoites escaping from the ingested sarcocysts invade the intestinal epithelium, where they become male (micro) and female (macro) gamonts. Fusion of male and female gametes results in production of a zygote, which upon secreting a cyst wall is known as an oocyst. The precise location in the intestinal epithelium where this occurs varies with the species of parasite. In some species it is within enterocytes; in others it is in goblet cells. Ultimately, the oocysts undergo sporulation in the lamina propria of the intestinal wall, resulting in the production of two sporocysts, each of which contains four sporozoites. These mature oocysts have a thin wall that ruptures easily when they enter the intestinal lumen. Both intact oocysts and individual sporocysts are found in feces. The time lapse between ingestion of sarcocysts and production of oocysts usually ranges from one to two weeks.

Ingestion by the intermediate hosts of infective sporocysts or oocysts in contaminated food or water results in the liberation of sporozoites. Although the life cycle is not precisely known for most animal species, it appears that the initial invasion of the endothelium of small arteries in mesenteric lymph nodes is followed by a process of asexual multiplication known as schizogony (or merogony). Merozoites are produced and then invade the endothelial lining of capillaries and small arteries throughout the body, starting a second generation of schizogony. Merozoites from these schizonts invade skeletal and striated muscle cells, where they begin the process of tissue cyst formation that leads to sarcocysts. Although two generations of schizogony appear to be characteristic for larger domestic animals, smaller animals have only one generation before sarcocyst development. Invasion of muscle cells by merozoites initiates sarcocyst formation. Merozoites develop initially as metrocytes and then mature into bradyzoites, which divide by endodyogeny and produce the tissue cysts. Although sarcocysts can survive for the lifetime of the host, many persist for only several months. Diagnosis of enteric infection requires demonstration of oocysts or sporocysts in feces. To diagnose tissue infection, characteristic sarcocysts must be found in histologic sections of muscle tissue.

Pathology and Clinical Manifestations

When humans serve as definitive hosts for *S. hominis* and *S. suihominis*, infections often appear to be asymptomatic and clear spontaneously. In other instances, however, mild fever, acute diarrhea, chills, vomiting, and respiratory difficulties develop. Symptomatology generally lasts for a day or less and abates spontaneously. *Sarcocystis suihominis* appears to be more pathogenic than *S. hominis*. Given the wide prevalence of sarcocysts in food animals, transient diarrhea caused by these or other as yet undescribed species may be more frequent than reported in the literature. In the human host, sarcocysts generally have not been associated with pathologic conditions, although individuals with such infections occasionally have reported myalgia, muscle weakness, and transitory edema. Experimental infections of food animals with various species of *Sarcocystis* have demonstrated varying degrees of pathogenicity. In some animals, few clinical manifestations are noted; in others, anemia, eosinophilic myositis, tissue necrosis, and abortions and fetal deaths occur.

Parasite Morphology

Sporulated oocysts of *S. hominis* measure approximately 13 to 16 µm long by 16 to 21 µm wide, with the individual sporocysts measuring 13 to 16 µm long by 8 to 11 µm wide. In the other human species, *S. suihominis*, the oocysts are slightly smaller (13 by 19 µm), with individual sporocysts measuring 13 by 10 µm. Many species of *Sarcocystis* occur in canine and feline hosts. In general, the sporocysts passed in canid feces measure approximately 15 by 10 µm, whereas those in felines are slightly smaller, about 12 by 10 µm (➡ 10).

Several morphologic types of sarcocysts have been observed in skeletal and myocardial tissues. Grossly, sarcocysts in skeletal muscle tend to be elongated or spindle shaped, tapering at the ends, whereas the cysts in cardiac muscle are more rounded. Depending on their age in the tissue, the cysts may attain lengths of several millimeters and may have diameters of up to 200 µm or more. Tissue cysts in myocardial tissue tend to be small (Plate 9:14), less than 100 µm in diameter. In some animal hosts, such as cattle, tissue cysts reach lengths of 8 mm and have diameters of 1 mm. Sarcocysts in human tissues are often identical to cysts found in the tissues of primates and other animals, which are the hosts most likely to be ingested by the definitive predator hosts.

In histologic sections, the sarcocyst wall varies among species, from thin and smooth to thick and striated (Plate 10:1–4). Some bear projections (often called cytophaneres), which may be of different shapes, ranging from thick and villous to hairlike (Plate 10:2). The internal part of the cyst may or may not be divided into compartments by septa (Plate 9:1–3, 5). The bradyzoites inside the cysts typically are banana shaped and measure between 3 and 6 µm long by 1 to 3 µm wide (Plate 10:5 & 6).

Sarcocysts are most likely to be confused with the tissue cysts of *Toxoplasma* and *Neospora*. However, the sarcocysts are often much larger and can be visualized grossly. In histologic sections, sarcocysts usually have thicker walls and may be striated. The cyst is often compartmentalized. The bradyzoites of *Sarcocystis* are larger and more prominent. In *Toxoplasma,* the entire bradyzoite (except the nucleus) is PAS positive; in *Sarcocystis,* areas in the cytoplasm are PAS negative.

References

Beaver PC, Gadgil RK, Morera P. *Sarcocystis* in man: a review and report of five cases. *Am J Trop Med Hyg.* 1979;28:819-844.

Dubey JP. *Toxoplasma, Neospora, Sarcocystis,* and other tissue cyst-forming coccidia of humans and animals. In: Kreier JP, ed. *Parasitic Protozoa, Vol VI.* 2nd ed. San Diego, Calif: Academic Press Inc; 1993.

Pamphlett R, O'Donoghue P. *Sarcocystis* infection of human muscle. *Aust N Z J Med.* 1990;20:705-707.

Wong KT, Clarke G, Pathmanathan R, et al. Light microscopic and three-dimensional morphology of the human muscular sarcocyst. *Parasitol Res.* 1994;80:138-140.

Wong KT, Pathmanathan R. Ultrastructure of the human skeletal muscle sarcocyst. *J Parasitol.* 1994;80:327-330.

Sarcocystis species

Image 1

Sarcocysts of an unidentified *Sarcocystis* species are evident in this section of human deltoid muscle. The cyst is divided into compartments by septa, but the individual bradyzoites within the compartments are not evident at this magnification (H&E, 200x). (Case courtesy of R. Pamphlett.)

Image 2

At high magnification, the compartmentalization of one of the sarcocysts is evident. The primary cyst wall is 50 to 60 μm thick, and the individual bradyzoites are numerous and small within irregularly shaped compartments (H&E, 500x). (Courtesy of R. Pamphlett.)

Image 3

Cross-section of a sarcocyst in the arm muscle of an Indian. The cyst wall is thin and smooth. Many small bradyzoites are seen within the cyst. Tissue cysts similar to this one have been seen in rhesus monkeys from India (H&E, 750x).

Image 4

A small sarcocyst is visible in this section of cardiac muscle of a Costa Rican child. The cyst wall is thin, but the bradyzoites appear to be reasonably large. The species is unknown, but the cyst morphology is similar to that of *S. cruzi* (H&E, 500x).

Image 5

Another sarcocyst in a muscle biopsy specimen of an Indian. The grouping of the bradyzoites within the cyst suggests the presence of septa, although the walls cannot be seen. The cyst wall is thin and smooth (H&E, 1000x).

Image 6

Transverse section through the muscle of a patient who had lived in Asia. In this cyst of an unknown species of *Sarcocystis*, the wall appears thin and the individual bradyzoites appear as dotlike structures (PAS, 400x).

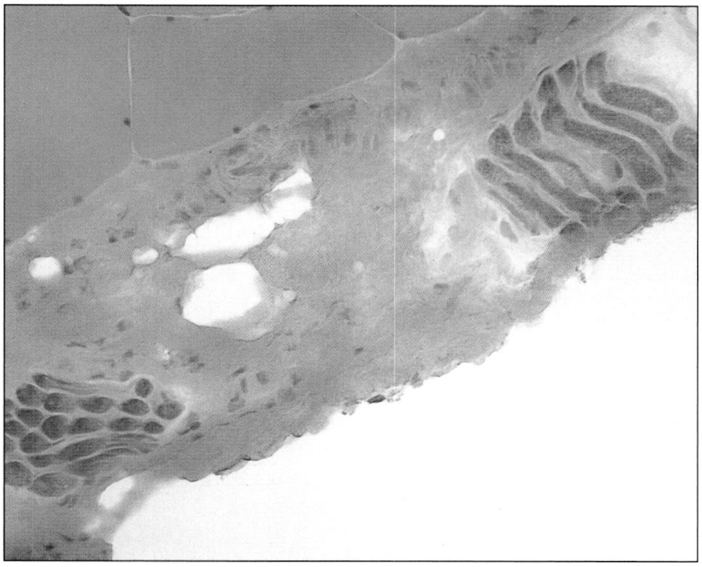
1

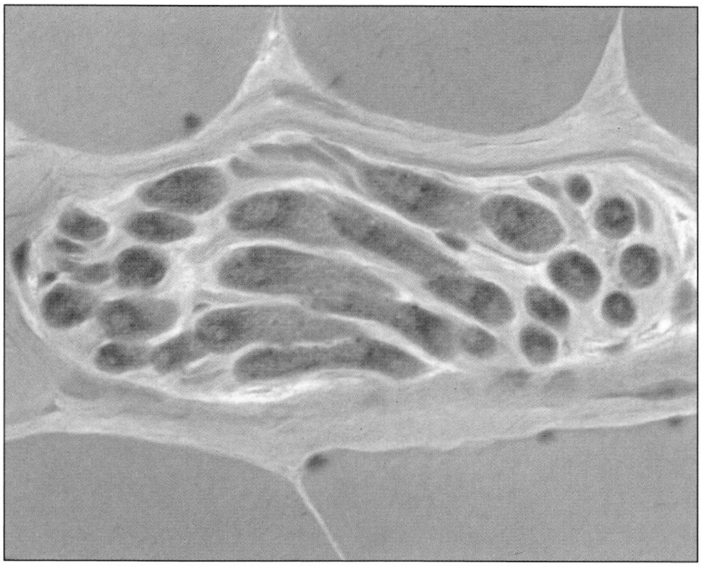
2

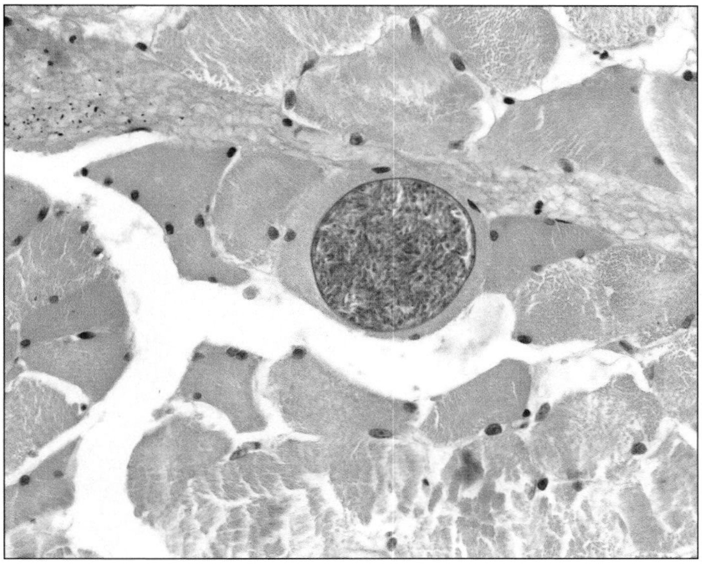
3

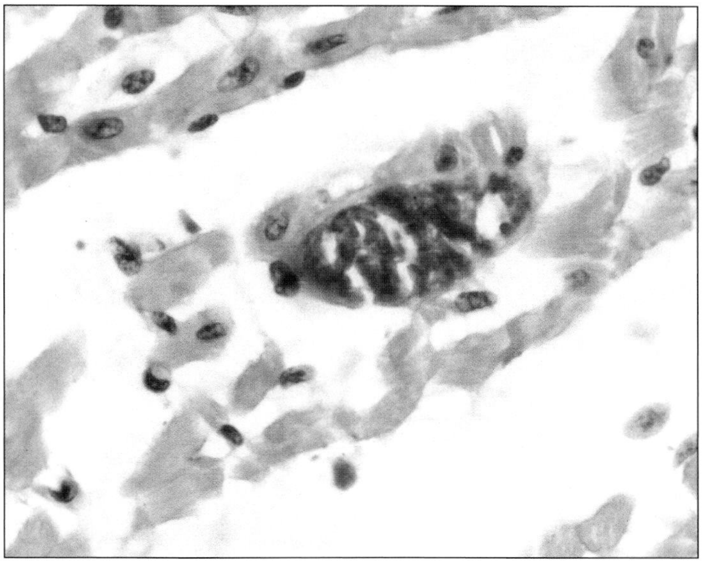
4

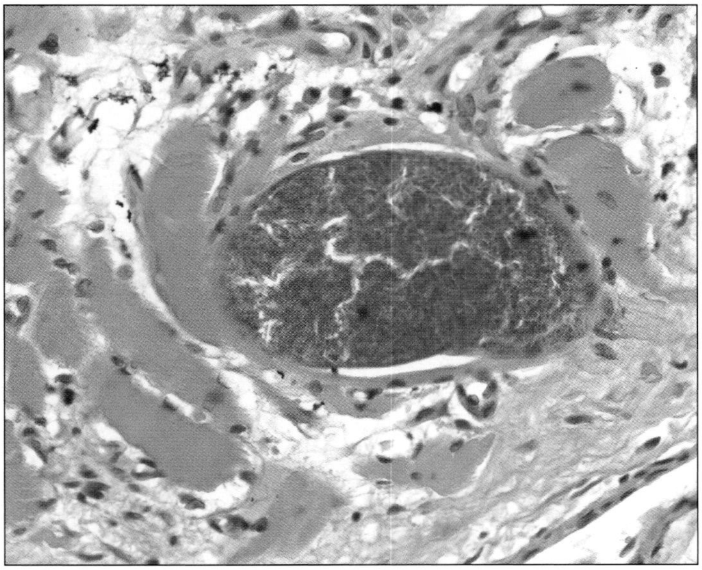
5

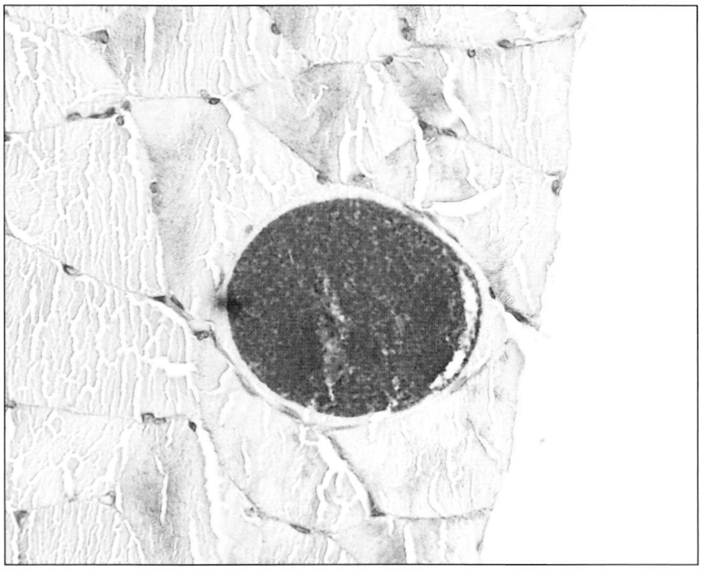
6

Plate 10

Sarcocystis species

Image 1

An unidentified species of sarcocyst in the leg muscle of an East African. This longitudinal section demonstrates a cyst with a thick surrounding wall and an internal mass divided into many compartments by septa (H&E, 50x).

Image 2

At higher magnification, the thick surrounding wall of this sarcocyst is seen to contain radiating processes on the outer surface. One can make out the septa (darts) forming the compartments, which contain some metrocytes and many bradyzoites. Individual bradyzoites measure 8 to 12 µm long and approximately 2 µm in diameter (H&E, 100x).

Image 3

A sarcocyst cut in cross section from the same case as Image 2. The sarcocyst is filled with bradyzoites (H&E, 500x).

Image 4

Another transverse section through a sarcocyst. The thick wall (arrow) of the cyst is evident, the compartments are polygonal, and septa are visible (H&E, 750x).

Image 5

Sarcocysts of *S. suihominis* in the tongue of a pig. Most of the elongated cysts are cut in transverse section and appear rounded. Bradyzoites are visible, but one cannot see their structural details at this magnification (H&E, 125x).

Image 6

At higher magnification, an elongated cyst of *S. suihominis* is seen. In pigs, sarcocysts are usually spindle shaped, reach lengths of 1 to 1.5 mm, have thick, striated walls, and are divided internally into compartments. Bradyzoites of this species are approximately 15 µm long by 4 µm to 5 µm wide. The septa are not apparent in this section of the sarcocyst (H&E, 500x).

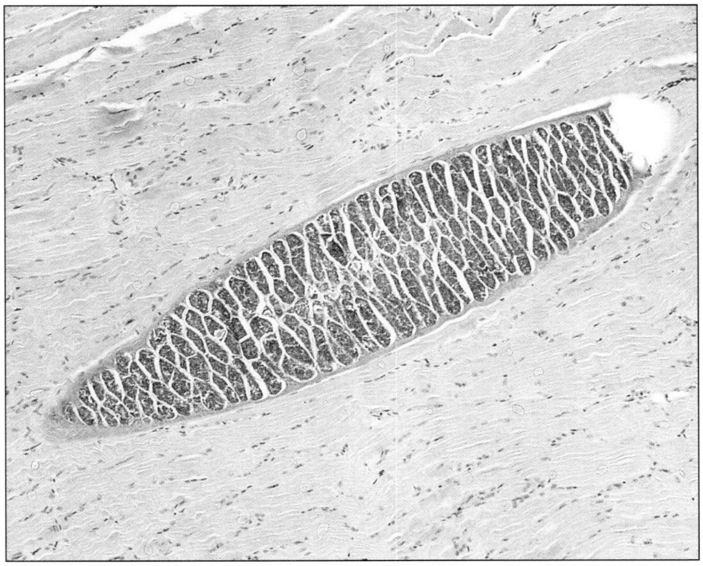
1

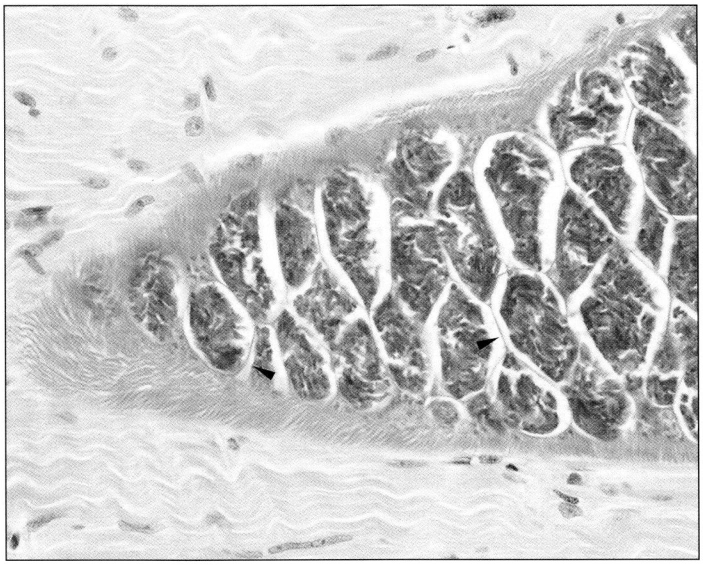
2

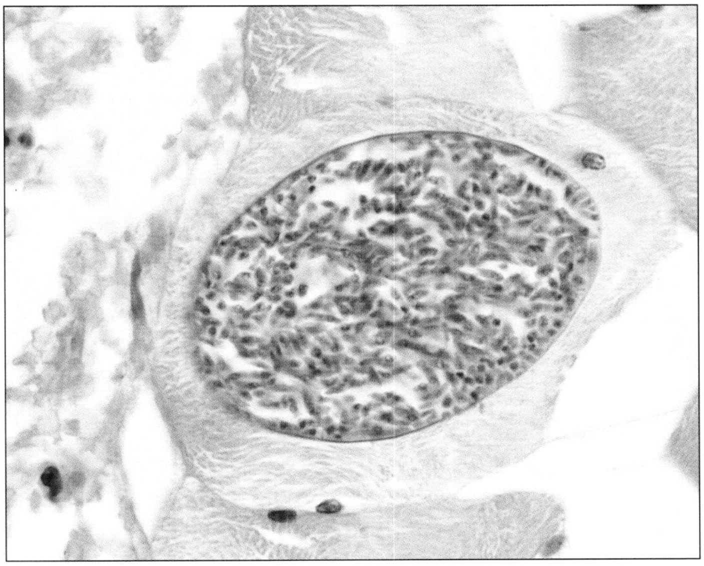
3

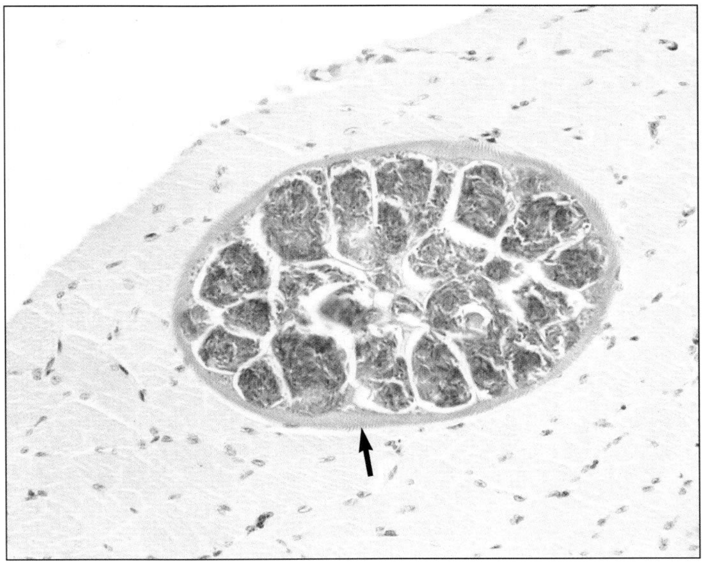
4

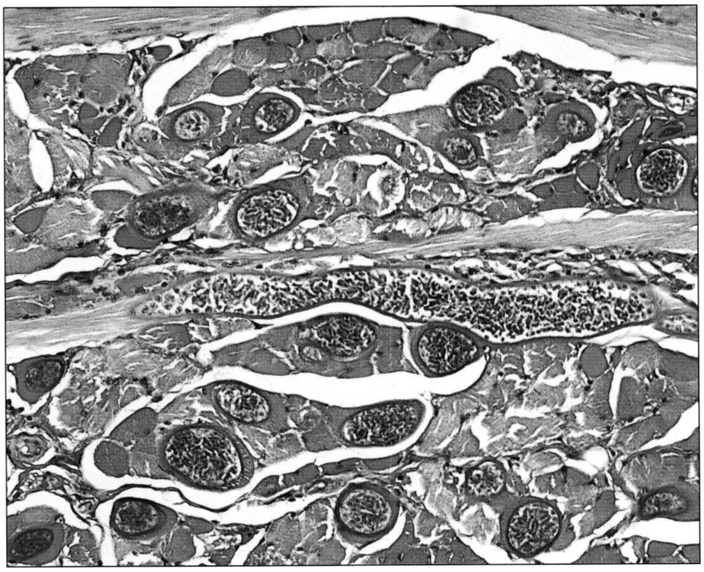
5

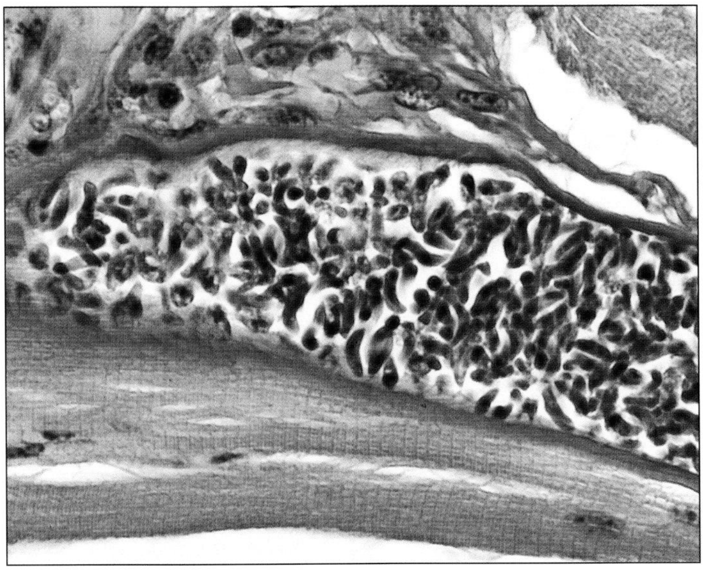
6

Toxoplasma gondii

Toxoplasmosis

Toxoplasma gondii is the best known and most important of the apicomplexan coccidian parasites that cause human disease. This parasite is prevalent throughout the world, with low to high seropositivity rates in humans, depending on diet and geographic location. Although congenital toxoplasmosis has long been recognized as one of the most important manifestations of this parasite, it also causes central nervous system disease in patients with AIDS and other immunosuppression conditions.

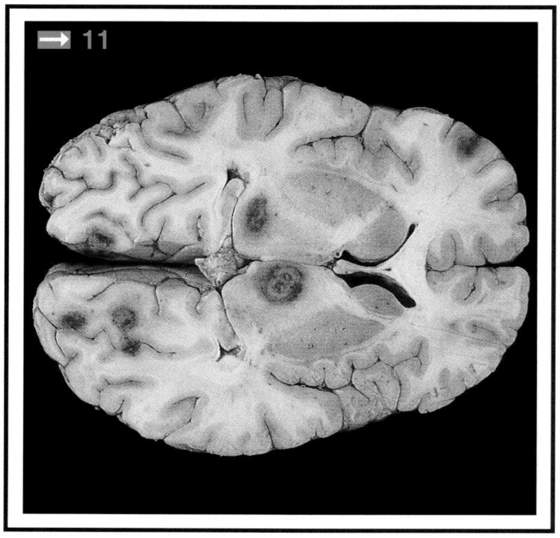

Biology and Life Cycle

Toxoplasma gondii is an intracellular parasite of humans and a wide range of mammalian and avian hosts. Domestic and wild felines are the only hosts in which sexual reproduction occurs in the intestinal epithelium, resulting in the passage of unsporulated oocysts in feces. In the external environment sporulation to the infective stage usually takes one to three days. The infective oocyst contains two sporocysts, each with four sporozoites. Oocyst production does not occur in any other mammalian or avian host, and tissue cysts are the end result.

In the mammalian host, asexual reproduction is by endodyogeny, a process of division in which two daughter organisms develop within the parent cell. The parent cell is destroyed when the daughter organisms are liberated. In early acute infections, the rapidly proliferating organisms are called tachyzoites, and they invade and multiply in every kind of mammalian cell except nonnucleated erythrocytes. These groups of tachyzoites are often referred to as pseudocysts or terminal colonies. After the extensive multiplication that is characteristic of acute infection, tissue cysts begin to form, signalling the chronic phase of infection. In tissue cysts, the organisms are called bradyzoites, and they multiply more slowly than do tachyzoites. Although tachyzoite multiplication occurs widely throughout the body, the tissue cysts of chronic infection are found most frequently in skeletal or cardiac muscle, the brain, and other tissues of the central nervous system. Humans can acquire infection in several ways: by ingesting sporulated oocysts, by consuming tissue cysts in undercooked meat (especially lamb and pork), by transplacental transmission from infected mother to fetus, by transfusion of packed leukocytes, and by organ transplantation from infected donors.

Pathology and Clinical Manifestations

In acute toxoplasmosis, rapidly multiplying tachyzoites cause the destruction of host cells, which leads to the production of diffuse or focal lesions. Such lesions in cardiac tissue, liver, lung, brain, and connective tissue result in myocarditis, hepatitis, pneumonia, and encephalitis. When toxoplasmosis is acquired for the first time by a pregnant woman, an approximately 35% chance exists for transplacental transmission of infection to the fetus. Pathologic abnormalities in the infected fetus are often related to the trimester in which infection is acquired. The most severe pathologic conditions usually result when infection is acquired during the first trimester. Manifestations include hydrocephalus, intracranial calcifications, and retinochoroiditis. Infections acquired late in pregnancy may not produce any overt manifestations in the fetus at birth. However, abnormalities such as impaired hearing, mental retardation, and ocular lesions may appear later in life.

In most immunocompetent individuals who acquire toxoplasmosis for the first time, clinical manifestations are often unrecognized or present as a flulike condition of a few days' duration. However, the tissue cysts that develop remain as a latent infection. Subsequent immunosuppression due to treatment for Hodgkin's disease or other malignancies, organ transplantation, or AIDS can reactivate the infection. Cerebral toxoplasmosis, a common complication in patients with AIDS, results from reactivation of latent tissue cysts. Pathologic abnormalities manifest as extensive necrotic foci (➡ 11). In general, the spectrum of clinical manifestations and pathologic conditions produced by *Toxoplasma* infection is great and depends on host factors and perhaps the strain of parasite involved.

Parasite Morphology

Oocysts excreted in feces are spherical, measuring 10 to 12 µm in diameter. When fully sporulated, they contain two sporocysts, each with four sporozoites. Tachyzoites are crescent shaped, taper at both ends, and measure approximately 6 by 2 µm (Plate 11:1). Bradyzoites differ only slightly from tachyzoites, being a bit smaller and more slender. The nucleus of both organisms is situated at or slightly posterior to the midbody. Both have complicated series of organelles in the anterior portion of the body, which are visible only by electron microscopy. Tissue cysts are spherical to subspherical, vary in size (from 5 to 100 µm or larger), and contain hundreds to thousands of bradyzoites (Plate 11:2–6; Plate 12:1–4).

Tachyzoites and bradyzoites are seen when ruptured from cells or cysts. With Giemsa stain, the nucleus is red.

Within cysts, the bradyzoites most frequently appear as many dark-staining nuclei without evident cytoplasm, although in some stained preparations it is possible to make out individual organisms. Bradyzoites within cysts are strongly PAS positive, whereas tachyzoites, free or in cells, are less so. Tissue cysts have a relatively thin wall (0.5 to 1.0 μm). This wall is eosinophilic with H&E stain, is only slightly PAS positive, and stains intensely black with silver stain.

The tissue cysts of *T. gondii* must be differentiated from those caused by species of *Sarcocystis* or other apicomplexan parasites. Tissue cysts of *Sarcocystis* are seen most frequently in skeletal or cardiac muscle, where they tend to be larger than those of *Toxoplasma*. The cyst wall of *Sarcocystis* species is usually thicker and may have striations and microvilli (cytophaneres). Within cysts, bradyzoites are formed within compartments, depending on the species.

In recent years, a new genus of apicomplexan parasite, *Neospora*, has been described in animals and must be differentiated from *Toxoplasma*. *Neospora caninum* produces paralysis and death in dogs. Similar parasites of the same or a different species have caused neonatal mortality and abortions in sheep, goats, cattle, and horses, but human infection is unknown. The life cycle of *Neospora* has not been described, and thus far transplacental transmission is the only known route of infection. Although tachyzoites of *Neospora* have been found in many organs and tissues, tissue cysts have only been described from neural tissues. In *Neospora* infection, tissue cysts are similar in size to those of *Toxoplasma,* the cyst wall is smooth and 1 to 4 μm in thickness, and the cyst is not divided into compartments (Plate 12:5 & 6). Although it is difficult to distinguish cysts of *N. caninum* from cysts of *Toxoplasma* with light microscopy, it is possible to distinguish them using electron microscopy and immunohistochemical procedures. *Neospora* does not react with antisera raised against *T. gondii*. Ultrastructurally, the rhoptries in *Neospora* bradyzoites are more numerous and do not form a meshlike structure as in *T. gondii.* It is likely that tissue cysts of other as yet undescribed coccidian parasites will turn up in animal and human tissues and require identification.

References

Chabotar B, Scholtyseck E. Ultrastructure. In: Long PL, ed. *The Biology of the Coccidia*. Baltimore, Md: University Park Press; 1982:101-165.

Conrad PA, Barr BC, Sverlow KW, et al. In vitro isolation and characterization of a *Neospora* species from aborted bovine foetuses. *Parasitology*. 1993;106:239-249.

Dubey JP. A review of *Neospora caninum* and *Neospora*-like infections in animals. *J Protozool Res*. 1992;2:40-52.

Dubey JP. *Toxoplasma, Neospora, Sarcocystis,* and other tissue cyst-forming coccidia of humans and animals. In: Kreier JP, ed. *Parasitic Protozoa, Vol VI.* 2nd ed. San Diego, Calif: Academic Press Inc; 1993.

Ferguson DJP, Hutchison WM. An ultrastructural study of the early development and tissue cyst formation of *Toxoplasma gondii* in the brains of mice. *Parasitol Res*. 1987;73:483-491.

Gherardi R, Baudrimont M, Lionnet F, et al. Skeletal muscle toxoplasmosis in patients with acquired immunodeficiency syndrome: a clinical and pathological study. *Ann Neurol*. 1992;32:535-542.

Grossniklaus HE, Specht CS, Allaire G, et al. *Toxoplasma gondii* retinochoroiditis and optic neuritis in acquired immune deficiency syndrome: report of a case. *Ophthalmology*. 1990;97:1342-1346.

Ho-Yen DO, Joss AWL, eds. *Human Toxoplasmosis*. Oxford, England: Oxford University Press; 1992.

Jautzke G, Sell M, Thalmann U, et al. Extracerebral toxoplasmosis in AIDS: histological and immu nohistological findings based on 80 autopsy cases. *Path Res Pract*. 1993;189:428-436.

Nash G, Kershmann RL, Herndier B, et al. The pathological manifestations of pulmonary toxoplasmosis in the acquired immunodeficiency syndrome. *Hum Pathol*. 1994;25:652-658.

Pavesio CEN, Chiappino ML, Setzer PY, et al. *Toxoplasma gondii*: differentiation and death of bradyzoites. *Parasitol Res*. 1992;78:1-9.

Plate 11

Toxoplasma gondii

Image 1

Leukocyte infected with *T. gondii.* Paired tachyzoites resulting from the asexual process of multiplication known as endodyogeny are seen within the cell (Giemsa, 1000x). (Case courtesy of J. Remington.)

Image 2

Two typical tissue cysts of *Toxoplasma* are seen in this section of mouse brain. At this magnification, the bradyzoites within the cysts appear as dark-staining dots. Some shrinkage of the cysts is apparent, and the thin cyst wall is not readily seen (H&E, 500x).

Image 3

In a smear made from brain tissue, a large (45 µm) tissue cyst is seen. Many bradyzoites can be seen within the cyst (Giemsa, 500x).

Image 4

From a brain biopsy, this smear demonstrates a typical cyst with recognizable individual bradyzoites (Giemsa, 1000x). (Case courtesy of M. Zeuthen.)

Image 5

Phase-contrast microscopy illustrates tissue cysts in brain (400x). (Courtesy of W. Hutchison.)

Image 6

A tissue cyst in a smear of infected mouse brain visualized using a peroxidase-antiperoxidase stain (250x). (Courtesy of J. Remington.)

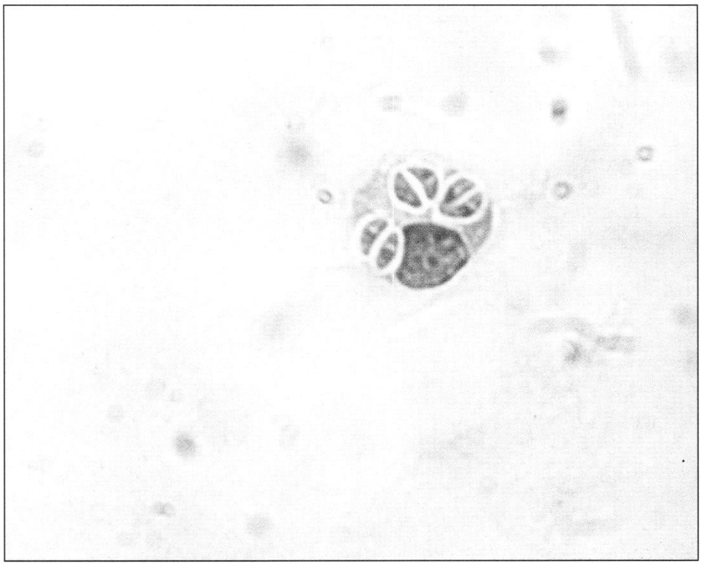
1

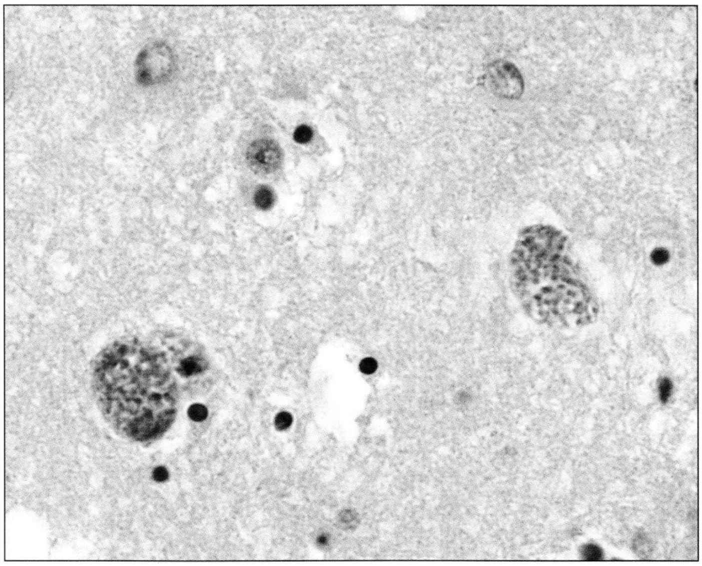
2

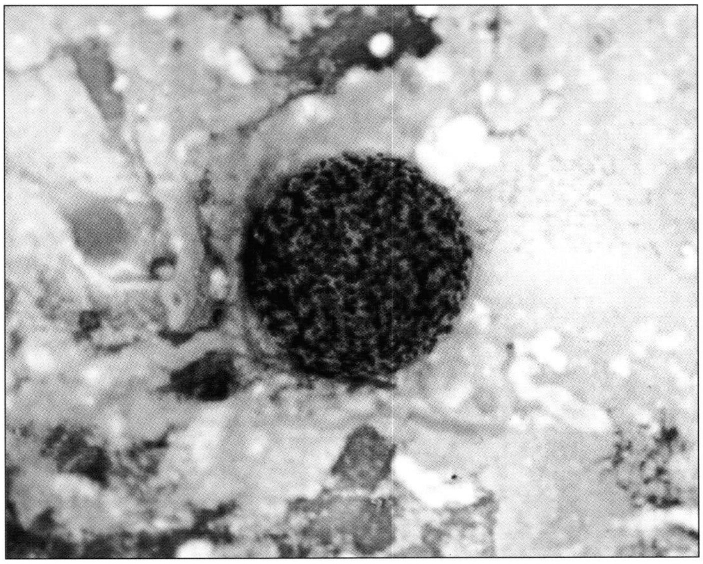
3

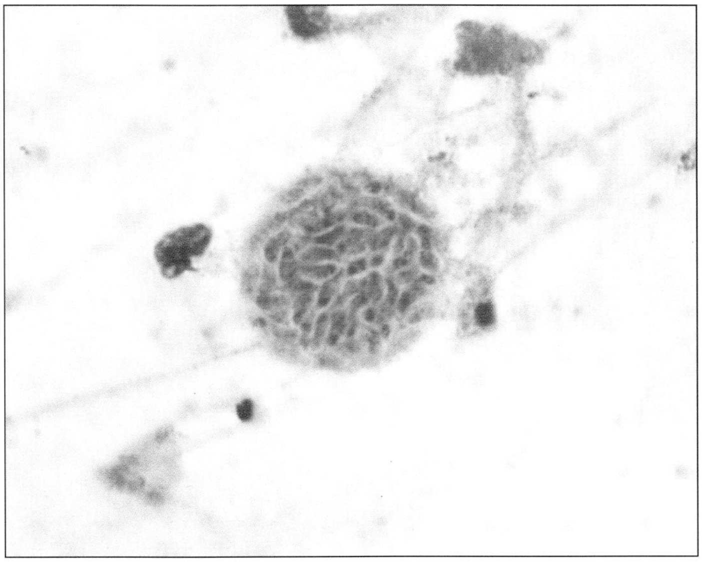
4

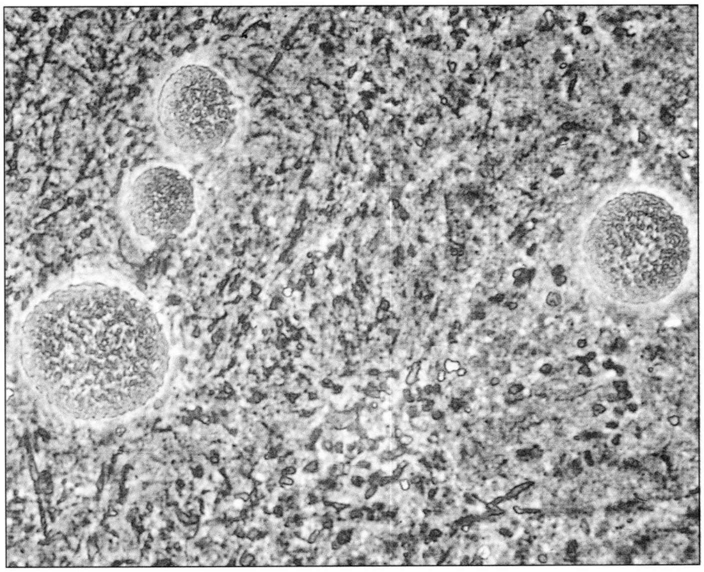
5

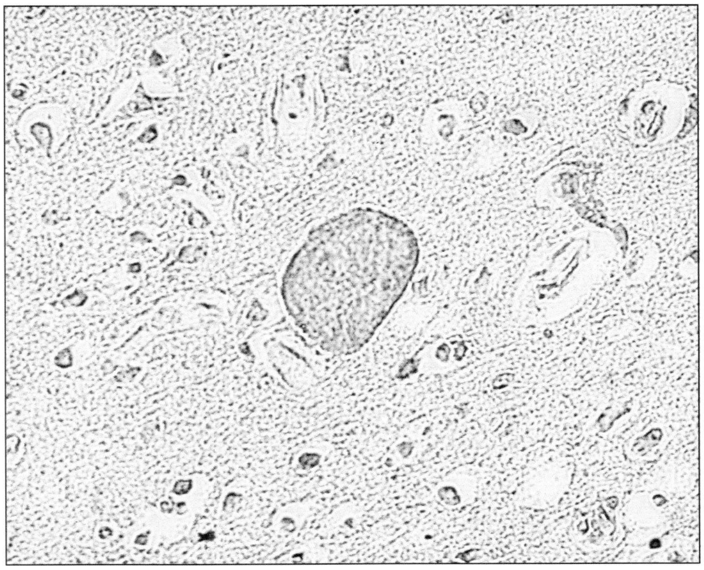
6

Plate 12

Toxoplasma gondii

Image 1

Brain biopsy specimen from a patient with AIDS. Note the rupturing cyst of *Toxoplasma.* Bradyzoites are being liberated (H&E, 1125x).

Image 2

A typical cyst of *Toxoplasma* is seen in the ganglion cell layer of a human retina. Individual bradyzoites are brown (PAP, 1000x). (Courtesy of G. Dutton.)

Image 3

A small cyst containing tachyzoites is evident in this section of human lung. Nuclei of the organisms are seen as small, dark-staining spots (H&E, 750x).

Image 4

A small tissue cyst in the kidney. Nuclei of the organisms appear as dark-staining spots (H&E, 500x).

Image 5

Two tissue cysts of *Neospora caninum* in a dog cerebrum. The cysts closely resemble the tissue cysts of *Toxoplasma. Neospora* infection has been misdiagnosed as toxoplasmosis in many instances. At the light-microscopic level, it is difficult if not impossible to clearly distinguish the cysts of *Neospora* or *Neospora*-like organisms from those of *Toxoplasma* (H&E, 750x). (Case courtesy of J. Dubey.)

Image 6

Neospora in the spinal cord of a calf. Whether this is *N. caninum* or a related species of the genus is not known. In this cyst the individual bradyzoites can be clearly seen. The cyst wall is thicker than typically seen in toxoplasmosis, but this does not appear to be a consistent feature (H&E, 750x). (Case courtesy of J. Dubey.)

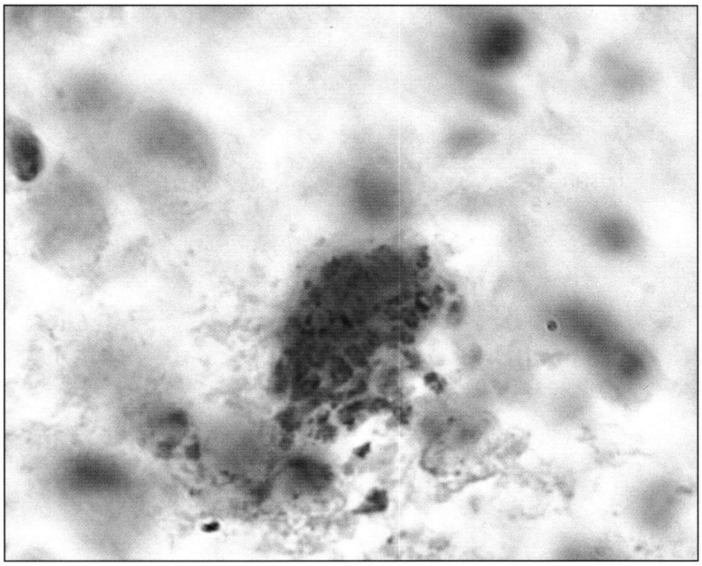
1

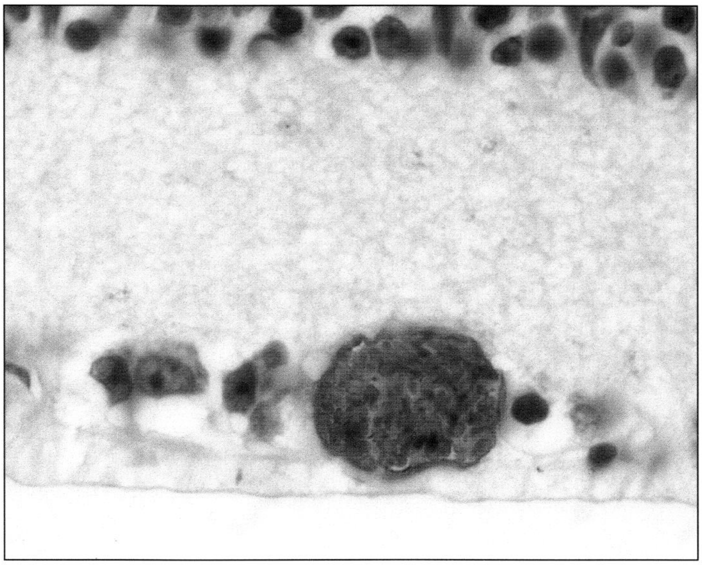
2

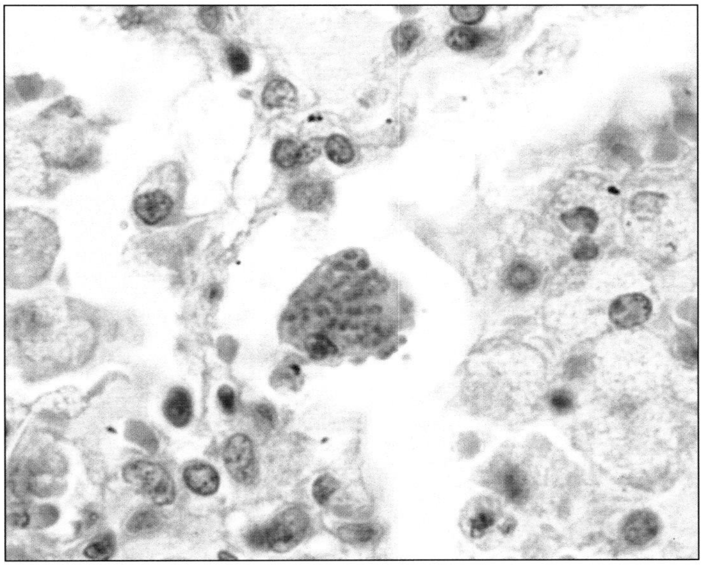
3

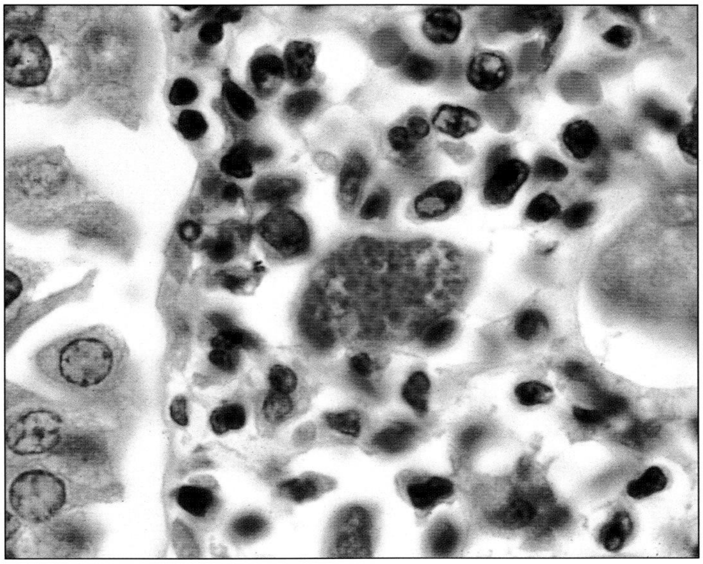
4

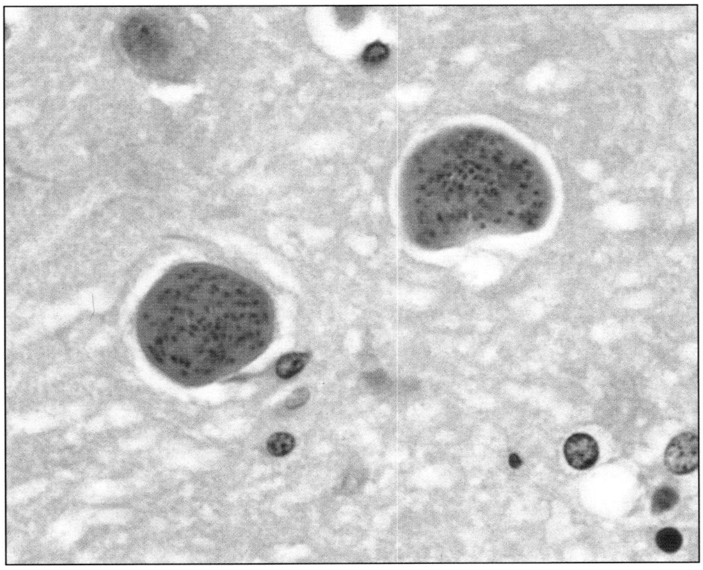
5

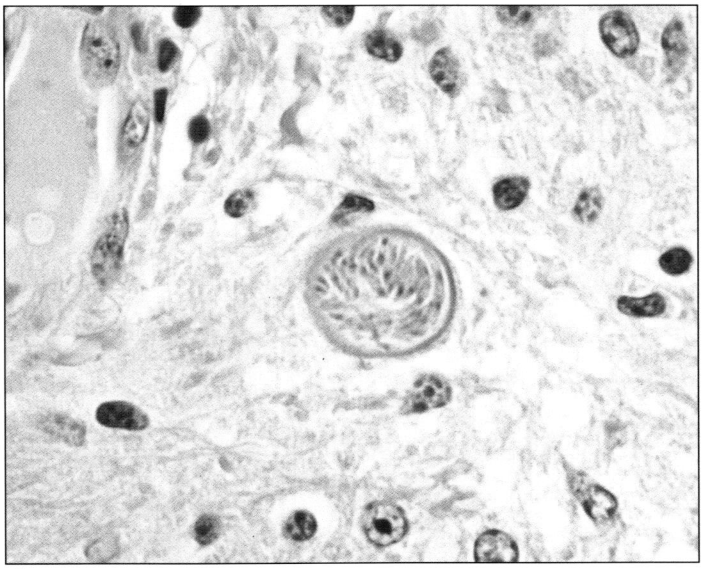
6

Encephalitozoon species, *Enterocytozoon bieneusi, Nosema* species, *Pleistophora* species, *Septata intestinalis*

Microsporidiosis

Members of the phylum Microspora have only recently assumed prominence as human parasites. Although early sporadic human cases of microsporidiosis have been reported, the organisms have been described with increasing frequency as the source of opportunistic infections in patients with AIDS. In 1985 *Enterocytozoon bieneusi* in the intestinal tract was described as a cause of diarrhea in immunocompromised patients, and since then it has been shown to infect the liver and lungs as well. A second microsporidian that also causes diarrhea in patients with AIDS was described in 1993 as both a new genus and a new species, *Septata intestinalis.*

Although two species of *Encephalitozoon, E. cuniculi* and *E. hellem*, have been reported to cause human infections, the latter has been found principally in the corneal and conjunctival epithelium of patients with AIDS. Evidence suggests that although these two species are morphologically identical, *E. hellem* is antigenically and biochemically different from *E. cuniculi.* Possibly the earlier reports of *E. cuniculi* in humans were in fact *E. hellem*. Two species of the genus *Nosema, N. connori* and *N. corneum*, and an unnamed species of *Pleistophora* have also been reported as agents of human infection.

In several cases of human microsporidiosis, organisms have been attributed to several species and have been assigned collectively to the genus *Microsporidium.* Although hundreds of species of microsporidian parasites have been described from all vertebrate groups as well as from many insects and other invertebrates, the small sizes of these mammalian parasites make it especially difficult to work with them. Most of our information about species that cause human disease has been obtained within the last decade, and the diagnosis of these infections has been achieved primarily through the use of electron microscopy and immunofluorescent antibody tests. As the procedures for the isolation and identification of species from human hosts improve, additional known or unknown species will undoubtedly be described as agents of disease.

Biology and Life Cycle

Microsporidia are obligate, intracellular protozoan parasites characterized chiefly by the production of spores. All of the species known to infect humans produce spores of similar size, usually 1 to 5 µm in diameter. Spores contain a coiled polar tubule that everts after ingestion and penetrates into a host intestinal epithelial cell. The contents of the spore are then injected via the tubule into the cytoplasm of the host cell (Plate 14:6). Intracellular division of the microsporidia is a complex process that varies among the different genera and species and includes a proliferative stage of multiplication followed by a phase of sporogony leading to spore formation. This asexual multiplication occurs either within a parasitophorous vacuole, which isolates the organisms from the host cell cytoplasm, or with the organisms in direct contact with the host cell cytoplasm. The end result of both methods is spore formation, with the newly formed spores disseminating to other parts of the host body or passing into the external environment via feces, urine, or the respiratory tract. For many species, survival of the spores and duration of infectivity in the external environment are imperfectly known, but some species have been shown to survive and remain infective for months to a year or longer.

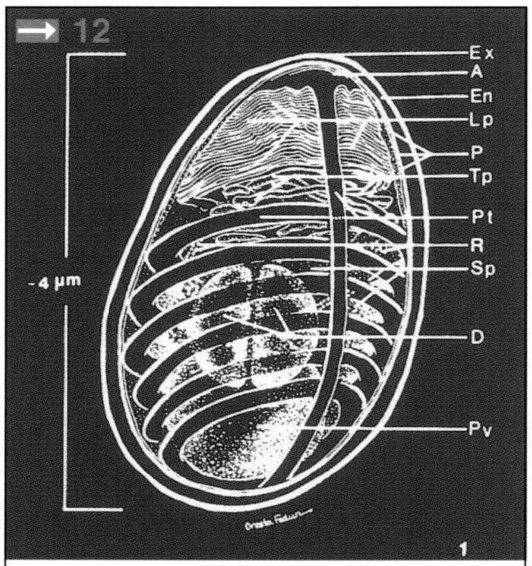

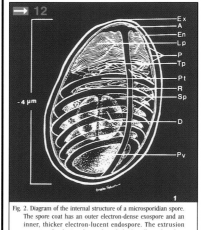

Fig. 2. Diagram of the internal structure of a microsporidian spore. The spore coat has an outer electron-dense exospore and an inner, thicker electron-lucent endospore. The extrusion apparatus (anchoring disc, polar tubule, lamellar polaroplast, and tubular polaroplast) dominates the spore contents and is diagnostic for microsporidia. The number of polar tubule coils depends on the particular species and can vary from a few to over 30. Key: Ex = exospore, En = endospore, P = unit membrane, A = anchoring disc, Pt = polar tubule, Lp = lamellar polaroplast, Tp = tubular polaroplast, Pv = posterior vacuole, R = ribosomes, D = diplokaryon nuclei, sp = sporoplasm.

Most infections are acquired orally. However, ocular infections may result from spores being directly introduced into the eye rather than disseminating from other sites in the body. Experimental instillation of spores into the nose has produced infections, which indicates that aspiration or inhalation of spores is a possible mode of infection. Transplacental transmission has been reported for *E. cuniculi* infection. Most detailed observations on the morphology and reproduction of these organisms have resulted from electron microscopy studies. Although *Enterocytozoon bieneusi, Encephalitozoon hellem*, and *Septata intestinalis* have thus far been described only in humans, these and the other microsporidian genera and species may also represent zoonotic infections.

Pathology and Clinical Manifestations

Intestinal microsporidiosis is caused by *E. bieneusi* and *S. intestinalis*, usually occurs in patients with AIDS, and is associated with a profuse chronic diarrhea and wasting. *Enterocytozoon* is found most frequently in the jejunum and distal duodenum. Histologically, the villi may be blunted, with many individual enterocytes undergoing degeneration. The cytoplasm is vacuolated and contains spores as well as other stages of the organism in the process of multiplication. Sloughing cells containing spores can often be found in the lumen. Although *S. intestinalis* causes a similar chronic diarrhea and weight loss, organisms are seen within enterocytes and also found in macrophages, fibroblasts, and endothelial cells of the lamina propria. Both *Enterocytozoon* and *Septata* have been shown to disseminate to other parts of the body. The former has been found in the liver and lungs, whereas the latter has been demonstrated in the gallbladder and kidney. Spores of *Enterocytozoon* have been found in bile, and the infection has been associated with sclerosing cholangitis. Spores of this organism have also been found in bronchoalveolar lavage and transbronchial biopsy material. Spores of *Septata* have been found in the urine of patients with severe tubulonephritis, as well as in nonparenchymal cells of the liver and bronchial epithelium. Both organisms may ultimately be found to disseminate to other organs and tissues as well. Several cases described in the early literature as *Encephalitozoon cuniculi* infection involved the central nervous system of humans and nonhuman primates. Spores were found both in the brain and in urine. Subsequently a new species, *E. hellem,* was described in several human cases. The organisms produced epithelial infection of the cornea, the conjunctiva, or both, with associated keratoconjunctivitis. Spores could also be demonstrated in urine. Whether these two are a single species has not yet been resolved.

Microsporidial spores in the corneal stroma of several individuals who did not have AIDS but were otherwise immunocompromised have been identified as belonging to the genus *Nosema. Nosema corneum* was reported only from the eye, but a second species, *N. connori,* produced a fatal case in which spores disseminated to all organs and tissues. Species of the microsporidian genus *Pleistophora* usually occur in insects and fish, but two human infections by undescribed species have been reported. In both cases myositis was produced. One of the individuals was HIV positive and the other was HIV negative.

Parasite Morphology

Although microsporidial spores range from 1 to 12 μm, those infecting humans are oval, pyriform, or elongated and usually have diameters of 1 to 5 μm (Plate 13:1–4; Plate 14:3). Spores are thick walled and contain the characteristic coiled polar tubule (➡ 12). The number of coils within each spore varies among genera and species, ranging from a few to more than 30. The sporoplasm within the spore contains one or two nuclei depending on the species. Other specific morphologic characteristics are discernible with electron microscopy.

Although spores and plasmodial stages within tissues can be recognized using light microscopy (Plate 14:1, 5, & 6; Plate 15:1 & 5), their small size has necessitated that they be studied by electron microscopy (Plate 14:2; Plate 15:2). Routine H&E stain demonstrates spores in tissue (Plate 13:5 & 6); however, various special stains such as tissue Gram stains (Brown-Hopps or Brown and Brenn methods) (Plate 14:4; Plate 15:6), Grocott's staining method for fungi (GMS), and the Ziehl-Neelsen acid-fast stain (Plate 15:4) are often more useful. If plastic-embedded tissue is sectioned at 1 μm and stained, the spores and multinucleate sporogonial plasmodial stages are more readily seen (Plate 15:3). Other stains, including Giemsa, PAS, and toluidine blue, are also useful. In particular, a PAS-positive granule present in the anterior end of mature spores is diagnostic for microsporidial infection. Electron microscopy facilitates specific identification by revealing morphologic features such as the number of coils of the polar tubule, the thickness of the spore wall, and the exact location in the cell of the plasmodial stages.

Specific identification and differentiation of microsporidia species require electron microscopy, tissue culture, immunofluorescent study, and perhaps, in the future, polymerase chain reaction methodology. At the light-microscopic level, it is possible to distinguish spores of microsporidia occurring in feces from bacteria and yeasts because microsporidia are smaller. Unfortunately, new species of microsporidia are continually being discovered in the same tissues from which other species have already been described, which suggests that diagnosis will continue to pose a problem in the future.

References

Cali A, Kotler DP, Orenstein JM. *Septata intestinalis,* n.g., n.sp., an intestinal microsporidian associated with chronic diarrhea and dissemination in AIDS patients. *J Euk Microbiol.* 1993;40:101-112.

Call A, et al: Corneal microsporidiosis *Am J Trop Med Hyg* ; 44(5): 463–468, 1991.

Chupp GL, Alroy J, Adelman LS, et al. Myositis due to *Pleistophora* (Microsporidia) in a patient with AIDS. *Clin Infect Dis.* 1993;16:15-21.

Field AS, Hing MC, Milliken ST, et al. Microsporidia in the small intestine of HIV-infected patients: a new diagnostic technique and a new species. *Med J Austral.* 1993;158:390-394.

Kotler DP, Giang TT, Garro ML, et al. Light microscopic diagnosis of microsporidiosis in patients with AIDS. *Am J Gastroenterol.* 1994;89:540-544.

Orenstein JM. Microsporidiosis in the acquired immunodeficiency syndrome. *J Parasitol.* 1991;77:843-864.

Orenstein JM, Tenner M, Cali A, et al. A microsporidian previously undescribed in humans, infecting enterocytes and macrophages, and associated with diarrhea in an acquired immunodeficiency syndrome patient. *Hum Pathol.* 1992;23:722-728.

Peacock CS, Blanshard C, Tovey DG, et al. Histological diagnosis of intestinal microsporidiosis in patients with AIDS. *J Clin Pathol.* 1991;44: 558-563.

Schwartz DA, Bryan RT, Hewan-Lowe KO, et al. Disseminated microsporidiosis (*Encephalitozoon hellem*) and acquired immunodeficiency syndrome: autopsy evidence for respiratory acquisition. *Arch Pathol Lab Med.* 1992;116:660-668.

Schwartz DA, Visvesvara GS, Diesenhouse MC, et al. Pathologic features and immunofluorescent antibody demonstration of ocular microsporidiosis (*Encephalitozoon hellem*) in seven patients with acquired immunodeficiency syndrome. *Am J Ophthalmol.* 1993;115:285-292.

Weber R, Kuster H, Visvesvara G, et al. Disseminated microsporidiosis due to *Encephalitozoon hellem*: pulmonary colonization, microhematuria, and mild conjunctivitis in a patient with AIDS. *Clin Infect Dis.* 1993;17:415-419.

Enterocytozoon bieneusi

Image 1

Direct fecal smear from an unconcentrated formalin suspension demonstrates many minute, pink-red–staining spores of *E. bieneusi.* These microsporidial spores are approximately 1.5 by 0.9 µm (modified trichrome, 1250x).

Image 2

Spores of *E. bieneusi* concentrated from unfixed duodenal aspirate material from a patient with AIDS. A characteristic beltlike structure running diagonally or equatorially is visible in some of the spores (Gram, 1250x).

Image 3

Gram-positive microsporidial spores of *E. bieneusi* from a patient with AIDS are seen in this smear of bronchoalveolar lavage material. Dissemination of this infection from the intestinal tract is being seen with increased frequency in immunocompromised patients (Gram, 1250x).

Image 4

Smear of enterocytes from the small intestine of a patient with AIDS. The multinucleated sporogonial plasmodial stage of *E. bieneusi* (ie, the proliferative stage of the life cycle) is seen (Giemsa, 1250x). (Courtesy of E. Canning.)

Image 5

Thin section from the small intestine of a patient with AIDS. Two small clusters of developing microsporidial spores (darts) are seen within enterocytes (H&E, 1000x). (Courtesy of B. Gazzard.)

Image 6

Infective spores are seen within enterocytes (same case as Image 5). One infected enterocyte (dart) has already been sloughed into the lumen, and others appear to be in different stages of breaking away from the intestinal epithelium. The extremely small size of the spores when viewed with light microscopy easily differentiates them from other small intestinal parasites such as *Cryptosporidium* (H&E, 1000x). (Courtesy of B. Gazzard.)

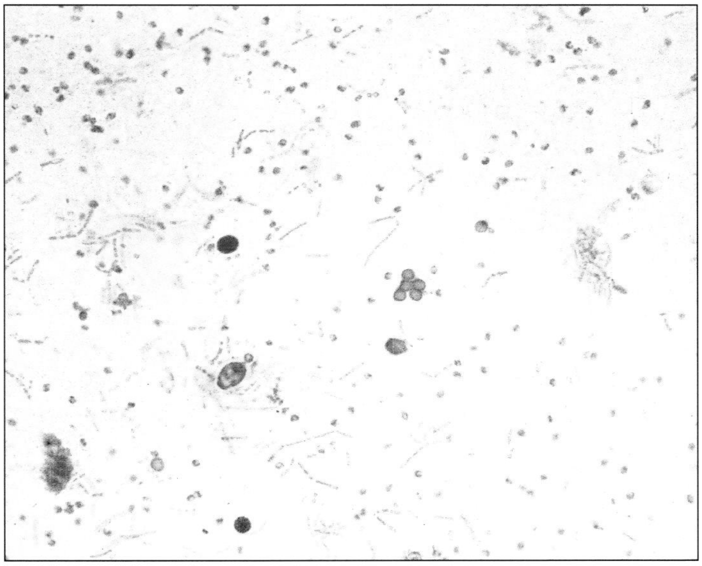

1

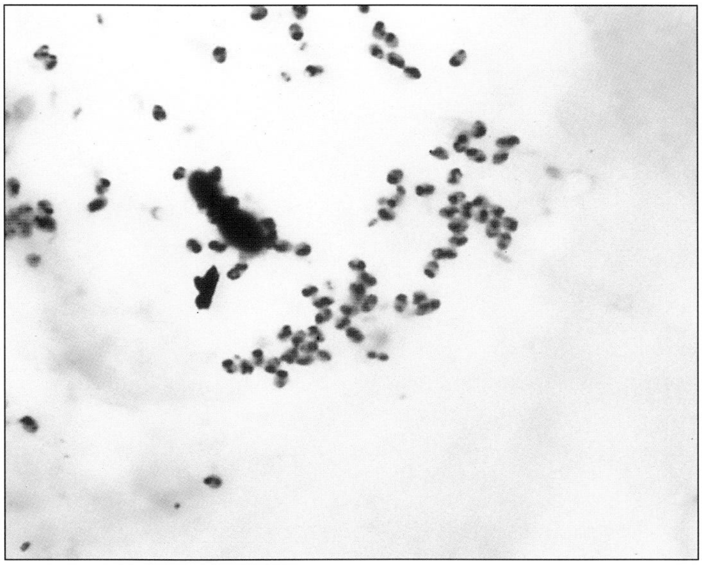

2

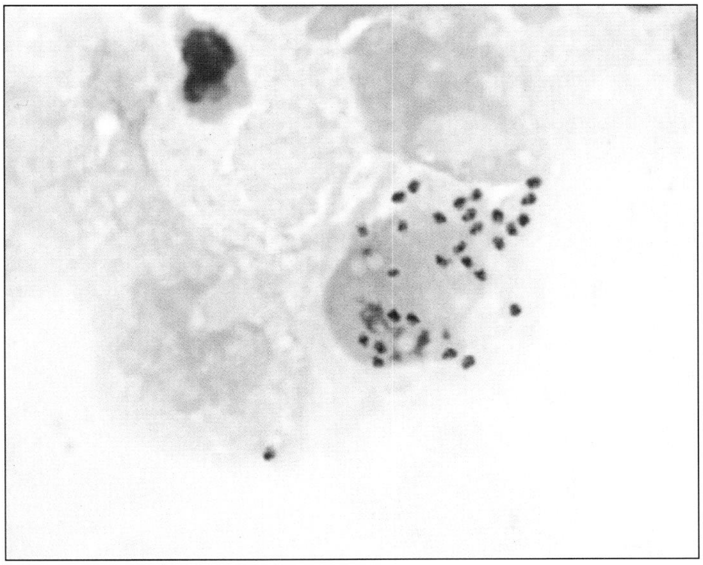

3

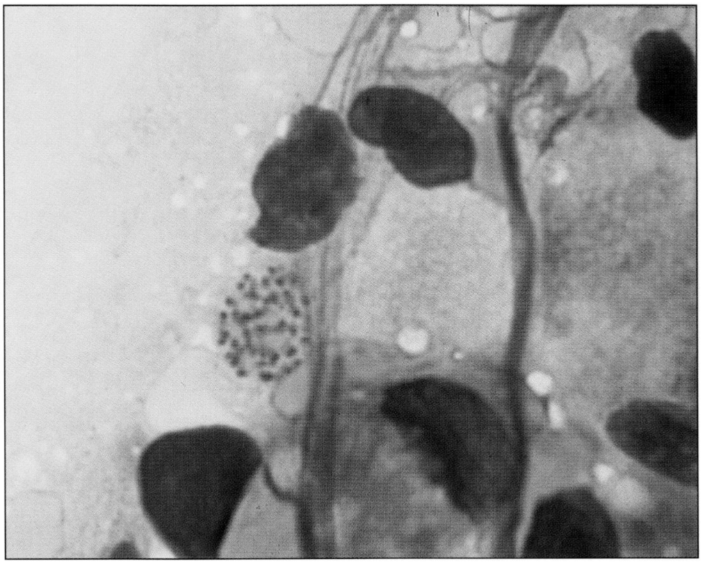

4

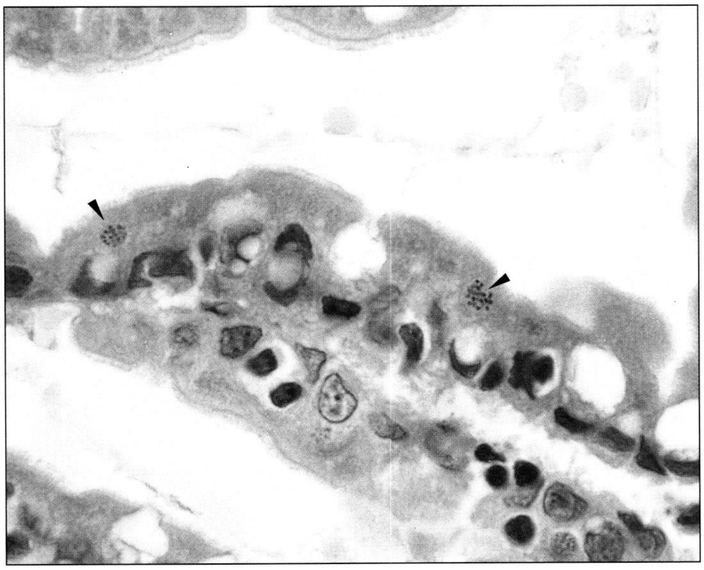

5

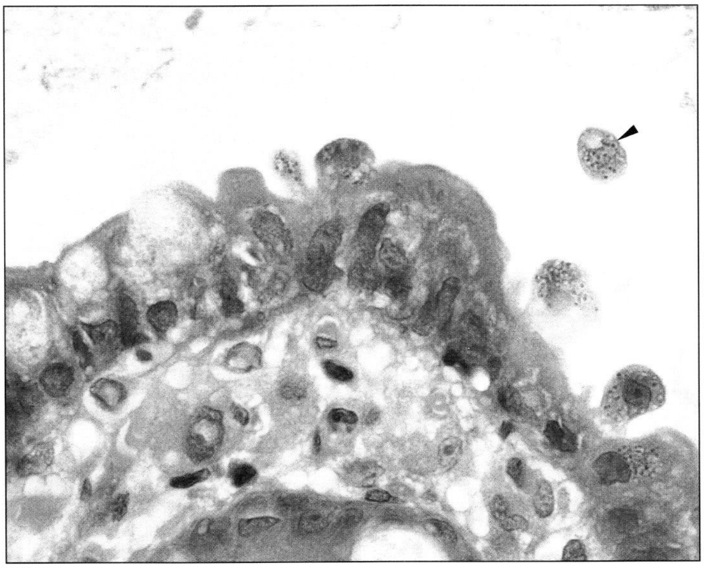

6

Plate 14

Enterocytozoon bieneusi and *Encephalitozoon hellem*

Image 1

Intestinal biopsy specimen from a patient with AIDS. Four small clusters of spores of *E. bieneusi* are within separate enterocytes (keyline) (PAS, 1000x).

Image 2

Transmission electron micrograph of two spores of *E. bieneusi* in a biopsy specimen of small intestine from a patient with AIDS. Two groups of five coils (darts); each of the polar tubules are clearly seen. (Courtesy of B. Gazzard.)

Image 3

Urinary sediment from a patient with disseminated *E. hellem* infection. The spores stand out as blue-staining oval objects (Gram, 1250x). (Courtesy of R. Bryan.)

Image 4

Oval, brown-staining spores of *E. hellem* stand out in the renal cortex of a patient with AIDS (Brown-Hopps tissue Gram, 1000x). (Courtesy of R. Bryan.)

Image 5

Spores of *E. hellem* immunofluoresce brilliantly in the renal cortex of a patient with AIDS (1250x). (Courtesy of G. Visvesvara.)

Image 6

Using immunofluorescence, extruded polar tubules can be seen in two of the spores of *E. hellem* (1250x). (Courtesy of E. Didier.)

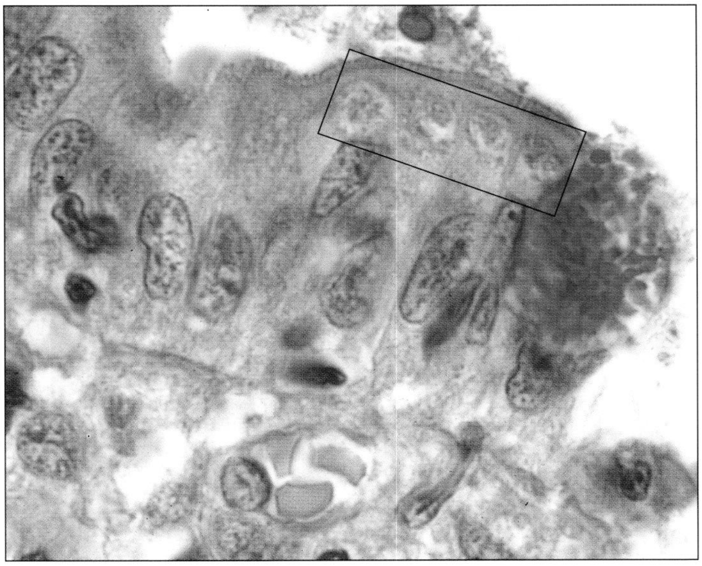

1

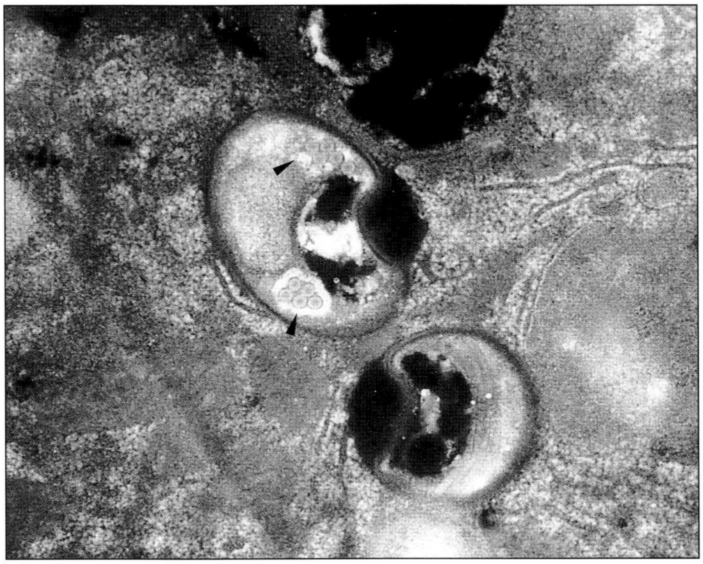

2

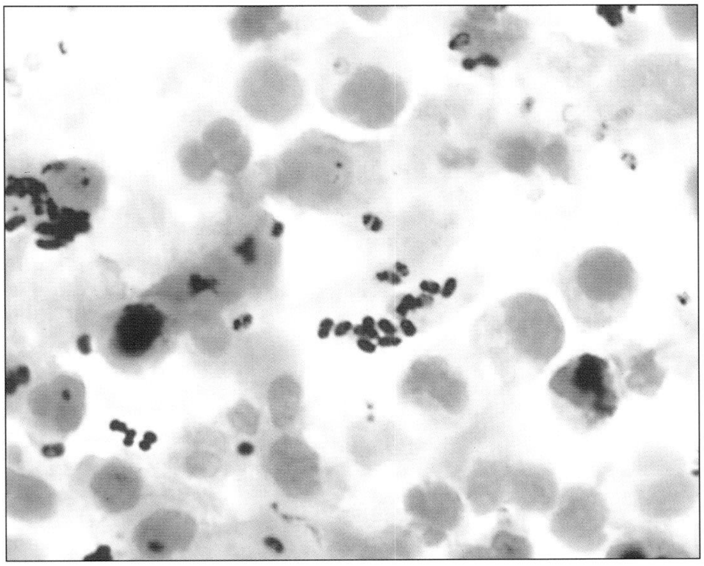

3

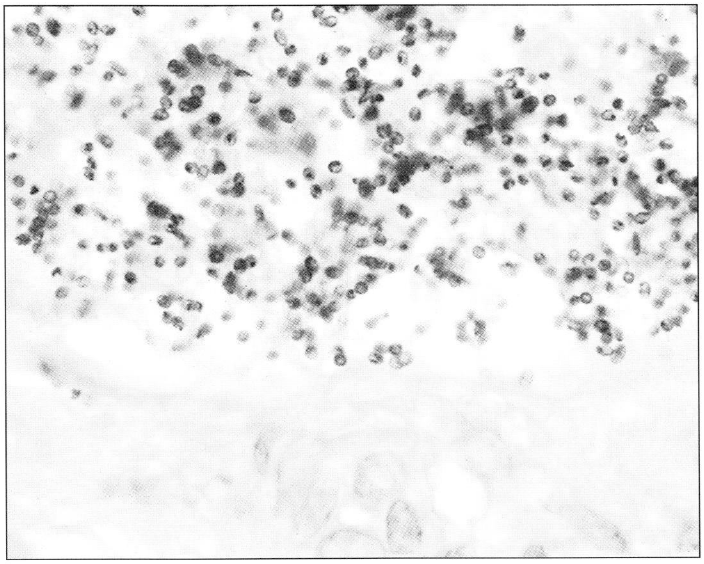

4

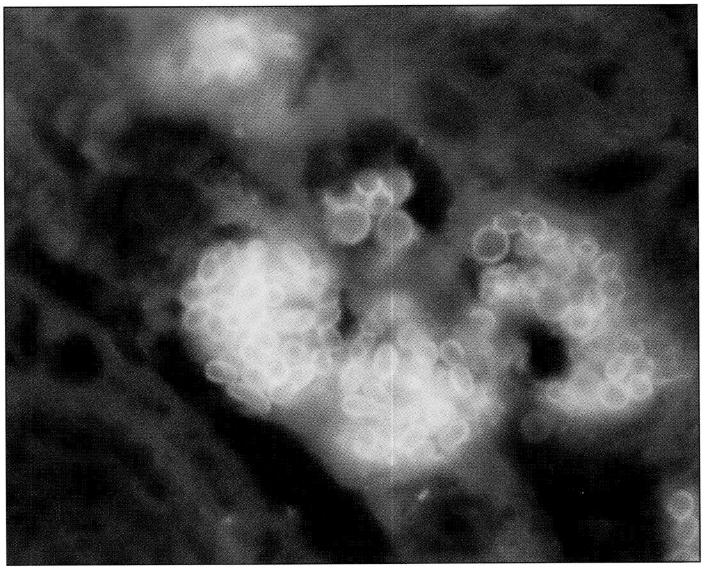

5

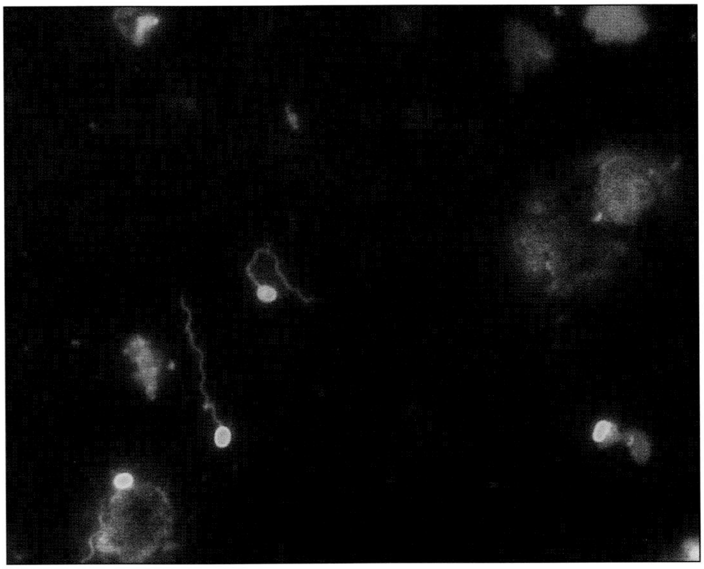

6

Plate 15

Encephalitozoon hellem, Nosema **species,** ***Pleistophora*** **species**

Image 1

In this scraping from human corneal epithelium, small, oval, intracellular, gram-positive spores are seen. This is probably *E. hellem* infection (Gram, 1000x). (Courtesy of R. Bryan.)

Image 2

Transmission electron micrograph of a conjunctival epithelial cell containing numerous spores that were reported to be *E. cuniculi*. In retrospect, however, this infection was probably caused by *E. hellem,* which has been chiefly responsible for keratoconjunctivitis in patients with AIDS. The organisms vary in appearance, which probably reflects different stages of development (5600x). (Courtesy of B. Gazzard.)

Image 3

In this resin-embedded section (1 µm) of muscle from a patient with AIDS and myositis, dark-staining spores of a species of the microsporidian genus *Pleistophora* are easily seen (Toluidine blue, 1250x).

Image 4

Spores of a species of *Pleistophora* are readily visualized in this field from an immunosuppressed HIV-negative patient with myositis (Ziehl-Neelsen, 1000x). (Courtesy of R. Bryan; attributed to AFIP.)

Image 5

In this case of myositis caused by *Pleistophora* species, spores are easily seen (Giemsa, 1000x). (Courtesy of R. Bryan; attributed to AFIP.)

Image 6

Red-staining spores (thought to be *Nosema* species) seen in this corneal biopsy specimen from an HIV-negative, immunocompetent patient with ocular microsporidiosis (Brown-Hopps tissue Gram, 1250x). (Courtesy of R. Bryan.)

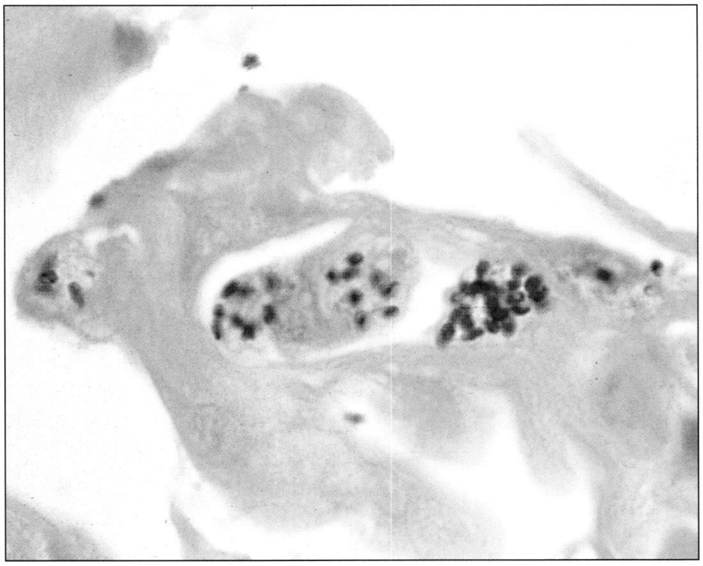
1

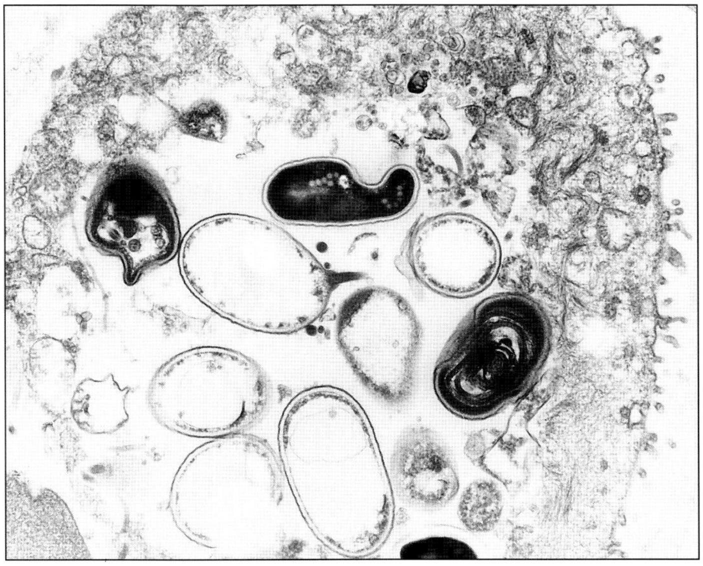
2

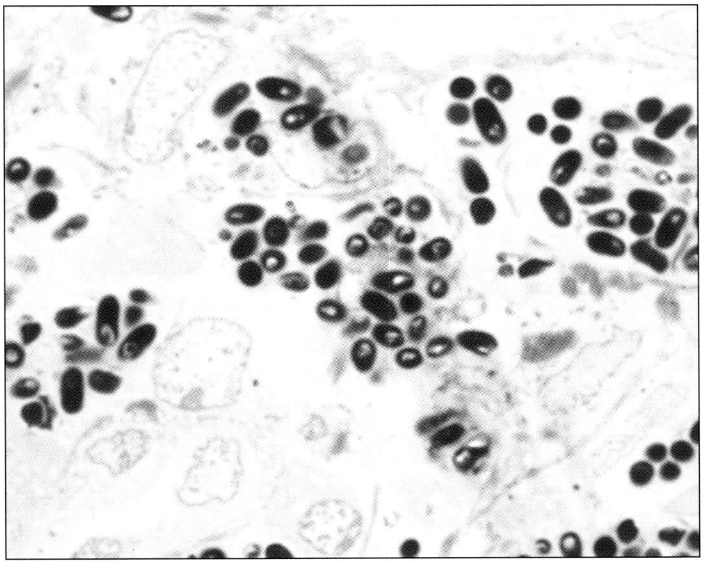
3

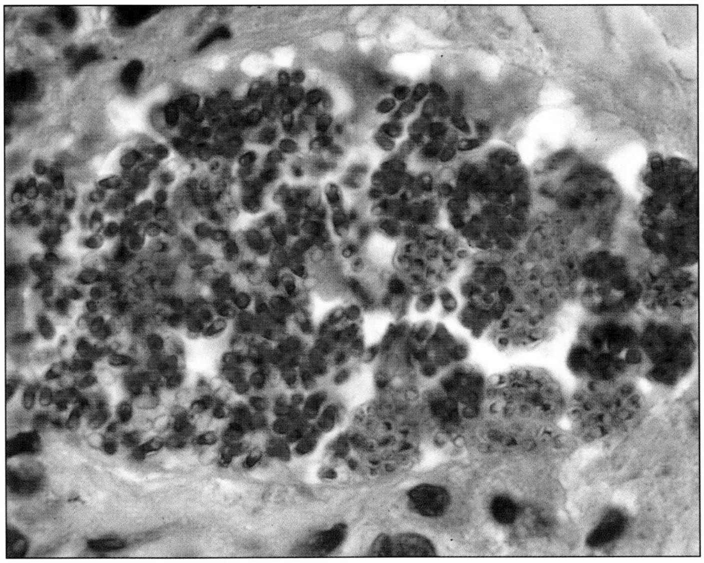
4

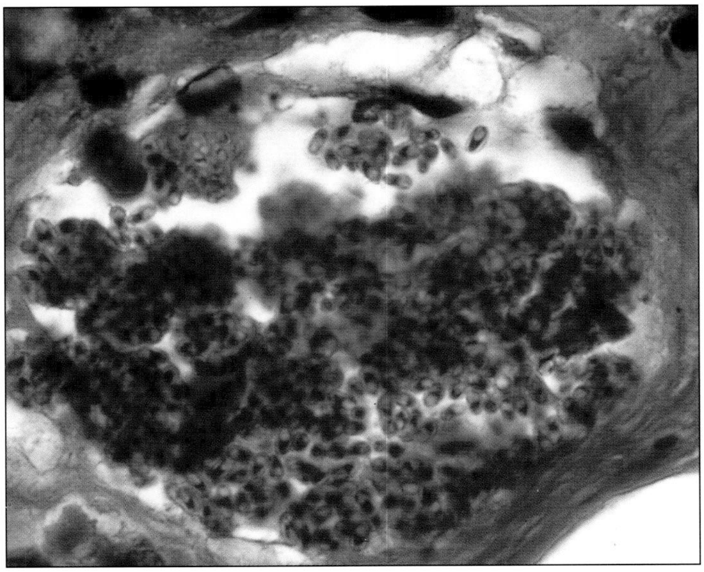
5

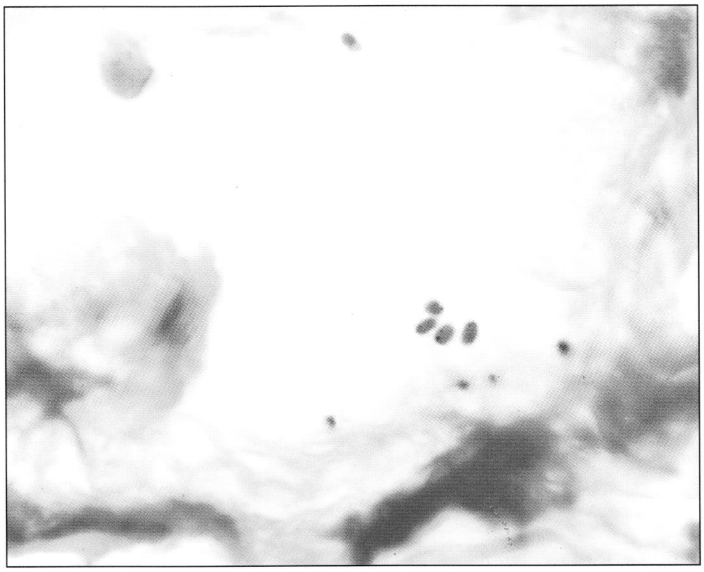
6

Plasmodium falciparum

Falciparum Malaria

Malaria remains the single most important human parasitic disease. As many as 200 to 300 million cases occur each year, most in the tropical areas of Asia, Africa, and Latin America, with an annual mortality of over one million people. Four species of *Plasmodium—P. falciparum, P. vivax, P. malariae,* and *P. ovale*—are responsible for human disease, but *P. falciparum* is the most widespread and pathogenic. Diagnosis of infection still rests principally on the demonstration of malarial parasites within erythrocytes in stained thick and thin blood films. Tissue stages of malarial parasites in human hosts generally involve the liver, where preerythrocytic stages of every species develop, and blood vessels, where malarial pigment is present in *P. falciparum* infections.

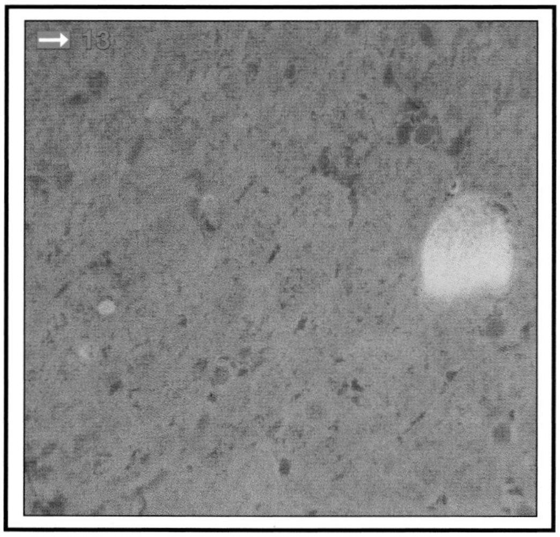

Biology and Life Cycle

Human malaria is biologically transmitted by female mosquitoes of various species of *Anopheles.* Mosquitoes become infected when they take a blood meal containing male and female gametocytes from a person with malaria. Within the mosquito, cycles of sexual and asexual reproduction result in the production of sporozoites, the infective stage for the human host. The time required for sporozoite development in mosquitoes varies depending on the species of malaria, the temperature, and the humidity. A period of one to two weeks is typical. After inoculation, the sporozoites rapidly leave the bloodstream and enter parenchymal cells of the liver. In the hepatic cells, schizogony occurs and results in the development of exoerythrocytic schizonts (➡ 13). Development of mature tissue schizonts usually takes 1 to 2 weeks (Plate 16:1 & 2). Rupture of these mature schizonts liberates merozoites into the bloodstream; the merozoites then invade red blood cells and initiate the erythrocytic phase of the malarial life cycle. The incubation period for infection is approximately two weeks for *P. vivax, P. falciparum,* and *P. ovale* and one month for *P. malariae.* Morphologic stages of the malarial parasites in red blood cells include trophozoites, schizonts, and gametocytes.

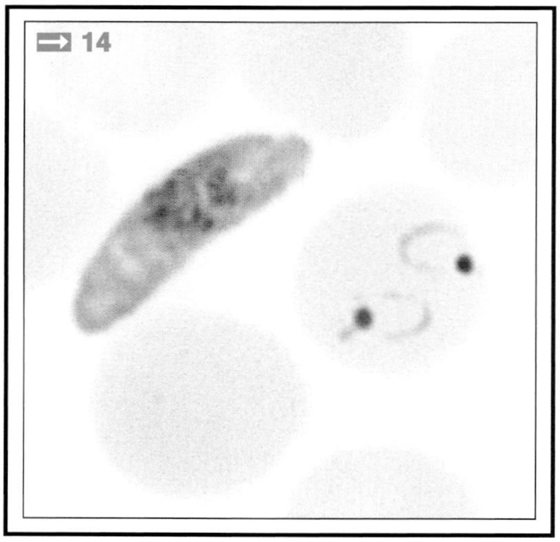

Pathology and Clinical Manifestations

Clinical symptomatology of malaria infection usually includes the classic paroxysm of chills, fever, and profuse sweating. Generalized aching, malaise, vomiting, diarrhea, and respiratory symptoms are seen with all species. Coma, convulsions, and heart failure are rarely seen in species other than *P. falciparum*. Attachment of *P. falciparum*–infected erythrocytes to the endothelial lining of blood vessels results in thrombosis of these vessels and accounts for much of the disease caused by this infection. In histologic sections, the most common findings in *P. falciparum* infections are malarial pigment and infected red blood cells in thrombosed blood vessels. Among the organs and tissues most frequently studied for pathologic changes due to *P. falciparum* infection are the brain (Plate 16:4), spleen (Plate 16:5), liver (Plate 16:3), kidney, and placenta (Plate 16:6). We focus primarily on the exoerythrocytic stages in hepatic cells and the presence of malarial pigment in tissues.

Parasite Morphology

Merozoites within exoerythrocytic schizonts are small (1.0 to 1.5 µm) and have a nucleus surrounded by a small amount of cytoplasm. The morphology of the subsequent bloodstream stages of *P. falciparum* (➡ 14) and other malarial species has been well described.

The size of exoerythrocytic schizonts developing in parenchymal cells of the liver and the amount of time required for development vary according to the species. Mature tissue schizonts measure from 45 to 80 µm and contain from a few thousand to 40,000 or more merozoites, depending on the species. The exoerythrocytic schizonts have thin walls and displace the nucleus of the liver cell toward the periphery. Hosts do not react to their presence. Hypnozoites, the persistent and latent liver stages that occur in *P. vivax* and *P. ovale,* are almost impossible to see with standard tissue stains but can be demonstrated with immunofluorescent staining. Malarial pigment can be observed in parasitized red blood cells, free in blood vessels, and within histiocytes.

Malaria is usually diagnosed clinically, and tissues are not often referred for examination without malaria at least being suspected. In tissue sections, the bloodstream stages of malaria parasites are usually not seen with standard tissue stains. Pigment in blood vessels can be seen with routine tissue stains, but the use of polarized light may also be helpful in demonstrating the birefringent granules of malarial pigment.

References

Bulmer JN, Rasheed FN, Francis N, et al. Placental malaria, I: pathological classification. *Histopathology*. 1993;22:211-218.

Cogswell FB. The hypnozoite and relapse in primate malaria. *Clin Microbiol Rev*. 1992;5:26-35.

Hidayat AA, Nalbandian RM, Sammons DW, et al. The diagnostic histopathologic features of ocular malaria. *Ophthalmology*. 1993;100:1183-1186.

Krotoski WA. The hypnozoite and malarial relapse. *Prog Clin Parasitol*. 1989;1:1-19.

Ranque P. A simple method for postmortem confirmation of the diagnosis of cerebral malaria: transethmoidal puncture of the brain. *Trans R Soc Trop Med Hyg*. 1986;80:663.

Plate 16

Plasmodium species

Image 1

Three dark-staining exoerythrocytic schizonts of *P. cynomolgi* can be seen in liver tissue from an experimentally infected monkey (H&E, 125x).

Image 2

At higher magnification, a single exoerythrocytic schizont is seen. The merozoites appear as small dotlike structures within the schizont, which helps in distinguishing an exoerythrocytic schizont of malaria from a tissue cyst of *Toxoplasma.* Merozoites of malarial species are much smaller than tachyzoites or bradyzoites (H&E, 500x).

Image 3

In a section of human liver from a fatal case of malaria, pigment deposition is seen as black granules in the Kupffer cells (H&E, 125x).

Image 4

Characteristic appearance of malarial pigment in blood vessels in the brain (fatal *P. falciparum* infection) (H&E, 400x).

Image 5

The spleen is usually enlarged and dark in *P. falciparum* infection in spleen. Note the accumulation of pigment (ie, hemozoin) (H&E, 500x).

Image 6

Malarial pigment resulting from a *P. falciparum* infection as seen in a section of human placenta (H&E, 500x).

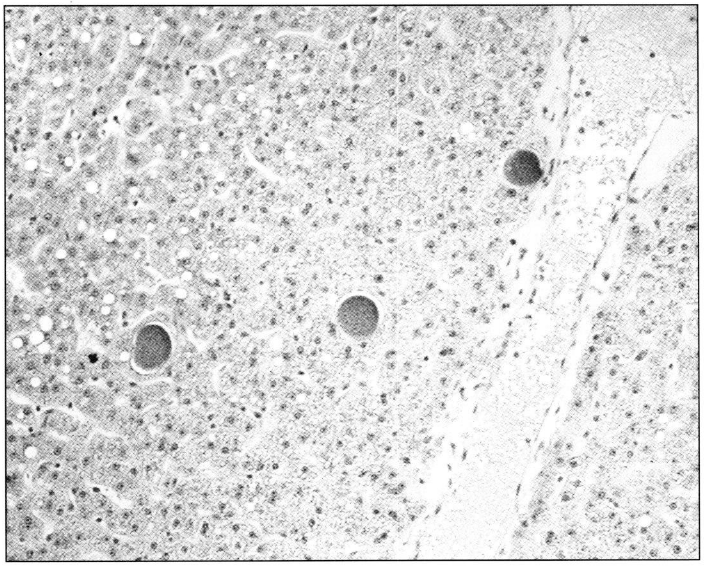
1

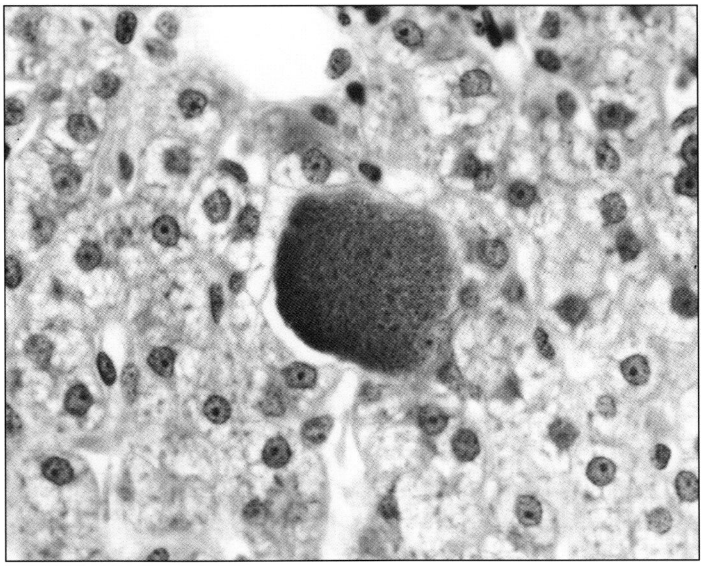
2

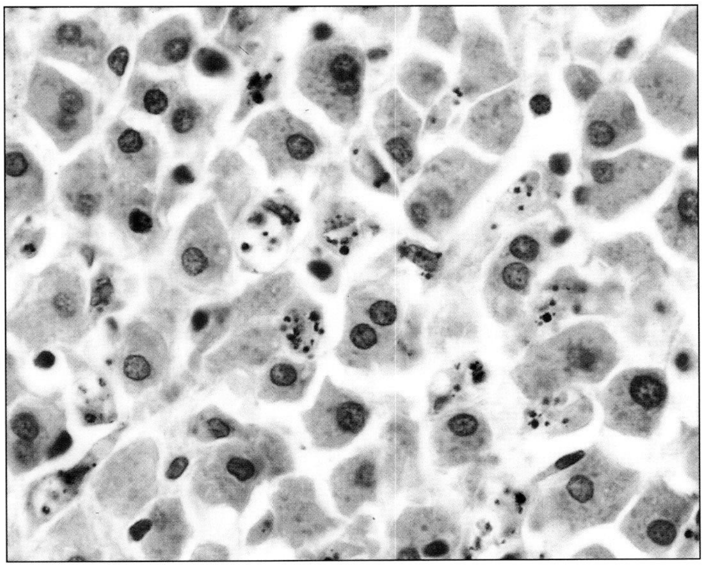
3

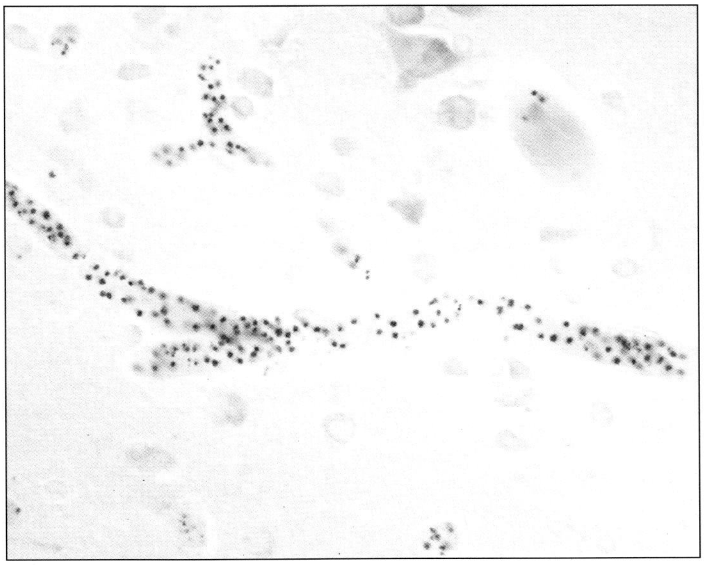
4

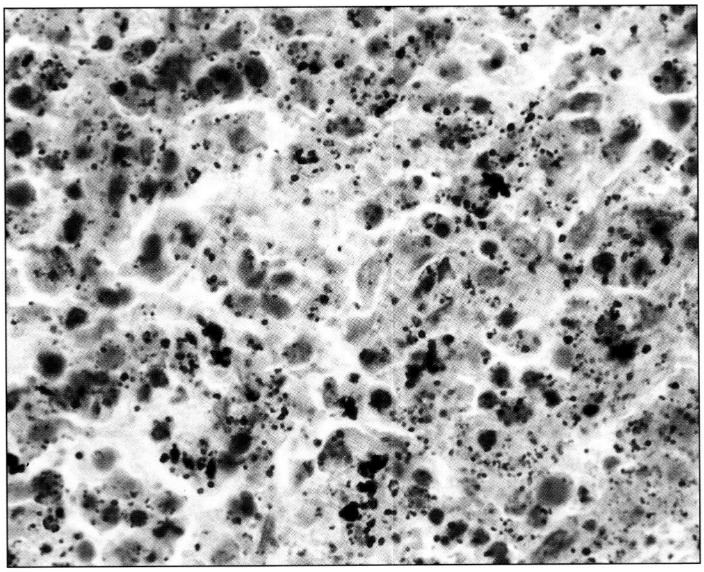
5

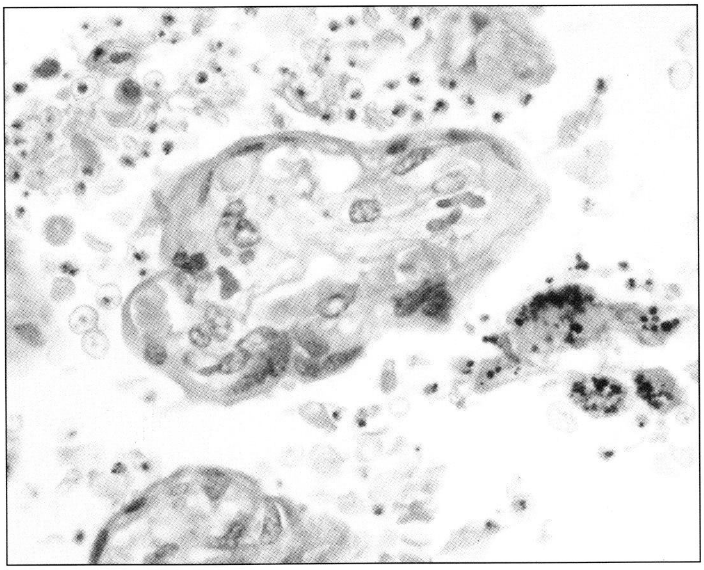
6

Leishmania species

Leishmaniasis

Species of *Leishmania* are known as hemoflagellates and are responsible for cutaneous, mucocutaneous, and visceral leishmaniasis. These diseases occur in tropical regions of the Indian subcontinent, Africa, and the Americas; subtropical areas of Asia; and islands in and countries bordering on the Mediterranean Sea. The World Health Organization estimates that 1.5 million new cases occur annually, with one third due to the often fatal, visceral form of the disease. Numerous species cause human and animal disease, and their taxonomy and classification have changed significantly in recent years. Visceral disease (kala-azar) is caused by *Leishmania donovani, L. chagasi,* and *L. infantum.* Some researchers believe that rather than classifying these as three separate species, they should be referred to as three subspecies within an *L. donovani* complex. In the Americas, *L. mexicana* and several other species cause cutaneous disease, while *L. braziliensis* is the primary cause of cutaneous and mucocutaneous disease. Cutaneous disease has been found in Texas in recent years, which indicates that *L. mexicana* infection has extended northward from Mexico. In Africa and parts of Asia, the primary etiologic agents of cutaneous leishmaniasis are *L. tropica, L. major,* and *L. aethiopica.*

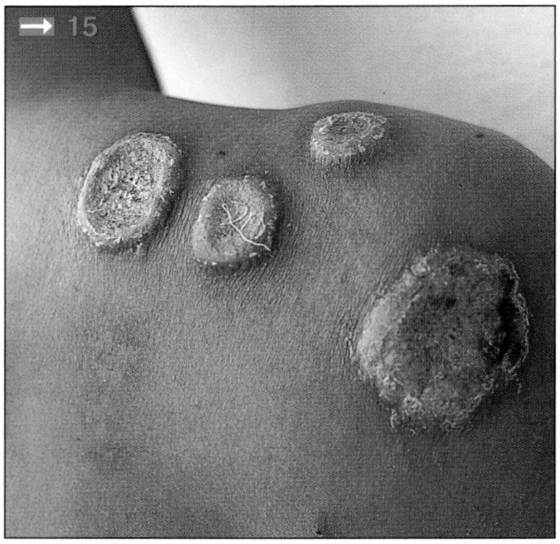

Biology and Life Cycle

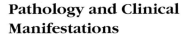

Leishmania comprises only two morphologic stages: amastigotes and promastigotes. Amastigotes occur only in the vertebrate host, promastigotes are the developmental and infective stage, which occurs only in the insect vector. Female phlebotomine flies (sandflies) of the genera *Phlebotomus* (Old World) and *Lutzomyia* (New World) are the required intermediate hosts. Amastigotes within macrophages or other cells of the reticuloendothelial system are ingested during the probing process before flies take a blood meal. In the alimentary tract, amastigotes undergo morphologic change to become flagellated forms—promastigotes—that then multiply and eventually migrate to the proboscis where, in the infective stage, they are injected by the sandfly during its feeding process. In all forms of leishmaniasis, the promastigotes are engulfed by macrophages in the skin and immediately transform into amastigotes. Division of amastigotes ultimately results in rupture of the cells, releasing amastigotes that then enter new macrophages. In cutaneous disease, amastigotes usually remain in the skin but may migrate to other cutaneous areas via the lymphatics. In some cutaneous species (eg, *L. tropica*), visceral involvement occasionally occurs. In the mucocutaneous forms of the disease, amastigotes typically migrate to the naso-oropharyngeal area and cause disfiguring ulcerations. In visceral leishmaniasis, after initial multiplication in the skin, amastigotes migrate within monocytes in the bloodstream to the spleen, liver, and bone marrow, where they continue to multiply.

Pathology and Clinical Manifestations

The different forms of leishmaniasis have various clinical manifestations, including the development of self-limiting cutaneous ulcers, metastasis, the formation of destructive lesions in naso-oronasopharyngeal locations, and systemic visceral disease, which results in hepatosplenomegaly, weight loss, leukopenia, and ultimately death if untreated. Cutaneous disease may result in one or more ulcers (➡ 15), usually of limited duration, which generally produce immunity to reinfection with the homologous strain but not other strains or species. The immunologic status of the host—in particular, whether the host is capable of a normal cell-mediated immune response—is highly important in determining its response to infection. Cutaneous lesions begin as small papules on exposed areas of the body and progress to ulcers over a period of several weeks to two months or more. These ulcers persist for up to a year or longer. Histologically, cutaneous leishmaniasis manifests as a granulomatous lesion with many macrophages and varying numbers of lymphocytes, plasma cells, and polymorphonuclear leukocytes (Plate 17:3). Infected cells containing amastigotes may be numerous or few.

Although mucocutaneous disease (espundia) is primarily caused by members of the *L. braziliensis* complex, *L. tropica* and subspecies of *L. mexicana* also cause this clinical manifestation. Mucocutaneous lesions usually represent secondary spread from cutaneous ulcers, although the metastasis occurs after the skin ulcers have healed. Tissue destruction in mucocutaneous disease is typically limited to the nasal septum, but in more severe cases the entire nose may be destroyed and the upper lip and hard and soft palate may also be involved. Facial disfiguration is often extensive, because the combination of leishmanial organisms and secondary bacterial infection can cause a significant amount of tissue destruction.

Visceral leishmaniasis has an incubation period of weeks to months and sometimes occurs in epidemic fashion. Fever, sweating, weakness, weight loss, anemia, and gradual enlargement of the liver and spleen are typical manifestations of the disease. Although kala-azar in Asia, India, and central Africa affects people of all ages, in Latin America and along the Mediterranean littoral the disease primarily involves children. Pathologically, the liver, spleen, bone marrow, and other parts of the reticuloendothelial system are affected in visceral disease. The spleen may be enormously enlarged and contain many infected macrophages. Hepatomegaly is primarily caused by hyperplasia of Kupffer's cells, which are packed with amastigotes. Parenchymal liver cells are rarely parasitized. Skin nodules containing amastigotes are seen in the early as well as the later stages of visceral leishmaniasis. Involvement of the intestinal tract in kala-azar appears to be uncommon, but rectal biopsy in such cases has revealed the presence of amastigotes in macrophages within the lamina propria. Given the association in some areas of the world between visceral leishmaniasis and AIDS, rectal biopsies may prove useful in detecting unsuspected or chronic disease.

Parasite Morphology

Amastigotes of most of the human leishmanial organisms are round to ovoid and measure 2 to 4 µm long by 1 to 3 µm wide. In Giemsa-stained preparations, they have a large nucleus, a prominent ovoid or rod-shaped kinetoplast, and a short axoneme that is difficult to see by light microscopy (Plate 17:1, 2, 4, & 5). They have no external flagellum. Promastigotes are not seen in the vertebrate host but they can be found in the insect vector or in culture media, because this stage is readily cultured. Promastigotes are usually elongated, measuring 10 to 15 µm long by 1.5 to 3.5 µm wide. They have a large central nucleus and a kinetoplast near the anterior end, and they possess a single flagellum that emerges at the anterior end and is as long or longer than the body.

Because of shrinkage during tissue processing, amastigotes in histologic section are even smaller than what is ordinarily seen in impression smears or touch preparations. They are only 1 to 3 µm, and it is extremely difficult to see both the kinetoplast and nucleus, which are the morphologic criteria used for confirming identifications of leishmanial organisms. In many tissue sections, the amastigotes appear as dotlike structures within macrophages, and morphologic features are hardly evident.

Amastigotes of *Leishmania* species must be distinguished from the amastigote stage of *Trypanosoma cruzi* infection, from *Toxoplasma gondii,* and from various fungi, including *Histoplasma.* In general, the localization of amastigotes of *T. cruzi* is principally in the heart, brain, tissues of the gastrointestinal tract, and placenta. Amastigotes of *Leishmania* are more commonly encountered in the skin, spleen, liver, and other cells of the reticuloendothelial system. Differentiation between *Leishmania* and *T. gondii* is based on recognition of characteristic amastigote morphology. In histoplasmosis, the fungal cells are 2 to 4 µm long and the cytoplasm of the cell is retracted from the thick, poorly staining cell wall to produce a halolike effect. Unlike amastigotes, no kinetoplast is present (Plate 17:6). In addition, cells of *Histoplasma* stain positively with PAS and silver methenamine, whereas amastigotes stain negatively. The granulomatous lesions produced by leishmanial infection must be distinguished from similar lesions frequently seen in lepromatous leprosy.

References

Furner BB. Cutaneous leishmaniasis in Texas: report of a case and review of the literature. *J Am Acad Dermatol.* 1990;23:368-371.

Idoate MA, Vazquez JJ, Civeira P. Rectal biopsy as a diagnostic procedure of chronic visceral leishmaniasis. *Histopathology.* 1993;22:589-590.

Magill AJ, Grogl M, Gasser RA Jr, et al. Visceral infection caused by *Leishmania tropica* in veterans of Operation Desert Storm. *N Engl J Med.* 1993;328:1383-1387.

Melby PC, Kreutzer RD, McMahon-Pratt D, et al. Cutaneous leishmaniasis: review of 59 cases seen at the National Institutes of Health. *Clin Infect Dis.* 1992;15:924-937.

Leishmania species

Image 1

Amastigotes of *L. (Viannia) braziliensis* are seen within a macrophage. The nucleus of the organisms (arrow) is clearly visible, but the rod-shaped kinetoplast is only evident in a few organisms (dart) (Giemsa, 1250x).

Image 2

Amastigotes are seen in an impression smear made from a patient infected with *L. mexicana.* Although the magnification in this image is somewhat lower than that in Image 1, it is still possible to identify both a nucleus and a kinetoplast in several of the organisms (darts)(Giemsa, 1000x).

Image 3

Section of a skin biopsy specimen in a Texan infected with *L. mexicana.* Amastigotes cannot be recognized within these histiocytes. A diffuse cellular infiltrate is present in the dermis and is composed predominately of histiocytes, but also comprises many lymphocytes and plasma cells (H&E, 125x). (Case courtesy of B. Furner.)

Image 4

At higher magnification, amastigotes within vacuolated histiocytes (keyline) can be recognized. It is difficult to distinguish nuclei and kinetoplasts in the organisms (H&E, 1250x).

Image 5

A section of liver from a case of visceral leishmaniasis. A Kupffer cell containing many amastigotes is seen, but again, it is difficult to recognize nuclei and kinetoplasts in these organisms (H&E, 1250x).

Image 6

In this smear from human bone marrow (taken from a California patient thought to have kala-azar), one can see a monocyte that contains organisms. However, the organisms seen are not leishmanial amastigotes but spores of *Histoplasma.* The cells are similar in size to those of amastigotes, but a "halolike" effect around the thick cell wall and the lack of a kinetoplast in any of the cells confirm a diagnosis of histoplasmosis (Giemsa, 1250x).

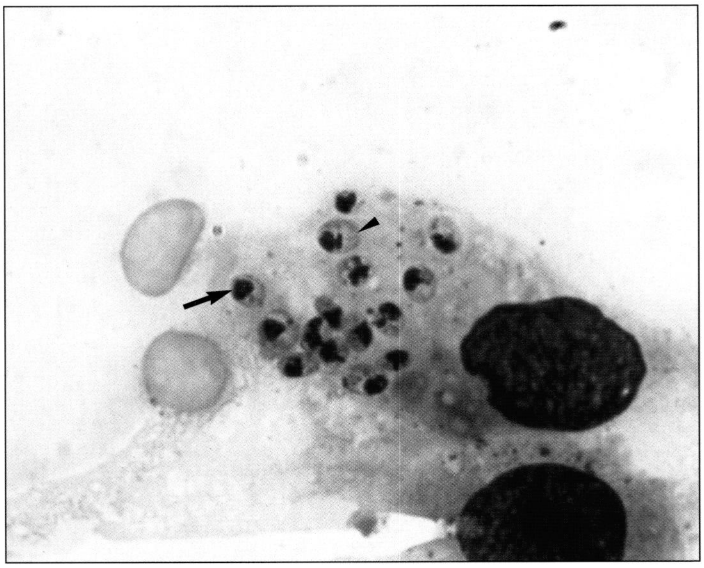
1

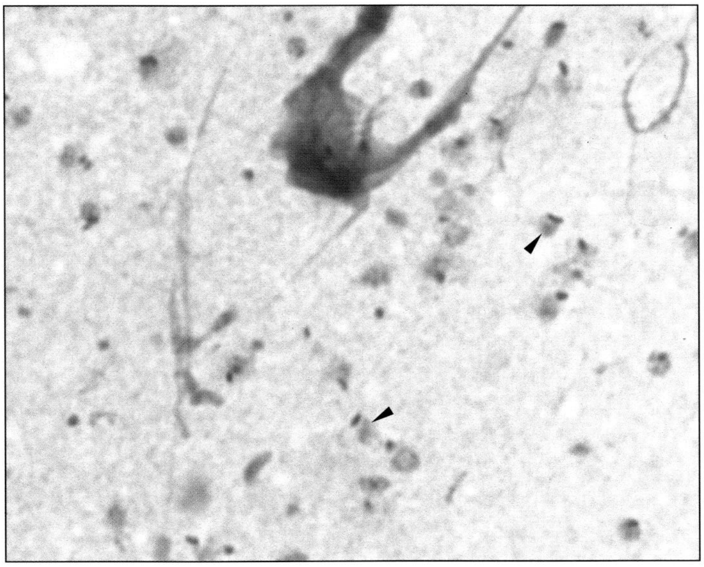
2

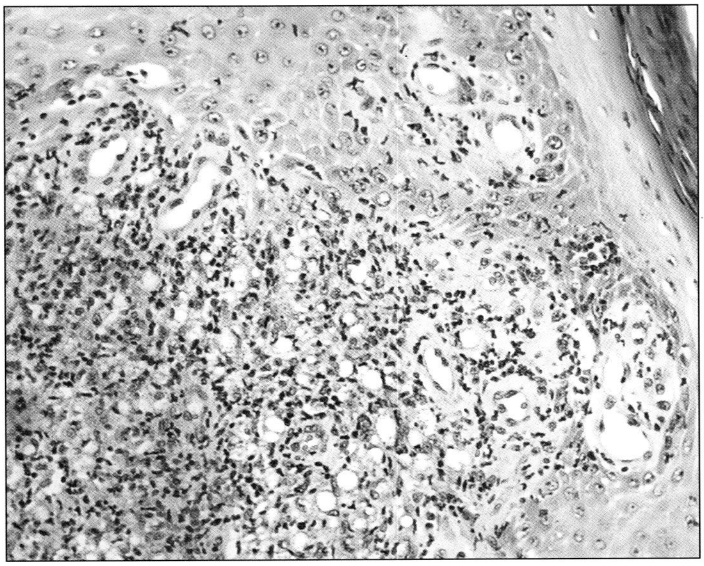
3

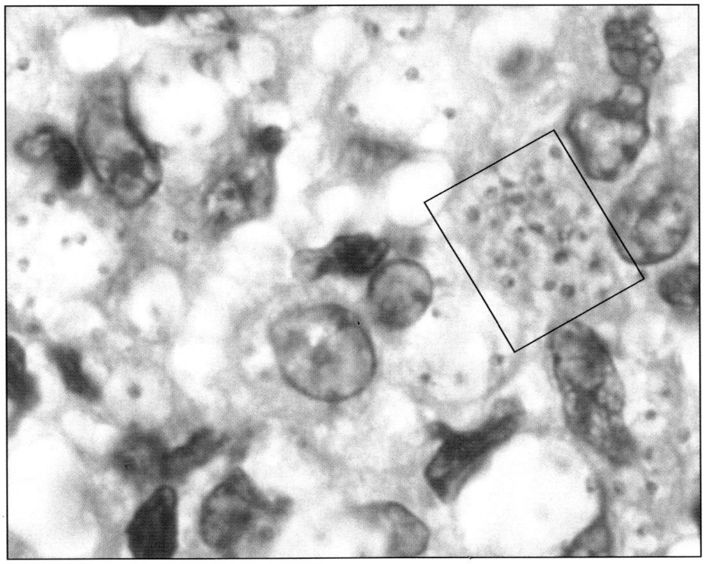
4

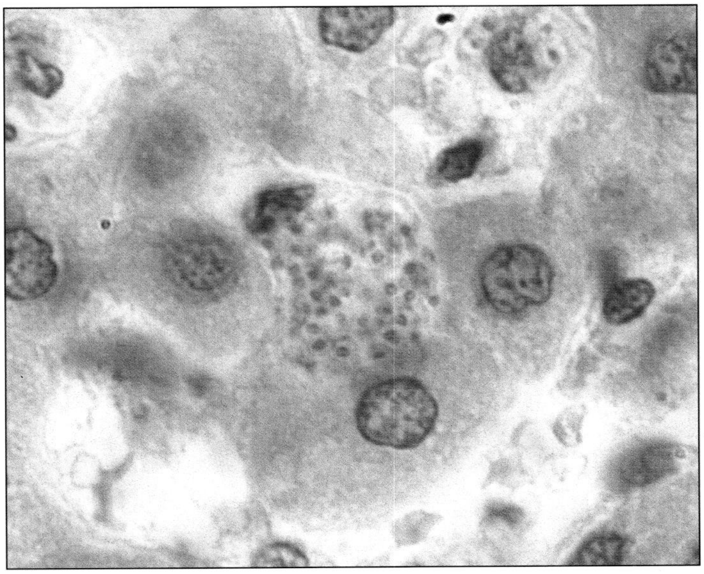
5

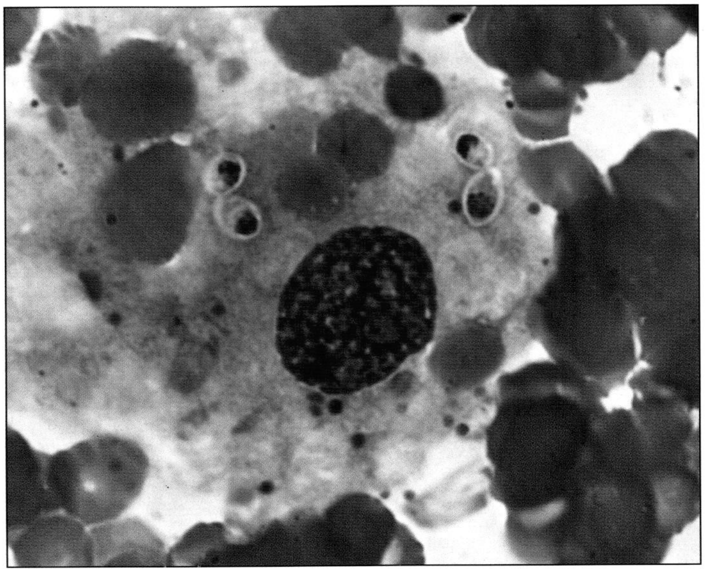
6

Trypanosoma cruzi, T. brucei gambiense, and *T. brucei rhodesiense*

Chagas' Disease

American trypanosomiasis, which is usually referred to as Chagas' disease, is caused by the blood and tissue flagellate *Trypanosoma cruzi.* This parasite is endemic only in the Western Hemisphere and can be found from the United States southward to Argentina. The disease is an important public health problem in South and Central America. The World Health Organization estimates that approximately 16 to 18 million people are infected with the parasite and that about twice that number are at risk of becoming infected. The annual incidence of infection is estimated at one million people, and approximately 45,000 deaths per year are attributed to the disease. *Trypanosoma cruzi* infects a diverse and large group of feral and domestic mammalian hosts and is difficult to control. Spread of infection is usually directly attributable to poor socioeconomic conditions, which allow for exposure to the triatomid vector of the parasite. Because the parasite is present in the bloodstream (➡ 16), however, transmission via blood transfusion is an important mechanism for human infection. In recent years, *T. cruzi* has been increasingly associated with encephalitis as an opportunistic infection in patients with AIDS. Chronic infections may last for many decades. Unfortunately, no effective chemotherapy is available for the disease.

➡ 16

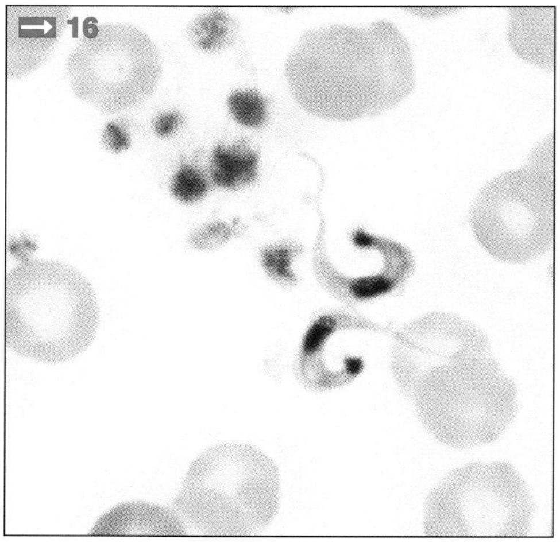

African Trypanosomiasis

African trypanosomiasis, which is caused by *Trypanosoma brucei gambiense* and *T. brucei rhodesiense* and transmitted by tsetse flies of the genus *Glossina*, is restricted to the African continent. These parasites are detected and identified primarily by demonstration of trypomastigotes in the bloodstream or in cerebrospinal fluid. Tissue stages are not usually reported, other than demonstrations of trypomastigotes in fine needle aspirates from lymph nodes in early infections. Although a characteristic disease may be produced in the central nervous system and other tissues, organisms generally cannot be found in tissues. Therefore, we do not cover them except to illustrate trypomastigotes (➡ 17).

➡ 17

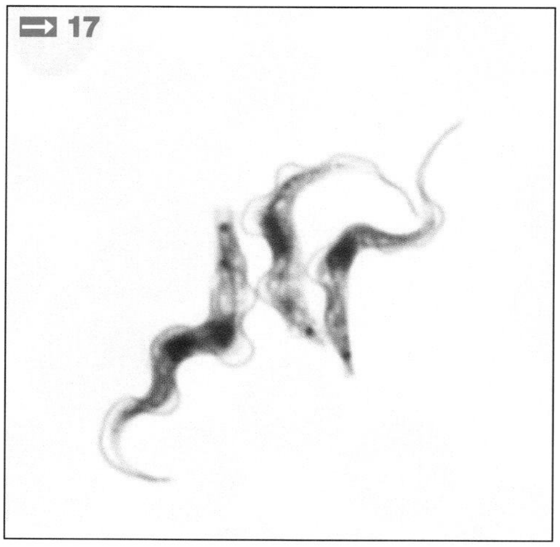

Biology and Life Cycle

Trypanosoma cruzi infection is transmitted by various species of triatomid bugs—*Rhodnius, Triatoma,* and *Panstrongylus*— which are commonly referred to as kissing bugs. Trypomastigotes circulating in the peripheral blood are taken up by the bugs while they are feeding on infected human or animal hosts. In the midgut of the bug, the trypomastigotes transform to an epimastigote stage, which is followed by extensive multiplication. Epimastigotes migrate to the rectal region of the bug and transform into infective, metacyclic trypomastigotes 6 to 15 days after the bug became infected. Although infection is passed on to the human host when triatomids take their next blood meal, it is not transmitted via the biting process. Instead, the infective metacyclic trypomastigotes are excreted in the liquid feces of the bug, which is deposited on the skin after completion of feeding. Subsequent inadvertent rubbing of this fecal material results in the introduction of trypomastigotes into the host, through either the bite wound or other skin abrasions that might be present. Trypomastigotes do not multiply in the vertebrate bloodstream; instead, they invade cardiac and smooth muscle cells, glial cells, and mononuclear phagocytic cells, among others. In these cells, the trypomastigotes transform into amastigotes and multiply by binary division, forming nests of amasti-gotes, which are sometimes referred to as pseudocysts (Plate 18:1–3). Rupture of these cells liberates the amastigotes (as well as some transitional promastigote and epimastigote forms), which transform into trypomastigotes in the bloodstream. Two types of trypomastigotes can be found in the peripheral blood: a slender form that is associated with acute infection and a more stumpy form that is associated with chronic infection and appears to be more infective to the insect vector.

Pathology and Clinical Manifestations

Acute infection with *T. cruzi* may go unnoticed, although a skin granuloma (chagoma) and a unilateral periorbital edema (Romaña's sign) are frequent manifestations of early infection. Symptomatology associated with acute infection includes fever, increased pulse rate, and hepatosplenomegaly. Acute infections are not usually fatal, but when fatalities occur the principal causes are myocarditis or encephalitis. Acute infection progresses to chronic disease, which primarily involves damage to heart muscle through the inflammatory response to amastigote multiplication in cardiac cells. The prolonged myocarditis ultimately results in heart failure in individuals between 25 and 50 years of age.

Other important manifestations of chronic infection include dilation of the esophagus or colon, which produces the syndromes of megaesophagus or megacolon, respectively. These conditions are caused by amastigotes multiplying in peripheral autonomic nerve ganglia. Recently, in immunosuppressed patients such as those with AIDS, *T. cruzi* has been found to produce brain lesions (Plate 18:4–6). Given the large numbers of HIV-infected patients in Brazil and other Latin American countries where Chagas' disease is highly endemic, the potential for *T. cruzi* to behave as an opportunistic infection along with other fungal, protozoal, or microbial organisms is great. Histologic sections of cardiac muscle, gastrointestinal tract, and brain readily demonstrate amastigotes in large nests or in individual cells. Chagas' disease also causes congenital infection: amastigotes can be found in placental villi as well as in many organs of the fetus.

Parasite Morphology

Trypomastigotes of *T. cruzi* range from 12 to 30 µm long (mean, 20 µm) and taper at the ends (➡ 16). They have a large, bulging subterminal kinetoplast at the pointed posterior end and a long flagellum that courses forward to emerge at the anterior end as a free flagellum. An undulating membrane is present. A large central nucleus in midbody typically stains red or violet with Giemsa. In stained preparations, trypomastigotes typically assume a C shape. Amastigotes are round or ovoid, measuring 1.5 to 4.0 µm in diameter. As with amastigotes of other hemoflagellates, a nucleus and a rod-shaped kinetoplast are present.

Amastigotes undergo some shrinkage during tissue processing, from 1 to 3 µm in diameter. Although both the nucleus and kinetoplast can be seen in some amastigotes in tissue section, usually these two structures are not clear.

Amastigotes of *Leishmania* species are similar to those of *T. cruzi*, but the organs and tissues in which amastigotes of these genera might be found differ considerably. Amastigotes of *T. cruzi* are more likely to be found in the brain and in cardiac and smooth muscle cells, whereas leishmanial amastigotes are found more frequently in the skin, liver, and spleen. Nests of amastigotes are more prominent in *T. cruzi* infection. Although *Toxoplasma* and *Histoplasma* might also be confused with *T. cruzi* amastigotes, both of these organisms lack a kinetoplast. Trypomastigotes of *T. cruzi* must be distinguished from those of the human African trypanosomes as well as from *T. rangeli*, a species found in humans in South America. *Trypanosoma cruzi* trypomastigotes have a large, bulging kinetoplast and do not divide in the peripheral blood, whereas the African trypanosomes, *T. b. gambiense* and *T. b. rhodesiense*, have small kinetoplasts and can be found dividing in the bloodstream (➡ 17). *Trypanosoma rangeli* is longer than *T. cruzi* (mean, 30 µm) and does not assume a C shape in blood smears.

References

Gluckstein D, Ciferri F, Ruskin J. Chagas' disease: another cause of cerebral mass in the acquired immunodeficiency syndrome. *Am J Med.* 1992;92:429-432.

Hoare CA. *The Trypanosomes of Mammals: A Zoological Monograph.* Oxford, England: Blackwell Scientific Publications; 1972.

Pittella JEH. Central nervous system involvement in Chagas' disease: an update. *Rev Inst Med Trop São Paulo.* 1993;35:111-116.

Rocha A, DeMeneses ACO, DaSilva AM, et al. Pathology of patients with Chagas' disease and acquired immunodeficiency syndrome. *Am J Trop Med Hyg.* 1994;50:261-268.

Shapiro SZ, Thulin JD, Morton DG. Periocular and urogenital lesions in mice (*Mus musculus*) chronically infected with *Trypanosoma brucei. Lab An Sci.* 1994;44:76-78.

Tanowitz HB, Kirchhoff LV, Simon D, et al. Chagas' disease. *Clin Microbiol Rev.* 1992;5:400-419.

Vickerman K, Preston TM. Comparative cell biology of the kinetoplastid flagellates. In: Lumsden WHR, Evans DA. *Biology of the Kinetoplastida.* London, England: Academic Press; 1976:35-130.

Plate 18

Trypanosoma cruzi

Image 1

In this section of heart tissue, the typical inflammatory reaction is seen. At this relatively low magnification, numerous nests of amastigotes (keyline) in cardiac muscle cells are seen (H&E, 125x).

Image 2

Two nests of *T. cruzi* amastigotes are seen in this section of cardiac muscle. At this magnification, one sees the nucleus and kinetoplast in some of the organisms (H&E, 1250x).

Image 3

In another section of cardiac tissue, a more elongated nest of *T. cruzi* amastigotes is seen. Again, in a few of these both the nucleus and kinetoplast are visible (H&E, 1250x).

Image 4

In a section of brain from an Ecuadorian who died of AIDS, one sees large numbers of *T. cruzi* amastigotes in glial cells (keyline), even at low magnification (H&E, 250x).

Image 5

At higher magnification, the nucleus and kinetoplast of a number of the *T. cruzi* amastigotes in glial cells of the brain are clearly seen (keyline) (H&E, 1250x).

Image 6

The morphologic features of amastigotes easily separate them from apicomplexan organisms such as *Toxoplasma* (H&E, 1250x).

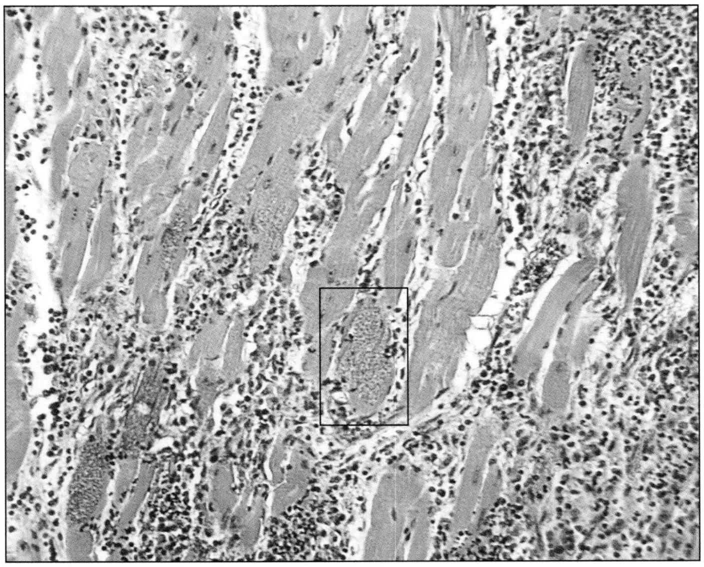
1

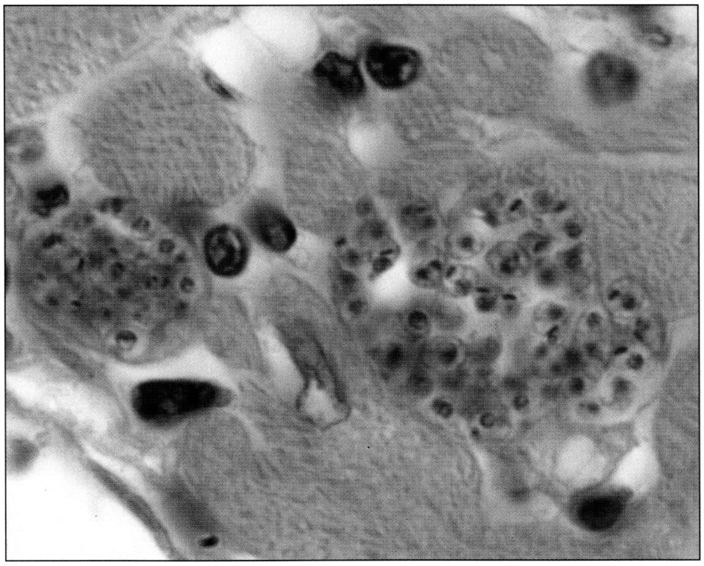
2

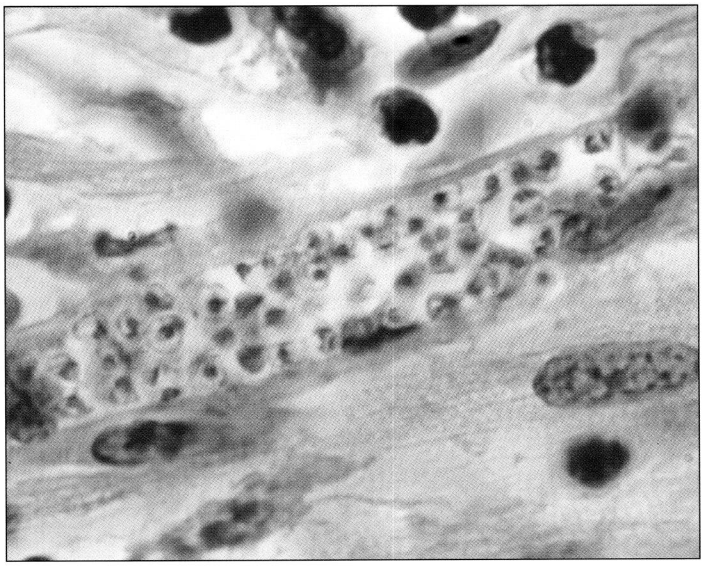
3

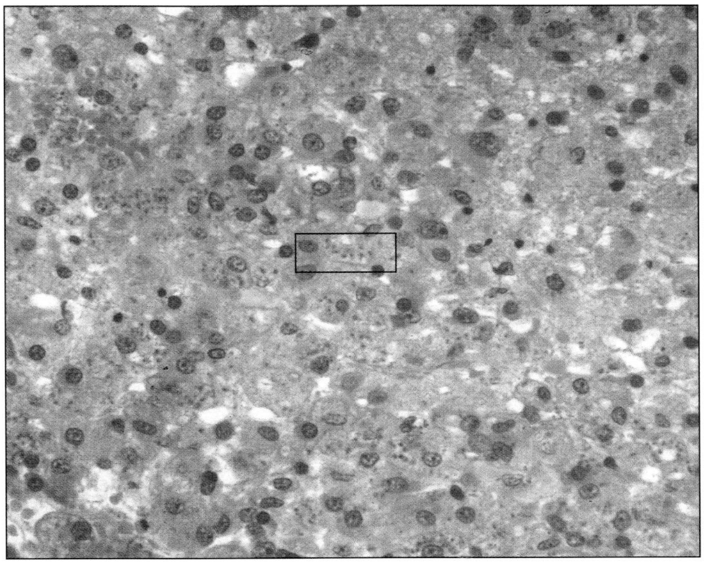
4

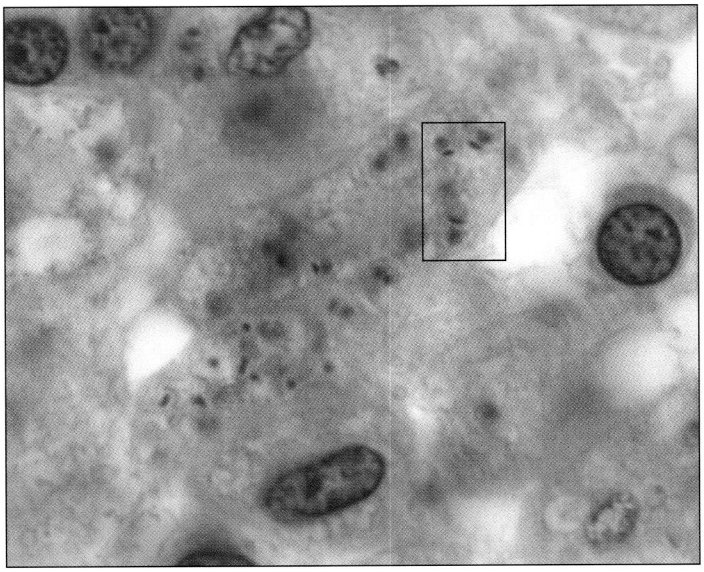
5

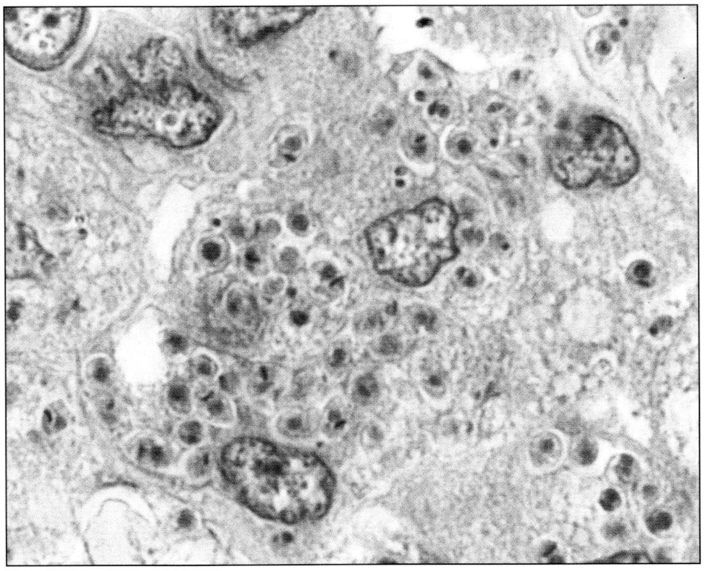
6

Pneumocystis carinii

Pneumocystosis

Pneumocystis carinii was first described in 1909 in the lungs of guinea pigs. It was first recognized as an important cause of human disease when it was found to produce an interstitial plasma cell pneumonia in malnourished and otherwise debilitated children from Europe following World War II. It assumed new importance in the 1960s, when it was found to cause pneumonia in patients who were receiving corticosteroids and various forms of immunosuppressive therapy. With the advent of the AIDS epidemic in the early 1980s, *P. carinii* became recognized as the most common and medically important opportunistic infection producing morbidity and mortality in patients with AIDS.

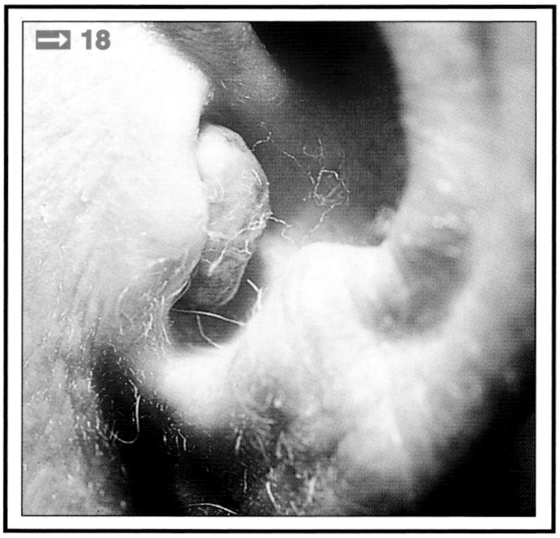

Despite extensive research, *P. carinii* remains an enigmatic organism. Controversy still exists regarding whether it should be classified as a protozoan or as a fungus. The organism has characteristics of both protozoa and fungi, although through the use of molecular technology it appears to have stronger affinities to the fungi. However, becasue of its importance in AIDS and its still questionable taxonomic classification, we continue to treat *P. carinii* as a protozoan parasite.

Biology and Life Cycle

The life cycle of *P. carinii* is not fully understood. Descriptions of the trophozoite, precyst, and cyst stages of the parasite have been derived from ultrastructural studies on infected human and rat lung sections. Both sexual and asexual cycles of reproduction have been described, but questions still are raised regarding whether a sexual cycle exists. Infection with the organism is widespread, and most individuals appear to be serologically positive after the first several years of life. The parasite appears to exist in the environment. Although experimental studies have demonstrated that infection is spread via the respiratory route, the infective stage has not been identified. Disease in the human host appears to develop from latent infections already present as a consequence of immunosuppression or various forms of debilitation. All stages of the organism can be found within alveoli, where they are suspended in a frothy, honeycombed exudate. Cysts contain eight intracystic bodies. After the cysts rupture, trophozoites are liberated and undergo extensive multiplication by binary division or initiate a sexual cycle of reproduction. Efforts to fully unravel the life cycle of *P. carinii* have been considerably hampered by the inability to establish continuous cell cultures of the organism

Pathology and Clinical Manifestations

The clinical picture of *P. carinii* infection varies according to the host and type of immunosuppression. In debilitated and malnourished infants, epidemic interstitial plasma cell pneumonitis remains a problem in many developing countries but is rare in the developed world. Disease onset, which occurs during the first year of life, is insidious: respiratory symptomatology develops slowly and is characterized by dyspnea, tachypnea, and cyanosis. In about 25% of cases, the disease follows a fulminating course, with death occurring several days after the onset of symptoms. Pathologically, the lungs are firm and enlarged, the interstitial septa are thickened and heavily infiltrated with plasma cells and lymphocytes, and the alveolar lumen is filled with the typical frothy exudate composed of desquamated epithelial cells, alveolar macrophages, and pneumocystis organisms.

Pneumocystosis has assumed its greatest importance as a fatal opportunistic infection in patients with AIDS and in other immunocompromised hosts. Fever, dyspnea, and a nonproductive cough are the most common manifestations. In patients with AIDS, the onset is gradual, with nonspecific symptoms, weight loss, fatigue, and night sweats. Disease progression includes increasing respiratory difficulty, shortness of breath, and cyanosis. The disease can be fulminating and fatal when untreated. Diffuse pneumocystosis affects all lobes of the lungs and histologically shows interstitial thickening of the alveolar septa and frothy honeycombed material in the alveoli. Organisms appear to be more numerous in patients with AIDS than in other immunocompromised hosts. Cellular infiltration of the septa is usually not marked. Lung infections that manifest as single nodules or granulomatous lesions have been infrequently described. Extrapulmonary pneumocystosis has been reported in almost all organs and tissues. Dissemination appears to be by both hematogenous and lymphatic routes. The most common sites of dissemination are the lymph nodes, spleen, liver, and bone marrow. Ocular infection usually involves the choroid. Cutaneous involvement has been reported, including the development of bilateral polypoid nodules in the external auditory ear canals (18; Plate 20:4).

Parasite Morphology

The trophozoite is pleomorphic and ranges from 1 to 5 µm in size. In Giemsa-stained preparations of lung material, the trophozoites appear ameboid. Their delicate cytoplasm stains a pale blue, and they have a red dotlike nucleus (Plate 19:3 & 4). The precyst is oval and measures betwen 4 and 6 µm. It does not contain intracystic bodies but may have one or more nuclei. The cyst is thick walled, spherical, 5 to 8 µm, and contains eight intracystic bodies (sometimes referred to as sporozoites) (Plate 19:1–5; Plate 20:1–5). Both thin- and thick-walled cysts have been described. Thin-walled cysts are believed to rupture and liberate sporozoites in the tissues. The sporozoites are 1 to 2 µm and contain a nucleus.

Trophozoites are difficult to identify in routine histologic section. Their nuclei appear as small dotlike structures in the alveolar exudate. With tissue imprints, Giemsa, Wright's, or Diff-Quik® stains demonstrate trophozoites and intracystic bodies within cysts, but the cyst wall does not stain (Plate 19:1 & 2). Trophozoites are not stained by silver stains or PAS. A variety of stains are useful for demonstrating cysts in tissue. Grocott's modification of GMS stain demonstrates cysts in tissue or in imprints as black-staining, collapsed, cup-shaped bodies. Other useful cyst wall stains include toluidine blue O, Gram-Weigert, and PAS. Cysts fluoresce when ultraviolet light is used with Papanicolaou-stained smears.

Pneumocystis must be differentiated from yeasts, fungi, and other organisms. The cysts of *Pneumocystis* are characteristic in their morphologic and staining properties. In addition, unlike many fungi, *Pneumocystis* does not undergo budding in the tissues.

References

Bedrossian CWM. Ultrastructure of *Pneumocystis carinii*: a review of internal and surface characteristics. *Semin Diagn Pathol.* 1989;6:212-237.

Bedrossian CWM, Mason MR, Gupta PK. Rapid cytologic diagnosis of *Pneumocystis*: a comparison of effective techniques. *Semin Diagn Pathol.* 1989;6:245-261.

Hennessey NP, Parro EL, Cockerell CJ. Cutaneous *Pneumocystis carinii* infection in patients with acquired immunodeficiency syndrome. *Arch Dermatol.* 1991;127:1699-1701.

Lipschik GY, Masur H. *Pneumocystis carinii* pneumonia (PCP). *Prog Clin Parasitol.* 1991;2:27-71.

Murray CE, Schmidt RA. Tissue invasion by *Pnemocystis carinii*: a possible cause of cavitary pneumonia and pneumothorax. *Hum Pathol.* 1992;23:1380-1387.

Orozco-Florian R, Trillo A. Identification of *Pneumocystis carinii* by quick hematoxylin and eosin smear. *J Histotech.* 1991;14:179-180.

Pfitzer, P: Fluorescence microscopy of Papanicolaou-stained bronchoalveolar lavage specimens in the diagnosis of *Pneumocystis carinii*. *Acta Cytol.* 1989;33(4):557-559.

Pohlmeyer G, Deerberg F. Nude rats as a model of natural *Pneumocystis carinii* pnemonia: sequential morphological study of lung lesions. *J Comp Path.* 1993;109:217-230.

Witt K, Nielsen TN, Junge J. Dissemination of *Pneumocystis carinii* in patients with AIDS. *Scand J Infect Dis.* 1991;23:691-695.

Plate 19

Pneumocystis carinii

Image 1

One centrally positioned cyst (dart) and many minute trophozoites, which appear as purple dots, can be seen in this smear prepared from rat lung. The wall of the cyst does not stain with Giemsa, but the intracystic bodies are clearly seen. Even with oil immersion, it is difficult to make out morphologic details of the trophozoites (Giemsa, 1250x).

Image 2

In another smear of rat lung, many cysts (darts) containing intracystic bodies can be seen. Few trophozoites are visible (Giemsa, 1250x).

Image 3

In a smear of bronchoalveolar lavage material, many *P. carinii* trophozoites are visible. It is difficult to define the limits of individual organisms, but two of those present are indicated (darts) (Giemsa, 1000x).

Image 4

In a smear from human lung, two dark-staining cysts are clearly seen. Cysts typically have a cup-shaped or collapsed appearance. The prominent black dots in each cyst are part of the cyst wall (GMS, 1250x).

Image 5

In this section of human lung, cysts are in various stages of collapse; however, many have the typical cup-shaped appearance (Toluidine blue O, 500x).

Image 6

The alveoli in this section of human lung are filled with purple-staining, foamy exudate (EX). With H&E stain, however, it is usually not possible to see either trophozoites or cysts of *P. carinii* (H&E, 250x).

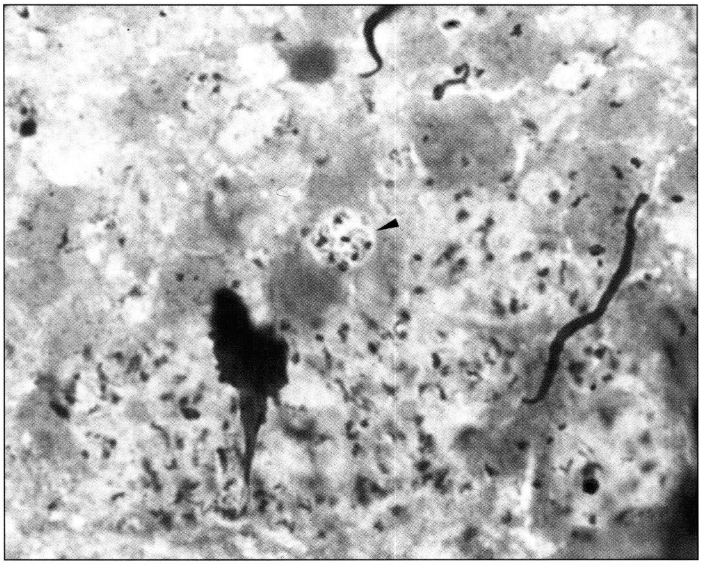

1

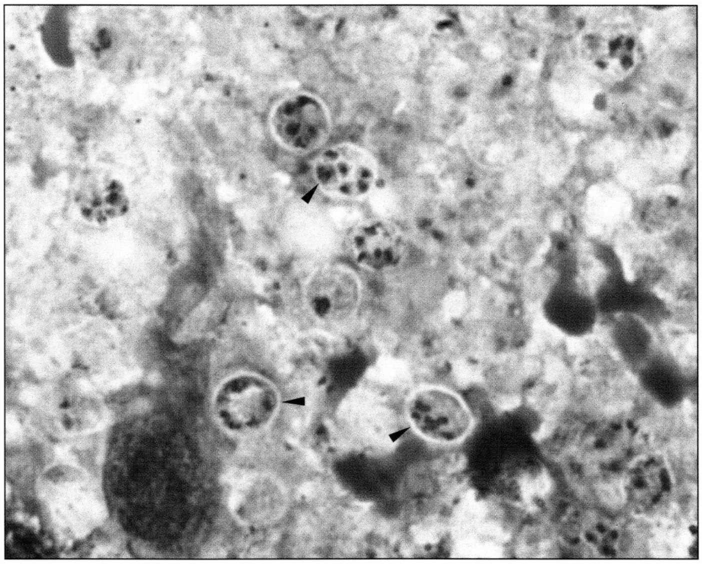

2

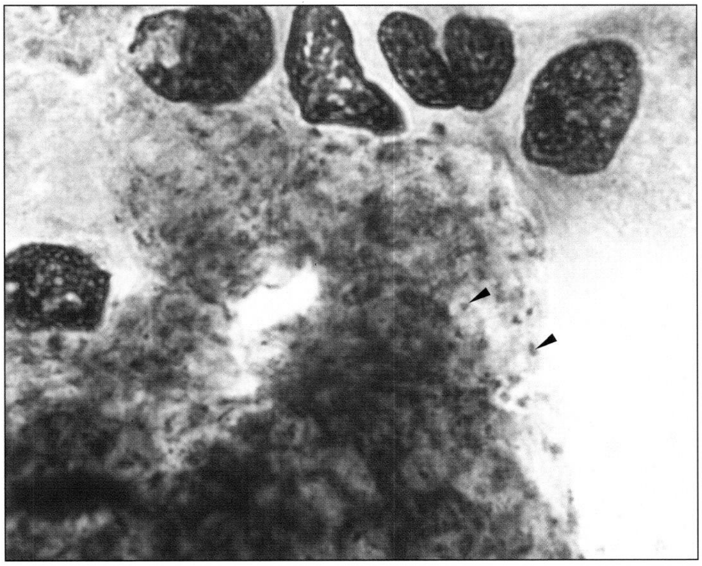

3

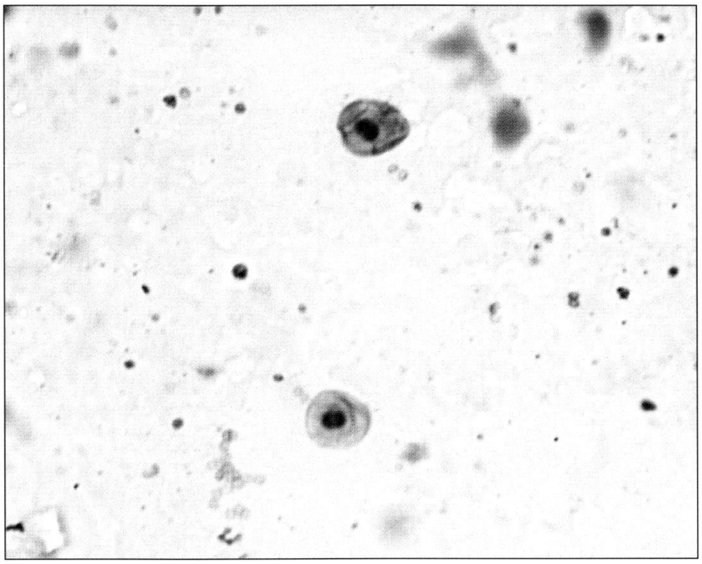

4

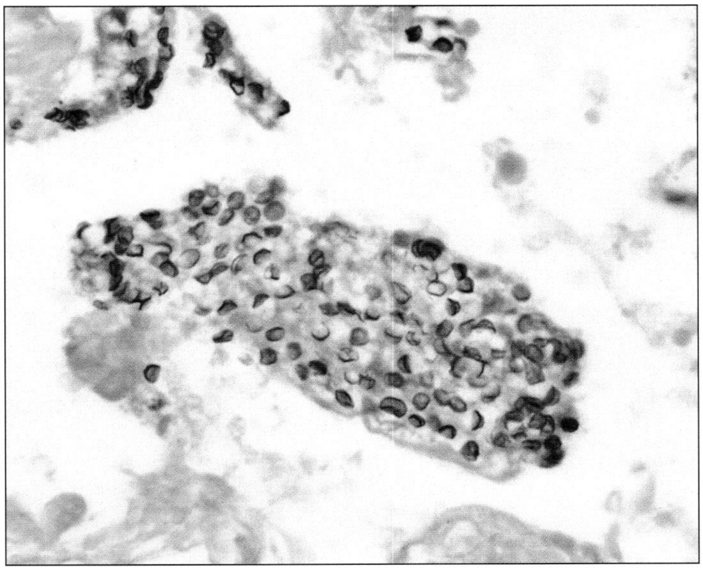

5

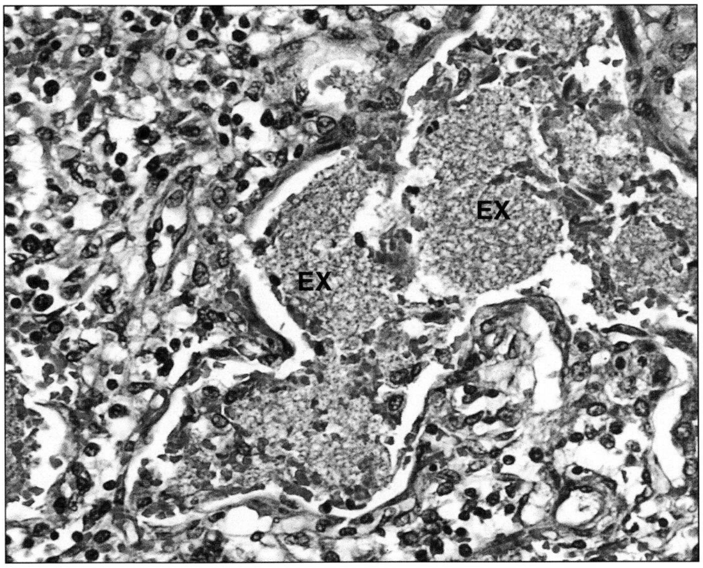

6

Plate 20

Pneumocystis carinii

Image 1

A small cluster of *P. carinii* are visible in this Papanicolaou-stained bronchoalveolar lavage specimen viewed with fluorescent illumination (1200x). (Courtesy of P. Pfitzer.)

Image 2

The cyst walls of *P. carinii* (keyline) can be seen in this immunostained preparation from human lung (Papanicolaou, 180x). (Courtesy of C. Bedrossian.)

Image 3

In a smear made from lung biopsy tissue fixed with cytosol spray, a cyst and intracystic bodies of *P. carinii* can be seen (dart). Although H&E used on tissue sections does not demonstrate the organisms, its use on smear preparations results in staining of both cysts and trophozoites (H&E, 1000x). (Courtesy of R. Orozco-Florian.)

Image 4

This section of a polypoid nodule from the external auditory ear canal of a patient with AIDS shows typical dark-staining cysts of *P. carinii* (keyline), which are scattered throughout the tissue (GMS, 100x). (Courtesy of I. Greene.)

Image 5

A section of liver tissue from a patient with AIDS . Two foci of infection on either side of normal lobular architecture are seen. At this relatively low magnification, one can detect black-staining cysts in the affected areas (GMS, 125x.)

Image 6

At high magnification, the characteristic cup-shaped cysts are clearly seen (GMS, 750x). (Case courtesy of M. Sohn.)

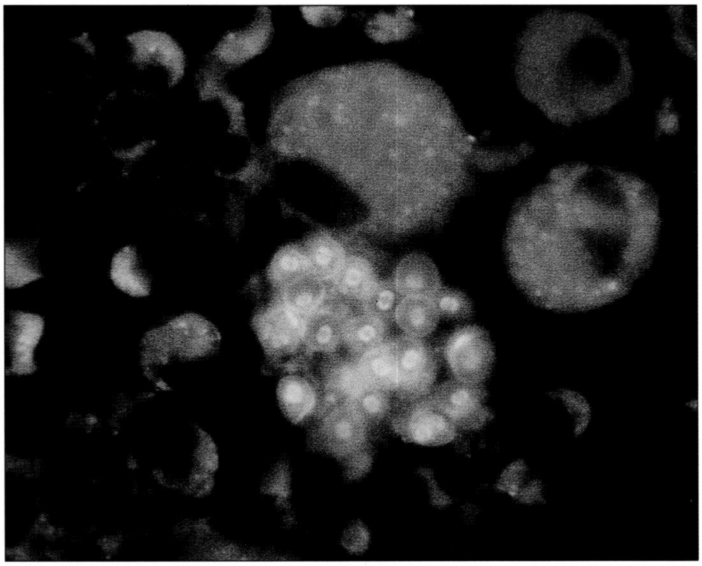

1

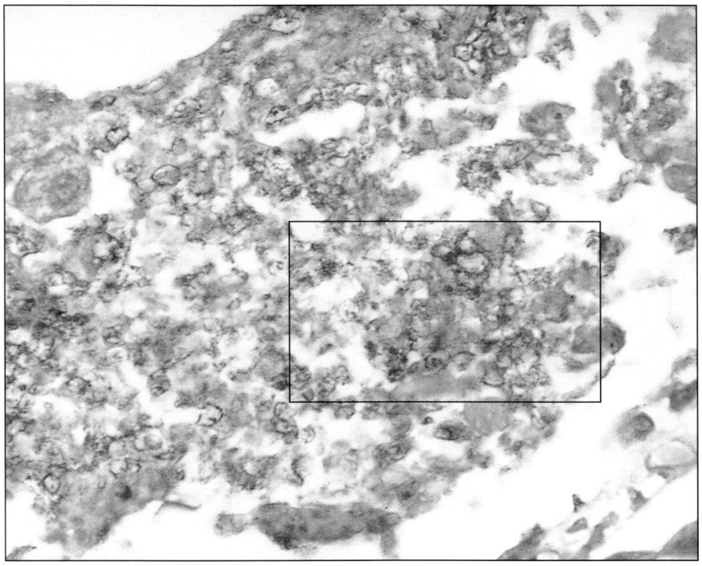

2

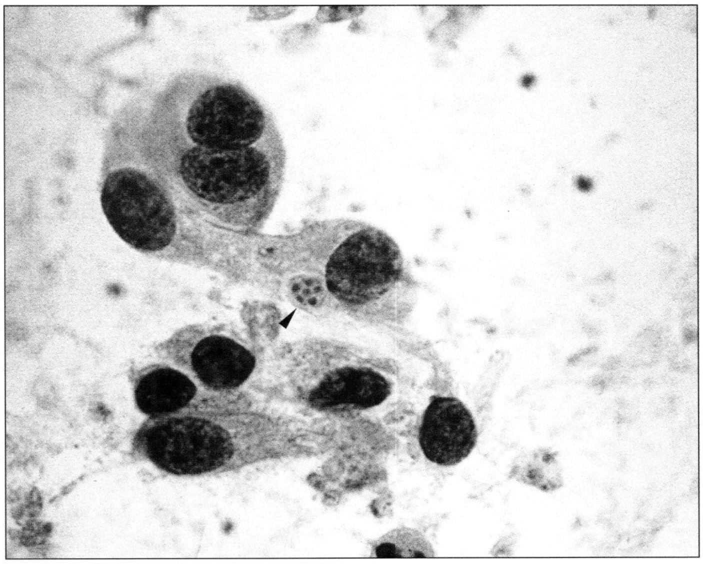

3

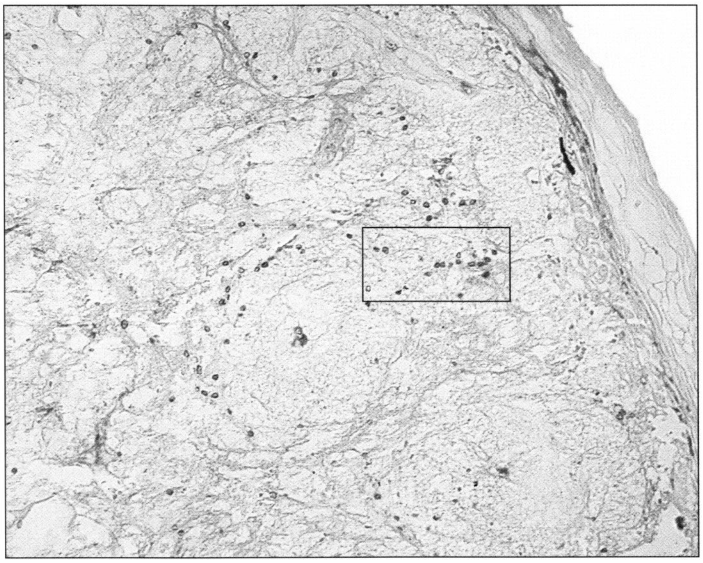

4

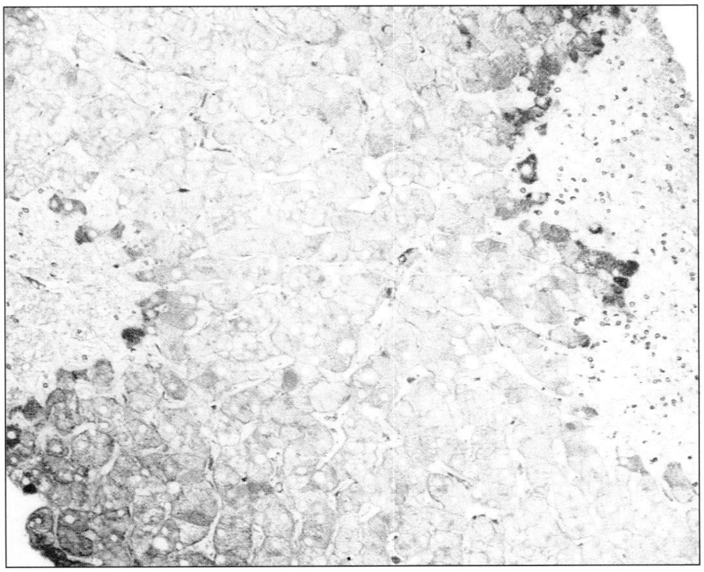

5

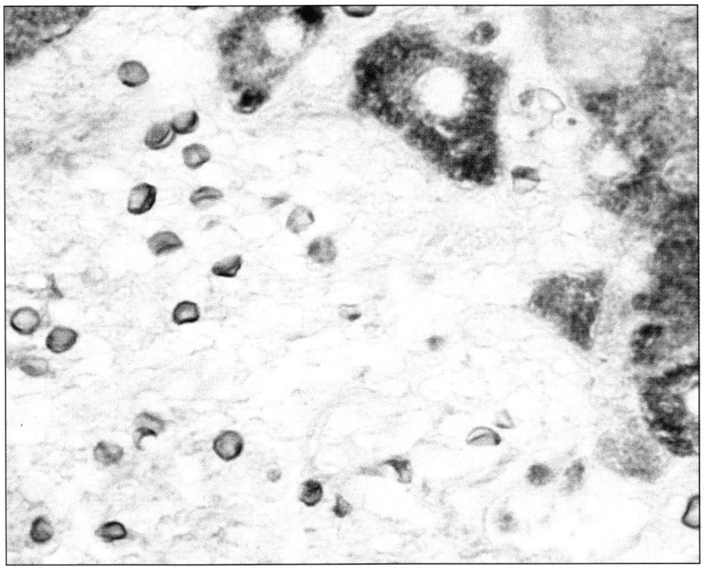

6

Nematoda

More than 16,000 species of nematodes have been described in the literature, and more than twice that number of undescribed species are believed to exist. Of the approximately 2300 genera that have been described, about one-third are parasites of vertebrates. The vast majority are secernenteans (Anderson, 1992). Coombs and Crompton (1991) compiled a list of 138 nematode species belonging to 62 genera that have been found in humans. However, the actual number of species may vary considerably; synonyms, errors in original identifications, pseudoparasitism, and recent reports of heretofore undescribed cases of zoonotic parasites must also be taken into account. Of the 138 species of nematodes listed by Coombs and Crompton, a much smaller number are actually tissue dwellers, although most are intimately involved with tissues and organs. We discuss all of those species that in one stage or another appear in human tissues likely to be subject to pathologic examination.

It is important to have some insight into the interrelationships among the nematode groups and the variations in their structure and biology. As an introduction, we provide an overview of the life histories of nematodes, the relationships and differences among groups, and the basic microscopic anatomy of the parasites, stressing those morphologic features that are most useful in identifying parasites in tissue.

Nematode Life Cycles

The life cycles of the nematodes vary widely. Some life cycles are simple and direct. For example, eggs of *Enterobius*, the pinworm, are deposited on the perianal skin and are almost immediately infective. They are mechanically transmitted to a new host, and upon ingestion, the larva immediately begins its maturation to the adult stage.

The eggs of the so-called soil-transmitted nematodes, such as *Ascaris* and *Trichuris*, are deposited on soil where they develop to an infective larval stage. In the case of *Trichuris*, infective eggs hatch in the intestine of the new host, and the larva that emerges migrates to an appropriate level of the gut to complete its development and maturation to an adult. The ingested infective eggs of *Ascaris*, by contrast, hatch in the gut, and the larva migrates through the liver and lungs before taking up permanent residence in the intestine, where it completes its development.

Another soil-transmitted nematode, the hookworm, discharges eggs in feces. When these eggs are deposited on soil, they develop rapidly. The rhabditoid larva that hatches in the soil develops to the infective stage, penetrates the skin of a new host, migrates to the lung, and then passes on into the intestine to complete development to the adult stage.

Strongyloides exemplifies yet another variation in the life cycle of a soil-transmitted nematode. This parasite produces rhabditoid larvae that are discharged in feces. Upon reaching the soil, the rhabditoid larvae may alternate generations whereby they develop to infective (filariform) larvae and gain entry to a new host by skin penetration. Conversely, the rhabditoid larvae may develop into free-living adults, ultimately producing rhabditoid larvae that become infective (filariform) larvae and infect new hosts by skin penetration. The larvae of *Strongyloides* and hookworms enter the skin and migrate to the lung before returning to the gut for final maturation to the adult stage.

Other nematodes use intermediate hosts that support development of the parasite to the third (infective) stage. These include coprophagous insects, aquatic crustaceans, and various blood-sucking insects, which are known as vectors. An intermediate host serves many functions. It protects the larval parasite from the hazards of the external environment; it may remove some uncertainties of transmission by actually directing the infective stage of the parasite to a new host through its own food preferences; and it provides the larva with a nutrient-rich environment (Anderson, 1992). Examples include those filariae whose microfilariae in the blood are ingested in the course of the vector's feeding and then develop to the infective stage over a period of several days or weeks. Subsequent blood feedings by the vector give the parasite a new host and fulfill the nutritional needs of the vector.

Other nematodes require two intermediate hosts to reach the infective stage (eg, *Gnathostoma*). In still other nematode groups, the parasite uses additional hosts in its infective stage, during which little or no growth or further development occurs until a natural definitive host is encountered (eg, various ascaridoids). This process is called paratenesis, and the hosts are called paratenic hosts.

An accurate knowledge of the parasite's life cycle provides clues as to how the accidental human host may have acquired infection.

Nematode Relationships

The taxonomic schemes used to illustrate the relationships among nematodes vary somewhat from one author to another, although they tend to be similar in perspective. The most widely accepted view is to regard the nematodes as a phylum that is divided into two major groups or classes.

Class Secernentea

Characteristics of the secernenteans, the larger group, include an excretory system with lateral canals and a terminal excretory duct lined with cuticle, phasmids, and an esophagus that, although variable in its structure, never has a stichosome. The third larval stage is usually infective to the final host. Many subdivisions exist among the secernenteans, including those superfamilies whose members have been found in human tissues.

Nematode Taxonomy

Secernentea

Order Ascaridida
- Superfamily Ascaridoidea
  - *Ascaris*
  - *Toxocara*
  - *Baylisascaris*
  - *Lagochilascaris*
  - *Anisakis*
  - *Pseudoterranova*

Order Oxyurida
- Superfamily Oxyuroidea
  - *Enterobius*

Order Strongylida
- Superfamily Ancylostomatoidea
  - *Ancylostoma*
  - *Necator*
- Superfamily Strongyloidea
  - *Oesophagostomum*
  - *Mammomonogamus*
- Superfamily Metastrongyloidea
  - *Angiostrongylus*

Order Spirurida
- Superfamily Gnathostomatoidea
  - *Gnathostoma*
- Superfamily Physalopteroidea
  - *Physaloptera*
- Superfamily Rictularioidea
  - *Rictularia*
- Superfamily Thelazioidea
  - *Thelazia*
- Superfamily Spiruroidea
  - *Gongylonema*
  - *Spirocerca*
- Superfamily Filarioidea
  - *Wuchereria*
  - *Brugia*
  - *Onchocerca*
  - *Loa*
  - *Mansonella*
  - *Dirofilaria*
  - *Loaina*
  - *Meningonema*
- Superfamily Dracunculoidea
  - *Dracunculus*

Order Rhabditida
- Superfamily Rhabditoidea
  - *Strongyloides*
  - *Pelodera*
  - *Halicephalobus*

Adenophorea

Order Enoplida
- Superfamily Trichinelloidea
  - *Trichuris*
  - *Trichinella*
  - *Capillaria* (*C. philippinensis*)
  - *Eucoleus* (*C. aerophila*)
  - *Calodium* (*C. hepatica*)
  - *Anatrichosoma*
- Superfamily Dioctophymoidea
  - *Dioctophyme*
  - *Eustrongylides*

Ascaridoidea

The parasites in this group are large, robust worms that basically parasitize the intestinal tract of amphibians, reptiles, birds, and mammals, including humans. Morphologically, they are characterized by three large lips and a club-shaped esophagus, which in some species may have an esophageal diverticulum or intestinal cecum (eg, *Anisakis*, *Contracaecum*, *Pseudoterranova*).

These parasites include species such as *Ascaris* and *Toxocara*, which are soil transmitted, and others such as *Anisakis*, which have one or more intermediate hosts. The genera considered here include *Ascaris*, *Toxocara*, *Baylisascaris*, *Lagochilascaris*, *Anisakis*, and *Pseudoterranova*.

Oxyuroidea

These nematodes are usually referred to as pinworms. They are intestinal parasites that generally have a simple, direct life cycle, with an egg that contains the infective stage. The human pinworm, *Enterobius vermicularis*, is the only species we discuss.

Ancylostomatoidea

The members of this superfamily are commonly referred to as hookworms. They are parasites of the intestinal tract of amphibians, reptiles, and a wide range of mammals. Morphologically, they are recognized by their distinctive buccal capsule, which is heavily sclerotized and contains either teeth or cutting plates; the male is recognized by a well-developed bursa at the posterior end. These soil-transmitted parasites are able to penetrate intact skin or mucous membranes to gain entry into the definitive host. *Ancylostoma duodenale* and *Necator americanus* are species of special interest, as are the species of *Ancylostoma* found in cats and dogs, which are agents of "creeping eruption" in humans.

Strongyloidea

These are primarily intestinal parasites that include several species of veterinary and medical importance. The adults have complex buccal structures that lack the teeth and cutting plates of the ancylostomes but often have the stoma protected by a corona radiata, a series of leaflike elements that surround the lips. Typically, the adult esophagus is cylindroid or clavate shaped. Males have a well-developed bursa and paired, equal spicules. Females produce eggs resembling those of hookworms, which embryonate in the soil. The oesophagostomes or nodular worms (*Oesophagostomum*) are of particular interest because of their involvement with the tissues. *Mammomonogamus* is mentioned briefly in our discussion.

Metastrongyloidea

These slender, filiform worms have a reduced or rudimentary buccal cavity and a reduced bursa. As adults, they live in the pulmonary or mesenteric arteries of their mammalian hosts, produce first-stage larvae that are excreted in the feces, and utilize a molluscan intermediate host. The species that infect humans include *Angiostrongylus cantonensis* and *A. costaricensis*.

Gnathostomatoidea

This group of nematodes comprises only a few genera that for the most part are parasites of lower vertebrates. An exception is the genus *Gnathostoma,* which is found in mammals and has been well studied because of its importance in animal and human health. The gnathostomes are small, robust worms that parasitize a variety of carnivorous and omnivorous animals (felines, raccoons, otters, opossums, and domestic and wild pigs) that feed on cold-blooded vertebrates. The adult worms are found embedded in the gastric mucosa, where they produce nodules or tumors. Their most striking gross morphologic feature is an inflatable head bulb armed with numerous rows of hooks. The surface of the body is covered in whole or in part by spines. The gnathostomes have two intermediate hosts: the first an aquatic crustacean, a copepod; the second includes various amphibians, reptiles, and fishes, which may serve additionally as paratenic hosts.

We focus on the species that accidentally infect humans, *Gnathostoma spinigerum*, *G. hispidum*, *G. doloresi,* and *G. nipponicum.*

Physalopteroidea

The physalopterids parasitize a wide range of lower vertebrates, including fish, amphibians, reptiles, some birds, and mammals. With some exceptions, members of this group have a cuticular collarette on the anterior extremity that surrounds the large lateral lips. Males have large caudal alae supported by long slender papillae, which have the appearance of a bursa. These gross features facilitate a quick identification of the parasite. The worms are usually found in the stomach or intestine of their hosts and produce typical spiruroid eggs (ie, thick shelled with a larva). Their life cycles are not well known, but it is believed that they may have more than one intermediate host as well as paratenic hosts. Two species have been reported from humans, *Physaloptera caucasica* and *P. transfuga.*

Rictularoidea

These nematodes are intestinal parasites found in a variety of mammals including rodents, insectivores, bats, and carnivores. Their distinguishing morphologic features include a well-developed buccal capsule with teeth and spines at its base. The oral opening is usually displaced to the dorsal side of the anterior extremity of the worm. The presence of rows of spines or combs along the length of the body aid in rapid identification of these parasites either grossly or in sections of tissue. They use insects as intermediate hosts. The only member of this group that we will consider is a species of Rictularia that has been recovered from human tissues.

Thelazioidea

This group includes the eyeworms of birds and mammals. The parasites live in the orbit, conjunctivae, and lacrimal ducts and glands of their hosts. They produce larvae or eggs containing a larva and are transmitted by muscid and other flies. Numerous wild and domestic animals are infected, and humans occasionally acquire infection from accidental contact with infected flies. Our primary interest is in the species of *Thelazia, T. californiensis* and *T. callipaeda,* that infrequently infect humans.

Spiruroidea

Authorities disagree on how this group is constituted. We view it as including four subgroups that are mainly parasites of the anterior gut of birds and mammals. Almost all of the species produce an embryonated egg and use an insect as the intermediate host as well as paratenic hosts that feed on these insects. Of special interest are the species of *Gongylonema* that burrow in the mucosa and submucosa of the pharynx, esophagus, and stomach. Morphologically, they all have plaques or bosses on the cuticle of the anterior extremity. They tend to be long and filiform, resembling some filariid species. Additionally, species of *Spirocerca* are found in tumors in the walls of the esophagus, stomach, and aorta of their final host (eg, dogs). We describe the features of *Gongylonema* species and *Spirocerca lupi,* which have been found in human tissues.

Filarioidea

The filariae parasitize the tissues of a great variety of animals ranging from amphibians to mammals, with numerous species afflicting humans. All use a blood-sucking arthropod as a vector. Adult worms vary considerably in size. They tend to be long, slender, delicate worms with a simple, unadorned anterior end. The esophagus is usually divided into anterior muscular and posterior glandular parts. The intestine is a simple tube. The female has an anteriorly placed vulva. The male has paired complex spicules and a tail that bears papillae and often caudal alae. The female produces a larva called a microfilaria, which circulates in the blood or is found in the skin. Species of special interest include *Wuchereria bancrofti*, *Brugia malayi* and other *Brugia* species, *Loa loa*, *Onchocerca volvulus* and other *Onchocerca* species, *Dirofilaria* species, *Mansonella perstans* and *M. streptocerca*, *Loaina* species, and *Meningonema peruzzi.*

Dracunculoidea

Dracunculoids parasitize animal tissues, including the tissues of fish, reptiles, and mammals. The group is best known for the species *Dracunculus medinensis,* which has been an important human parasite for millennia. Adult female worms tend to be large; males are much smaller. The female produces larvae that are discharged into an aquatic environment. Small crustaceans, copepods, serve as intermediate hosts. We consider only *Dracunculus medinensis.*

Rhabditoidea

This group includes species that are free-living, saprophagous forms as well as truly parasitic forms. Our interests include certain of the free-living species—namely *Halicephalobus* and *Pelodera*, which on rare occasions can parasitize vertebrates, including humans—and the truly parasitic forms such as *Strongyloides* species.

Rhabditoid species such as *Pelodera* are found in rotting vegetation, nests of rodents, and on body surfaces of animals soiled with manure. Their relationship to animals is fortuitous. Their presence may produce a dermatitis.

Halicephalobus (= *Micronema*), another saprophytic organism, may also invade human tissues, especially the nervous system. Males are unknown; females are assumed to reproduce by parthenogenesis. This parasite possesses a rhabditoid-type esophagus, is monodelphic, and produces only one egg at a time.

Another group within the superfamily is typified by *Strongyloides* species, which have free-living and parasitic generations. The parasitic generation includes only hermaphroditic females.

We will discuss *Strongyloides stercoralis, Halicephalobus deletrix,* and *Pelodera strongyloides.*

Class Adenophorea

This major nematode group is characterized by having an excretory system that lacks lateral canals and has a terminal excretory duct without a cuticular lining. Phasmids are absent. The esophagus is either cylindrical or it has esophogeal glands that form a stichosome and lie within the pseudocoelom. Caudal alae are absent or few. The first-stage larva is typically infective to the final host. Eggs have bipolar prominences and usually are in the one-cell stage, or they may develop and hatch in utero. The majority are monodelphic.

Trichinelloidea

The members of this group include the trichuroids (*Trichuris*) or whipworms, which are found in the large intestine of mammals; the capillarids, which are found in many organs (eg, gut, urinary tract, respiratory system, liver, and skin of most vertebrate groups); the trichosomoids, which live in the digestive system and bladder epithelium of mammals; and the trichinelloids, which are widely dispersed in wild and domestic animals. *Trichinella* species have been studied intensively because of their medical importance. We discuss *Trichuris trichiura, Capillaria* (= *Calodium*) *hepatica, C. philippinensis, C.* (= *Eucoleus*) *aerophila, Anatrichosoma* species, and *Trichinella* species.

Dioctophymoidea

This unusual group includes only four genera of parasites, two of which are especially interesting, *Dioctophyme* and *Eustrongylides*. Unlike other adenophoreans, these parasites have a well-developed cylindrical esophagus rather than a stichosome. Additionally, the male tail is modified to form a ventral sucker. Females are monodelphic. Species of *Dioctophyme* parasitize wild mustelids and canines; adult *Eustrongylides* are found in piscivorous birds.

Nematode Morphology

The nematodes are remarkably consistent in their basic anatomic features, yet diverse in structural detail. They are vermiform, unsegmented, bilaterally symmetrical, and pseudocoelomate organisms. They have four main longitudinal hypodermal chords, a triradiate esophagus, and a circumesophageal nerve ring. They have neither a circulatory nor a respiratory system. They have one or two gonads that open at the vulva in the female and into the rectum in the male.

We review the organ systems and some of the common variations within each. Again, our account is not exhaustive; it is merely intended to provide enough information to facilitate recognition of the individual group in tissues at the histologic level.

Cuticle

The nematode cuticle is a three-layered structure. The layers or "zones," as they are often termed, are, from the surface inward, cortical, median, and basal. In addition, the surface of the cuticle is often covered by a thin epicuticle. The three major layers are usually divided further into additional sublayers, which vary considerably in number among species. The layers of the cuticle are not always discernible in stained sections under light microscopy. The cuticle varies considerably in thickness among nematode species, ranging from 0.20 µm to more than 50 µm. The surface of the cuticle may include various markings, which are useful not only to taxonomists but also to those examining worms in tissues.

The cuticle of most nematodes has transverse markings called striae or annulations, depending on their width and depth, which often give the impression of segmentation. The widths of these transverse markings often vary within a single organism and among organisms as well as among species. In addition, longitudinal striae may impart a blocklike appearance to the surface of the cuticle. Generally, the transverse striations are visible in longitudinal sections of the worm.

The surface of the cuticle may bear conspicuous longitudinal ridges that cover most of the body length on all surfaces (Plate 21a:1). These ridges are especially common in trichostrongyles and certain species of *Dirofilaria* (Plate 58:4; Plate 62:6). Other longitudinal ridges in the lateral fields are called alae. In the anterior extremity these are called cervical alae; through most of the body length, they are referred to as longitudinal alae; posteriorly they are called caudal alae. They may be single (Plate 21a:2), double (Plate 34:5), or triple. In some species, they involve the cortical and medial layers and may have internal structural supports (Plate 21a:3). Alae are seen in adult and larval stages. The presence or absence of alae as well as their forms are especially useful in identifying some nematode species in tissues.

Additionally, the surface of the cuticle may have inflations or blisterlike structures called bosses or plaques, which assist in identifying species such as *Gongylonema* (Plate 21a:3) and *Loa* (Plate 54:4). Other cuticular adornments seen in nematodes include a variety of spines (Plate 21a:4), combs (Plate 42:1 & 2), and spiral rings (Plate 52:4). The cuticle may also have lateral internal cuticular ridges, which are useful in identifying certain species of filariae (eg, *Dirofilaria*) (Plate 57:6).

In degenerating worms, the layering of the cuticle often becomes more evident and even exaggerated in its appearance. Changes in some of the markings also become exaggerated and make recognition easier (Plates 60:4 & 6). Because of some features of the cuticle (eg, longitudinal ridges), a generic identification (eg, *Dirofilaria*) can be made solely from study of the degenerating fragments or remnants of the cuticle (Plate 59).

Hypodermis

The hypodermis is a layer or sheet of cells that lies between the cuticle and the muscles and projects into the pseudocoelom at the dorsal, ventral, and lateral positions to form the four chords (Plate 22:1B). These chords also divide the muscle layer into quadrants. The hypodermis secretes the cuticle. It is often and perhaps more commonly referred to as the epidermis. We have decided to use the term hypodermis because it is so widely used by parasitologists; however, the terms hypodermis and epidermis are synonymous. In secernentean nematodes, the hypodermis is syncytial in adults but may be partly cellular in larval stages. In some species, subsidiary chords may be located between the four main chords. In adenophorean nematodes (eg, *Trichuris*), the hypodermis is cellular, and hypodermal gland cells along with specialized regions of the cuticle form the bacillary band (Plate 23:1A; Plate 68:3).

The lateral chords are the most conspicuous. They take various forms that sometimes are characteristic for the genera or species. Some are large and protrude deeply into the pseudocoelom (Plate 21a:5). Others have a peculiar shape (Plate 21a:6). In still others, one chord may be larger than the other (Plate 21a:3). In some groups, the lateral secretory/excretory columns lie within or associated with the lateral chords (eg, *Ascaris*) (Plate 21a:5).

In secernenteans, the hypodermal nuclei are confined mostly to the lateral chords, although some may be seen in the dorsal and ventral chords. Nuclei are essentially absent from the interchordal areas. Their distribution within the lateral chords may be random or it may appear to have consistent patterns of arrangement. The dorsal and ventral chords are less conspicuous than the lateral ones (Plate 22:1A & B) and may even be difficult to identify in sections of worm.

Musculature

Body muscles may be divided into two types: somatic and specialized. The somatic muscles are elongate, spindle-shaped cells. They lie in rows under the hypodermis and are parallel to and usually overlap each other. Each cell is composed of a basal, contractile portion and a cytoplasmic, noncontractile portion. We use the terms contractile and cytoplasmic. If the contractile portion of the cell is wide and shallow and lies close to the hypodermis, it is described as platymyarian (Plate 21a:8; Plate 34:2). If the contractile portion is U shaped and extends up the sides of the cell, it is described as coelomyarian (Plate 21b:9). Some variation may occur in shapes among coelomyarian muscle cells (Plate 21b:9 & 10). When the cytoplasm is entirely surrounded by the contractile portion of the cell, it is called circomyarian. If the number of rows of muscle cells does not exceed two, it is holomyarian; if it is between two and five, it is meromyarian; and if it is more than five, it is polymyarian. Typically, polymyarian forms are coelomyarian, and meromyarian and holomyarian forms tend to be platymyarian. Numerous exceptions exist, however, and muscle cell counts are difficult because the individual muscle cells tend to overlap.

In addition to the somatic muscles, specialized muscles are associated with the digestive system (esophagus, intestine, rectum) and reproductive systems (with the female's vulva, ovejector, uterine tubes, etc, and with the male's spicules, bursa, etc), which are usually of limited or no value in identifying parasitic worms in the tissues (see Bird and Bird, 1991).

Digestive System

The nematode digestive system is composed of the mouth or stoma, the buccal cavity, the esophagus, the intestine, and the rectum, exiting the body via the anus. The mouth may be simple or surrounded by lips that vary in number and appearance in different groups. The buccal cavity is variable as well: it may be vestigial or absent in the typical filaria or large and complex in the hookworms (Plate 34:1). The esophagus, also referred to as the pharynx, is a pumping organ with a triradiate, cuticle-lined lumen (Plate 21b:11 & 12). Various forms of the esophagus exist, with variations within each form. An esophagus that can be divided into corpus, isthmus, and bulb is commonly referred to as the rhabditiform type (eg, *Halicephalobus* and *Pelodera*). Another type of esophagus is basically cylindroid and may be divided into anterior muscular and posterior glandular parts; this type is seen in many parasites, including spiruroids and filariae (Plate 21b:11 & 12). A third type, seen in strongyles such as the hookworms, may be clavate or club shaped (Plate 34:1). A fourth type is seen in adenophoreans such as *Trichuris*, *Capillaria*, and *Anatrichosoma*. This type of esophagus is tubular and embedded in a row of block-shaped cells called the stichosome; the individual cells in the stichosome are called stichocytes (Plate 23:1A & B; Plate 68:2; Plate 72:2). The lumen of this esophagus may be tubular rather than triradiate. In certain anisakine ascarids, modifications of the terminal portion of the esophagus and anterior part of the intestine occur, with formation of an appendix derived from the esophagus and a cecum that is an outgrowth of the intestine. The presence or absence of these structures is used in identifying generic groups. An esophago-intestinal valve links the esophagus with the intestine and may at times be seen in appropriate sections of a nematode.

The intestine is a simple tube lined by a layer of epithelial cells that vary in number, form, and presence of cellular inclusions. The lumen of the intestine is equally variable in shape. The intestinal cells are usually uninucleate (Plate 21b:13 & 14) but may be multinucleate

(Plate 21b:16), and they vary in height from cuboidal to columnar (Plate 21b:13 & 14), even within the same organ (Plate 21b:16). The luminal border of the cell is usually covered with microvilli, which are frequently conspicuous (Plate 21b:15). A variety of inclusions, including glycogen granules, lipid droplets, and spherocrystals, may be seen. The morphology of the intestine frequently is an important key to identification of the parasite. The intestine leads directly into the rectum through an intestinal or rectal valve. This portion of the gut is usually lined with cuticle and leads directly to the anus.

Reproductive Systems

In most nematodes, the sexes are separate. The reproductive systems are simple tubular structures. Among the secernenteans, the male usually has only one testis and the female has two ovaries.

Male

The tubular male organ is divided into three parts: the testis, seminal vesicle, and vas deferens. Most parasites of animals and humans have only one testis. Among the secernenteans, the testis is telegonic (ie, spermatogonia are generated from the end of the testis), and it is usually flexed or coiled. The testis is divided into germinal and growth zones and is covered with an epithelium that is continuous with the seminal vesicle, where sperm are stored. The seminal vesicle is dilated and lined by cuboidal to columnar epithelium. The vas deferens is the longest portion of the system and is usually modified or divided into tubular and glandular regions. Often its terminal region is covered by a layer of muscle and functions as the ejaculatory duct. The vas deferens enters the ventral side of the rectum, forming a cloaca. A spicular pouch enters the cloaca from the dorsal surface. It contains the spicules, usually two but in some species only one or none. The spicules are cuticularized, yellow to dark brown or black, and easily recognized in tissue sections (Plate 29:5; Plate 35:5). They may or may not be equal in size and sometimes have dissimilar structures.

On the male tail, caudal alae may be supported by papillae of various sizes and shapes, which are easily recognized in sections of the posterior end (Plate 54:5 & 6). In others, such as the strongyles, the caudal alae may be expanded and supported by modified caudal papillae referred to as rays, which are also easily recognized in sections of the male worm. In addition, other sclerotized cuticular structures, such as the gubernaculum and telemon, are present in some species. These accessory sex structures are also used in taxonomy but are usually difficult to identify in sections of tissue. The number, type, and arrangement of papillae and the morphology of the spicules are widely used taxonomic characters as well. Reconstructing spicules from sections of worm is difficult and unwarranted; sections of worm provide some idea of the structure of spicules (Plate 35:5).

Female

This system usually has two ovaries, each divided into germinal and growth zones among telegonic forms. They typically are long and highly coiled, and within a single transverse section of female worm cut at the appropriate level there are often several sections of ovary (Plate 46:5). The ovaries lead into the usually muscular oviducts, which typically have tall epithelium (Plate 46:4; Plate 53:3). Eggs are often found within the oviducts, which lead into the two uterine tubes. In the mature female, the terminal portion of each uterine tube serves as a seminal receptacle and is usually filled with sperm and a few eggs (Plate 48:3). The uterine branches and their placement in the body are frequently used in taxonomy. The uteri are termed amphidelphic if they go in opposite directions, prodelphic if they are parallel and directed anteriorly from their point of origin, and opisthodelphic if they are parallel and directed posteriorly from their origin. The paired uterine tubes empty into the vagina uterina and then the vagina vera, which is usually lined with cuticle and most terminally a muscular, sometimes branched ovejector (Plate 29:3). In females seen in transverse sections, one can determine whether they are mature (functioning ovaries) (Plate 46:5; Plate 58:6); whether they have been inseminated (presence of sperm in the seminal receptacles) (Plate 48:3); and whether they are reproductive (presence of developing or maturing eggs or microfilariae) (Plate 50:3 & 4). Fully developed eggs in utero often make a specific diagnosis possible (Plate 24:6; Plate 32:5; Plate 71:4; Plate 72:4).

Nervous System

The nervous system of nematodes is complex and not well described. Interestingly, the nervous system of *Caenorhabditis elegans* has been the most exhaustively studied among all animals and, as stated by Bird and Bird (1991), "...may well become a reference point for research into the nervous systems of all secernentean nematodes." For our purposes, structural details of the system are of little value in identification. We can view the system as a circumesophageal ring of nerve ganglia from which six nerve trunks pass anteriorly and four posteriorly. In addition, numerous special nerve branches lead to sensory papillae, setae, and chemoreceptors such as the amphids anteriorly and the phasmids (in secernenteans) posteriorly.

Excretory System

The excretory system, frequently referred to as the secretory/excretory (S/E) system, varies considerably in structure and function among the nematodes and is distinctly different in secernenteans and adenophoreans. The S/E system in adenophoreans is composed of a single large gland cell that opens to the exterior via a duct in the ventral midline of the worm, usually near the anterior end in the region of the nerve ring. The S/E system in secernenteans is more complex and variable in its structure. In its most primitive form, it is H shaped, with one or two renette cells from which tubular canals run anteriorly or posteriorly in the lateral chords (Plate 21a:5) or, in some larvae, appear to be free in the pseudocoelom (eg, *Toxocara*) (Plate 27:3). This may be modified to an inverted U shape, or the tube may remain on one side of the body only. The system opens to the exterior via a duct to the excretory pore.

Pseudocoelom

Because of its germ cell origin, the body cavity in nematodes is not regarded as a true body cavity—-hence its designation, pseudocoelom. However, more recent cell lineage studies cast some doubt on the validity of that term. At any rate, the body cavity in nematodes is filled with fluid that bathes the organs. Special cells called coelomocytes are found in the body cavity of both secernenteans and adenophoreans. Coelomocytes, along with crystalloid bodies, are of unknown function.

References

Anderson RC. *Nematode Parasites of Vertebrates: Their Development and Transmission.* Wallingford, England: CAB International; 1992.

Bird AF, Bird J. *The Structure of Nematodes.* 2nd ed. San Diego, Calif: Academic Press Inc; 1991.

Chitwood BG, Chitwood MB. *An Introduction to Nematology.* Baltimore, Md: Monumental Printing Co; 1950.

Coombs I, Crompton DWT. *A Guide to Human Helminths.* London, England: Taylor and Francis; 1991.

Rupert EE. Introduction to the Aschelminth phyla: a consideration of mesoderm, body cavities, and cuticle. In: Harrison FW, Ruppert EE, eds. *Microscopic Anatomy of Invertebrates, Vol IV: Aschelminthes.* New York, NY: Wiley-Liss Inc; 1991.

Wright KA. Nematoda. In: Harrison FW, Ruppert EE, eds. *Microscopic Anatomy of Invertebrates, Vol IV: Aschelminthes.* New York, NY: Wiley-Liss Inc; 1991.

Plate 21a

Nematode Anatomy, Structural Variations

Image 1

Dirofilaria corynodes. Transverse section through the cuticle illustrates longitudinal ridges on the surface (Trichrome).

Image 2

Lagochilascaris species, lateral ala. Note the prominent lateral chord (LC) (H&E).

Image 3

Gongylonema species. Transverse section through anterior extremity shows the large cuticular bosses (arrows) and cervical alae (darts). The alae have internal structural supports. Note also the different sizes of the lateral chords (LC) (H&E).

Image 4

Gnathostoma procyonis. Cuticular spines are seen on the surface of the cuticle (H&E).

Image 5

Ascaris lumbricoides. Transverse section shows large lateral chord and excretory canal (EC) (H&E).

Image 6

Anisakis species. Transverse section through the body shows large, Y-shaped lateral chord (LC) (H&E).

Image 7

Dioctophyme species. Transverse section through the body wall shows the conspicuous ventral hypodermal chord (dart), with nuclei assuming a U-shaped arrangement in the cytoplasm (H&E).

Image 8

Nochtia nochti. Transverse section shows the typical platymyarian muscle cells (unknown stain).

1

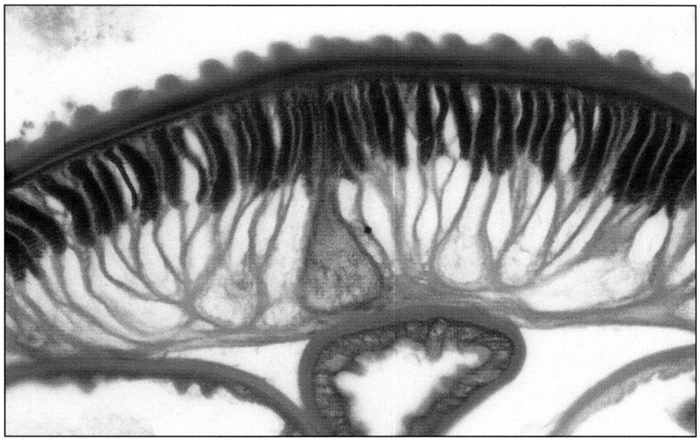

2

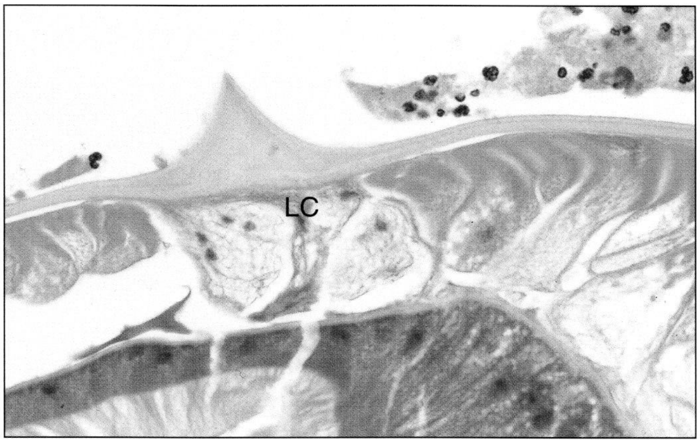

3

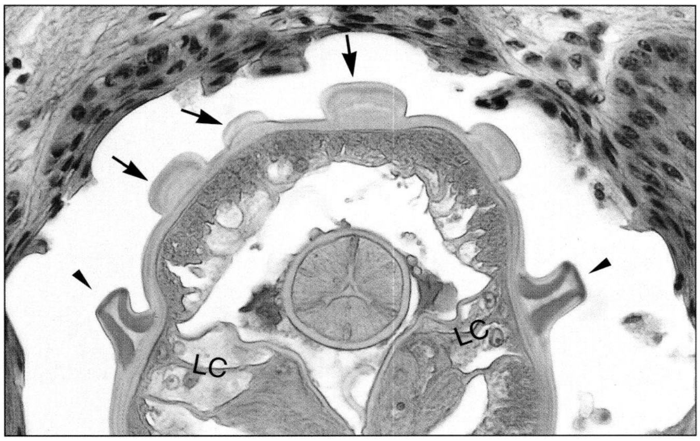

4

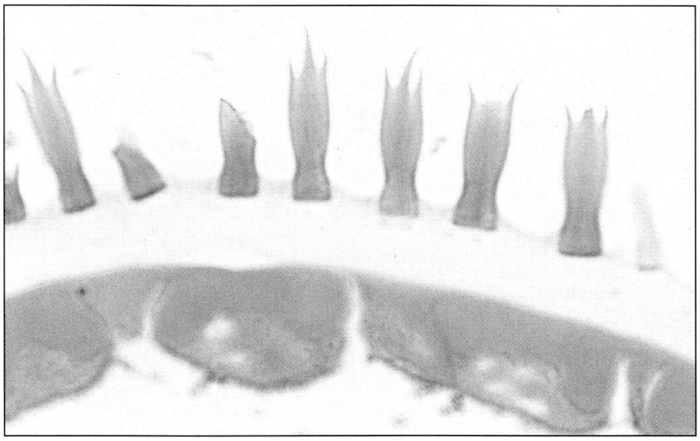

5

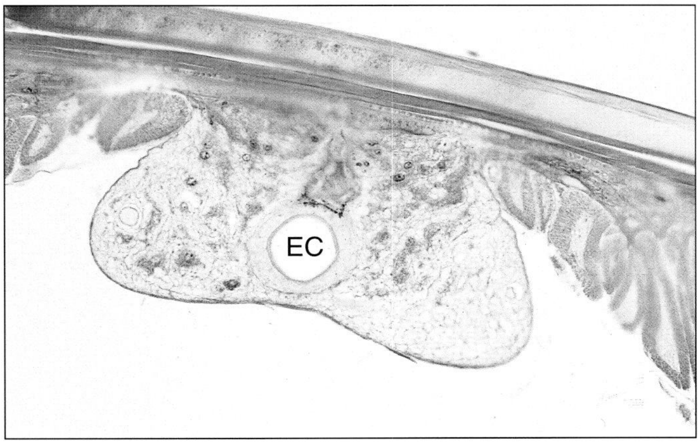

6

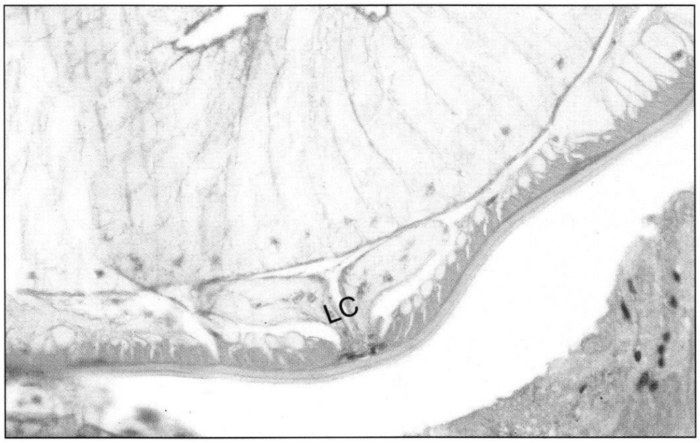

7

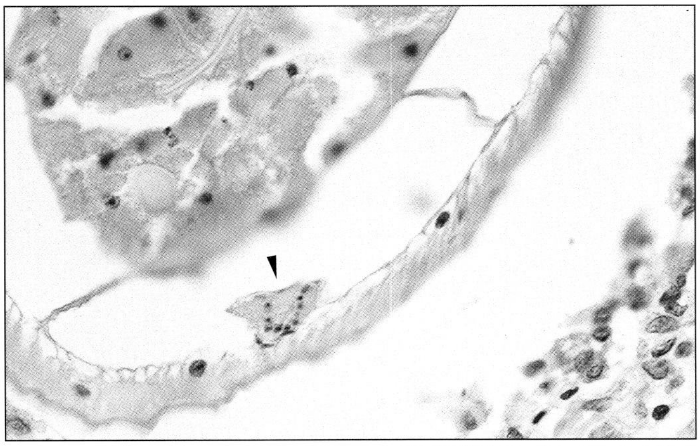

8

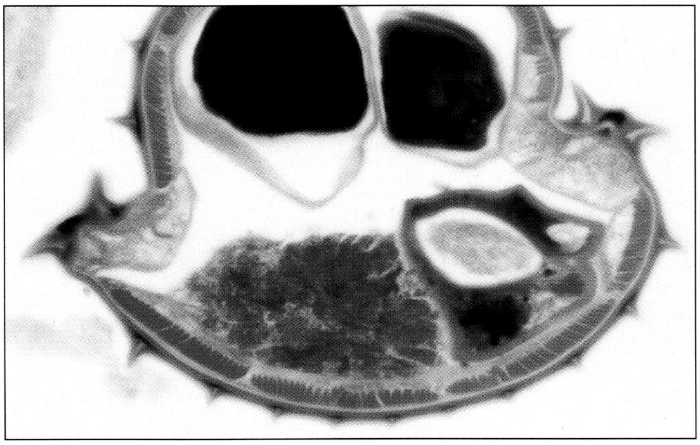

Plate 21b

Nematode Anatomy, Structural Variations

Image 9

Loa loa. Transverse section through the body wall shows a variation in the morphology of a coelomyarian muscle cell. Note the heavier contractile elements of the cell (Trichrome).

Image 10

Dirofilaria repens. Transverse section through the body wall shows a typical coelomyarian muscle cell. Note the cell nucleus in the protoplasmic portion of the cell. The thin, pink-staining hypodermis is especially clearly delineated in this section (HY) (Trichrome).

Image 11

Gongylonema species. Transverse section through the muscular region of the esophagus. Note the triradiate, cuticularized lumen (dart) (H&E).

Image 12

Gongylonema species. Transverse section through the glandular region of the esophagus. Note the triradiate lumen and concentration of glandular elements (H&E).

Image 13

Dirofilaria corynodes. Transverse section through intestine. Intestinal epithelium is composed of numerous cells, each with a single nucleus. Microvilli are visible as well (Trichrome).

Image 14

Eustrongylides ignotus. Transverse section through intestine shows the numerous tall, slender columnar epithelial cells. Note the uniform position of the nuclei near the base of the cell (H&E).

Image 15

Oesophagostomum species. Transverse section through the intestine shows its syncytial structure. The microvillus (MV) border is prominent (H&E).

Image 16

Gnathostoma species. Transverse section through the intestine demonstrates the varying heights of the individual intestinal epithelial cells and their multinucleated condition. The microvillus border is conspicuous (H&E).

9

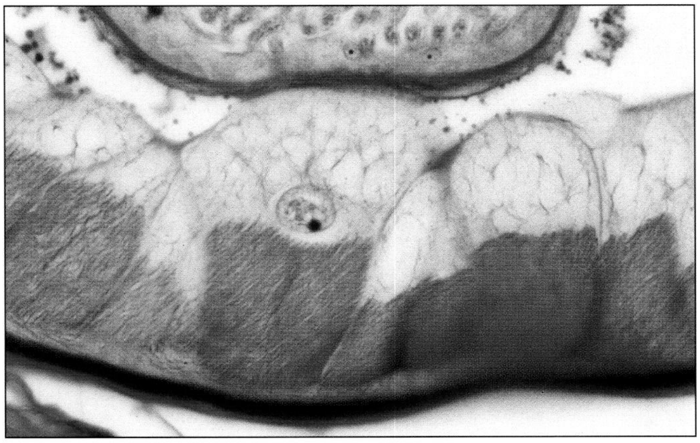

10

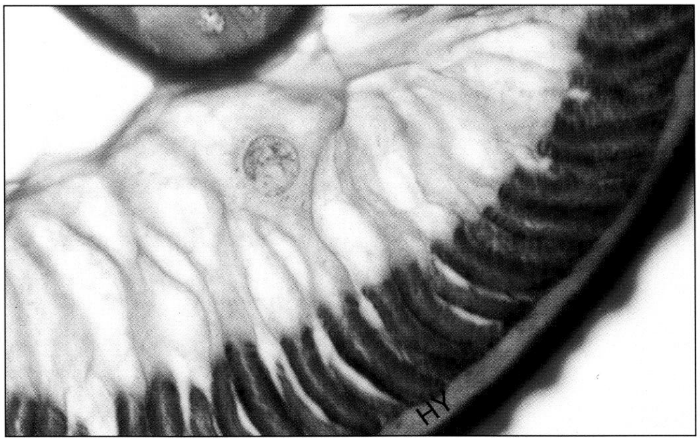

11

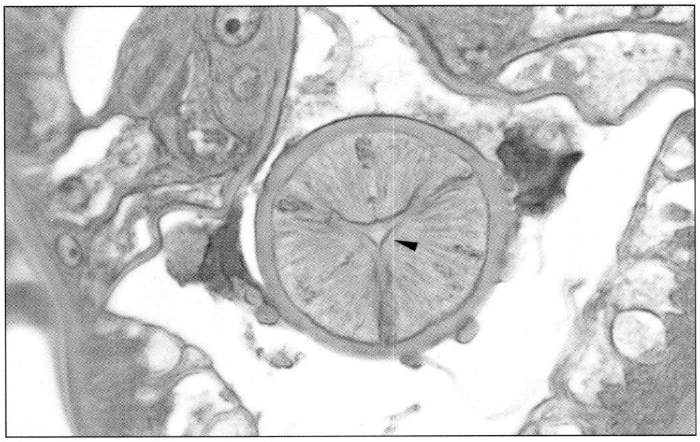

12

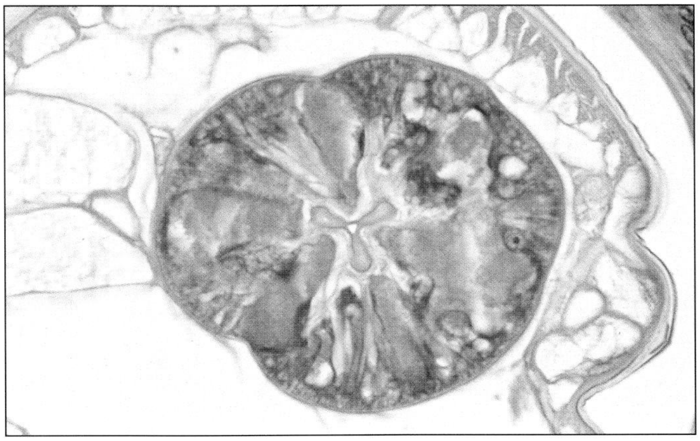

13

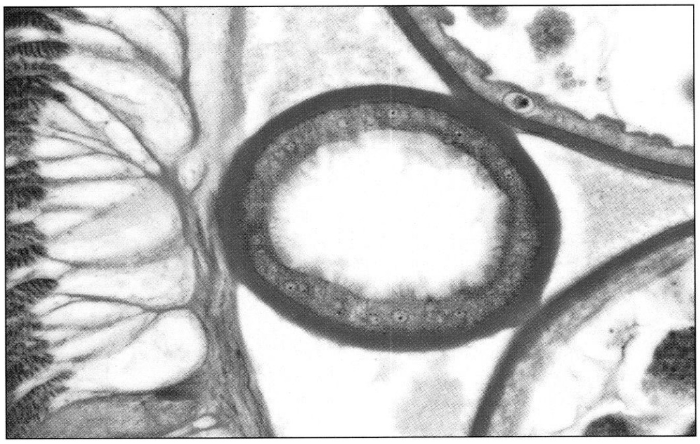

14

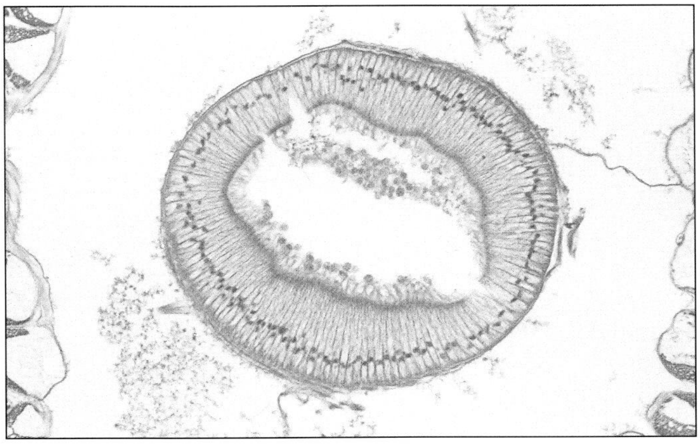

15

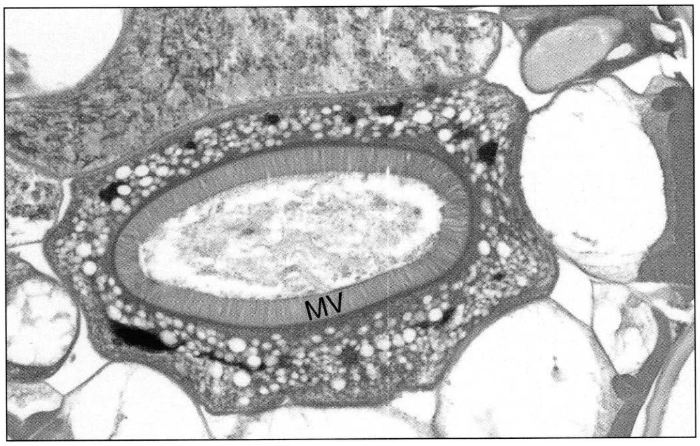

16

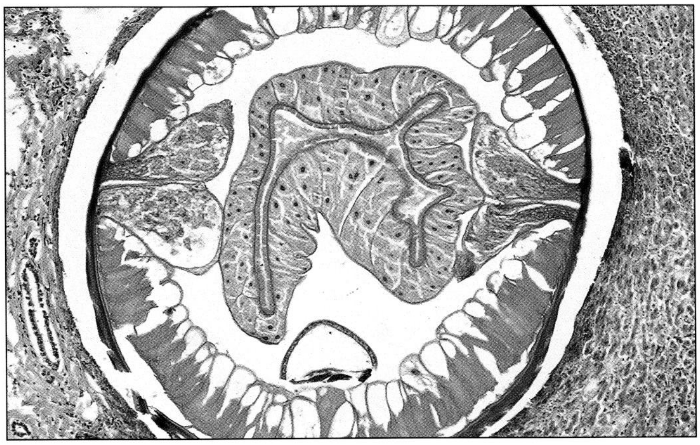

Secernentea Anatomy

Image 1

A. Transverse section through a female *Loa loa* illustrates the principal morphologic features of a secernentean nematode. Note particularly the cuticle (C), the lateral (LC) and dorsal/ventral (D/VC) (see also Plate 22:1B) hypodermal chords, and the well-developed muscle layer, which is divided into four bands by the chords. These coelomyarian muscles have well-defined cytoplasmic (CM) and contractile (fibrillar) (FM) parts. Within the pseudocoelom (PC), the intestine (IN) and the reproductive tubes, eg, uterine branches (UT), seminal receptacles (SR), as well as other parts not present in this section, may be seen (Trichrome).

B. Transverse section through a male *Loa loa* illustrates the male reproductive tube—in this case, the seminal vesicle (SV). MU = muscle, HY = thin hypodermis (Trichrome).

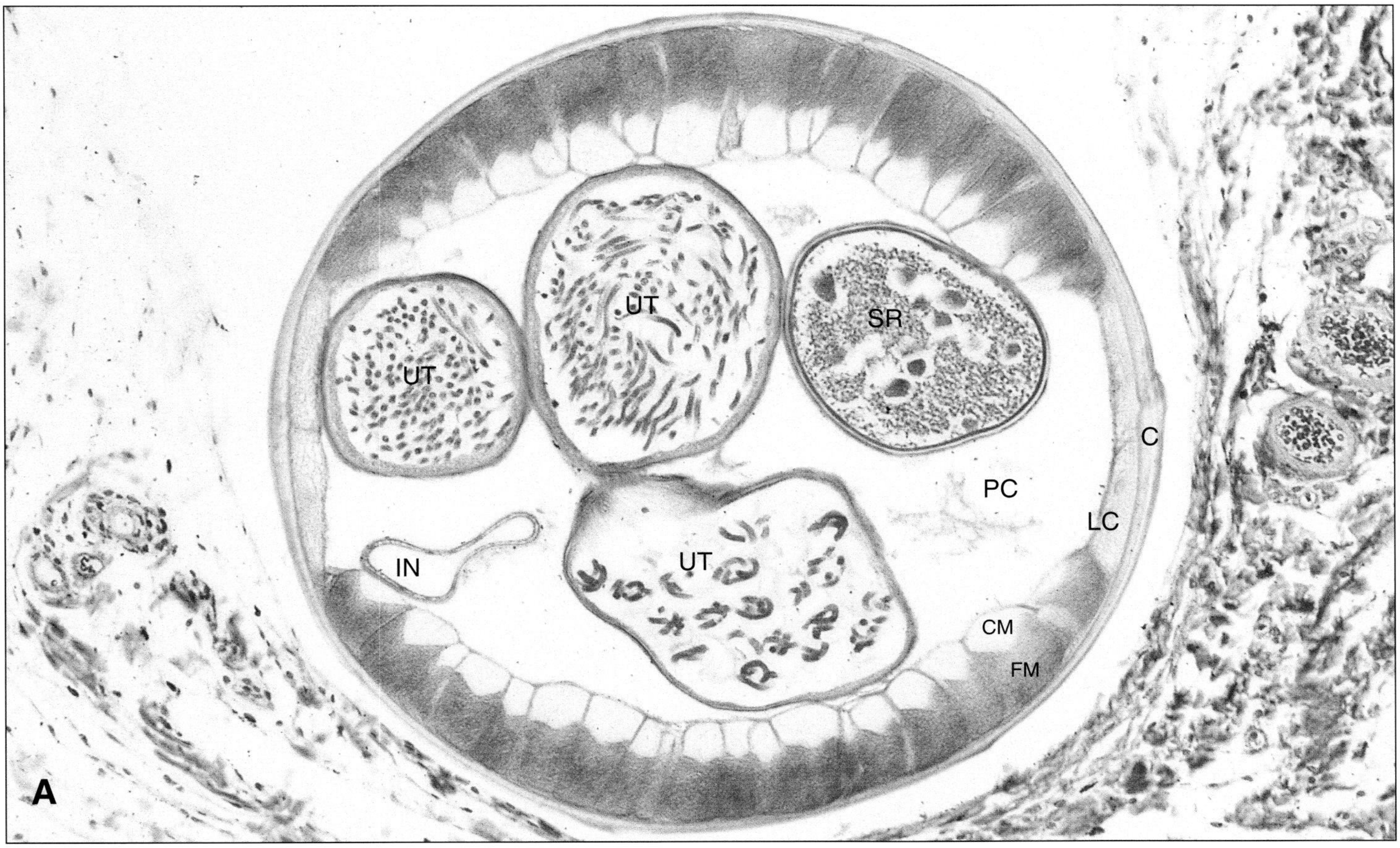
A
UT
UT
SR
C
PC
LC
IN
UT
CM
FM

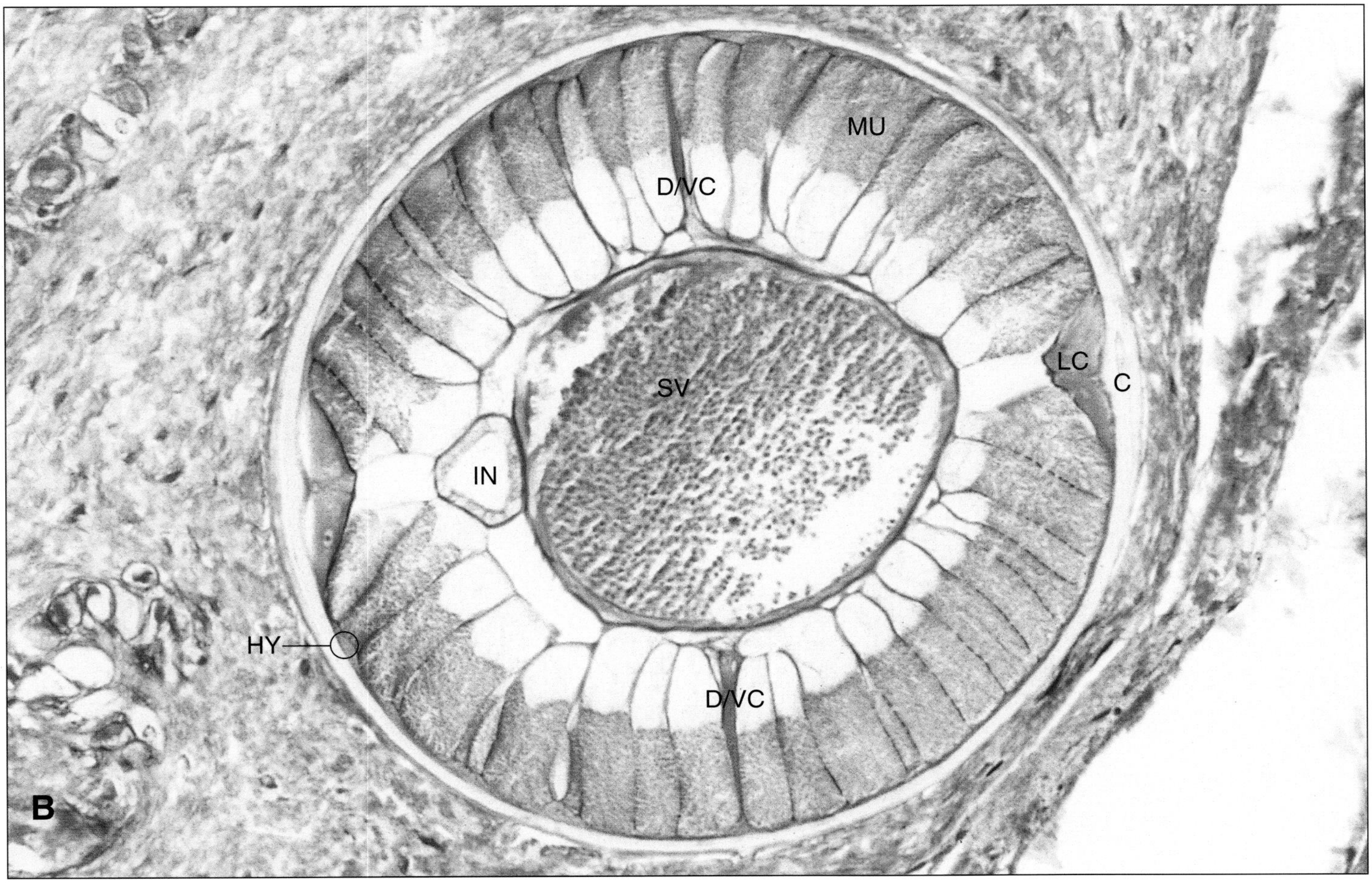
B
MU
D/VC
LC
C
SV
IN
HY
D/VC

Plate 23

Adenophorea Anatomy

Image 1

Morphologic features of adenophorean nematodes seen in transverse and longitudinal sections.

A. Transverse section through the anterior part of the body of *Trichuris trichiura*. The structure of the body wall is well delineated. Note the thick cuticle (C) and the underlying cellular hypodermis (arrows), which together form the bacillary band (BB); the well-developed coelomyarian muscles (MU); the large stichocyte (ST); and the small esophageal tube (dart) within the pseudocoelom (PC).

B. Section through *Anatrichosoma* species. A stichocyte (ST), with its large nucleus (NU) and small dotlike nucleolus, almost surrounds the small thin-walled esophageal tube (dart).

C. Section through *T. trichiura* shows a portion of the linear row of stichocytes (ST) that make up the stichosome.

D. Section through the body wall of *T. trichiura* at high magnification provides a better view of the coelomyarian muscles (MU). The cellular hypodermis (HY) and the thick cuticle (C) are also well defined.

E. Section through the postesophageal region of a male *Anatrichosoma* shows paired bacillary bands (arrows) separating well-developed muscles, a small tubular intestine (IN), and the two sections of reproductive tube.

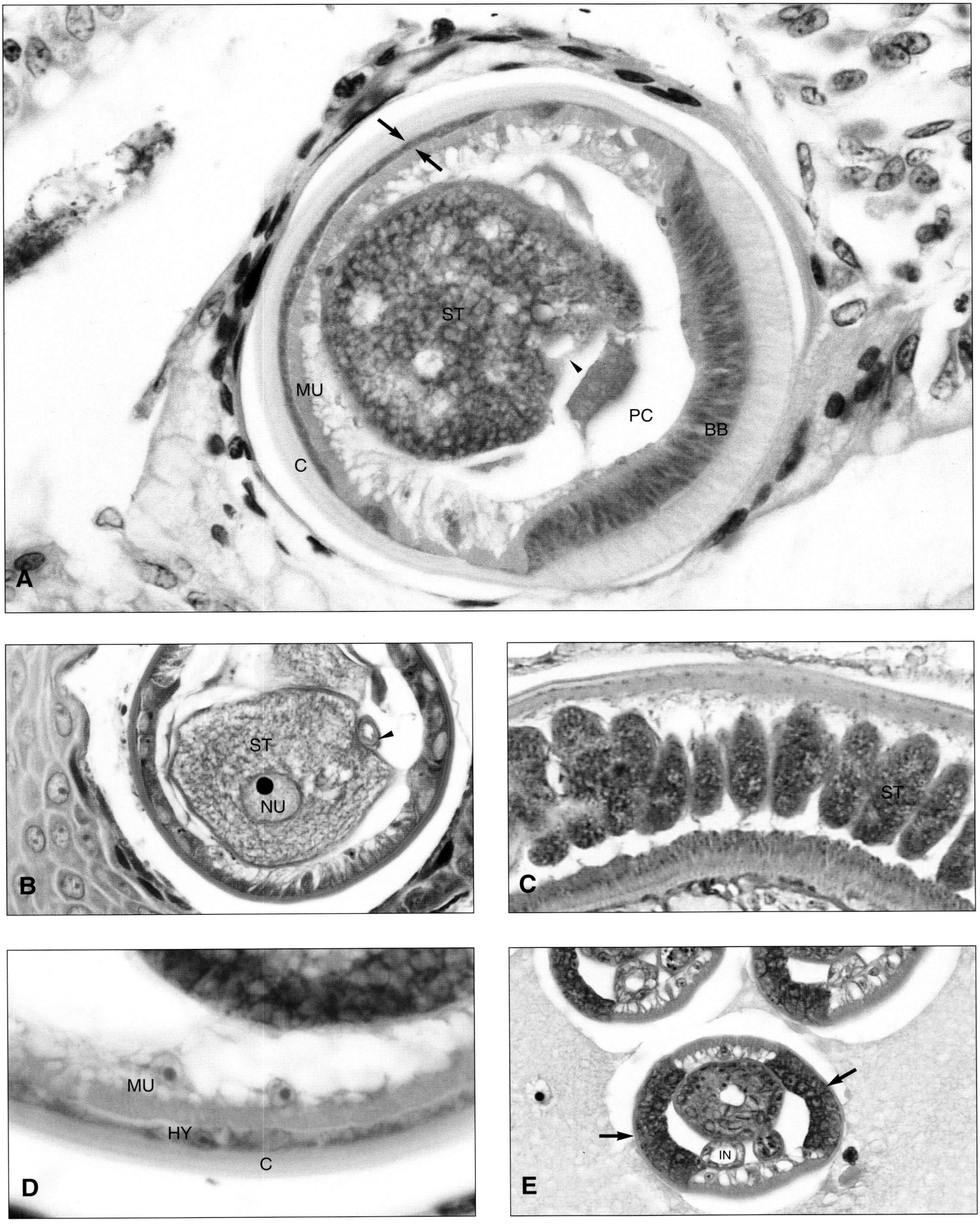

ST
MU
PC
BB
C
A
ST
NU
B
ST
C
MU
HY
C
D
IN
E

Ascaris lumbricoides

Ascaris lumbricoides, the giant intestinal roundworm, is regarded as the most common helminth parasite of humans. Approximately one billion people worldwide are infected with the parasite. Although *A. lumbricoides* is a lumen dweller, larval stages are found in tissues (liver and lung) as the parasite undergoes its development to the adult stage. Because adult worms have a penchant for entering orifices communicating with the gut lumen, they often block or partially obstruct structures such as biliary and pancreatic ducts, the appendix, etc. Although it is not difficult to identify adults encountered in tissues, recognizing dead, disintegrating worms in which normal body architecture has been lost is a greater challenge. Migratory larval stages must be differentiated from other species (some similar) that may occur in the same tissues.

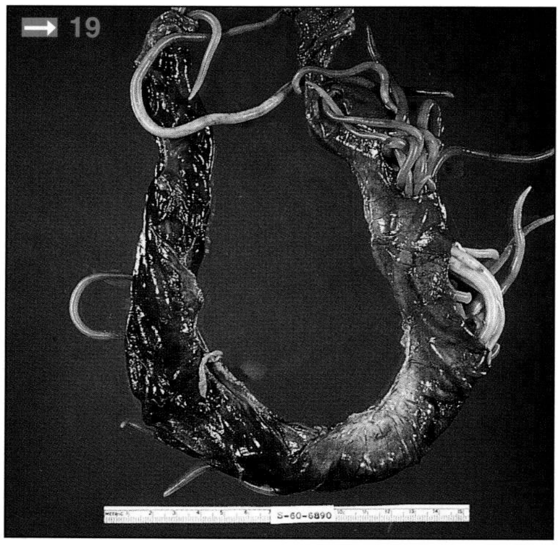

Biology and Life Cycle

Ascaris lumbricoides infects humans in temperate and tropical regions where sanitation is substandard. This nematode is a soil-transmitted species–that is, eggs liberated in feces develop in soil to the infective stage. When ingested by people, the fully embryonated eggs hatch in the gut, and the larvae enter the bloodstream or lymphatics, then migrate to the liver, the heart, and the pulmonary arteries. The larvae break out of the capillaries, enter the alveolar spaces, and migrate through the bronchi to the trachea and into the esophagus. Larvae molt to the third stage while in the lungs. Once in the esophagus, larvae are swallowed and ultimately settle in the intestine, most frequently in the jejunum, where they undergo two additional molts and mature to the adult stage. The adult worms live for about one year and they are spontaneously expelled from the body. In the patent period, each female produces many eggs (up to 200,000 per day), which are discharged from the body in feces. Eggs in the soil remain viable and infective for weeks, months, or even years if environmental conditions are suitable.

Pathology and Clinical Manifestations

Ascaris lumbricoides is well adapted to the human host and ordinarily causes few symptoms, usually only vague abdominal pain. When the worm burden is heavy, however, infected individuals may experience nausea, vomiting, abdominal discomfort, and anorexia. The presence of many worms creates the danger of intestinal obstruction (➡ 19); worms could also enter the biliary and pancreatic ducts and the appendix, with possibly serious consequences. Worms can penetrate into the liver parenchyma and produce abscesses. On rare occasions, young worms emerge from the nares and lacrimal ducts or are coughed up and discharged from the mouth. Even less commonly, worms may perforate the diseased intestinal wall and migrate into the abdominal cavity, causing peritonitis. Adult *Ascaris* worms are frequently found in ectopic sites in infected individuals at autopsy due to postmortem migration of the parasites, which can be confirmed by the absence of any histologic evidence of inflammatory changes in the tissues.

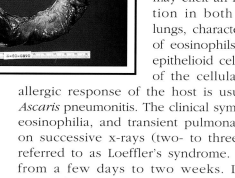

The passage of migrating larvae through the liver and the lungs may not cause any symptoms, particularly at the time of initial exposure to infection. However, subsequent migrations of larvae may elicit an intense cellular reaction in both the liver and the lungs, characterized by infiltration of eosinophils, macrophages, and epithelioid cells. The combination of the cellular response and an allergic response of the host is usually referred to as *Ascaris* pneumonitis. The clinical symptoms of bronchitis, eosinophilia, and transient pulmonary infiltrates visible on successive x-rays (two- to three-day intervals) are referred to as Loeffler's syndrome. Its duration ranges from a few days to two weeks. Larvae, along with eosinophils and Charcot-Leyden crystals, may be found in sputum or in gastric washings. *Ascaris* pneumonitis is seen more frequently in areas that have seasonal transmission rather than continuous transmission.

Parasite Morphology

Intact adult worms are easily identified regardless of their location in the host. They are large and robust, cylindrical in shape, and somewhat tapered at the extremities. The anterior end of the worm bears three fleshy lips, which are characteristic of the species. Females reach a length of 35 cm (sometimes longer) and have a maximum diameter of about 6 mm. Males are somewhat smaller, usually between 15 and 30 cm in length and up to 4 mm in diameter. The male tail typically is curved or hooked ventrad. In the female, the vulva is in the midventral line near the junction of the anterior and middle thirds of the body. In sections of host tissues, the adult *Ascaris* is recognized by its large size, even in an immature state (Plate 25:1). The body wall features a relatively thick, multilayered cuticle (Plate 24:4) and a fibrous-appearing hypodermis, which is thin in the submuscular areas but expands to form conspicuous lateral chords (Plate 24:3) and much less conspicuous dorsal and ventral chords. Large, lateral, excretory canals are seen embedded in the lateral chords (Plate 24:3). Many muscle cells are present in each quadrant of the body (Plate 24:1 & 2). They are tall, slender, and coelomyarian (Plate 24:4). The worms have a short, muscular esophagus and a simple intestinal tube with an irregular, often contorted lumen (Plate 24:1 & 2). The intestine is lined with tall, slender, columnar cells in which the nucleus is positioned near the base. The luminal margin of the cell has short microvilli (Plate 24:5). The female pseudocoelom is filled with the paired, extensively coiled genital tubes containing developing eggs (Plate 24:1). Within the paired uteri are maturing eggs, with their characteristic thick, mamillated outer coats (Plate 24:6). The male reproductive tube is also highly coiled (Plate 24:2).

Even dead adult worms in ectopic sites are easily recognized by their large size, multilayered cuticle (which may be swollen), and well-developed musculature and numerous reproductive tubes (Plate 25:2 & 3). Although the body wall of the worm may degenerate beyond recognition, eggs within the uterine tubes are often recognizable (Plate 25:3 & 4). Eggs in granulomatous lesions are recognized by their size, shape, shell, and contents (Plate 25:4–6).

Specific identification of the larval stages of *A. lumbricoides* in sections of tissue depends on relatively few morphologic features. In his classic studies on visceral larva migrans, Nichols (1956) states that "[a] single good transverse section of midbody levels (of a larva) may furnish sufficient material for specific recognition." Nichols showed that diagnostic features of several species of nematode larvae are based on the relative size of the larva, the type of intestine, the presence or absence and type of lateral alae, and the presence or absence and size of the excretory columns. The advanced second-stage larva of *A. lumbricoides*, which is about 300 µm in length, has a midbody diameter of 14 to 16 µm, prominent single lateral alae, an intestine that has a recognizable lumen and is composed of three cells, and small but well-defined excretory columns. The third-stage larva may grow to a length of 1.6 mm, with a diameter at the midbody level of 26 to 50 µm. This larva has larger excretory columns, with a cross-sectional area equal to or greater than the intestine, and as in the second stage, it possesses prominent alae and a patent gut, the lumen of which is lined with microvilli (Plate 26).

References

Beaver PC, Jung RC, Cupp EW. *Clinical Parasitology*. 9th ed. Philadelphia, Pa: Lea & Febiger; 1983.

Nichols RL. The etiology of visceral larva migrans, I: diagnostic morphology of infective second-stage *Toxocara* larvae. *J Parasitol.* 1956;42:349-362.

Nichols RL. The etiology of visceral larva migrans, II: comparative larval morphology of *Ascaris lumbricoides, Necator americanus, Strongyloides stercoralis* and *Ancylostoma caninum*. *J Parasitol.* 1956;42:363-399.

Ascaris lumbricoides

Image 1

Transverse section through the female worm shows typical structure of the body wall and body contents. Note the large intestinal tube. The remaining structures are part of the reproductive system (H&E, 9x).

Image 2

Transverse section through the male worm. Note the large, flattened intestine. Other tubes are part of the reproductive system (H&E, 9x).

Image 3

At high magnification, note the lateral chord that projects into the pseudocoelom and appears to have a fibrous matrix. A lateral excretory canal (dart) is embedded in the chord (H&E, 200x).

Image 4

At this magnification, the structure of the typical coelomyarian muscle cell (dart) and the cytoplasmic portion that also projects into the pseudocoelom can be clearly visualized. Note also the thick, multilayered cuticle (keyline) (H&E, 200x).

Image 5

A high-power view of the intestinal wall shows the numerous columnar cells, each with the nucleus positioned near the base and the low microvilli at the opposite luminal border (H&E, 200x).

Image 6

Maturing eggs within the uterine tube. These eggs already have the outer mamillated coating (H&E, 200x).

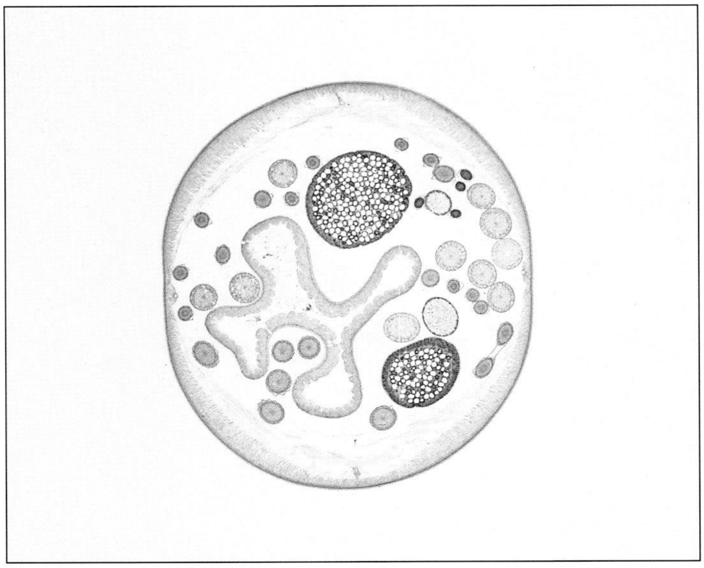
1

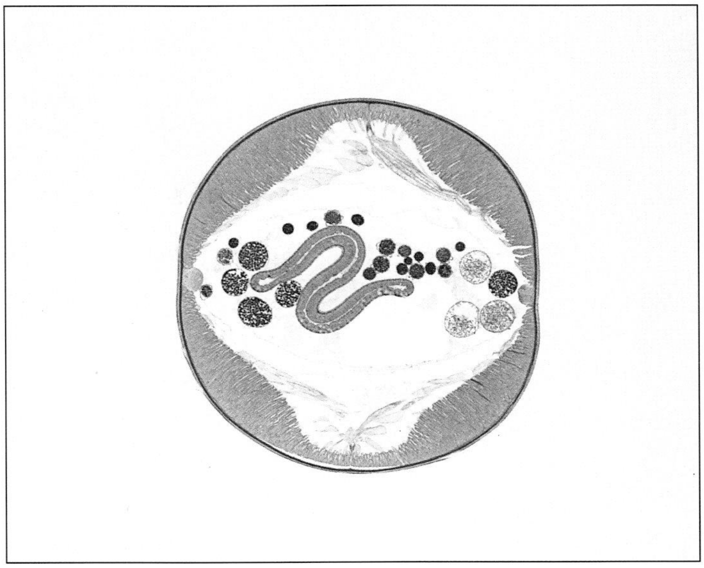
2

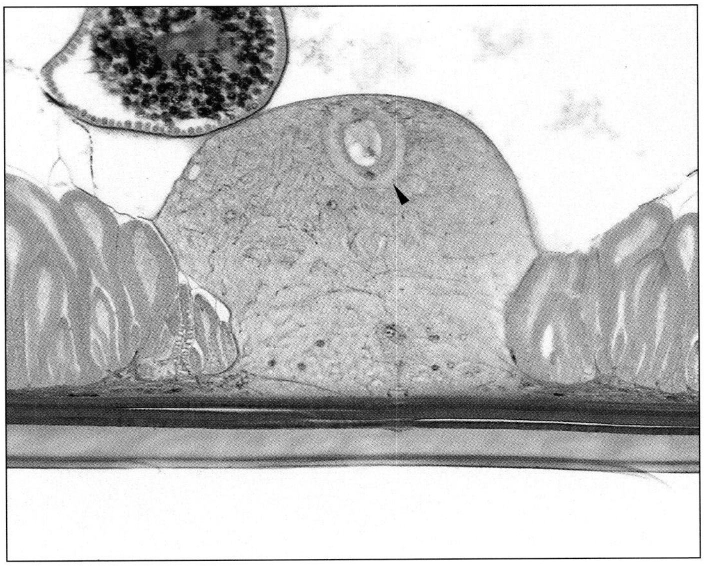
3

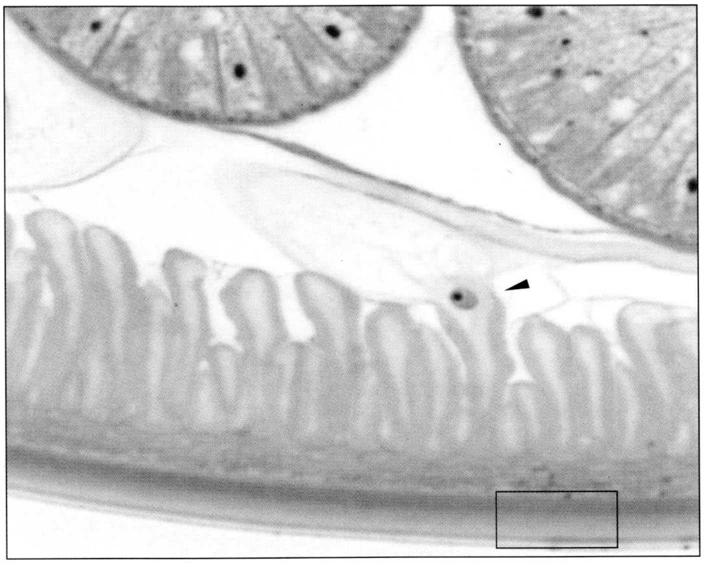
4

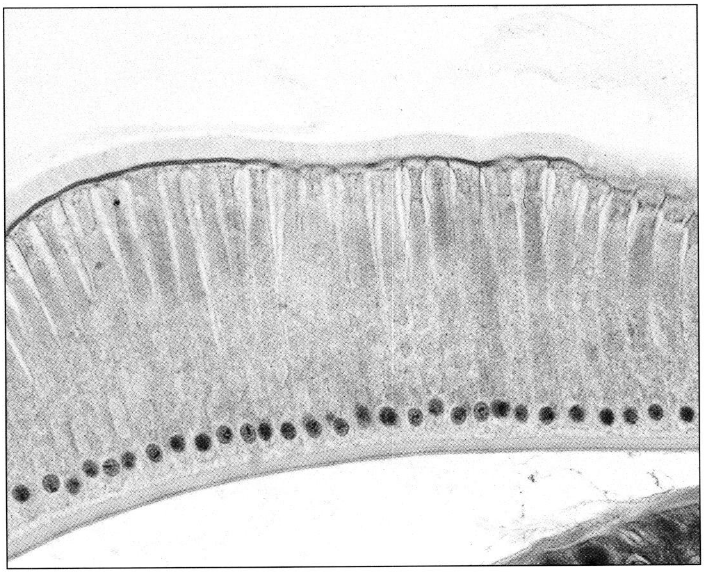
5

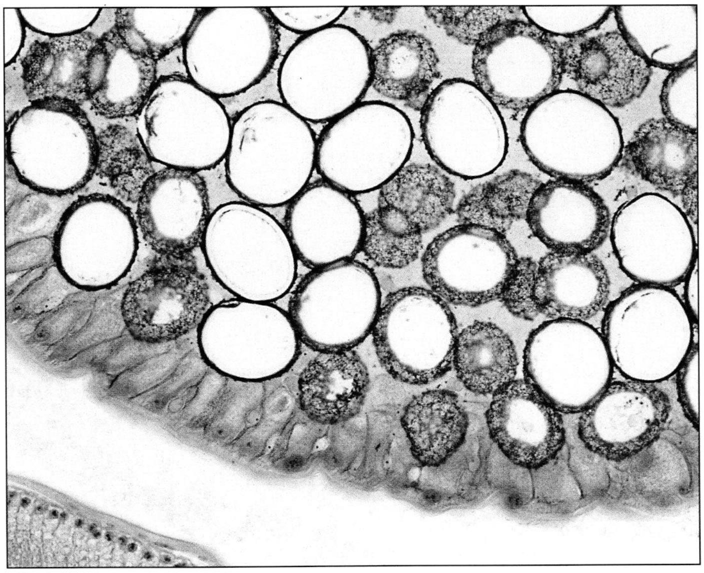
6

Plate 25

Ascaris lumbricoides

Image 1

Transverse section through the appendix shows two sections of an immature *Ascaris* in the lumen (H&E, 8x).

Image 2

Sections of a "stone" removed from the common bile duct of an individual. It is actually a dead, degenerated parasite, an immature *Ascaris* measuring about 1 mm in diameter. The cuticle is swollen and multilayered. The hypodermis is also thickened and degenerated (arrows). The normal architecture of the muscle layer is still recognizable (unknown stain, 40x).

Image 3

Elements of an *Ascaris* worm in an intrahepatic gallstone. Although the worm is hardly recognizable as such, numerous reproductive tubes can be seen, including a uterine branch (keyline) (H&E, 35x).

Image 4

High magnification of the area (keylined in Image 3) shows several eggs that are clearly those of *Ascaris lumbricoides* (H&E, 300x).

Image 5

At low magnification, this granulomatous mass removed from a patient's abdomen contains numerous egglike objects (darts) (H&E, 35x).

Image 6

At high magnification, it is evident from their size and structure that these are eggs of *Ascaris* and contain a single-cell ovum (darts) (H&E, 300x).

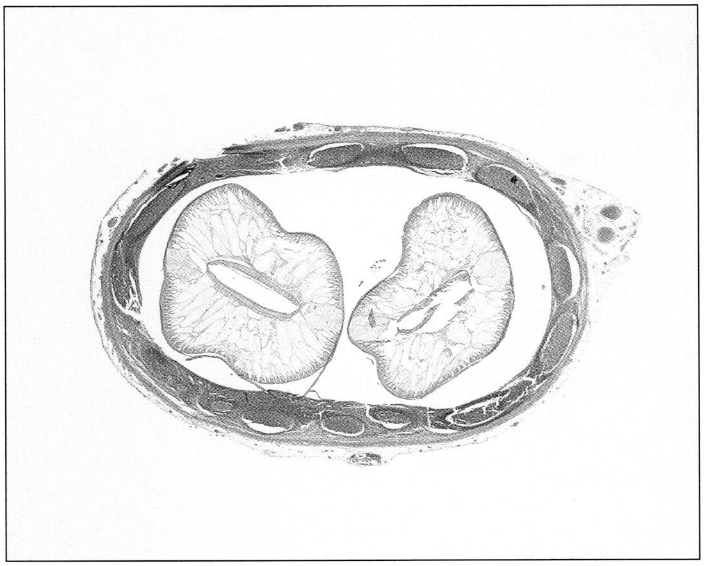

1

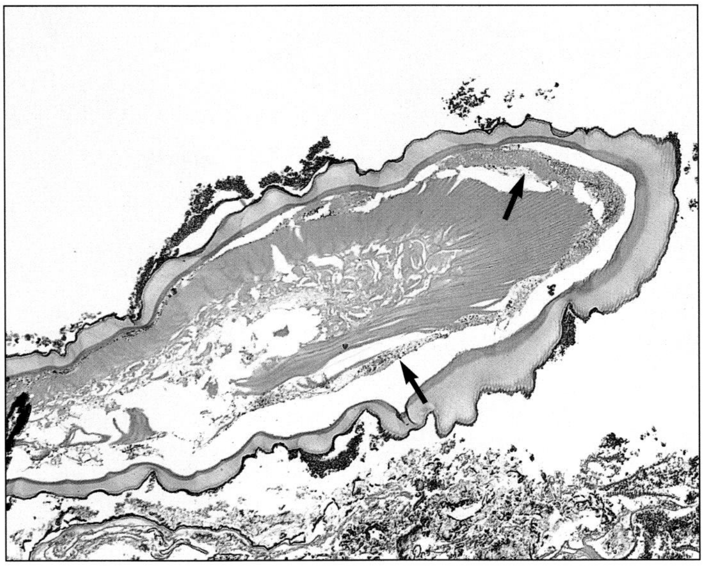

2

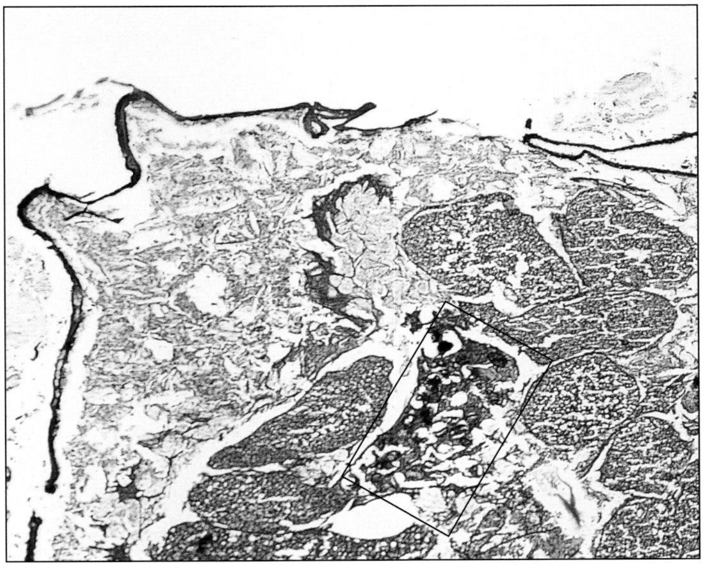

3

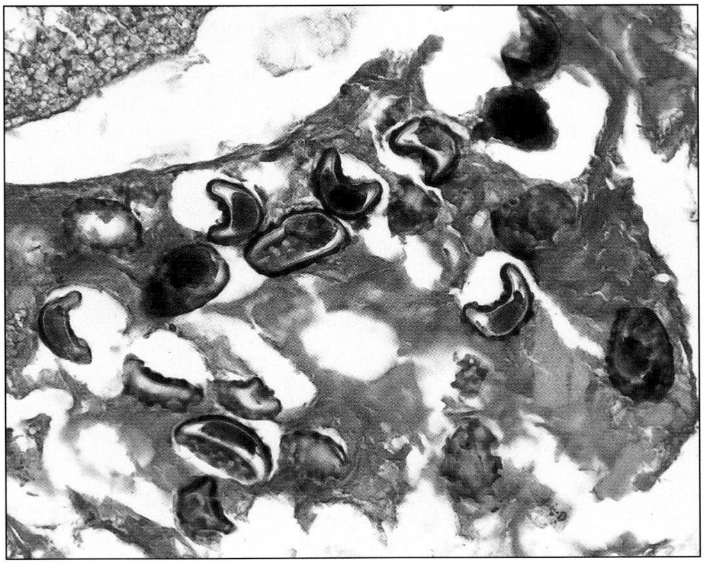

4

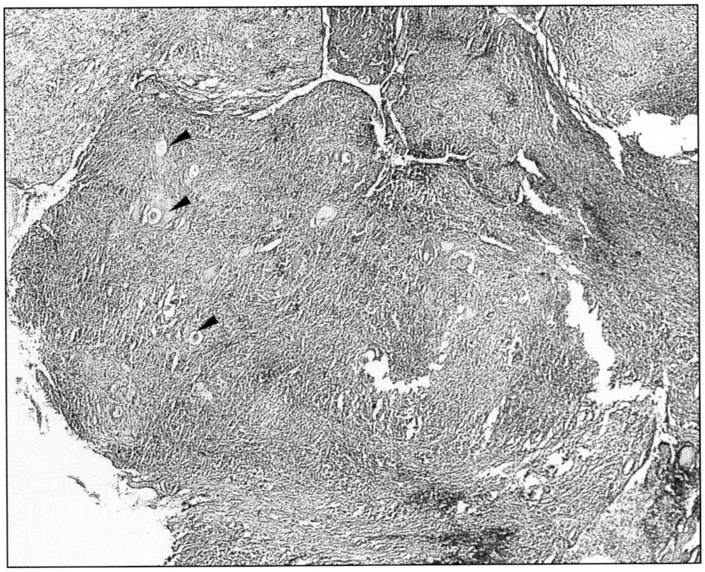

5

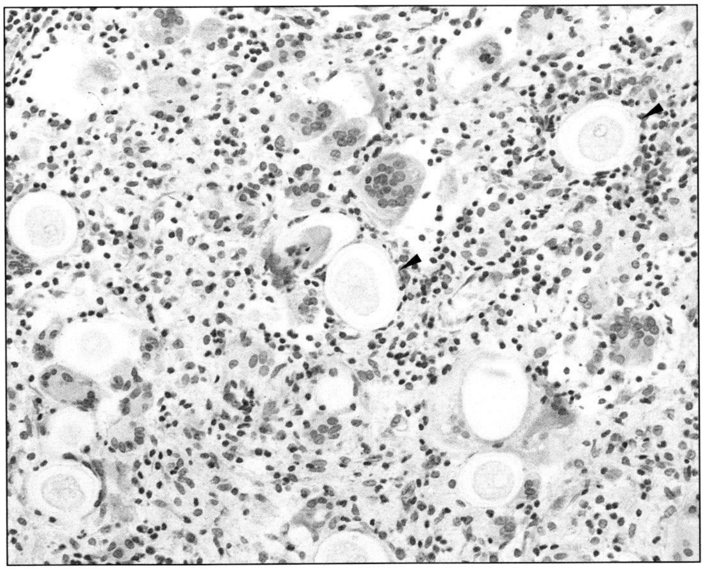

6

Plate 26

Ascaris lumbricoides

Image 1

Transverse section through one or more third-stage larvae in the bronchus of an experimentally infected mouse shows typical morphology of the larva. Note the prominent lateral alae (darts), the large excretory canals (EC), and the patent gut (H&E, 500x).

Image 2

At a more posterior level, alae (darts) are not as conspicuous but details of the body wall are evident. It is difficult to separate cuticle, hypodermis, and muscle cell boundaries. In lateral fields, hypodermal chords and their nuclei are distinct, and excretory canals are discernible (arrow). Muscle cells are few, and their nuclei lie in the cytoplasmic portion of the cell (H&E, 900x).

Images 3 and 4

Third-stage larvae in lung alveoli of a boy who died 48 hours after the onset of pneumonia. Larvae cut at different levels all have features characteristics of *A. lumbricoides* (H&E; 600x, 900x).

Image 5

Third-stage larvae (darts) in exudate of the lumen of a bronchus (H&E, 250x).

Image 6

Third-stage larvae found in alveolus of an individual at autopsy. Morphologic features are clearly those of *A. lumbricoides* (H&E, 500x).

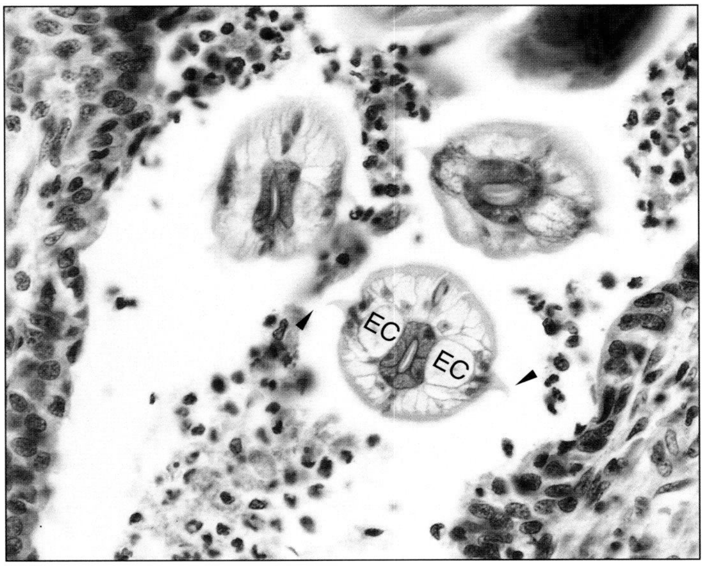

1

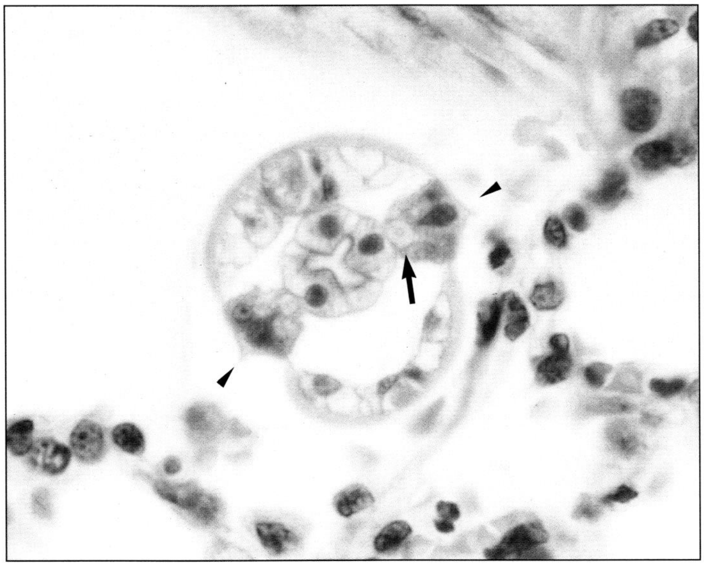

2

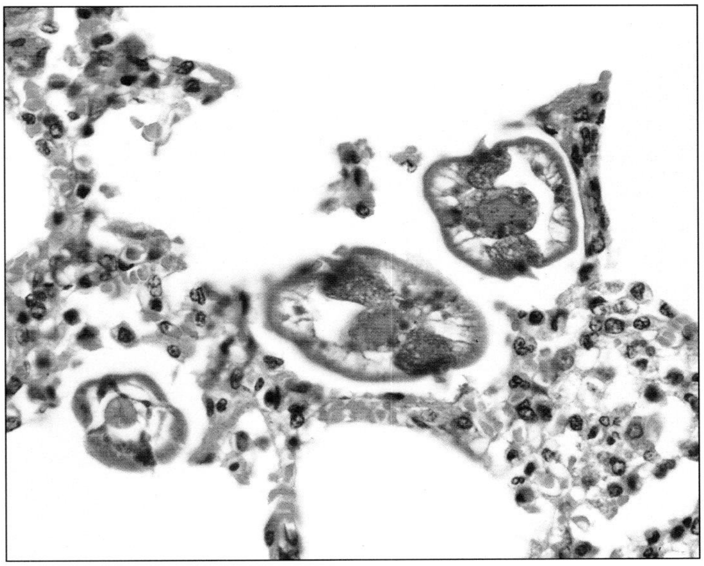

3

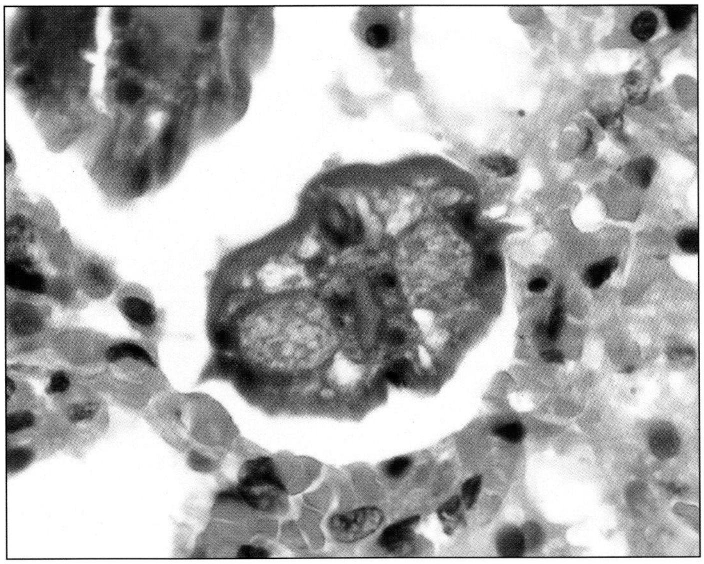

4

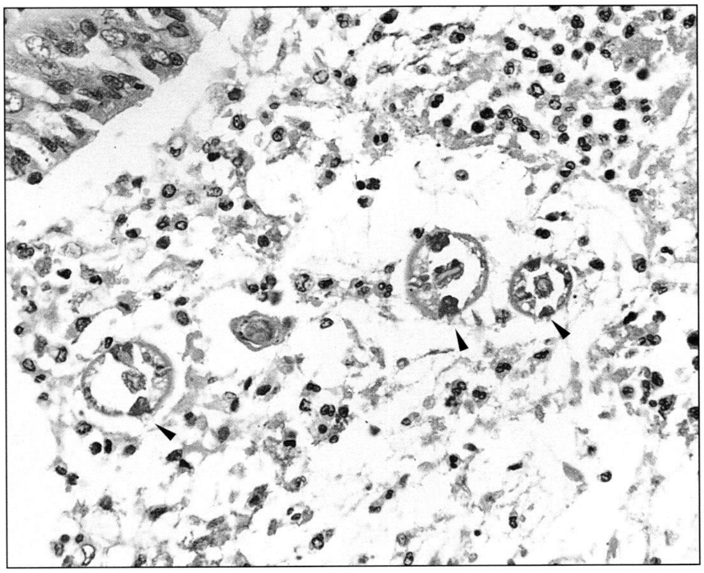

5

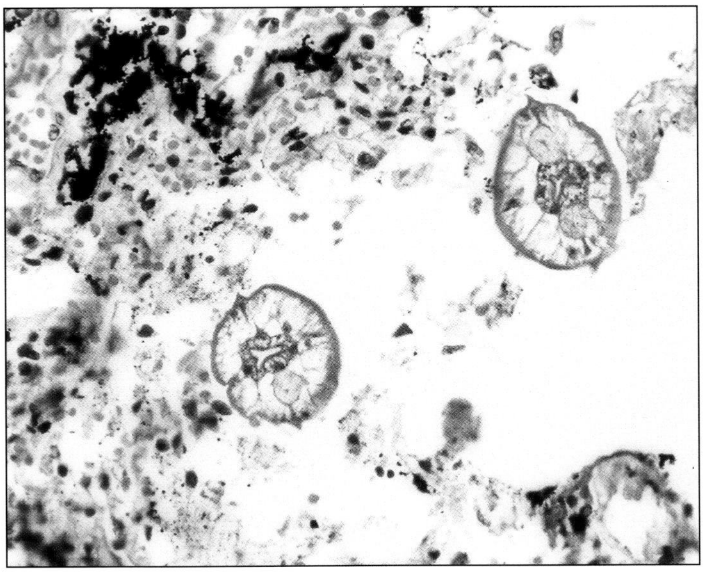

6

Toxocara and *Baylisascaris* species

Visceral Larva Migrans

Larval stages of the ascarid parasites of dogs, *Toxocara canis*, and cats, *Toxocara cati*, occasionally infect humans, especially children, in whom they undergo aberrant migrations in the tissues, producing a syndrome called visceral larva migrans (VLM). Both the parasites and the disease they produce are widely reported throughout the world. *Baylisascaris*, another ascarid found in raccoons in the United States and elsewhere, has been identified as the agent of at least two fatal human infections of the VLM type. (Other helminths involved in visceral larva migrans will be discussed elsewhere.)

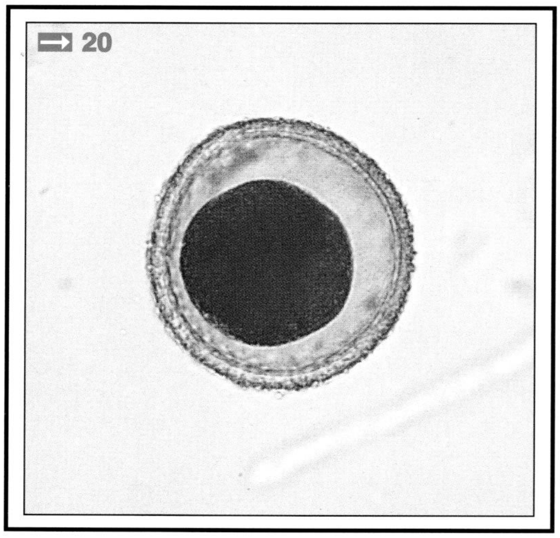

Biology and Life Cycle

Toxocara canis and *Toxocara cati* have a broader host range than just dogs and cats, but dogs and cats relate most closely to human disease problems. Human infections with adult *Toxocara* species, although reported in the literature on rare occasions, are questionable. In the natural hosts the adult worms inhabit the small intestine. The female worm produces a characteristic egg (⇨ 20), which is passed unembryonated in the feces. Eggs embryonate in the soil and reach infectivity in about three weeks. The second-stage larva within the egg is the infective stage. Infections are transmitted to a new host when the infective egg is ingested. The egg hatches in the gut, and the liberated larva undergoes a typical ascarid migratory pattern, moving through the liver and lungs. Thereafter, the parasites may show significant variation in their migratory behavior. In both the natural and accidental (paratenic) hosts, multiple routes of infection are well described.

Humans typically become infected by swallowing infective eggs from the soil or possibly via a paratenic host. Larvae hatched from the egg migrate to the liver, where most will remain, but others make their way to the lungs and even to the eye and central nervous system. They eventually become encapsulated in host tissues; however, before that and for periods of up to several weeks, they actively migrate through the tissues without further development, leaving trails of inflammatory reaction as testament to their presence. The *Toxocara* species most frequently involved in this aberrant migration in humans seems to be *T. canis*, although *T. cati* has been identified as well.

Baylisascaris procyonis, a common intestinal parasite of raccoons, has demonstrated its potential for extensive larval migration in rodent intermediate hosts and even in birds. In intermediate and accidental (aberrant) hosts, the parasite produces a usually fatal eosinophilic meningoencephalitis. It has also been identified as the cause of two fatal human cases, which involved severe visceral and central nervous system disease. Infection is produced by the ingestion of infective eggs from the soil or other sources contaminated by raccoon feces.

Pathology and Clinical Manifestations

Visceral larva migrans caused by *Toxocara* species is seen typically in young children in virtually all parts of the world and probably most commonly in the United States. Clinically, individuals may be asymptomatic; they may present with the typical syndrome of chronic hypereosinophilia, hepatomegaly, fever, cough, hyperglobulinemia, and moderate pulmonary infiltrates; or they may experience varying degrees of these symptoms. The liver contains the greatest concentration of larvae and is the organ primarily affected (Plate 27:1). However, almost any organ may be affected: lesions are found in the lungs (Plate 27:5), brain (Plate 28:3), eye (Plate 28:1 & 2), and heart (Plate 28:4) with significant frequency. The lesion seen early on in most organs is basically a granulomatous inflammatory process with an infiltrate of eosinophils, histiocytes, and lymphocytes surrounding a larva. The mature granuloma ultimately displays a necrotic center with an additional infiltrate of foreign body giant cells, epithelioid cells, and mononuclear and polymorphonuclear cells. The larva may be present, or it may not be seen unless serial sections through the granuloma are examined. Specific diagnosis depends on demonstration of the parasite in the tissues either by biopsy or at autopsy.

There is a dearth of critical information relating to the clinical presentations for baylisascariasis. Two human infections, both in young children and both fatal, have been reported. Both patients presented with an eosinophilic meningoencephalitis. In one child who had acute disease of eight days' duration, autopsy revealed congestion of the meninges and swelling and necrosis of the brain. Larvae in brain tissue were not encapsulated, although encapsulated larvae were found in small granulomas in other tissues and organs. The other case was chronic in its duration, lasting 14 months, and larvae were found encapsulated in the brain as well as in other tissues. In addition, in some cases *Baylisascaris* species has been suggested to be the agent of diffuse unilateral subacute neuritis (DUSN) and ocular larva migrans (OLM). Larval nematodes compatible with the gross morphologic features of *Baylisascaris* larvae have been reported in human cases of DUSN and OLM. The parasite has also been shown to cause OLM in experimentally infected primates.

Parasite Morphology

Adult worms play no part in human toxocariasis. Adult *T. canis* and *T. cati* are similar in their gross appearance to *A. lumbricoides* but have cervical alae and are substantially smaller.

The infective (second-stage) larvae of *T. canis* and *T. cati* are morphologically identical, except for their diameters. The larvae measure about 400 µm in length. *Toxocara canis* has a diameter of 18 to 21 µm, whereas *T. cati* has a diameter of 15 to 17 µm in the living state. Larvae in stained tissues are proportionately smaller. Based on reconstruction of larvae in tissue, they measure between 290 and 350 µm in length. *Toxocara canis* larvae remain about 18 to 21 µm in diameter, and *T. cati* are 16 µm or less in diameter. In transverse section the body wall has a thin cuticle and conspicuous single lateral alae (Plate 27:3). The cuticle adheres to the underlying hypodermis, from which it cannot be visually separated. Dorsal, ventral, and lateral chords are not evident, although their nuclei may be seen. There are a few muscle cells of the coelomyarian type in each body quadrant. Their nuclei are large, project into the pseudocoelom, and are often seen in transverse sections of the body (Plate 27:3). The muscular esophagus, which has a triradiate lumen, occupies about one-third of the total body length. The excretory system is a single cell. The excretory cell body is greatly elongated and has two long lateral columns that extend posteriorly well beyond the middle of the body on either side of the intestine and a short distance anteriorly in the esophageal region, giving it an H shape. Each excretory column has a small central canal, although it may not be well defined (Plate 27:3). The intestine is made up of seven linearly arranged cells and has no lumen. It is usually compressed laterally and forced dorsally by the excretory columns.

The diagnostic features of *Toxocara* larvae include a diameter of 17 to 21 µm, prominent single lateral alae, nonpatent intestine, and large, well-defined excretory columns that together occupy a greater portion of the body cavity than the intestine. Using these morphologic features, it is possible to identify *Toxocara* from a single transverse section through the body at the intestinal level.

Larvae of *Baylisascaris*, unlike those of *Toxocara*, undergo growth in the human host. Larvae of *B. procyonis* obtained from experimentally infected mice and in human tissues are much larger than *Toxocara*. The 14-day-old larva measures about 1.4 mm by 62 µm. The larva has characteristic morphologic features when viewed in transverse sections (Plate 28:5 & 6). The body wall has a thin cuticle with prominent single lateral alae, an underlying thin hypodermis, and well-developed muscles, although it is difficult to discern the natural boundaries between the three layers. The hypodermis is expanded laterally to form large lateral chords. Their boundaries are not sharp, but their nuclei can be seen near the base of the chords (Plate 28:5). Dorsal and ventral chords are usually not well defined. There are typically four to eight coelomyarian muscle cells in each quadrant of the body. The single-cell excretory system has paired columns, often irregular in shape, and each has a central canal, which is not always evident (Plate 28:5 & 6). The esophagus is cylindrical and muscular, with a triradiate lumen (Plate 28:5). The intestine is typically round to oval, with six to nine cells evident in each section (Plate 28:5 & 6). The intestinal lumen is lined by microvilli (Plate 28:6). Conspicuous basophilic inclusions are within the cytoplasm of the intestinal cells (Plate 28:6).

Larvae of *Baylisascaris* species, including *B. procyonis*, are quickly differentiated from larvae of *Toxocara* species by their much larger size, patent gut, and predilection for the central nervous system. *Baylisascaris* larvae have features like those of *Ascaris* but again, they are larger and have different tissue preferences.

References

Bowman DD. Diagnostic morphology of four larval ascaridoid nematodes that may cause visceral larva migrans: *Toxascaris leonina*, *Baylisascaris procyonis*, *Lagochilascaris sprenti* and *Hexametra leidyi*. *J Parasitol*. 1987;73:1198-1215.

Fox AS, Kazacos KR, Gould NS, et al. Fatal eosinophilic meningoencephalitis and visceral larva migrans caused by the raccoon ascarid *Baylisascaris procyonis*. *N Engl J Med*. 1985;312:1619-1623.

Glickman LT, Magnaval JF. Zoonotic roundworm infections. *Infect Dis Clinics N Amer*. 1993;7:717-732.

Nichols RL. The etiology of visceral larva migrans, I: diagnostic morphology of infective second-stage *Toxocara* larvae. *J Parasitol*. 1956;42:349-362.

Nichols RL. The etiology of visceral larva migrans, II: comparative larval morphology of *Ascaris lumbricoides*, *Necator americanus*, *Strongyloides stercoralis* and *Ancylostoma caninum*. *J Parasitol*. 1956;42:363-399.

Kazacos KR, Raymond LA, Kazacos EA, et al. The raccoon ascarid: a probable cause of human ocular larva migrans. *Ophthalmology*. 1985;92:1735-1743.

Plate 27

Visceral Larva Migrans

Image 1

Low-power view of granuloma produced by *Toxocara canis* in liver biopsy specimen from a child (H&E, 100x).

Image 2

Sections of the *T. canis* larva at high magnification. In the smaller transverse section, the single ala (arrow) and the intestinal cell (dart) are seen. In the other (tangential) section, the large excretory columns (EC) are most apparent (H&E, 1500x).

Image 3

High magnification of a typical *T. canis* larva from a liver biopsy specimen of a child from Indiana. The lateral alae (darts) and paired, large excretory columns (EC) are seen. The thin cuticle and well-developed musculature are evident. Specific identification can be made from morphologic features evident in this transverse section (H&E, 1500x).

Image 4

Transverse section of *T. cati* larva from the liver of an experimentally infected mouse. The larva of *T. cati* is smaller in diameter than *T. canis* but otherwise has identical morphologic features (H&E, 1500x).

Images 5 and 6

Heavily encapsulated *Toxocara* larva discovered in the lung of a 4-year-old child at autopsy. Higher magnification than that shown is required to visualize characteristic morphologic features of the larva (H&E; 100x, 400x).

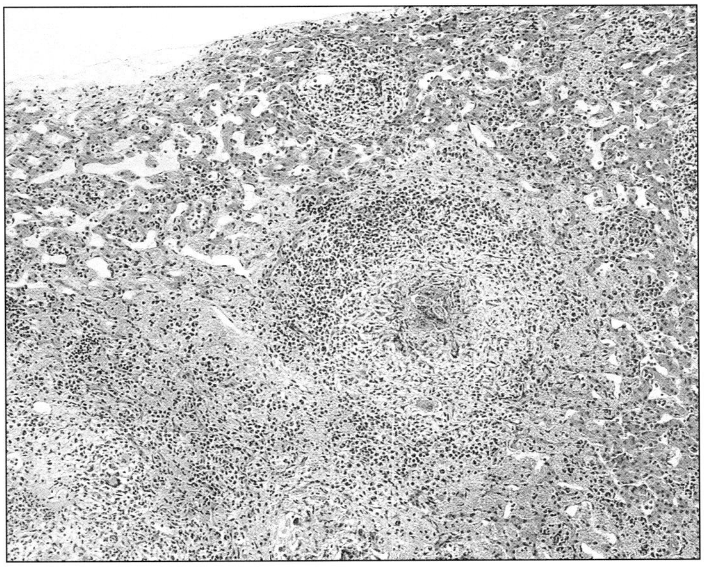

1

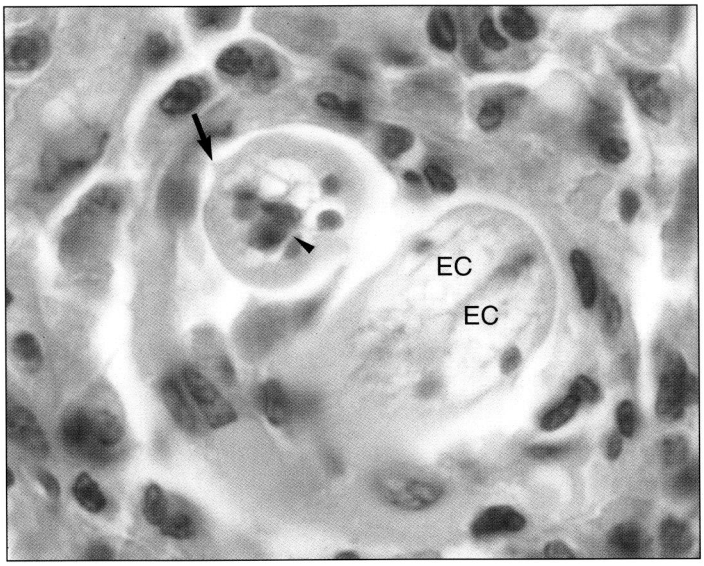

2

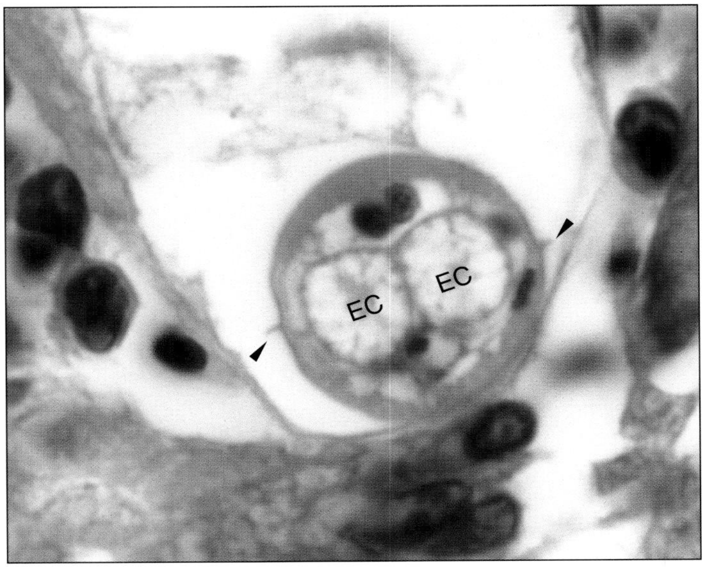

3

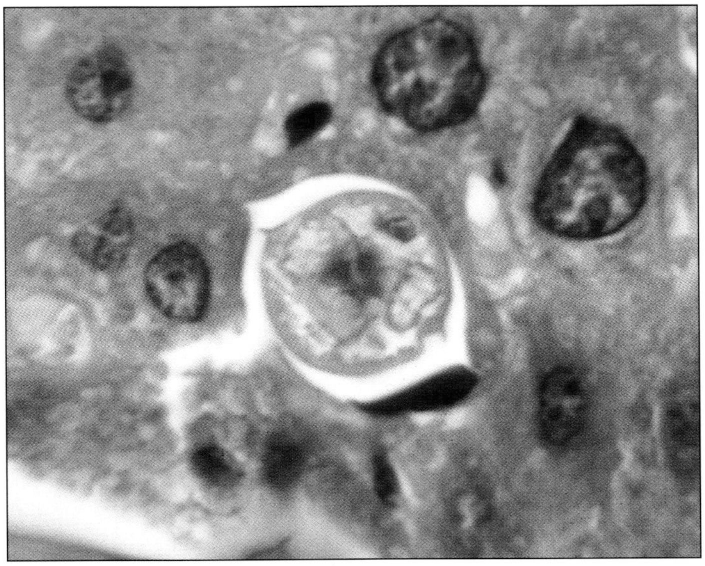

4

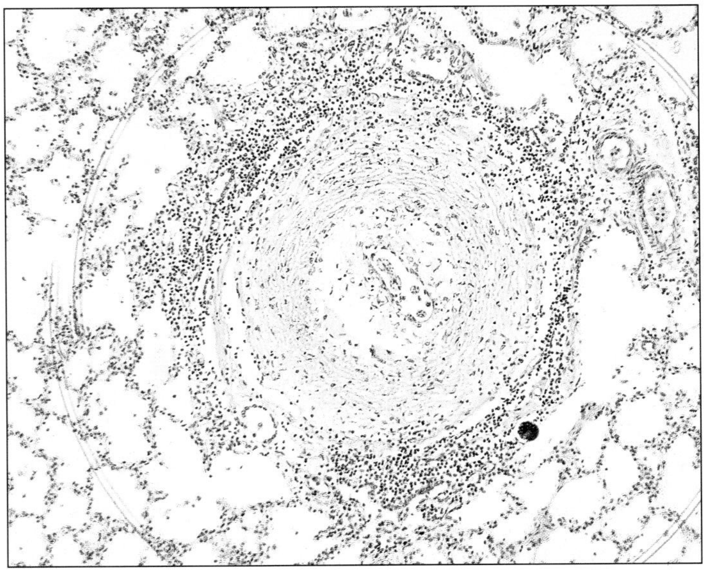

5

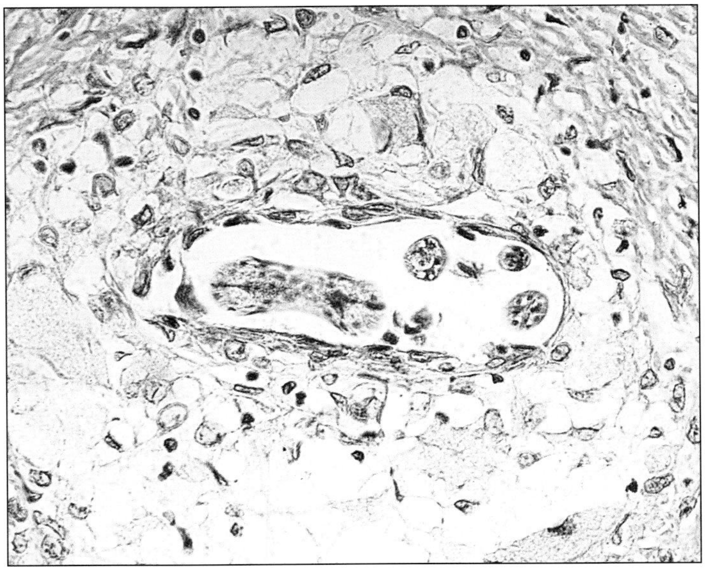

6

Visceral Larva Migrans

Images 1 and 2

Section through retina shows an inflammatory lesion in which portions of a larva (darts) identified as *T. canis* were identified at higher magnification (H&E; 40x, 500x).

Image 3

Transverse and longitudinal sections through a larva of *T. cati* in the brain of a 5-year-old Israeli child. The size of the larva, the slender, pointed lateral alae, and the body contents help identify the species of *Toxocara* (H&E, 1000x).

Image 4

Heavily encapsulated larva of *T. canis* discovered in the heart of a Colombian child at autopsy (H&E, 40x).

Image 5

Transverse sections of *Baylisascaris procyonis* in the brain of an experimentally infected mouse. One section is through the esophagus; the other is through the middle of the body and shows the intestine. At this magnification, the lateral alae (darts) and excretory columns (arrows) are conspicuous (H&E, 500x).

Image 6

Transverse section of *B. columnaris*, a parasite of the skunk (*Mephitis*), in the heart of an experimentally infected mouse. The intestine has a lumen, and the intestinal cells contain basophilic granules. The size of the larva and its patent gut along with conspicuous granules in intestinal cells help identify and differentiate it from larvae of *Ascaris* and *Toxocara*. Note the similarity of this species to *B. procyonis* in the previous image (H&E, 800x).

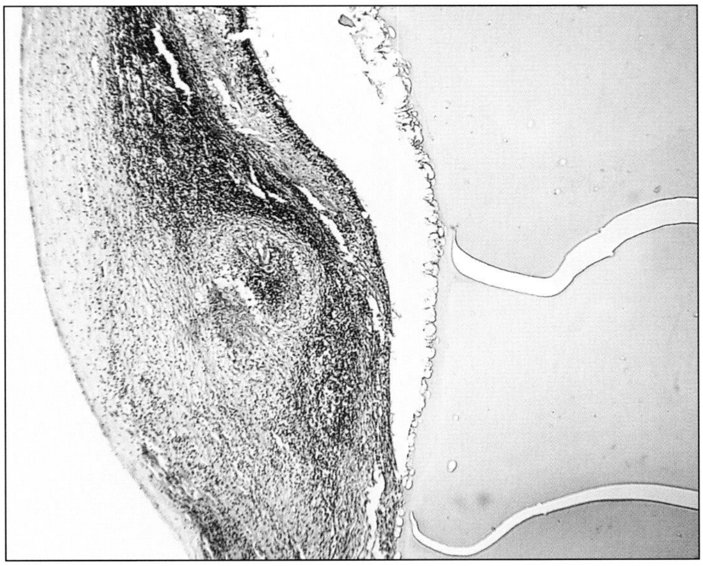

1

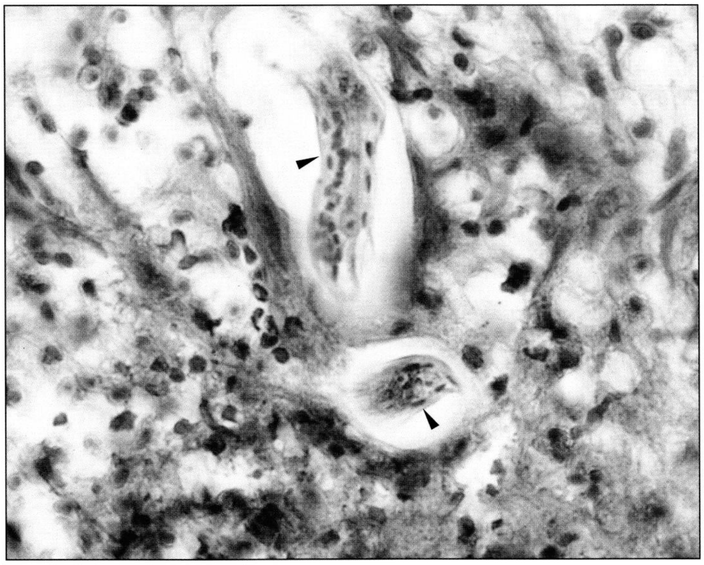

2

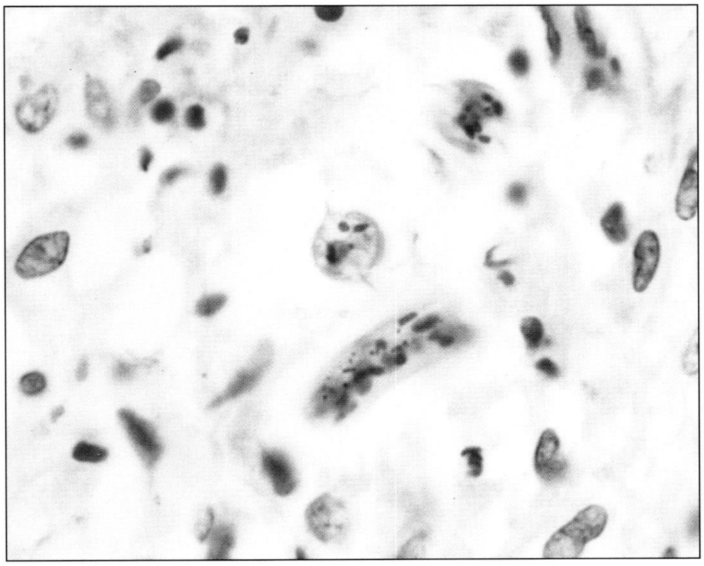

3

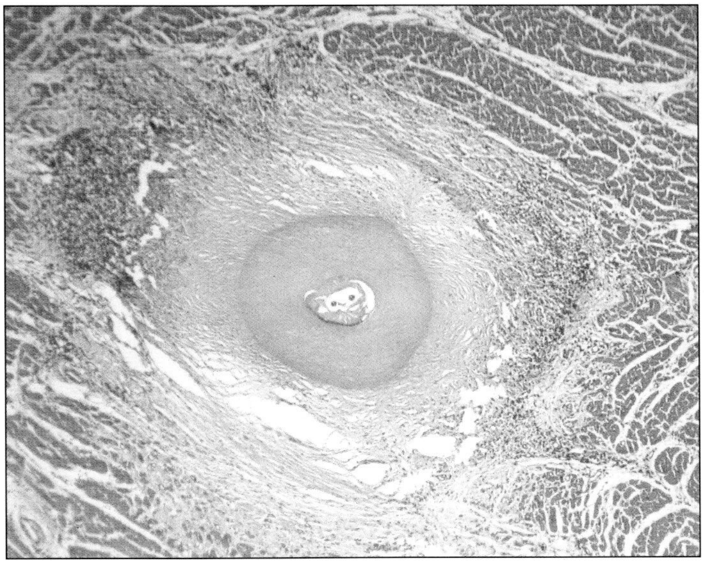

4

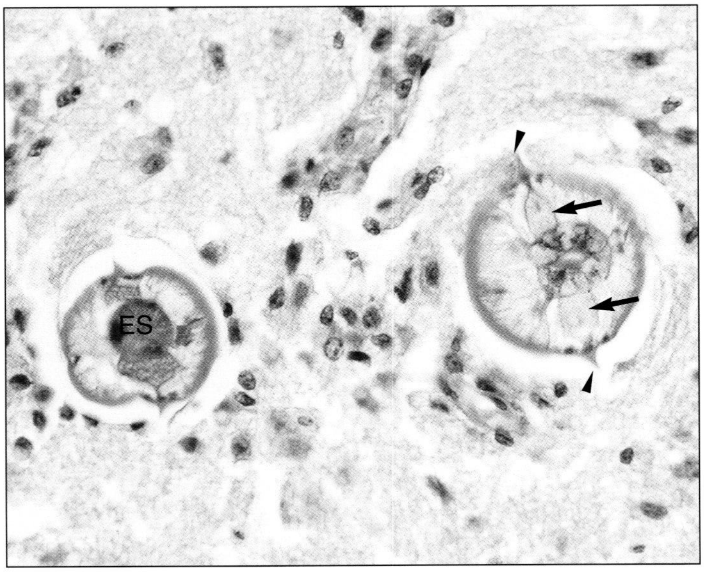

5

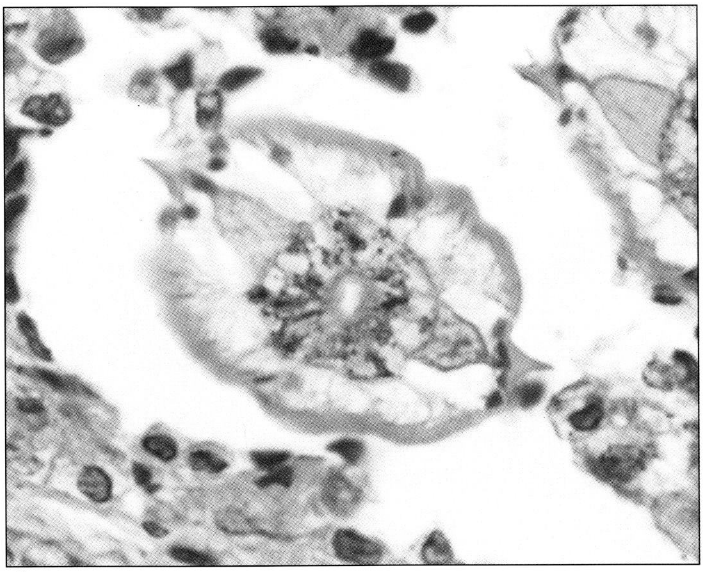

6

Lagochilascaris species

Lagochilascaris species are ascaridoid nematode parasites that are infrequently found in animals and humans. Only five species have been described: two from opossums in the Western Hemisphere, one from the lion in Africa, one from the American cougar, and one, *L. minor*, from humans in tropical America. The natural host for *L. minor* is assumed to be an as yet undetermined animal living in the region. Human infections typically present as deep, subcutaneous abscesses in the neck and pharynx (➡ 21). Larvae, adults, and eggs are discharged in pus from the lesions. Infections left untreated may persist for years. All human infections have been attributed to *L. minor* and all are from tropical America, with the majority of the 63 cases from Brazil. Others have been reported from Surinam (six), Trinidad (five), Tobago (one), Costa Rica (one), Venezuela (one), Mexico (one), and Colombia (two).

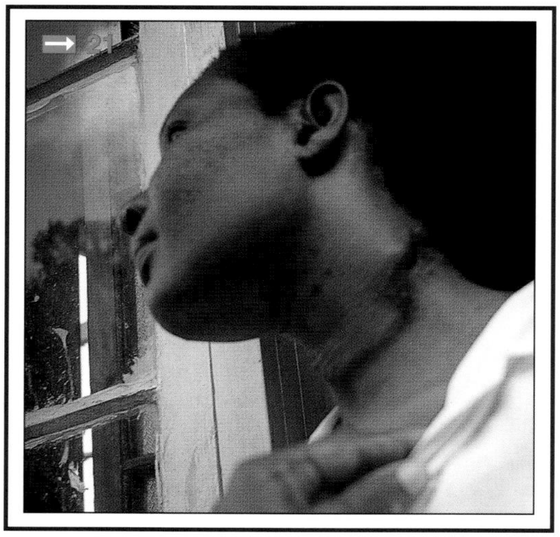

Biology and Life Cycle

The life cycle of *L. minor* is unknown, as is the mode of transmission to humans. Investigators suggest that the normal definitive host of *L. minor* must be an animal rather than a human, because the rarity of human infections would preclude maintenance of the parasite in nature. The life cycle of only one species, *L. sprenti* in the opossum, is known. *Lagochilascaris sprenti* has an obligatory, intermediate, mammalian host, probably a small rodent. Published reports suggest that humans may acquire infection by ingesting infective eggs or infective larvae encysted in the flesh of small wild animals. Left untreated, infections may persist for years with periodic elimination of adult worms. Investigators in Brazil, who observed embryonating eggs and young larvae in host tissues, suggest autoinfection in the human as an explanation for the long-term periodic discharge of adult worms.

Pathology and Clinical Manifestations

Patients usually present with a large, sometimes painful abscess on the neck (➡ 21). The worms are typically found in the soft tissues of the neck and pharynx, tonsils, mastoids, and paranasal sinuses, where they produce recurrent abscesses in the exudates of which worms and eggs may be found. Reports of a fatal pneumonitis and a fatal encephalopathy are attributed to *L. minor* as well.

Patients often complain of a crawling sensation in the throat and sometimes discharge worms through the mouth or nose. A feature common to almost all cases is that the patients have lived in a rural environment in relatively close contact with wild animals. In instances in which tissues such as tonsil were removed, larvae were seen in fibrous capsules in the submucosa of that organ. Autopsy findings in the case of fatal encephalopathy revealed diffuse foci of necrosis of the cerebral hemispheres and cerebellum as well as worms in the parenchyma and in the cisterns at the base of the brain. The lungs also contained hundreds of 2- to 5-mm abscesses scattered throughout the parenchyma. The majority of these abscesses contained advanced larvae, young adults, and mature adult worms.

Parasite Morphology

Most worms in these infections will be recovered intact from the lesions. The adults of *L. minor* are small, robust worms. Females measure up to 2.0 cm in length, with a maximum diameter of 0.81 mm, while males are slightly smaller, measuring up to 1.7 cm in length and 0.60 mm in diameter. Small but mature adults have been collected from tissues as well, with females and males measuring as little as 6.0 and 5.0 mm, respectively. The anterior end of the worm bears three large lips that are separated from the body by a deep, prominent, postlabial groove. Conspicuous lateral alae extend from the level of the nerve ring to near the anus (or cloaca). The cuticle also bears fine transverse striations. The tail of the female is short and sharply tapered. The vulva is usually located posterior to midbody. The male has a short, ventrally curved tail that is smooth and rounded. Up to 40 pairs of precloacal papillae and a variable but small number of postanal papillae are present. The paired spicules are alate in shape and measure up to 0.7 mm in length. The eggs produced by the female have an average size of 65 by 52 µm. The surface of the shell is sculptured with a reticulate pattern of irregularly shaped, saucerlike depressions.

Worms are occasionally encountered during histopathologic examination of tissues from surgical biopsies or at autopsy. However, little histologic material is available for the study of *L. minor* microscopically. The photomicrographs presented here are of *L. sprenti*; these have been compared with detailed descriptions and drawings of *L. minor* prepared by Sprent (1971) more than 20 years ago. The two species are similar at the microscopic level and will fully serve our needs.

The cuticle in both sexes is moderately thick, bears fine transverse striations, and has prominent lateral alae (Plate 29:1–3) supported by internal cuticular bars, which may or may not be visible in all sections. The alae as seen in intact worms extend along most of the length of the body from the level of the nerve ring posteriorly. The hypodermis is thin in the submuscular areas but expands laterally to form large lateral chords. The lateral chords vary in their configuration at different levels of the body—tall and slender at some levels (Plate 29:1 & 2) and flattened at others (Plate 29:3). Typically, up to four or more longitudinal rows of nuclei are in each sublateral sector of the chords. The dorsal and ventral chords tend to be inconspicuous. The musculature is coelomyarian and polymyarian. The individual muscle cell has a strong, contractile portion and a protoplasmic portion that varies in height at different levels of the body (Plate 29:2 & 3). The esophagus is cylindrical, somewhat thicker posteriorly, strongly muscular, and has a triradiate lumen (Plate 29:1). The wall of the intestine is made up of many tall, slender columnar cells in which the nuclei are positioned near the base of each cell. The luminal surface of the intestine has a tall, uniform, microvillus border (Plate 29:2). The shape of the intestinal lumen differs at different levels of the body (Plate 29:2 & 3).

The female reproductive system is similar to that of other nematodes and ascaridoids. The didelphic system and its parts are frequently coiled or looped, so that in any transverse section of a gravid female all or most components can be seen (Plate 29:3). The branched uterus in the mature female usually contains characteristic eggs, which aid in identifying the parasite (Plate 29:3). The male reproductive system is a single tube. The testis is usually coiled and occupies much of the anterior end of the worm, extending to the level of the esophago-intestinal junction. The testis leads to the vas efferens, which empties into the thin-walled seminal vesicle. The seminal vesicle leads into the vas deferens, with its thick-walled ejaculatory duct (Plate 29:4). The spicules in cross-section show the narrow shaft and the two wide alae, which give each their alate shape (Plate 29:5).

Larvae are not well characterized in tissue sections. Those of *L. sprenti*, as reported by Bowman (1987), have a maximum diameter of less than 200 µm. The cuticle is approximately 2 µm thick, the lateral alae are conspicuous, and the hypodermis is thin, with prominent lateral chords that are somewhat frothy in appearance. Muscle cells are coelomyarian and numerous. The intestine is tubular with an essential low columnar epithelium made up of 21 to 24 cells with a microvillus border (Plate 29:6). Diagnosis of *Lagochilascaris* infection will in most cases be based on clinical presentation and expulsion of worms from the lesion. However, the ascaridoid features of the worm, its size, the lateral alae on the lateral body surface, and the clinical history facilitate a correct identification.

References

Bowman DD. Diagnostic morphology of four larval ascaridoid nematodes that may cause visceral larva migrans: *Toxascaris leonina, Baylisascaris procyonis, Lagochilascaris sprenti* and *Hexametra leidyi*. *J Parasitol*. 1987;73:1198-1215.

Sprent JFA. Speciation and development in the genus *Lagochilascaris*. *Parasitology*. 1971;62:71-112.

Velosus MGP, Faria MCAR, de Freitas JD, et al. Lagoquilascariase humana sobre tres casos encontrados no distrito federal. *Braz Rev Inst Med Trop São Paulo*. 1992;34:587-591.

Plate 29

Lagochilascaris sprenti

Image 1

Section through the anterior end of a female worm at the level of the esophagus (ES). Note the lateral alae (darts) (H&E, 150x).

Image 2

Section through the anterior end of a female worm at the level of the intestine (IN). Note the irregular height of the intestinal epithelium (H&E, 150x).

Image 3

Section through the midbody of a female worm at the level of the vulva (dart). Note the ovejector (OJ), ovaries (OV), and the large uterine branches filled with eggs (H&E, 150x).

Image 4

Section through a male worm at the level of the ejaculatory duct (ED) (H&E, 150x).

Image 5

Section through the male tail illustrating the structure of the paired spicules (darts) and the cloaca (H&E, 150x).

Image 6

Transverse section through a larva shows lateral alae (darts), well-developed musculature, prominent lateral chords (keyline), and tubular intestine (IN) (H&E, 300x).

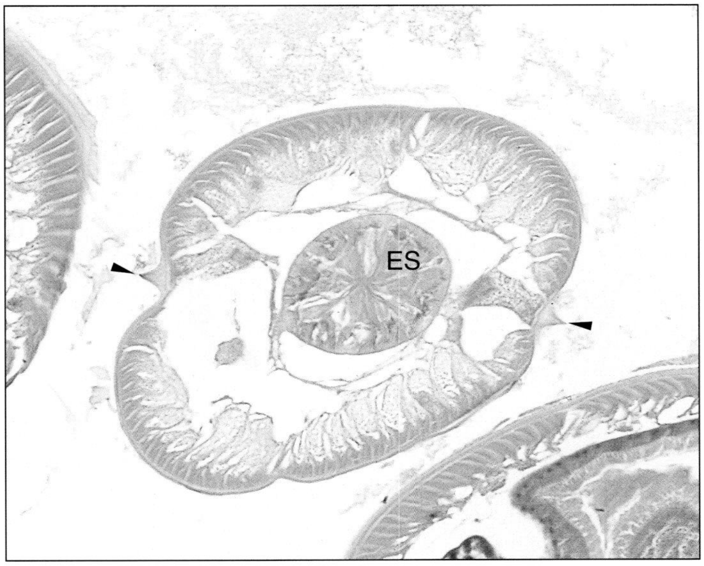

1

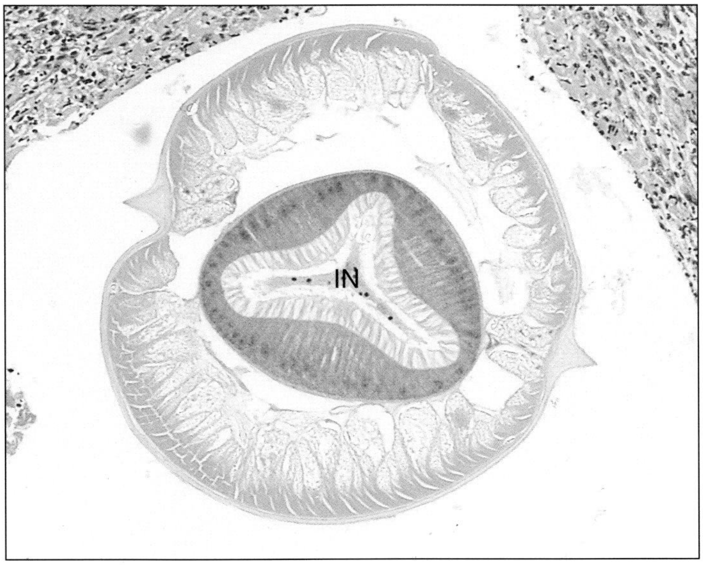

2

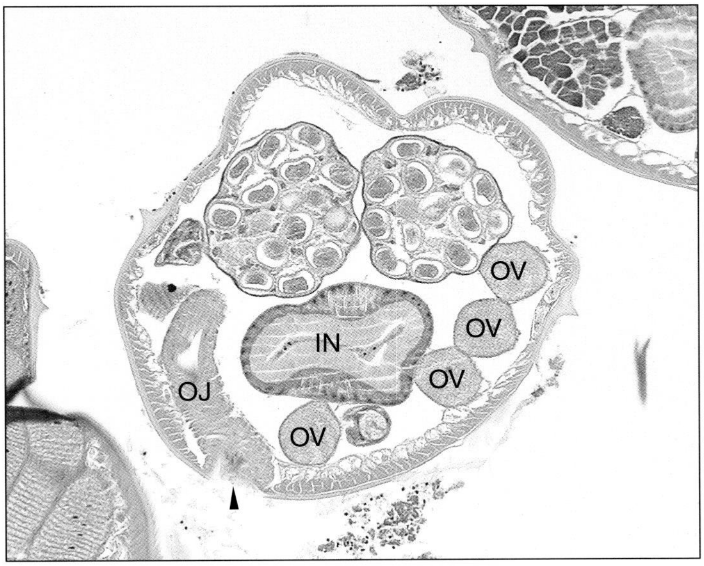

3

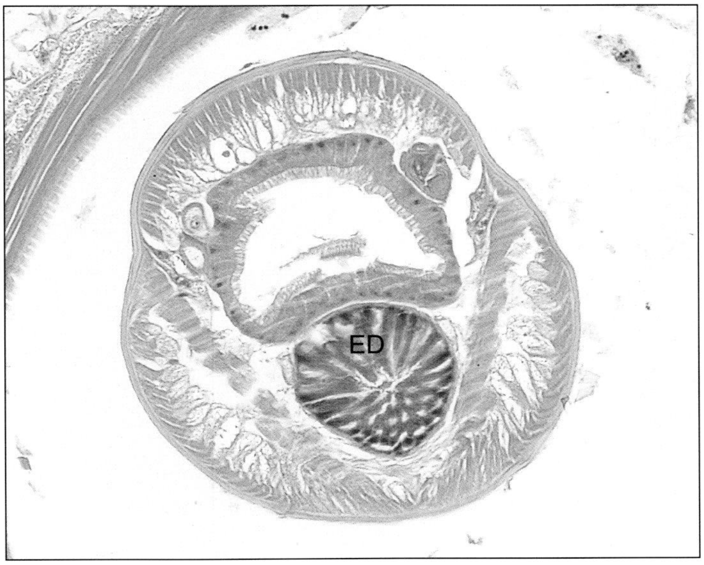

4

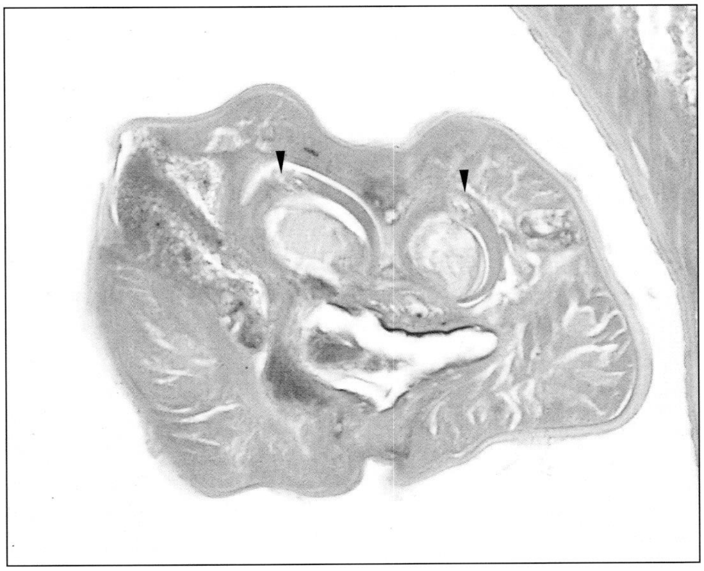

5

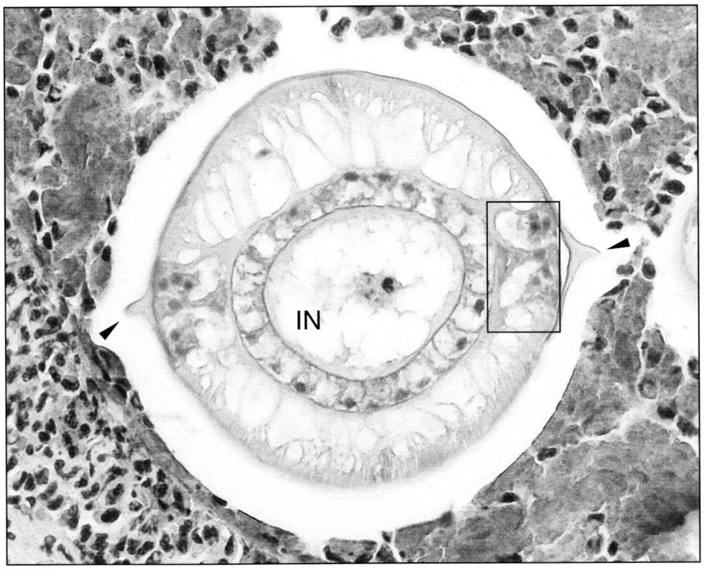

6

Anisakis and *Pseudoterranova* species

The increased popularity of eating raw or uncooked seafood has resulted in the proliferation of some human parasitic infections. One of the more important fish-transmitted infections is anisakiasis, which is caused primarily by nematodes of the genera *Anisakis* and *Pseudoterranova*. Although the taxonomy of the anisakids has changed frequently, two species of *Anisakis*, *A. simplex* and *A. physeteris*, and *Pseudoterranova decipiens* are responsible for most human infections. Anisakiasis was first recognized as an emerging public health problem in The Netherlands in the mid-1950s, but soon thereafter numerous cases were also reported in Japan. Since then, anisakiasis has become recognized as a potential parasitic disease problem in all areas of the world where people eat raw fish, including the United States. Many generic or regional raw fish dishes include sashimi, sushi, seviche, Tahitian salad, green herring, and others. Unfortunately, many individuals mistakenly believe that raw fish marinated in lime or lemon juices is safe to eat. Most such marinades do not kill nematode larvae in the flesh of fish. In the case of sashimi, the size of the fish pieces served may be so thick that larvae present in the flesh may not be seen during preparation. Many larval helminth parasites commonly occur in the flesh of both freshwater and marine fishes, and some may produce human disease.

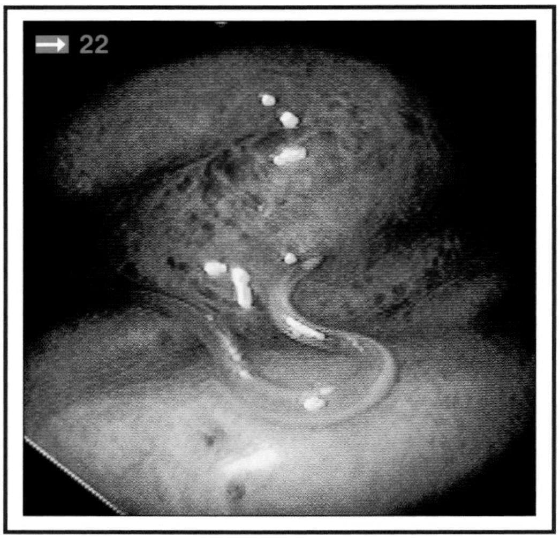

Biology and Life Cycle

The anisakid life cycle typically involves two intermediate hosts and the possibility of a wide range of paratenic hosts. Adult stages live in the stomach of marine mammals such as whales, porpoises, dolphins, seals, and sea lions. Eggs pass in feces into the water, where larval development and subsequent hatching occur over a period of one month or longer. Larvae are ingested by the first intermediate host, shrimplike crustaceans known as krill, in which essential development occurs. Fish and squid are second intermediate hosts. Although infected krill may be ingested by fish of all sizes, usually they are eaten by small fish, within which the larvae migrate into the body cavities or the musculature to undergo further development to mature third-stage larvae. These larvae are infective to the definitive cetacean or pinniped hosts, within which they mature to adult worms. However, because small fish frequently are eaten by progressively larger fish (the food chain), these larval stages have the ability to pass from one to the next, always reentering the body cavity or flesh to await ingestion by the proper definitive host. These fish are known as paratenic hosts, and they enhance the opportunity for the larval stages to ultimately infect the marine mammal host. Humans enter into this cycle by eating raw fish or squid containing infective larvae. Fish commonly infected with anisakid larvae include mackerel, haddock, herring, cod, halibut, rockfish, and pollack.

Pathology and Clinical Manifestations

Human infections result from eating living larvae in raw fish (often marinated, pickled, smoked, or salted). Within the human host, the larvae of *Anisakis* and *Pseudoterranova* behave somewhat differently. The larvae of *Anisakis* species may produce both gastric and intestinal disease, whereas *Pseudoterranova* infection is more often associated with invasion of the stomach wall. In some instances, after ingestion of larvae, these worms simply pass through the intestinal tract and are excreted in feces. In the United States, a common feature of *Pseudoterranova* infection is that larvae migrate out of the stomach after ingestion, crawl up the esophagus (which produces a tickling sensation), and are coughed up by the patient or extracted by a physician examining the throat. Occasionally, larvae will be found on the pillow in the morning after crawling out of the mouth of the sleeping patient.

Infection with *Anisakis* is more likely to result in invasion of gastric mucosa rather than the wall of the intestinal tract. Clinical symptomatology includes nausea, vomiting, and abdominal and epigastric pain. Low-grade fever, leukocytosis, and eosinophilia occur within the first few weeks of infection. Acute gastric anisakiasis is now diagnosed most frequently by endoscopy, which often allows for simultaneous extraction of the worm with biopsy forceps. The most frequent site for larval penetration in the stomach is the fundus (the greater curvature). Although any portion of the intestine may be a site of invasion, the terminal ileum is the most common. Penetration of the gastrointestinal wall into the abdominal cavity and subsequently into other organs is infrequent but may occur.

Histologically, the larva in acute anisakiasis is clearly recognizable as a nematode surrounded by many inflammatory cells, including numerous eosinophils. Some necrosis occurs in the surrounding tissue (Plate 30:2–6). More chronic lesions can be produced and reflect the duration of the infection. Abscesses surrounding dead and degenerating worms contain many eosinophils. Over time, these abscesses develop into granulomatous lesions within which the larva may totally degenerate. Portions of the cuticle and muscle may be seen, but internal anatomy may be unrecognizable (Plate 31:3–6). It may take six months or longer before such lesions resolve.

Parasite Morphology

Third- or early fourth-stage larvae of *Anisakis* species and *Pseudoterranova decipiens* range from 15 to 45 mm in length by 0.4 to 1.5 mm in width. Within the flesh or in the mesenteries of fish, the larvae of *Anisakis* species tend to be pink and are often tightly coiled; the larvae of *Pseudoterranova* are typically yellow-brown to brown and are loosely coiled. When viewed endoscopically, the larvae of *Anisakis* appear thin, milky-white, and stringlike; the larvae of *Pseudoterranova* are broader, thicker, and brown. By using endoscopy in early infections, it is often possible to see living worms on the surface of the gastric mucosa, where they will be actively moving, coiling and uncoiling (➡ 22).

When viewed grossly, the larvae have three lips, a small boring tooth at the anterior end, and a small spinelike structure (mucron) at the posterior end. The esophagus of anisakids typically has a long muscular portion and a shorter glandular portion, which is referred to as the ventriculus. The most important morphologic feature for differentiating between *Anisakis* and *Pseudoterranova* is an anteriorly directed cecum that arises from the ventriculus in *Pseudoterranova* but is absent in *Anisakis.* Other genera of anisakids can be distinguished from these two by the presence or absence of either a ventricular or an intestinal cecum or by the direction in which the cecum is oriented.

Anisakid larvae have a thick cuticle, between 5 and 13 µm in thickness (Plate 31:1 & 2). The musculature is polymyarian and coelomyarian, with the prominent cytoplasmic portions of the individual muscle cells extending into the pseudocoelom (Plate 30:5). In transverse section, the lateral chords are prominent and extend into the body cavity. In *Anisakis* species, the lateral chords are Y shaped, with a narrow base and pedunculate branches (Plate 30:3–5); in *Pseudoterranova,* the Y-shaped chords have a broader base and are more compact (Plate 31:1 & 2). In general, the lateral chords are taller anteriorly and more compressed posteriorly. In sections through the anterior portions of larvae, an excretory cell (renette cell) and excretory column are often prominent (Plate 30:5). In *Pseudoterranova* but not in *Anisakis* a section through the anterior end may show the ventricular cecum. The intestinal tract is composed of tall columnar cells with usually single nuclei at the base of the cells (Plate 30:4).

Morphologic details of the esophagus, intestine, and possible cecum, as well as features such as the excretory cell and column and the Y-shaped lateral chords, permit ready identification of the parasite as an anisakid. An accurate identification of genus may depend on suitable morphologic landmarks, but differentiation from other nematode larvae is usually not difficult.

References

Cheng TC. Anisakiasis. In: Steele JH, ed. *Parasitic Zoonoses, Vol II.* Boca Raton, Fla: CRC Press; 1982:37-54.

Ishikura H, Kikuchi K, Nagasawa K, et al. Anisakidae and anisakidosis. *Prog Clin Parasitol.* 1993;3:43-102.

Oshima T. Anisakis and anisakiasis in Japan and adjacent areas. *Prog Med Parasitol.* 1972;4:301-393.

Plate 30

Anisakis species

Image 1

The anterior portion of an anisakid, probably *Anisakis*, can be seen in oblique section. The worm is in the process of invading the wall of the stomach. The section of worm is cut near the esophageal-intestinal junction. The intestine (IN) and esophagus (ES) are seen at opposite ends of the worm (H&E, 60x).

Image 2

Section of anisakid in the wall of the stomach. Even at this low magnification, the typical intestine and one lateral chord (dart) of the parasite are seen (H&E, 35x).

Image 3

Section of human intestine shows two portions of the same worm. The intestine and Y-shaped lateral chords (darts) are visible (H&E, 40x).

Image 4

At higher magnification, note the tall columnar cells and the location of the nuclei near the base of the cells. Note also the Y-shaped lateral chords (darts). This worm had been identified as *Anisakis* species (H&E, 125x).

Image 5

Section of *Anisakis* species cut at the level of the muscular esophagus (ES). Note the well-developed musculature, portions of the Y-shaped lateral chords, and a portion of the excretory cell (dart). The esophagus has a well-defined triradiate lumen (H&E, 180x).

Image 6

Section of *Anisakis* species in the ileum of a Japanese. Note the morphologic characteristics of the intestine (IN), ie, tall, narrow, columnar cells with nuclei situated at the base of each cell. The lateral chords (keyline) and the smaller dorsal and ventral chords are also evident (H&E, 100x).

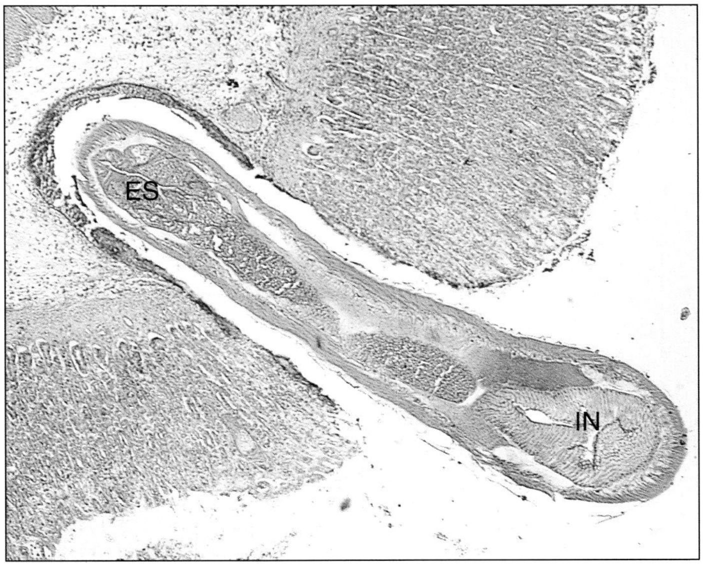

1

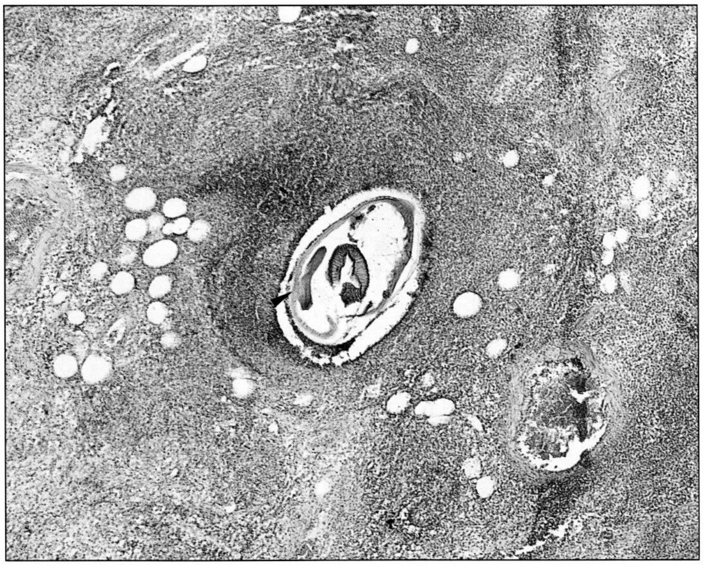

2

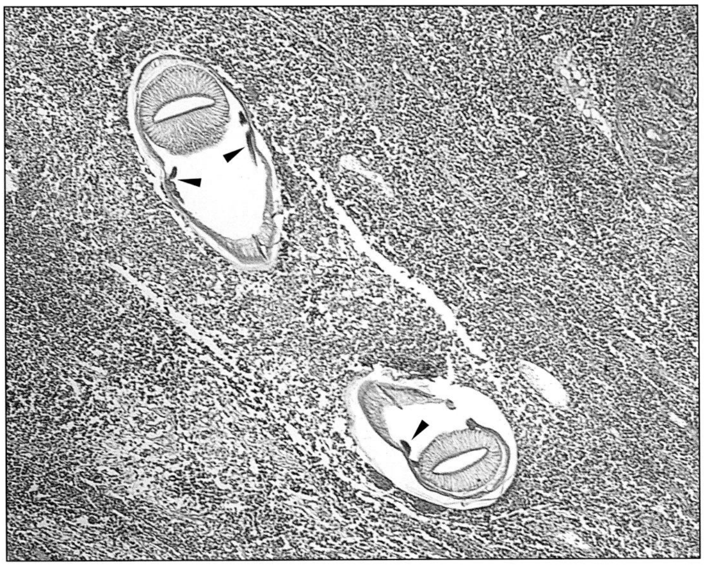

3

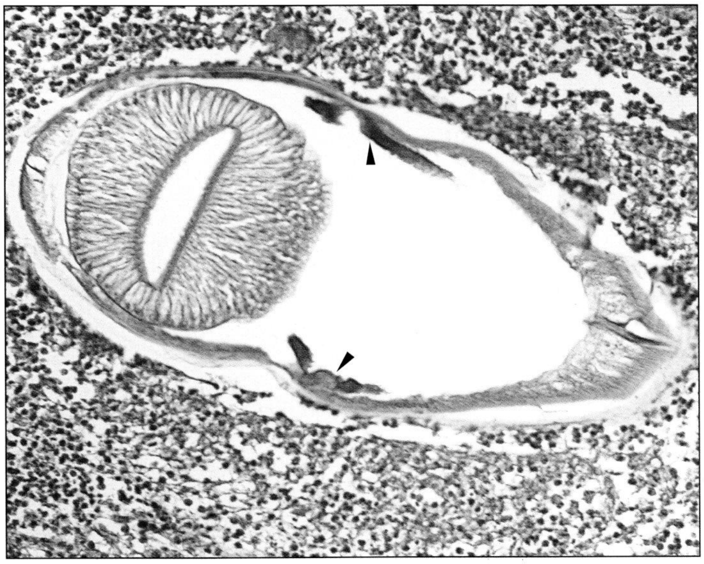

4

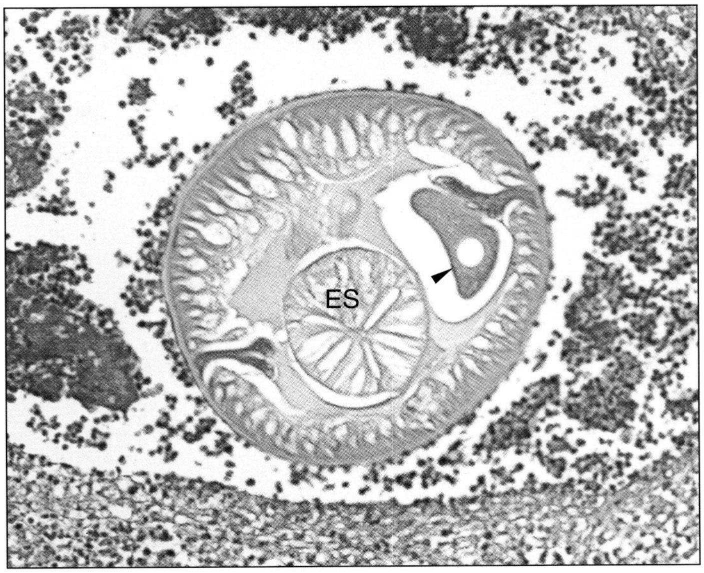

5

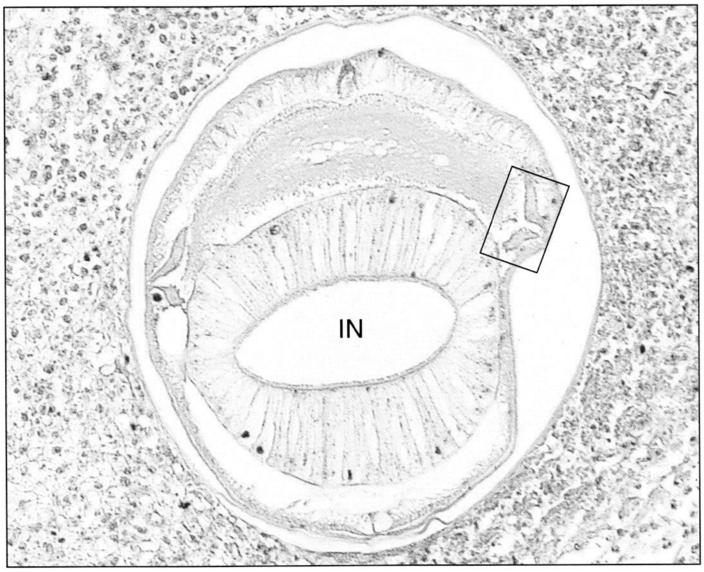

6

Plate 31

Anisakis and *Pseudoterranova* species

Image 1

Transverse section of an anisakid (probably *Pseudoterranova decipiens*) within paratesticular tissue of a Hispanic. This parasite was initially identified and described in the literature as a case of cysticercosis, but the worm is obviously an anisakid larva. The parasite is undergoing degeneration, but the cuticle (C), lateral chords (LC), and musculature (MU) are clear (H&E, 125x).

Image 2

At higher magnification, the morphologic features of the anisakid shown in Image 1 are more clearly seen. Even in the degenerated condition, the characteristic structure of the lateral chords is diagnostic for anisakid larvae (H&E, 250x).

Image 3

Two portions of an anisakid (widely separated in the original field) are shown here side by side. The anisakid was recovered from a woman with acute bowel obstruction. At this low magnification, little can be discerned about the parasite other than its resemblance to a nematode. Note the intense inflammatory reaction around the worm (H&E, 35x).

Image 4

Even though few morphologic features are clear, one of the Y-shaped lateral chords can be seen (keyline) at higher magnification (H&E, 200x).

Image 5

Section of an anisakid worm within an abscess in the stomach of a Japanese. Although a tumor was suspected before surgery, this parasite was found within a typical lesion associated with anisakiasis. It probably represents a species of *Anisakis* (H&E, 50x).

Image 6

At higher magnification, it is still possible to see the lateral chords (darts), although the other morphologic features have degenerated (H&E, 200x).

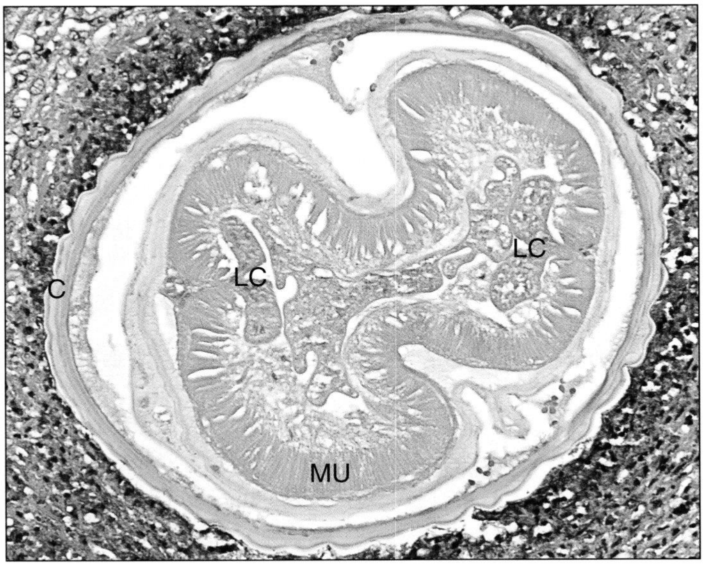

1

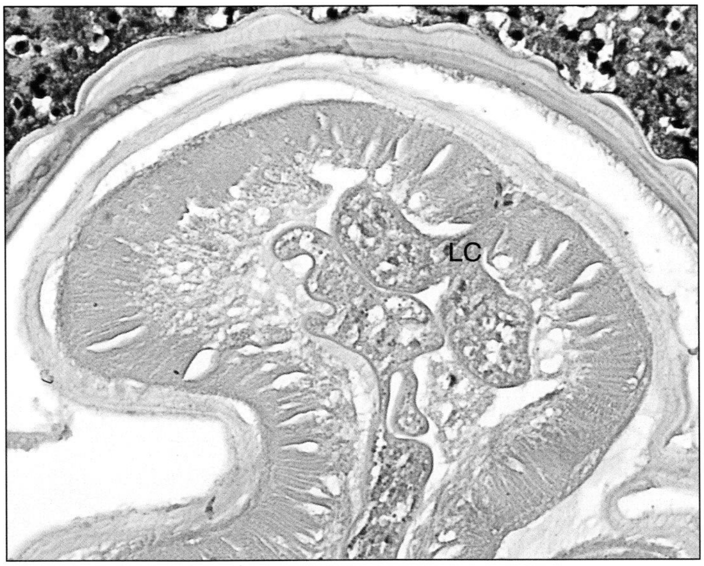

2

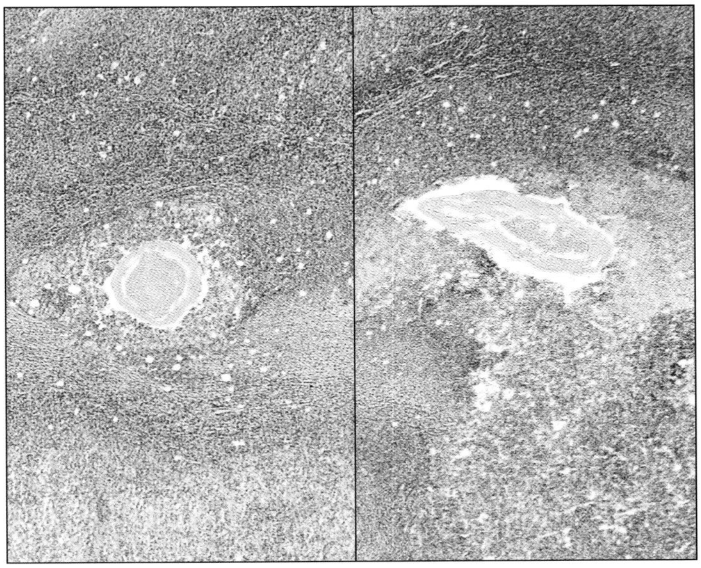
3

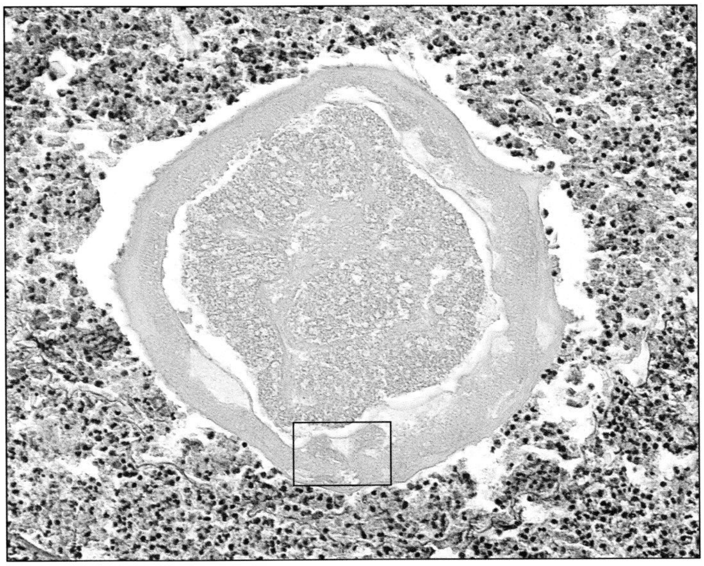
4

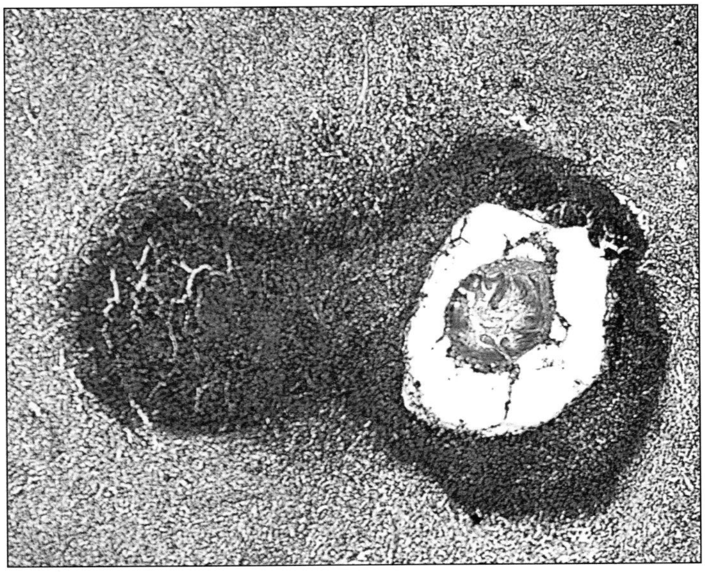
5

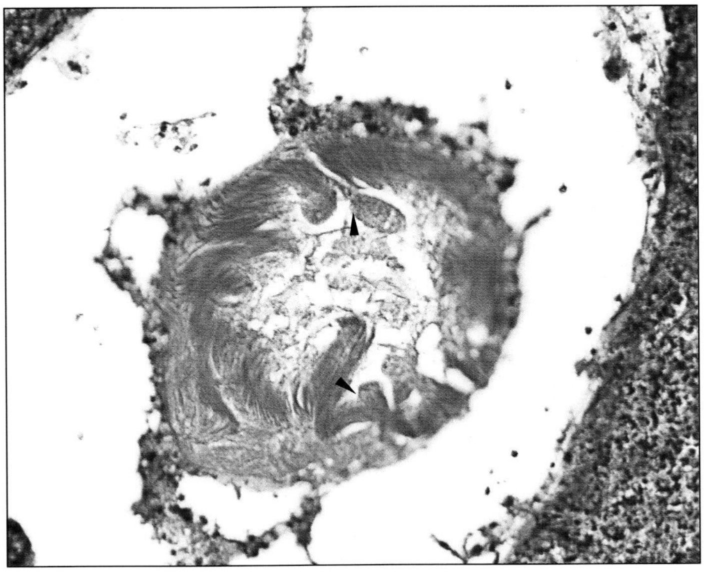
6

Enterobius vermicularis

The pinworm has a cosmopolitan distribution but is a more common human parasite in temperate regions of the world than in the tropics. Infections are more prevalent in children than adults and are encountered with greater frequency in institutional settings, especially where personal care and hygiene may be substandard.

Ordinarily, the pinworm causes discomfort; only rarely does it cause health problems. However, the female worm has a propensity for wandering in the body and is frequently found in lesions in unexpected locations.

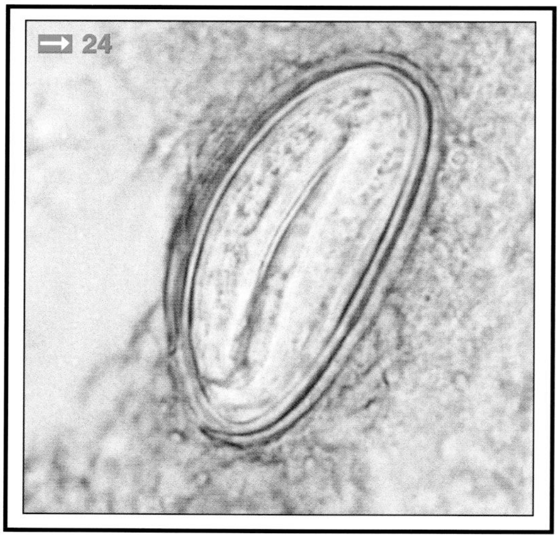

Biology and Life Cycle

The adult worms live primarily in the cecum but they also dwell in the appendix (Plate 32:1) and the colon. When female worms reach maturity, they migrate down the lower bowel to emerge at the anus and discharge their eggs on the perianal and perineal skin, usually at night while the host is asleep. Eggs deposited on the skin mature in a few hours and contain a fully developed larva (⇒ 24). Transmission to another host takes place when the eggs, clinging to various fomites, are ingested by another individual. Infections may possibly be airborne. The ingested eggs hatch in the intestine, and the liberated larvae move to the cecum and develop to adults in about three to four weeks, completing the cycle.

Pathology and Clinical Manifestations

Pruritus produced by the migration of the female worm out of the anus and onto the perianal skin is the cardinal symptom of pinworm infection, although in many instances patients may be asymptomatic. In female hosts the adult female worm may migrate into the reproductive tract and become encapsulated in the uterus or fallopian tubes. They may wander even farther to the peritoneal cavity, often becoming encapsulated in the mesenteries. They have also been found in the liver parenchyma, pulmonary nodules, spleen, lymph nodes, and ovaries. Pathologists will most often encounter adult worms in the lumen of the appendix, where little or no inflammation is present (Plate 32:1).

Parasite Morphology

Diagnosis of pinworm infection is based on the recovery and identification of the characteristic eggs from the perianal skin. The typical pinworm egg has a relatively thick but transparent and colorless shell that is smooth, oval, and flattened on one side. It contains a larva and measures 50 to 60 µm by 20 to 30 µm (⇒ 24). Eggs are obtained using the cellophane tape technique or some modification of it.

Recognizing the adult worm, particularly the female, and remnants of worms found in tissues is a greater concern. The worm can be identified by morphologic features or by eggs contained within the degenerating female worm. Adult worms are small but robust. Females measure up to 13 mm in length, have a diameter of 0.3 to 0.5 mm, and possess a long, pointed tail. Males are much smaller, with a length of about 2.5 mm; they have a blunt tail and only one spicule.

Some gross morphologic features characteristic of this species are equally evident in transverse sections of the parasite. The anterior end of both sexes has a cephalic inflation, which can be seen in sections through the anterior extremity. The lateral alae are conspicuous, especially in sectioned material (Plate 32:3–6). The esophagus is of the rhabditoid type, divided into corpus, isthmus, and bulb (Plate 32:2). Often, sections are seen through the muscular corpus in cuts through the anterior end of the worm (Plate 32:3). The intestine varies somewhat in its appearance. The lumen may range from tubular to narrow and irregular (Plate 32:4 & 6). The body wall has characteristic features: the cuticle is thin in the living worm (Plate 32:3–5), but may be swollen and much thicker in the dead worm (Plate 32:6). The lateral alae are conspicuous at all levels of the body (Plate 32:3–6). The hypodermis is thin and inconspicuous in the submuscular areas. The lateral chords are prominent but often have a highly vacuolated appearance (Plate 32:4), which makes them less evident. The muscles are platymyarian and meromyarian, and usually only two or three can be found in each quadrant of the body (Plate 32:4 & 6).

The female reproductive system is didelphic and amphidelphic and confined more or less to the middle half of the body. The vulva is positioned at the junction of the anterior and middle thirds of the body. As the female matures, the uterine branches become distended with eggs and fill almost the entire body cavity (Plate 32:5). The presence of the typical pinworm egg facilitates identification of the parasite. The male reproductive system is a single tube that occupies the posterior two thirds of the body. Typically, only the intestine and a genital tube are apparent in transverse section (Plate 32:6). However, because the testis is usually flexed, it and the seminal vesicle or some other segment of the tube can be seen. In ectopic sites, the worms are usually females and may be in an advanced stage of degeneration (Plate 33:1 & 3), so that diagnostic morphologic features may not be evident. However, the presence of typical eggs in utero aids diagnosis (Plate 33:2 & 4). In other cases, morphologic features of the worm itself confirm the identification (Plate 33:5 & 6). The structure of the body wall, especially the presence of lateral alae, the platymyarian musculature, and typical eggs in utero, make identification of *E. vermicularis* in tissues relatively straightforward.

Reference

Patterson LA, Abedi ST, Kottmeier PK, et al. Perforation of the ileum secondary to *Enterobius vermicularis*: report of a rare case. *Modern Pathol.* 1993;6:781-783.

Sinniah B, Leopairut J, Neafie RC, et al. Enterobiasis: a histological study of 259 patients. *Ann Trop Med Parasitol.* 1991;85:625-635.

Plate 32

Enterobius vermicularis

Image 1

Several transverse sections of adult worm in the lumen of an appendix (H&E, 10x).

Image 2

Longitudinal section through the anterior end of the body illustrates the structure of the esophagus: corpus, isthmus, and bulb. The cephalic inflation usually present at the anterior end is not evident in this image (H&E, 75x).

Image 3

Transverse section through the anterior end of the body at the level of the corpus of the esophagus. Note the prominent lateral alae (darts) (H&E, 200x).

Image 4

Transverse section through the body of a female worm illustrates the appearance of the body wall. Note the thin cuticle, platymyarian muscle cells (MU), and large lateral chords (LC). The intestine (IN) has an irregular lumen. Sections through the ovaries (OV) are also present (H&E, 200x).

Image 5

Transverse section through a gravid female worm whose uterine tubes (UT) are filled with developing eggs. Note the thin body wall with recognizable lateral chords (LC) and few muscle cells. The intestine (dart) with its irregular, narrow lumen can also be seen (H&E, 200x).

Image 6

Transverse section through a male worm found in a lymph node. The worm appears to be dead. The cuticle has begun to swell; the lateral alae are recognizable. In the pseudocoelom, the intestine (IN), with its irregular lining, and a reproductive tube containing spermatozoa are visible (H&E, 350x).

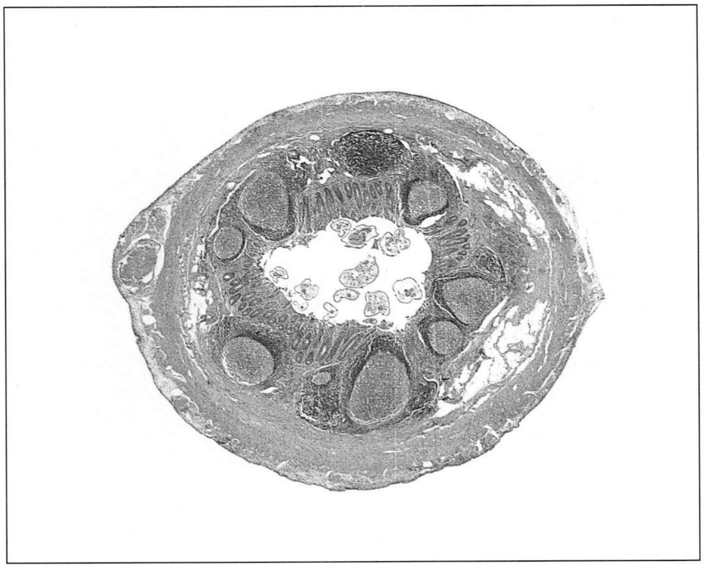

1

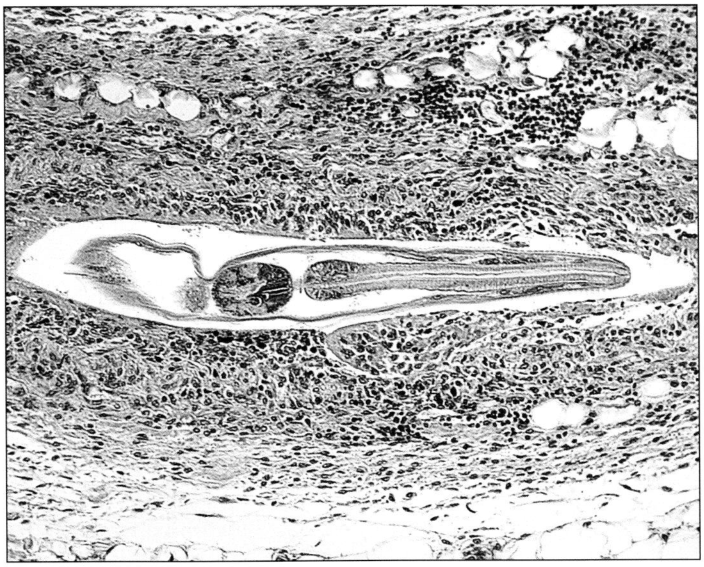

2

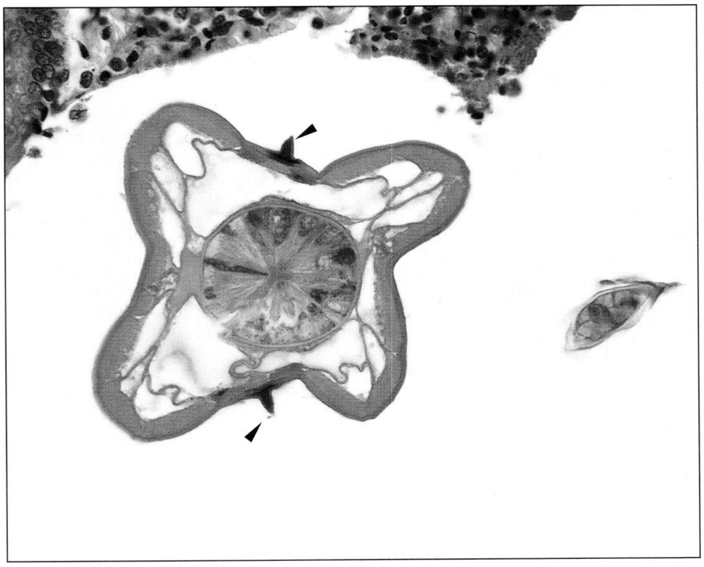

3

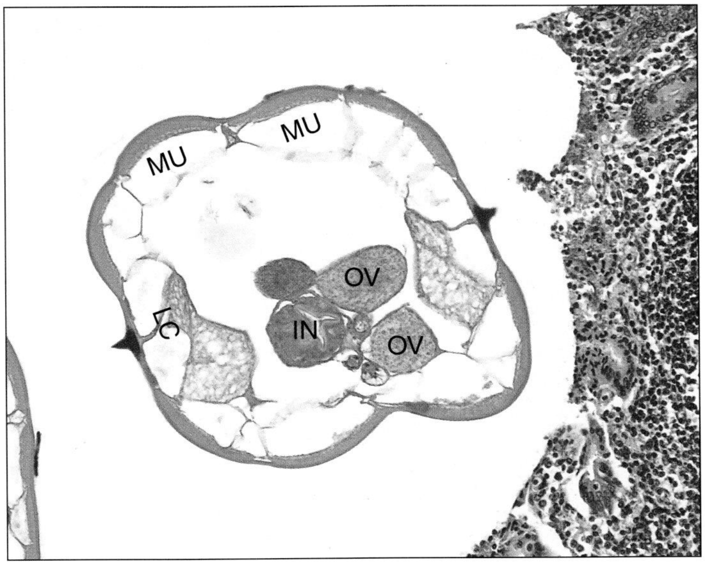

4

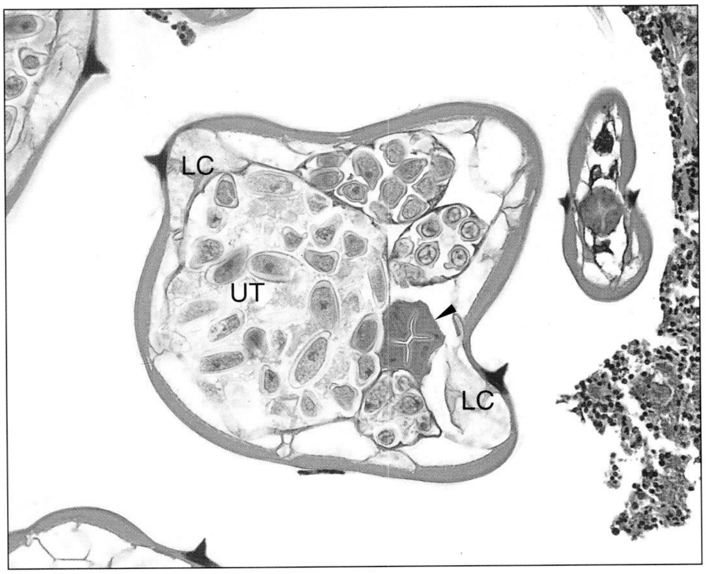

5

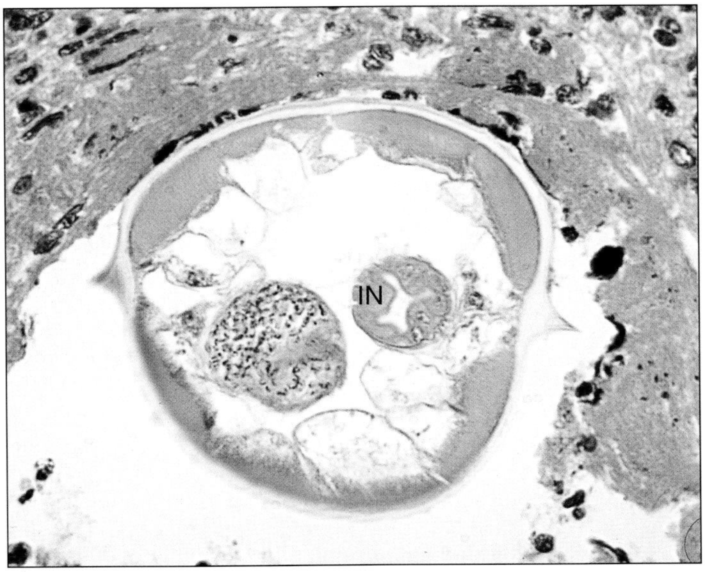

6

Plate 33

Enterobius vermicularis

Image 1

Section through a lesion on a human ovary. The body of the adult female worm has been destroyed, but remnants of the uterus (darts) filled with eggs remain (H&E, 40x).

Image 2

At high magnification, the morphology of the typical egg can still be seen. The eggs are unembryonated, but their shape and moderately thick shell, flattened on one side (dart), are evident (H&E, 500x).

Image 3

A female worm in a peritoneal granuloma. Although only a few remnants of the worm remain, many of the typical eggs contain developing larvae (H&E, 200x).

Image 4

At high magnification, several eggs can be seen in the process of maturation (H&E, 400x).

Image 5

Section through an aborted, dead fetus with a nematode worm (keyline) in the abdomen (H&E, 40x).

Image 6

At higher magnification, lateral alae, platymyarian muscle, and a uterine tube filled with eggs are recognizable as those of *E. vermicularis*. This female worm migrated into the uterus and into the fetal tissues after the fetus had died (H&E, 200x).

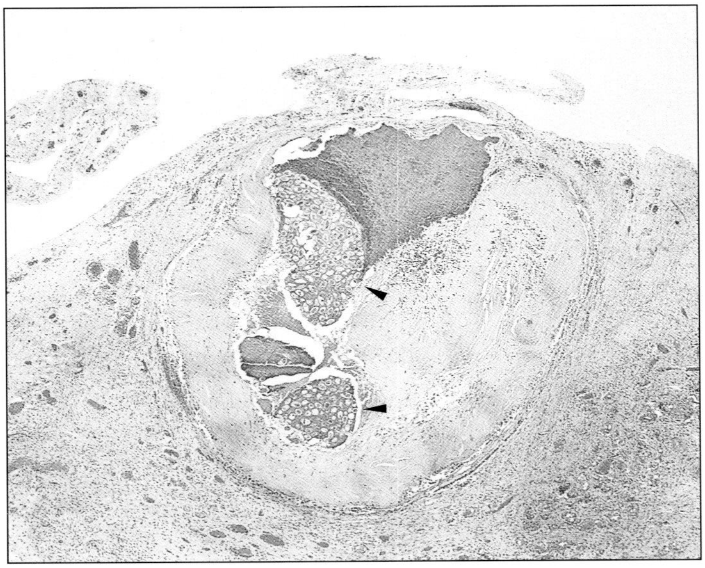

1

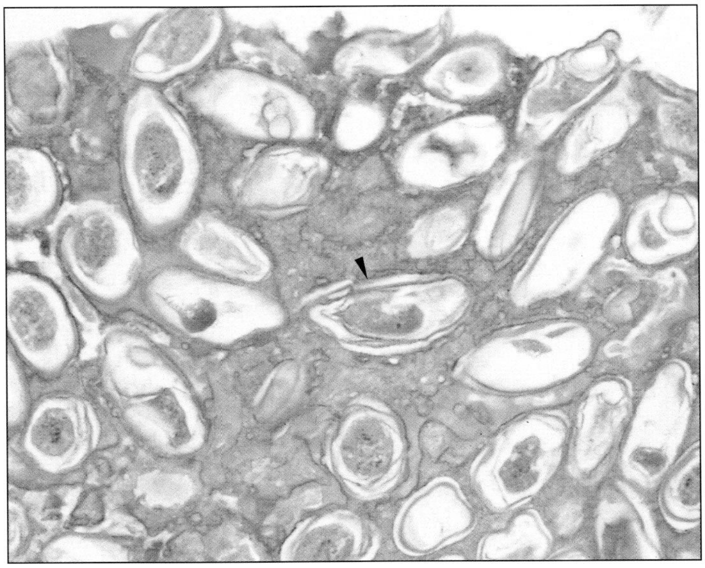

2

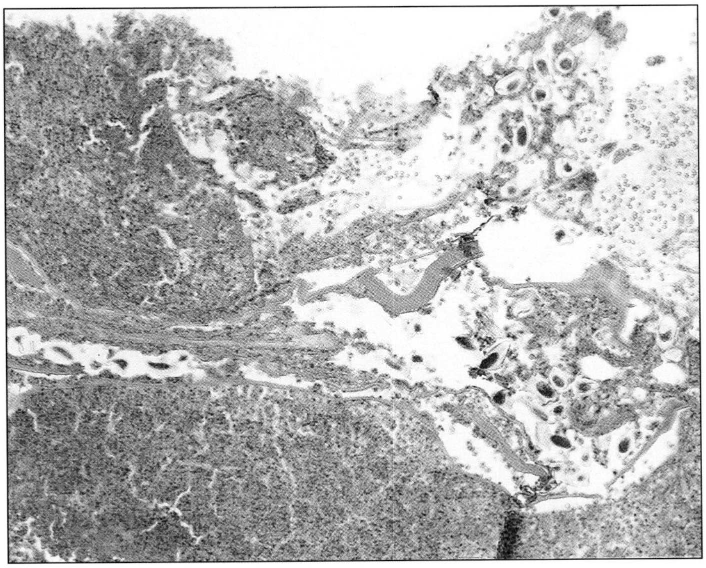

3

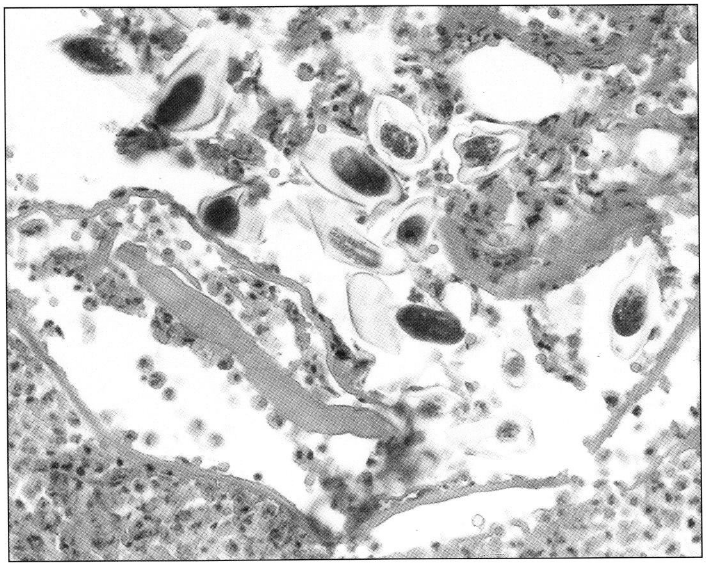

4

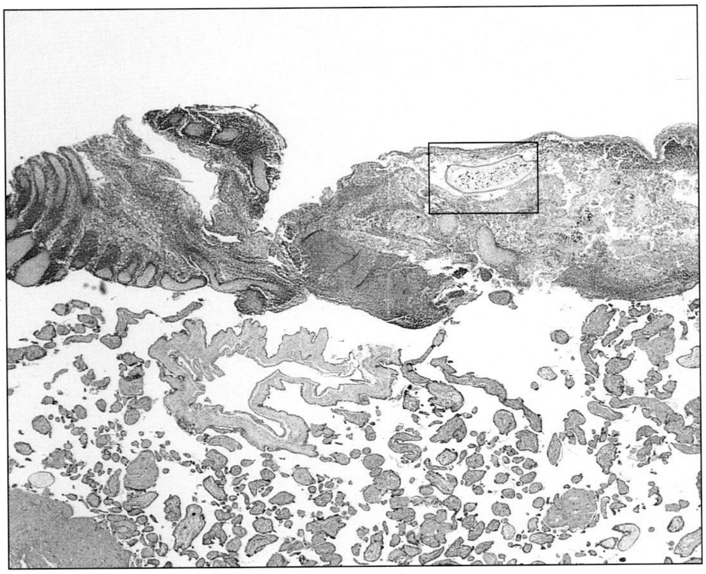

5

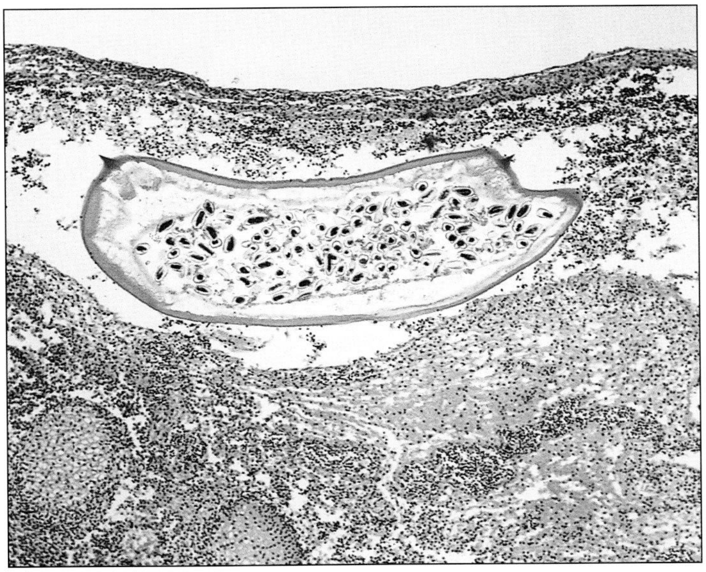

6

Ancylostoma and *Necator* species

Hookworms and Cutaneous Larva Migrans

The hookworms, *Ancylostoma duodenale* and *Necator americanus*, are among the most common parasites of humans and may cause significant human disease. More than 700 million people are estimated to be infected worldwide. Endemicity is limited for the most part to subtropical and tropical, nonarid, rural regions of the world with inadequate sanitation.

In addition to the species that infect humans, other species, found especially in dogs and cats, can invade human tissues. Because they are unable to complete their migration and development, they wander through the skin and produce a cutaneous larva migrans or creeping eruption (➡ 25).

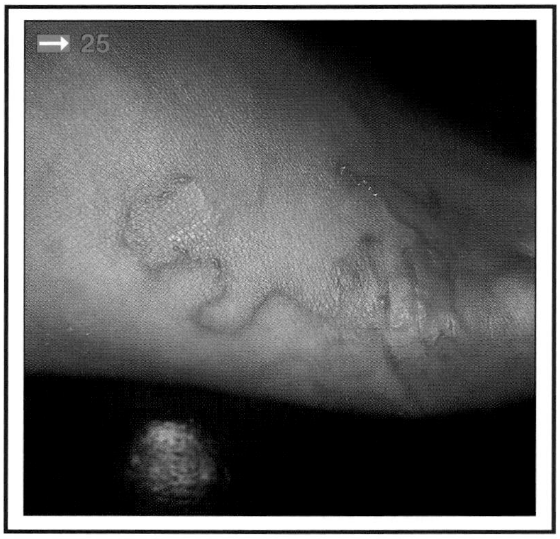

Biology and Life Cycle

Females of both *Ancylostoma duodenale* and *Necator americanus* produce eggs that measure approximately 60 to 75 µm and are in an early stage of cleavage when passed in feces (➡ 26). The species cannot be distinguished on the basis of egg morphology. Eggs that reach the soil will, under ideal circumstances, develop to rhabditoid larvae, hatch, and then develop to the infective (filariform) stage in about one week. The larvae of *Necator* penetrate the skin to infect humans; larvae of *Ancylostoma* are infective by both mouth and skin penetration. After entering the skin, larvae make a lung migration and then move from the alveoli and trachea to the esophagus and intestine, where they complete their maturation to the adult stage.

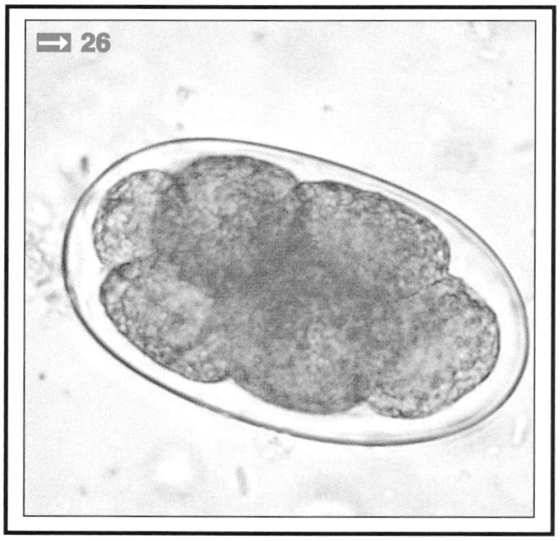

Prepatent development of *Necator* requires about six weeks, whereas that of *Ancylostoma* may range from several weeks to several months, because the larvae often remain in tissues for extended periods before completing migration to the intestine. Infections are diagnosed by finding eggs in feces.

The hookworms of dogs and cats (eg, *Ancylostoma braziliense* and *A. caninum* in the United States and other species in other parts of the world) have similar extrinsic development. Infective larvae are also found in warm, moist, shaded soil and, if they come into contact with exposed human skin, can penetrate and enter but are unable to migrate further. In Australia, recent studies have indicated that occult human infections with the dog hookworm, *A. caninum*, occur in northeast Queensland. Typically, the presence of a single adult worm is reported in these cases, which are characterized by eosinophilia, abdominal pain, and an eosinophilic enteritis (Croese et al, 1994).

Pathology and Clinical Manifestations

Itching, erythema, and vesiculation may develop at the site of skin penetration by the larvae. In the ensuing two weeks, mild and transitory pulmonary symptoms occur as the larvae pass through the lungs. When the larvae attach to the intestinal mucosa and complete their maturation, eosinophilia and abdominal symptoms such as dyspepsia, nausea, and epigastric discomfort may be present. Significant blood loss results from lacerations of the mucosa as worms detach, move, and reattach. Hemorrhage and blood loss tend to be directly proportional to the worm burden. In chronic infections, symptoms are essentially those of an iron-deficiency anemia. In light to moderate infections, blood loss can be compensated for by an adequate, iron-rich diet that includes other minerals, animal protein, and vitamin A. Heavy infections deplete body iron reserves and if left untreated may cause death, especially in infants.

Larvae of animal hookworms that have entered the epidermis of human skin are unable to pentrate more deeply into the tissues. Consequently, they wander through the epidermis, producing a cutaneous larva migrans or creeping eruption. Inflamed, superficial, serpiginous tracts develop and become edematous and pruritic. Old tracts begin to heal as new ones form. If left untreated, this creeping eruption can persist for several weeks.

Parasite Morphology

Hookworms are relatively small, robust worms that are found attached to the mucosa of the small intestine. They are characterized by a well-developed buccal capsule armed with teeth in *Ancylostoma* and cutting plates in

Necator. Males of both species have a well-developed copulatory bursa. Female *Ancylostoma* measure about 13.0 by 0.6 mm; males, 11.0 by 0.45 mm. Adult *Necator* are only slightly smaller. The diagnosis of hookworm infection rarely depends on identification of the adult worms in tissues. However, the adults may be found in sections of intestine of infected individuals. *Ancylostoma* and *Necator* adults in transverse sections are similar. The anterior end of the worm may be attached to the mucosa, with a tag of mucosa in the buccal capsule (Plate 34:1).

Morphologic features are similar in both species. The cuticle is thick, the hypodermis thin. Lateral hypodermal chords are usually easy to see, as are the much smaller dorsal and ventral chords (Plate 34:2), which divide the muscles into four bands. Usually three or four platymyarian muscles are apparent per quadrant (Plate 34:3). The globular buccal capsule (Plate 34:1) leads into the club-shaped, muscular esophagus (Plate 34:1 & 2), which possesses a triradiate lumen (Plate 34:2). The intestine is composed of a few multinucleate cells. Usually, several nuclei are visible in a transverse section of the intestine (Plate 34:4). The reproductive system of both sexes is typically confined to the posterior two-thirds of the body. The copulatory bursa is similar to that of *Oesophagostomum* species (Plate 35:6).

Skin biopsies are rarely performed to recover the larvae in cases of creeping eruption. Diagnosis is based on the patient's history and the clinical presentation. We will mention other agents of cutaneous larva migrans with the appropriate parasites.

References

Croese J, Loukas A, Opdebeeck J, et al. Human enteric infection with canine hookworms. *Ann Intern Med.* 1994;120:369-374.

Nichols RL. The etiology of visceral larva migrans, II: comparative larval morphology of *Ascaris lumbricoides, Necator americanus, Strongyloides stercoralis* and *Ancylostoma caninum*. *J Parasitol.* 1956;42:363-399.

Plate 34

Ancylostoma, Necator, and Cutaneous Larva Migrans

Image 1

Ancylostoma caninum. Longitudinal section through the anterior end of the body shows worm attached to the intestinal mucosa. Note the large buccal capsule (dart) and a segment of the long, club-shaped muscular esophagus (ES) (H&E, 100x).

Image 2

Ancylostoma caninum. Transverse section through the esophageal region shows the esophagus (ES) with its triradiate lumen and features of the body wall, including the thick cuticle, few muscle cells (MU), and lateral chords (LC) (H&E, 80x).

Image 3

Transverse section of *A. caninum.* Note the thick cuticle (CU), the platymyarian muscle cells (MU), and the very thin hypodermis between them (H&E, 200x).

Image 4

Ancylostoma caninum. At high magnification, the structure of the intestine is illustrated. Note the syncytial, multinucleated epithelial cells with a conspicuous microvillus border (MV) (H&E, 200x).

Image 5

Ancylostoma caninum larvae in the skin of a mouse illustrate the conspicuous double alae (darts) (H&E, 750x).

Image 6

Ancylostoma larva in epidermis of human skin barely demonstrates evidence of double alae (darts) (H&E, 750x).

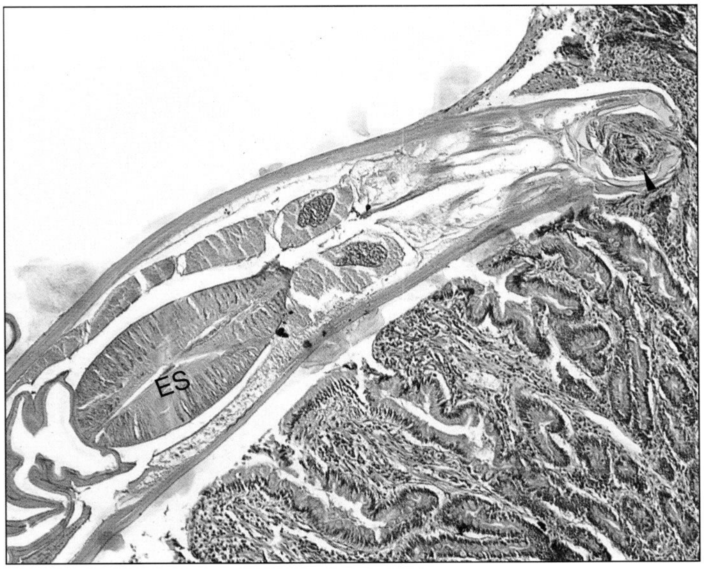

1

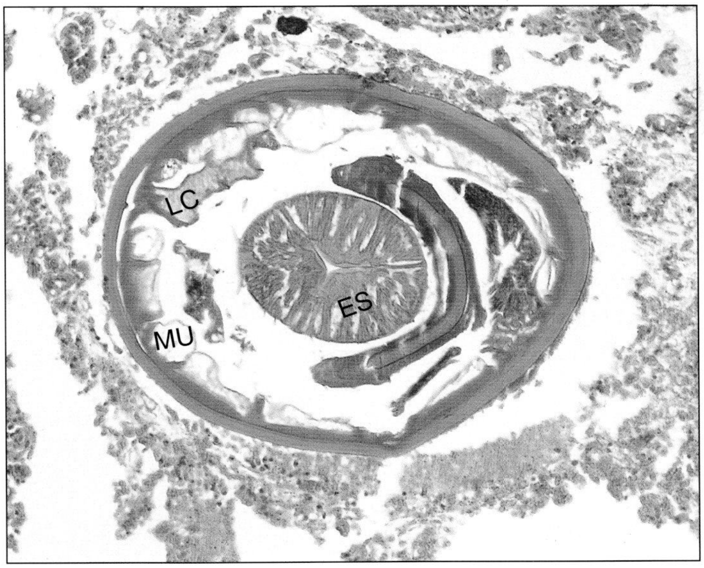

2

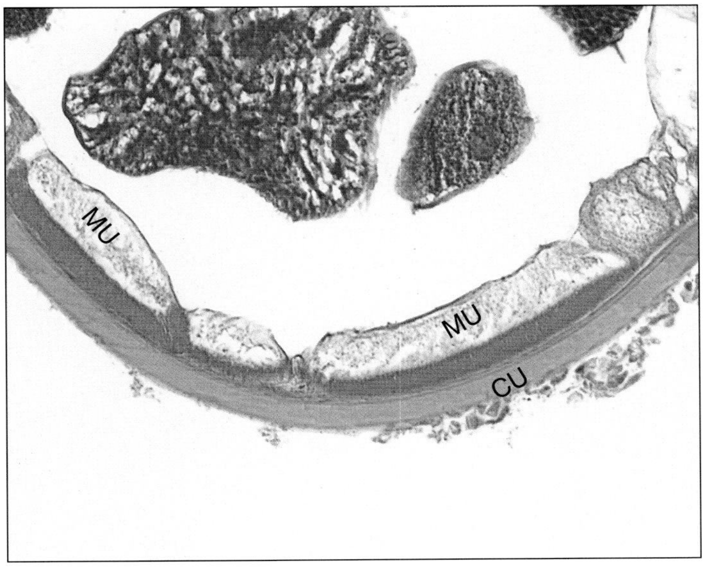

3

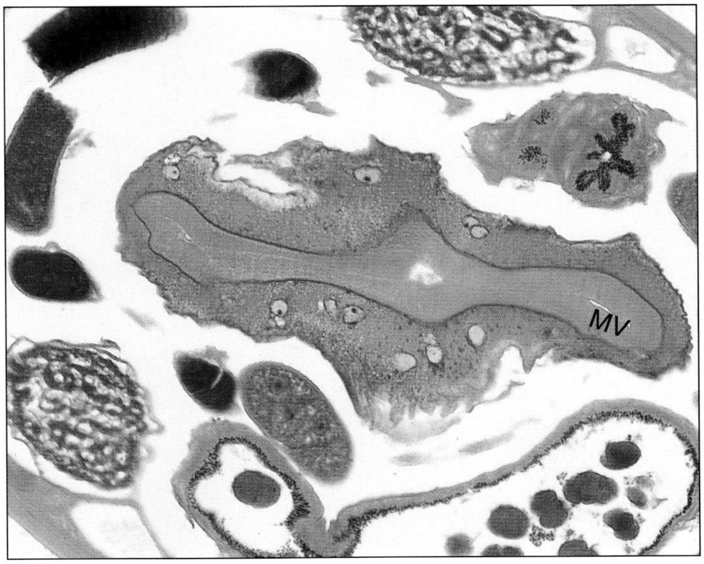

4

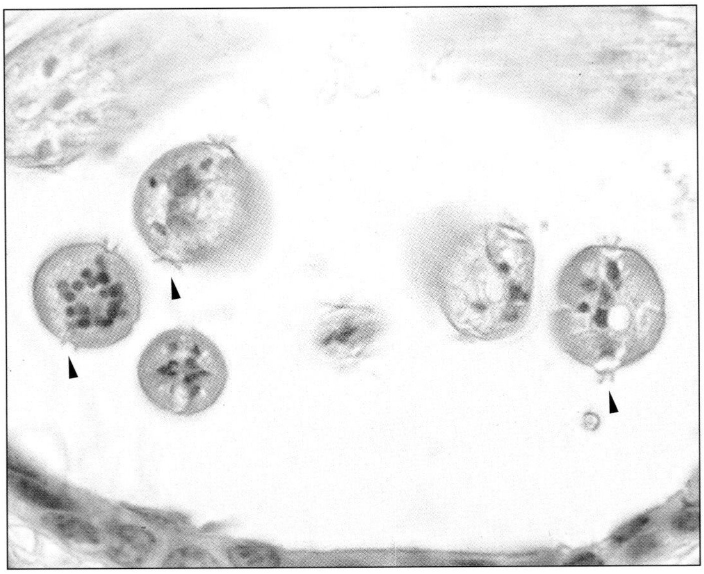

5

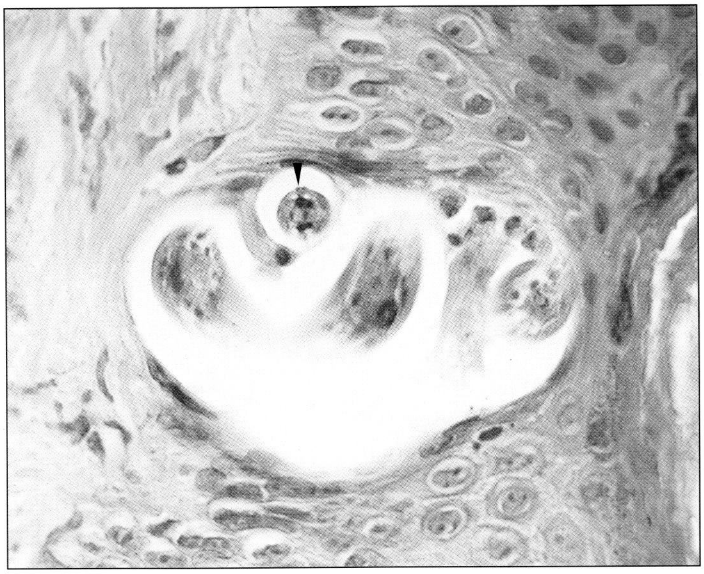

6

Oesophagostomum species

Oesophagostomes are bursate nematodes, related to the hookworms, and are common parasites of livestock (cattle, sheep, goats, and swine) and monkeys. These parasites have worldwide distribution. Oesophagostomes are also referred to as nodular worms because they produce nodulelike abscesses in the intestinal wall of the host while developing to the adult stage. Although human infections have always been regarded as accidental and rare, recent reports indicate that foci of human oesophagostomiasis are endemic to northern Togo and Ghana in West Africa. Several species of the parasites may be involved in human infections, which can produce serious medical problems.

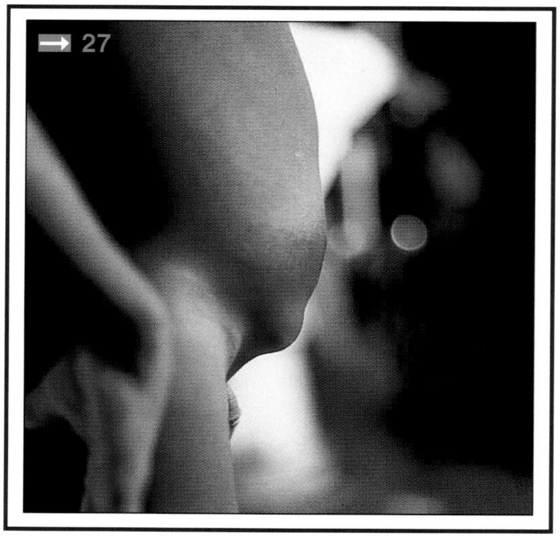

Biology and Life Cycle

The robust adult worms live in the large intestine of their hosts. Females are usually 1.5 to 3.0 cm long, while males are somewhat smaller. The females produce eggs that are virtually impossible to differentiate from those of hookworms. Coprocultures are typically used to distinguish the infective-stage larvae of the oesophagostomes from hookworm species. Eggs deposited on soil quickly embryonate and hatch. After several days, they molt twice to become infective larvae. Infections are transmitted orally when animals ingest larvae while grazing on vegetation. It is unclear how humans acquire infection, but it is probably by ingesting larvae on vegetable or plant products. Ingested larvae make their way to the large intestine where they burrow into the submucosa, quickly forming an inflammatory nodule and sterile abscess in which they complete their development (Plate 35:1). After the final molt, they typically reenter the lumen of the bowel, attach to the mucosa, and complete their maturation. In humans, the worms apparently are unable to complete their development and remain within the submucosal abscesses. However, under certain circumstances the cycle that occurs in natural hosts apparently can take place in humans. The actual prevalence of patent oesophagostomiasis in human populations is unknown but is likely to be masked by the similarity of oesophagostome eggs to those of hookworms that occur in the same area.

Pathology and Clinical Manifestations

With few exceptions (Indonesia, Brazil), the reports of human infections have come from rural areas of East and West Africa. No uniform clinical picture emerges, although most patients present with pain in the lower right quadrant, with one or more palpable abdominal masses (➡ 27). This condition frequently deteriorates, necessitating exploratory laparotomy. Surgery usually reveals a 4- to 6-cm mass in or attached to the bowel wall. Adhesions to adjacent tissues or the abdominal wall are not uncommon. Masses are most often found in the ileocecal region. The condition may imitate carcinoma, appendicitis, appendicular abscess, diverticular disease, amebiasis, etc. The bowel mucosa is typically intact; however, sequential tissue sections may reveal a worm tract from the nodule to the lumen. Opening the nodule usually reveals the young adult worm lying in thick pus. Histologically, an infiltrate of macrophages and eosinophils is present in early lesions; in older lesions, the cellular infiltrate is much greater and a rim or margin of epithelioid cells, macrophages, and eosinophils surrounds the central necrotic area.

Parasite Morphology

Intact worms retrieved from the contents of the nodule or from the lumen of the gut can be quickly identified on the basis of gross morphologic features. Females typically measure up to 3.0 cm in length with a maximum diameter of 800 to 900 µm depending on the species and stage of development. Males are somewhat shorter and have a smaller diameter. In both sexes, the anterior end has a cephalic inflation or vesicle, a ventral transverse groove, and an oral opening guarded by external and internal leaf crowns (Plate 35:2). In the female, the vulva is a short distance anterior to the anus. The tail is short and pointed. The male has a symmetrical bursa and paired, equal, rodlike spicules. The cephalic vesicle (Plate 35:2), the leaf crowns, and the muscular, club-shaped esophagus can be confirmed in tissue sections, depending on the cut. Transverse striations are also evident (Plate 35:2).

In transverse sections of the worm, the body wall has a characteristic appearance (Plate 35:3). The cuticle is moderately thick, and the hypodermis is thin and almost inapparent except for the large lateral chords. Muscle cells are platymyarian and meromyarian. The contractile portion of the muscle cell is well developed, and the cytoplasmic portion is highly vacuolated. Muscle cell nuclei are infrequently seen. Usually two and sometimes three muscle cells are in each quadrant. Lateral excretory canals can be seen in the lateral chords (Plate 35:3). The esophagus is grossly muscular and has a triradiate lumen. The intestine has a round to irregular lumen and is composed of a few multinucleate cells with a conspicuous, uniform, microvillus luminal border (Plate 35:3 & 4). Reproductive tubes are present in the pseudocoelomic cavity. In male worms cut near the posterior end, the paired spicules (Plate 35:5) and copulatory bursa (Plate 35:6) are usually evident.

The oesophagostomes can be differentiated from their close relatives, *Necator* and *Ancylostoma*, by habitat and tissue preference. Grossly, they are larger than either of the hookworms, lack the large globular buccal capsule armed with teeth or cutting plates, and have the conspicuous cephalic vesicle. Additionally, the vulva in the female oesophagostome is located posteriorly. In tissue sections, these same features and characteristics may also be evident. Oesophagostomes appear to have fewer muscle cells per body quadrant and are generally less mature reproductively than the hookworm.

Mammomonogamus (Syngamiasis)

Species of *Mammomonogamus* are common parasites of the respiratory tract of ruminants in the tropics. The adult female worm may reach 2 cm in length and is attached to the mucosa in the airways. The smaller male is attached to the female in permanent copula, forming a Y shape. Approximately 80 cases of human infection have been reported. The worms typically attach to the trachea and cause a chronic cough. Diagnosis is usually made from recovery of intact worms expelled during coughing episodes or by fiberoptic bronchoscopy. Eggs of the parasite may be found in feces as well. Most infections have been reported from tropical America.

References

Barrowclough H, Crome L. Oesophagostomiasis in man. *Trop Geogr Med.* 1979;31:133-138.

Blotkamp J, Krepel HP, Kumar V, et al. Observations on the morphology of adults and larval stages of *Oesophagostomum* sp. isolated from man in northern Togo and China. *J Helminth.* 1993;67:49-61.

Correa de Lara TA, Barbosa MA, Rodriguez de Oliveira M, et al. Human syngamosis: two cases of chronic cough caused by *Mammomonogamus laryngeus. Chest.* 1993;103:264-265.

Gardiner CH, Schantz PM. *Mammomonogamus* infection in a human: report of a case. *Am J Trop Med Hyg.* 1983;32:995-997.

Krepel HP, Baeta S, Polderman AM. Human *Oesophagostomum* infection in northern Togo and Ghana: epidemiological aspects. *Ann Trop Med Parasitol.* 1992;86:289-300.

Polderman AM, Krepel HP, Baeta S, et al. Oesophagostomiasis: a common infection of man in northern Togo and Ghana. *Am J Trop Med Hyg.* 1991;44:336-344.

Plate 35

Oesophagostomum species

Image 1

Section through a typical oesophagostome nodule in the colon of an African monkey. Three portions of the parasite lie in the necrotic contents of the lesion (H&E, 10x).

Image 2

A longitudinal section through the anterior end of an *Oesophagostomum* worm in a "cyst" removed from the umbilical region of an 8-year-old Ugandan girl. The cephalic vesicle (CV), shallow buccal cavity, and muscular esophagus (ES) are seen (H&E, 145x).

Image 3

Transverse section through an immature adult *Oesophagostomum* shows typical body wall structure. Note the cuticle (darts), lateral chords (LC), lateral body (arrow), and large platymyarian muscle cells (MU) (H&E, 230x).

Image 4

A high-power view of the intestine (IN) shows its syncytial structure, multinucleate condition, and the strong microvillus border (MV) (H&E, 400x).

Image 5

Transverse section through the posterior end of a male worm. In addition to the typical body wall features, the paired spicules (darts) are visible (H&E, 240x).

Image 6

Transverse section through the bursa (BU) of a male worm (H&E, 240x).

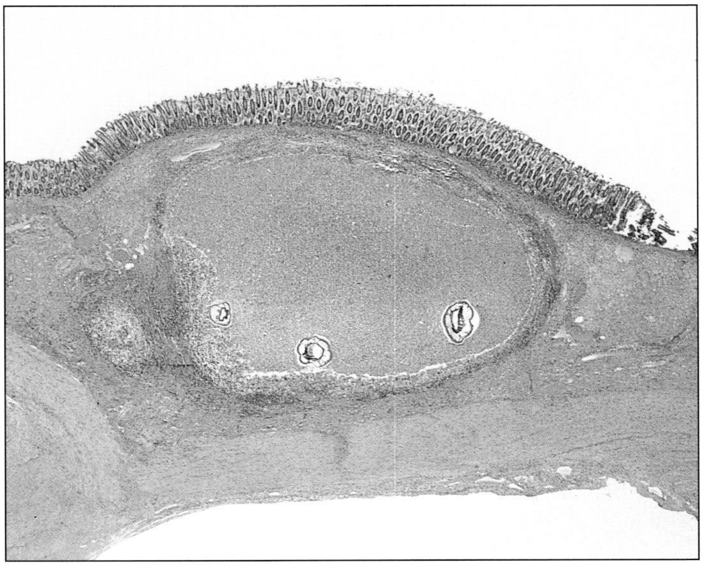

1

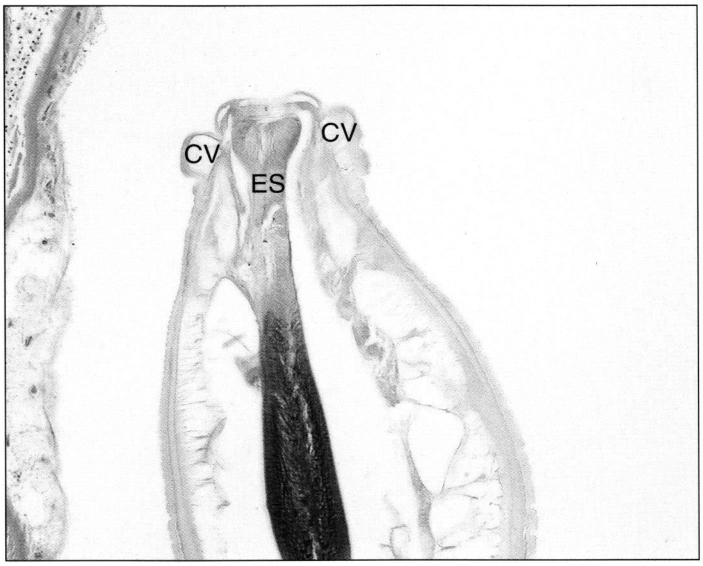

2

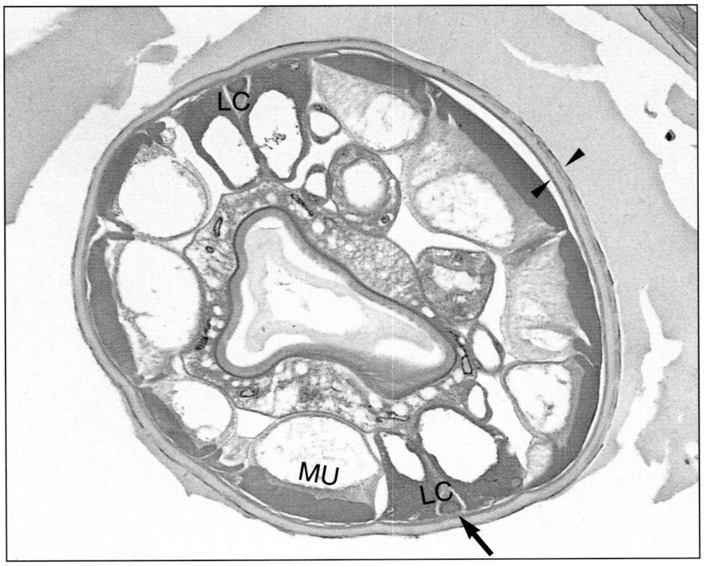

3

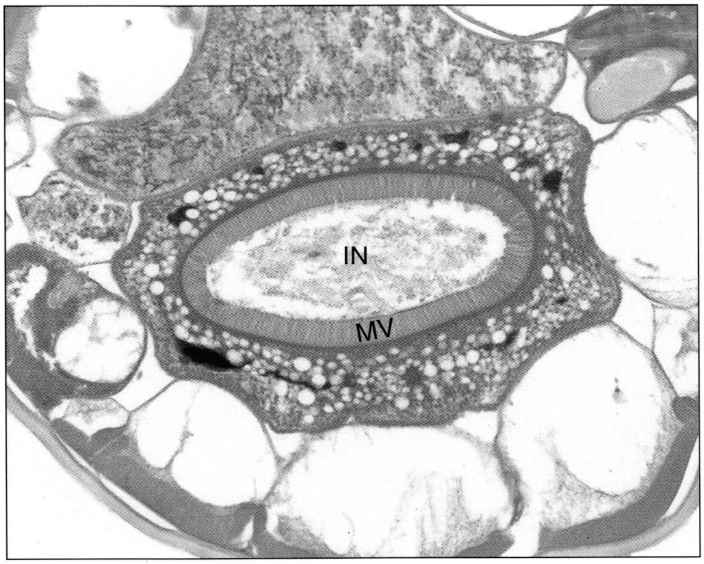

4

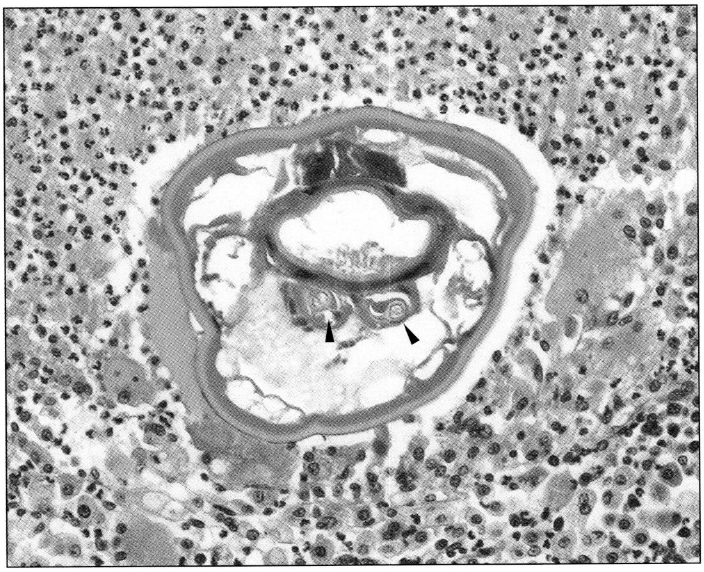

5

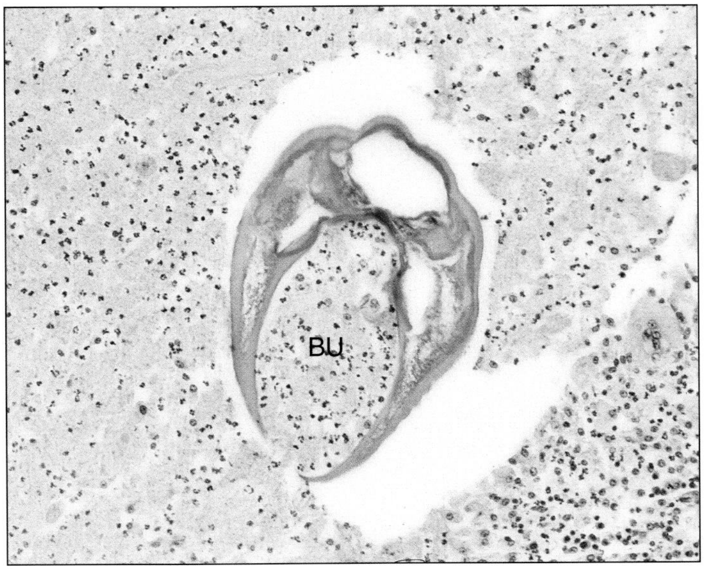

6

Angiostrongylus species

Metastrongylid nematodes are lungworms that parasitize a wide range of mammalian hosts and are economically important as disease-causing agents in domesticated animals. These bursate nematodes are related to hookworms and strongylid species. Metastrongyles do not normally parasitize humans, but two species of the genus *Angiostrongylus* are well known as significant agents of human disease. *Angiostrongylus cantonensis* causes eosinophilic meningitis or eosinophilic meningoencephalitis, and *A. costaricensis* produces abdominal angiostrongylosis. These parasites do not generally attain patency in human hosts.

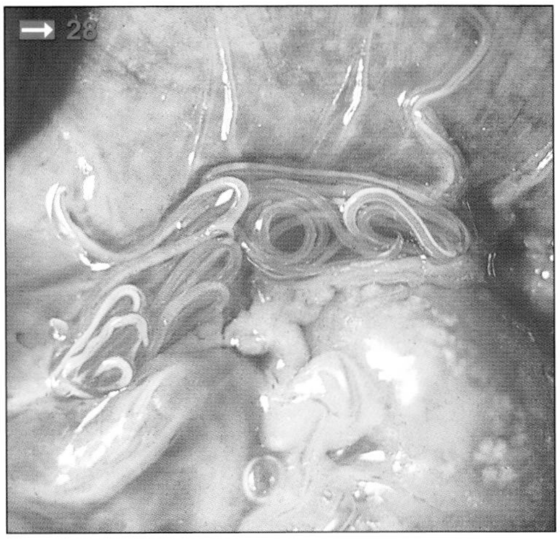

The number of geographic areas in which *A. cantonensis*, the rat lungworm, occurs appears to be expanding. Originally described from Tahiti and other Pacific islands, including Hawaii, the parasite has been reported as a major cause of human disease in Thailand and, to a lesser extent, in other parts of Asia including Taiwan, Malaysia, Vietnam, India, and Indonesia. Confirmed human cases in the Western Hemisphere have been reported from Cuba and a suspected case has been reported from Puerto Rico. In the United States, infections have been found only in rats and nonhuman primates. *Angiostrongylus costaricensis*, originally described from rodents and humans in Costa Rica, is found in Texas southward to Argentina, with cases reported from several countries in Central and South America. A single report of this parasite from Africa was based on identification of the organism in tissue sections, but adult parasites have not been reported from animals on that continent.

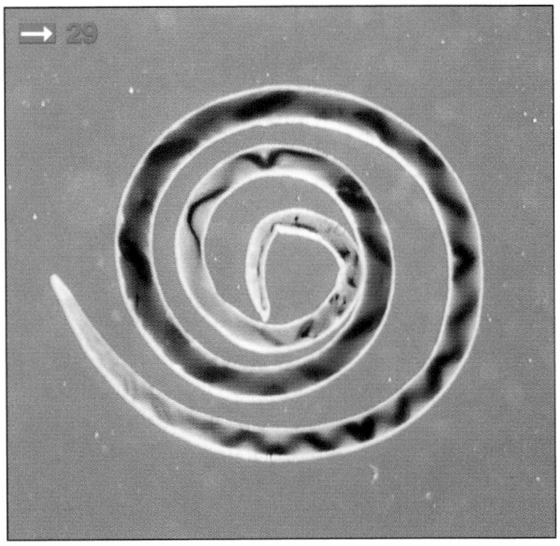

Biology and Life Cycle

Adults of *A. cantonensis* normally live in the pulmonary artery and right heart of the rodent host. Female worms discharge thin-shelled, unembryonated eggs into the bloodstream approximately five weeks after infecting the rat. These eggs are carried to the smaller blood vessels of the lung, where they lodge and begin to develop. First-stage larvae are produced by about the sixth week of infection. The larvae break out of the blood vessels, migrate into the bronchioles, and pass up into the trachea, where they are swallowed and subsequently excreted in feces. Sections of infected lung tissue demonstrate eggs in varying stages of development, larvae within eggs, and free larvae. In severe infections, rodent lung tissue may contain enormous numbers of eggs and larvae, and many larvae will be excreted. In the soil, first-stage larvae will directly penetrate or be ingested by terrestrial snails or slugs, which are the required intermediate hosts for this parasite. Development to the infective third-stage larva in the molluscan host takes approximately three weeks. The life cycle is completed when infected mollusks are ingested by rodents.

In the rodent host, larvae make an obligatory migration to the brain, where they develop to immature adults. Larvae initially develop in the parenchyma of the brain, but after 10 days they make their way to the surface of the organ where they come to lie beneath the meninges. The worms develop to immature adults and attain lengths of 1 to 2 mm in this site. Approximately one month after infection, they leave the subarachnoid space to enter the external jugular vein, travel to the heart, and move into the pulmonary artery where they reach maturity.

Angiostrongylus cantonensis makes extensive use of paratenic hosts during its life cycle, which gives it ample opportunity to infect humans through their food habits. When infected mollusks are ingested by terrestrial planarians, crabs, crayfish, fish, amphibians, reptiles, and even some mammals (in particular, calves), the third-stage larvae migrate into tissues where they await subsequent ingestion by humans or the rodent definitive host. In different geographic settings, acquisition of human infection depends on accidental ingestion of whole or partial molluscan intermediate hosts or the uncooked flesh of infected paratenic hosts.

Adult worms of *A. costaricensis* normally live in the mesenteric arteries and their branches in the intestinal wall of various rodents (➡ 28). Eggs discharged into the blood vessels embolize and embryonate in the intestinal wall. The first-stage larvae hatch, make their way to the lumen of the intestine, and are excreted in feces. Various slugs and terrestrial snails serve as the required intermediate hosts, and infective third-stage larvae develop in two to three weeks. Once rodents ingest infected mollusks, the infective larvae migrate rapidly to lymphatic vessels in the abdominal cavity, where they undergo limited development before migrating to their final location in the mesenteric arteries. Here, they develop to maturity and lay eggs approximately 24 days after infection. In humans who become accidentally infected by ingesting mollusks or paratenic hosts, larvae behave as they do in rodents (ie, by migrating to mesenteric arteries) (Plate 38:1). The parasites reach sexual maturity, mate, and the female worms lay eggs. Although these eggs may embryonate, first-stage larvae are not seen in the tissues or feces of humans.

Pathology and Clinical Manifestations

In humans, the infective-stage larvae of *A. cantonensis* behave as they do in their normal rodent host. The larvae enter the circulation, migrate to the brain, and undergo growth and development. The worms become immature adults and can attain a size similar to the size that they attain in rats. However, they may die within the brain parenchyma (Plate 37:3–6) or in the meninges during the course of the infection. These parasites rarely complete a migration to the lung in humans as they do in rats, but occasionally this does occur (Plate 36:3 & 6; Plate 37:1 & 2).

The length of time preceding the onset of meningeal symptoms in humans ranges from one day to three or more weeks. It appears to depend somewhat on the number of larvae ingested. Early clinical manifestations may include fever, vomiting, abdominal pain, flulike symptoms, and general malaise. Subsequent invasion of the brain by the larval parasite almost invariably results in a meningeal syndrome. Severe, bitemporal headache is the most prominent symptom, accompanied by nausea, vomiting, stiff neck, and an eosinophilic pleocytosis of the cerebrospinal fluid. The severe headaches may last several days or longer. A spinal tap can help determine the existence of a possible bacterial or viral etiology and provides relief from the headaches. In endemic areas where eosinophilic meningoencephalitis is well known, the combination of symptomatology and the eosinophilic pleocytosis readily suggests *A. cantonensis* infection.

Clinical manifestations appear to be directly related to the death of the larvae within the brain. In patients who become infected with few larvae, the course of the disease is self-limiting and is followed by spontaneous recovery within several weeks. In patients who ingest many larvae, disease manifestations may be more severe and prolonged, with occasional fatalities. Immunity to reinfection appears to be negligible, and individuals have had frequent recurrences of the disease after ingesting infective larvae. It is doubtful that worms live for long periods in the human brain. Based on experimental infections in nonhuman primates and other animals, the larvae may live for several weeks. In the few human cases where worms have migrated from the brain to the lung, the production of eggs has not been noted. In numerous cases, worms have migrated into the anterior or posterior chambers of the eye. These worms can be successfully removed through surgery. The use of spinal taps for diagnosing the type of meningitis has often resulted in the recovery of living immature adult worms from the cerebrospinal fluid.

Human infections of *A. costaricensis* are seen primarily in children. Symptomatology usually includes pain localized in the right flank and iliac fossa along with severe fever, anorexia, and vomiting. Physical examination frequently reveals an intra-abdominal mass, which can suggest appendicitis, malignancies, or other conditions. Eosinophilia is often prominent, reaching levels of 70% to 80% of 10,000 white blood cells. Histologically, the intestinal wall is thickened and hardened, which may result in partial or complete obstruction. Thin-shelled, unembryonated eggs are frequently seen in the intestinal wall, along with many eosinophils (Plate 38:5 & 6). Sections of adult worms may be observed in mesenteric arteries that are inflamed and thrombosed. Infections may be fatal.

Parasite Morphology

Adult worms of *A. cantonensis* from the heart and lungs of rats are usually larger than the immature adult worms seen in human tissues. In rats, adult female worms may attain sizes of 18 to 33 mm by 0.28 to 0.5 mm, whereas the immature female worms in humans probably do not exceed 12 mm in length. Adult male worms in rats measure from 15 to 25 mm by 0.25 to 0.35 mm, and the immature male worms in humans measure up to 11 mm. The cuticle of the female worm is smooth and transparent. The female's most prominent feature is the barber-pole-like appearance of its body, which is attributable to the milky-white, paired uterine branches that wind around the dark intestine in spirals (⇨ 29). The vagina is situated near the posterior end, slightly anterior to the anal opening. Male worms have a transparent cuticle, similar to that in females, through which slender, 1-mm spicules are readily visible. Males also have a well-developed bursa.

Adult females of *A. costaricensis* are similar in morphology to those of *A. cantonensis*, including the barber-pole-like appearance, but they may reach sizes of 40 to 45 mm by 0.13 to 0.35 mm. Males are similar in size to those of *A. cantonensis*, but their spicules are less than half the length, 0.31 to 0.38 mm long.

In sections of tissue, the cuticle of the immature adult *A. cantonensis* is thin (3 to 5 μm) and is either smooth or has fine transverse striations. Musculature is polymyarian and coelomyarian. Lateral chords are prominent, dome shaped, and usually taller than the adjacent muscle cells (Plate 36:5 & 6; Plate 37:2). The intestinal cells are few and multinucleated. With H&E stain, the nuclei are blue-purple with yellow granules in the cells, giving the metastrongylid intestine a distinctive appearance (Plate 37:2).

The histologic appearance of *A. costaricensis* adult worms in human tissues is similar to that of *A. cantonensis.* In humans, *A. cantonensis* is generally found within the brain and, less commonly, in the lung. The adults of *A. costaricensis*, by contrast, are found within the branches of the mesenteric arteries (Plate 38:1). It is also common to find the thin-shelled, unembryonated eggs of *A. costaricensis* within the wall of the intestine (Plate 38:5 & 6). The eggs of *A. cantonensis* have not been found in human tissues.

The presence of large, immature adult nematodes in the human central nervous system and brain is infrequent. In Thailand, not only *A. cantonensis* but also species of *Gnathostoma* may be found in humans. The morphologic appearance of *Angiostrongylus* and *Gnathostoma* in section is sufficiently distinct that it should not pose a diagnostic problem. However, *A. costaricensis* in the intestinal wall, especially when the nematode has died and undergone degenerative changes, may be difficult to distinguish from anisakids or other large nematodes that often invade the intestinal wall.

References

Cespedes R, Salas J, Mekbel S, et al. Granulomas entéricos y linfáticos con intensa eosinofilia tisular producidos por un estrongilideo (Strongylata), I: patología. *Acta Med Cost.* 1967;10:235-255.

Gardiner CH, Wells S, Gutter AE, et al. Eosinophilic meningoencephalitis due to *Angiostrongylus cantonensis* as the cause of death in captive nonhuman primates. *Am J Trop Med Hyg.* 1990;42:70-74.

Mackerras MJ, Sandars DF. The life history of the rat lungworm, *Angiostrongylus cantonensis* (Chen) (Nematoda: Metastrongylidae). *Austral J Zool.* 1956;3:1-21.

Morera P. Granulomas entéricos y linfáticos con intensa eosinofilia tisular producidos por un estrongilideo (Strongylata; Railliet y Henry, 1913), II: aspecto parasitológico (nota previa). *Acta Med Cost.* 1967;10:257-265.

Morera P. Life history and redescription of *Angiostrongylus costaricensis* Morera and Cespedes, 1971. *Am J Trop Med Hyg.* 1971;22:613-621.

Otsuru M. *Angiostrongylus cantonensis* and angiostrongyliasis in Japan, with those of neighboring Taiwan. *Prog Med Parasitol.* 1978;6:225-274.

Vazquez AJ, Boils PL, Sola JJ, et al. Angiostrongyliasis in a European patient: a rare cause of gangrenous ischemic enterocolitis. *Gastroenterology.* 1993;105:1544-1549.

Plate 36

Angiostrongylus cantonensis

Image 1

Section through the pulmonary artery of a rat infected with lungworms. Male and female worms are seen in transverse section. The larger transverse sections are female, and the smaller ones with single reproductive tubes are male. The surrounding lung tissue is filled with eggs and larvae of the parasite. An intense host response is evident (H&E, 35x).

Image 2

At higher magnification, the typical morphologic features of the cuticle, musculature, lateral chords (LC), intestine (IN), and single reproductive tube (RT) are visible in a transverse section of a male worm. The lateral chords are domelike, with only a single nucleus in each (H&E, 180x).

Image 3

Immature adult worms in a section of lung from a Taiwanese child. Migration to the lung is not a common feature of human infections with this parasite. No eggs or larvae can be seen in the surrounding lung parenchyma (H&E, 20x).

Image 4

From the same case, a thrombosed pulmonary artery shows several sections of immature adult female worms. Note the paired reproductive tubes. No eggs or larvae can be seen in the surrounding lung parenchyma (H&E, 50x).

Image 5

At higher magnification, a transverse section of an immature adult female worm is seen. The intestine (IN) is syncytial with nuclei scattered in the cytoplasm. Note the domelike lateral chords (darts) (H&E, 240x).

Image 6

At higher magnification of another transverse section, another immature adult female worm is shown. The lateral chords are characteristically domelike, the intestine (IN) appears to be syncytial, and the reproductive tubes contain developing eggs (H&E, 240x).

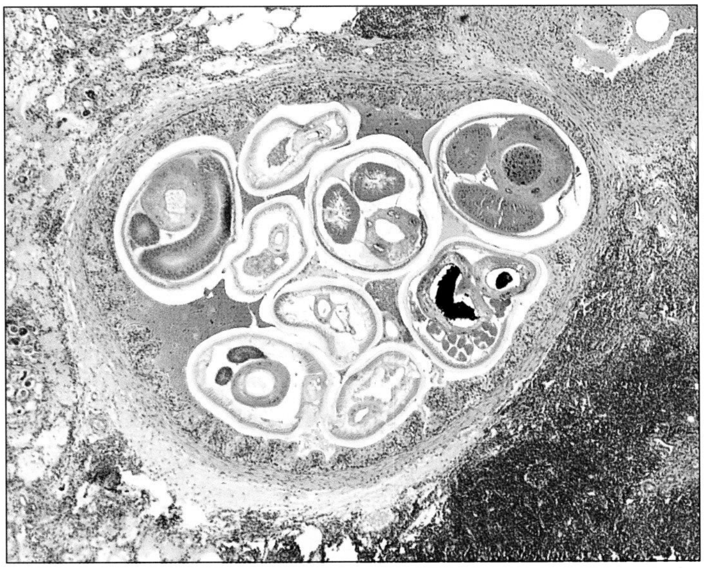
1

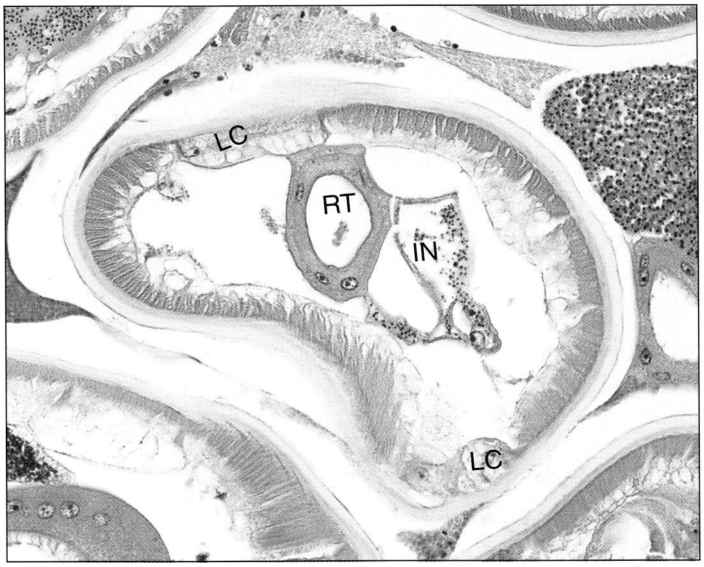

2

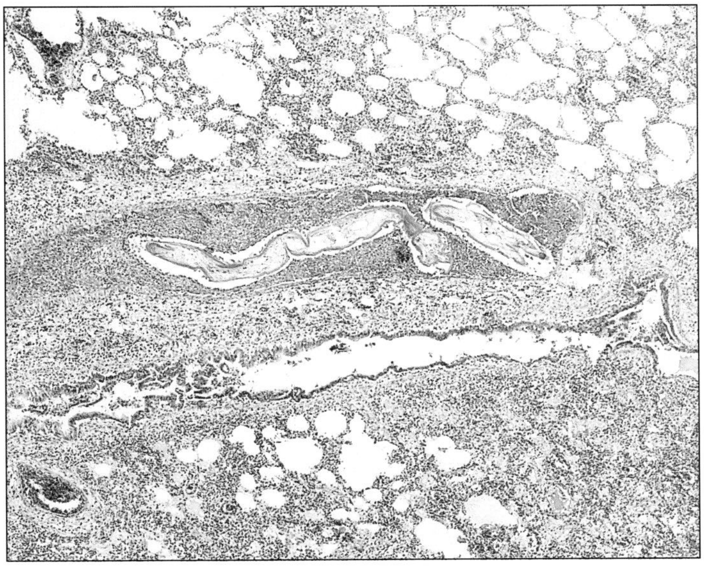
3

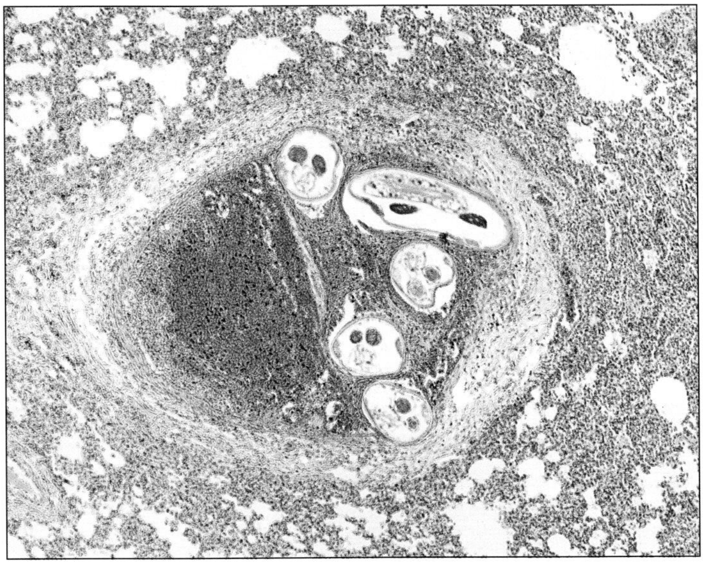
4

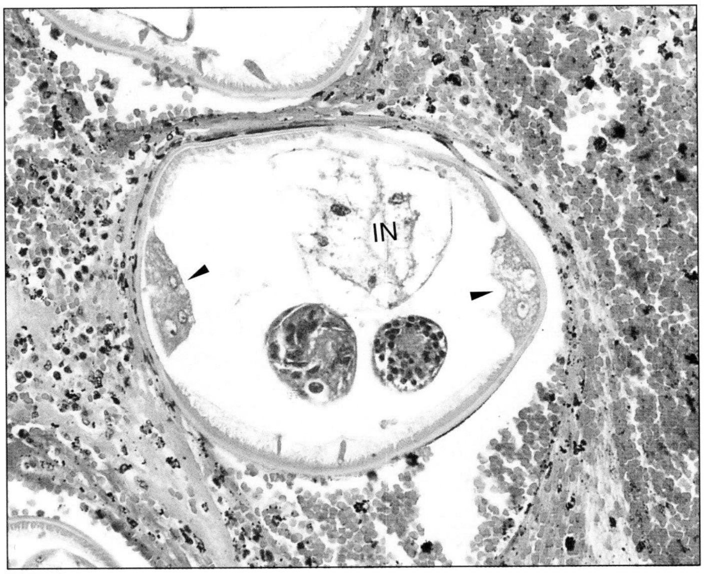

5

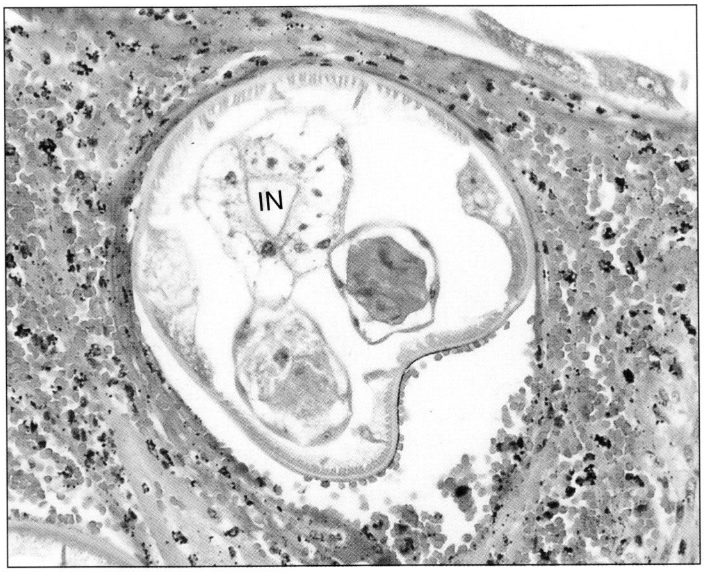

6

Plate 37

Angiostrongylus cantonensis

Image 1

Section of lung from a Taiwanese child (fatal case). Three sections of immature adult worms are seen within a branch of the pulmonary artery. At this magnification, the worms are difficult to diagnose as anything other than nematodes (H&E, 50x).

Image 2

A single section of an immature adult female worm in a different branch of the pulmonary artery. The intestine (dart) has all the characteristics of a metastrongylid intestine. Each cell has a single nucleus. The lateral chords (arrows) are evident but not prominent. The reproductive tubules are those of a female worm (H&E, 240x).

Image 3

Eosinophilic meningitis in a Thai woman (fatal case). A section of parasite can be seen in the midst of an abscess in the brain. Although the worm is visible, an identification cannot be made at this magnification. (H&E, 200x).

Image 4

At higher magnification, both lateral chords (darts) can be seen. The intestine is located in the middle of the section (H&E, 750x).

Image 5

A section of worm is seen in a brain abscess caused by a rat lungworm (fatal human case). At this magnification, it is difficult to make a specific identification (H&E, 125x).

Image 6

A dead and degenerated immature adult worm of *A. cantonensis,* from the first human case reported. All internal structures have been destroyed. Only remnants of the cuticle with surrounding inflammatory cells are visible. Identification of the parasite was made from intact worms recovered from the brain (H&E, 125x).

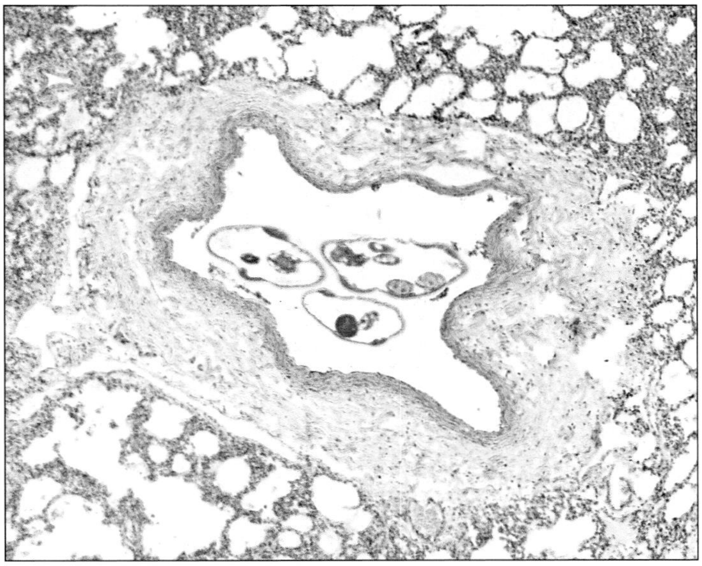
1

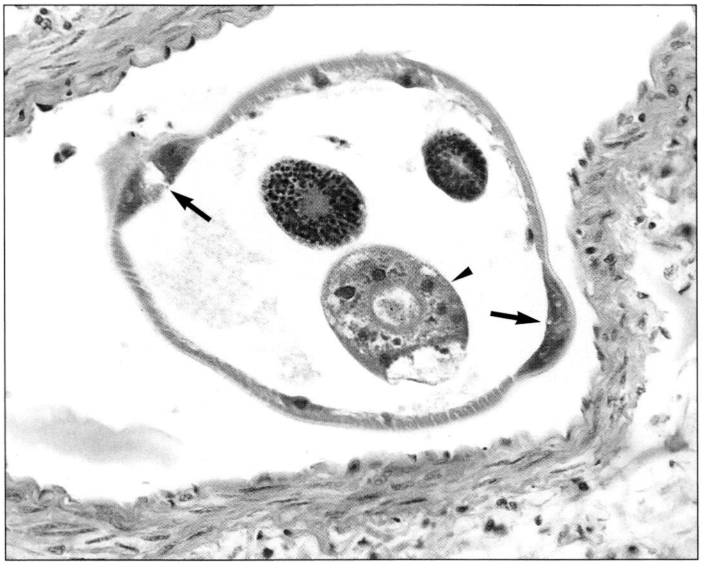
2

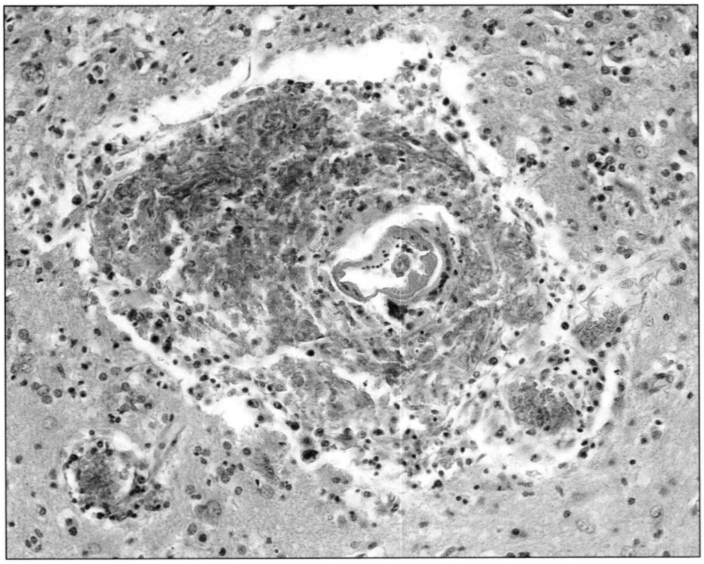
3

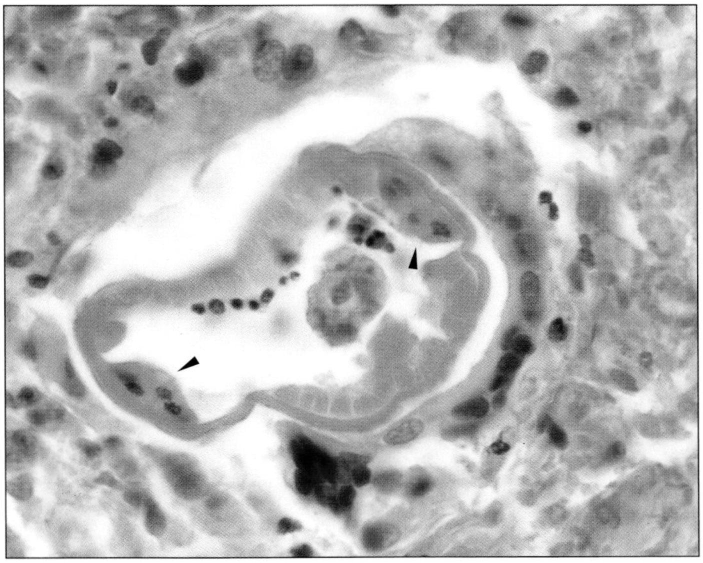
4

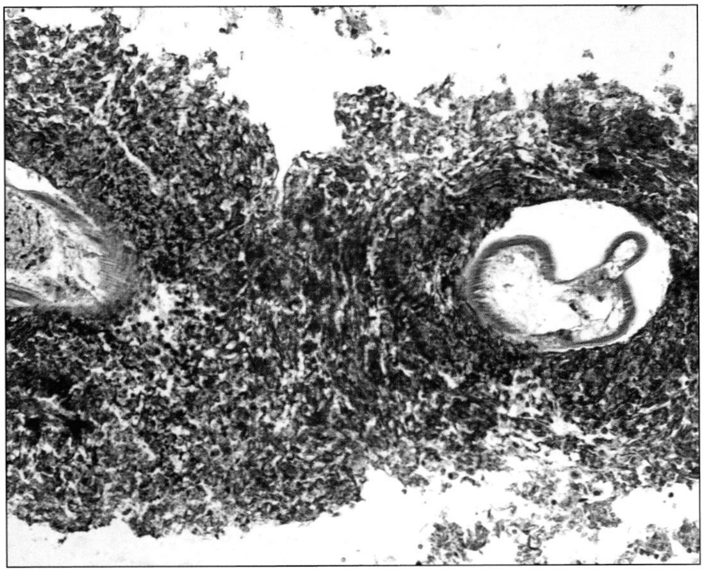
5

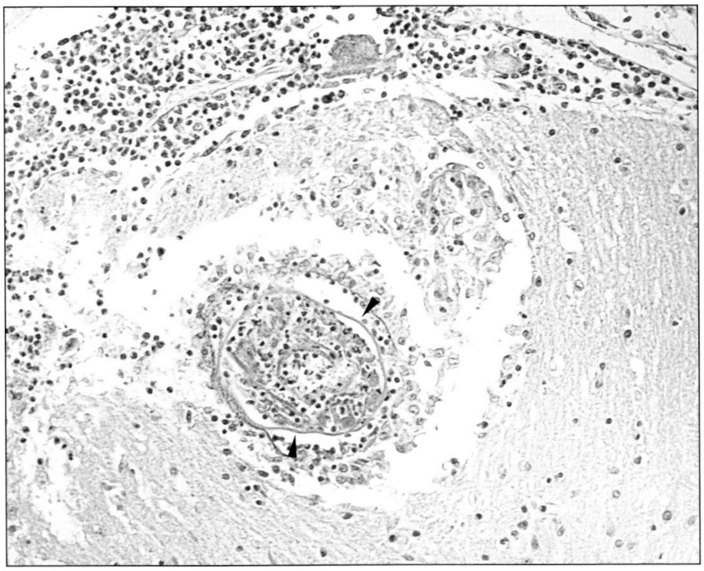
6

Plate 38

Angiostrongylus costaricensis

Image 1

Two sections of an adult worm are seen in this small artery in the intestinal wall of a Costa Rican. The size of the intestine differs according to the level in the body at which the section occurs (H&E, 100x).

Image 2

At higher magnification, the reproductive tubes of this female worm are more clearly seen. The lateral chords are not visible because they have been compressed by the intestine and reproductive structures. In general, however, the lateral chords are not as prominent in *A. costaricensis* as they are in *A. cantonensis* (H&E, 200x).

Image 3

Two sections of an adult worm are visible within a lymph node in the ileocecal region of a Costa Rican. Considerable inflammation surrounds the parasite (H&E, 65x).

Image 4

At higher magnification, one can see a single reproductive tube (RT) and the intestine (IN) of the male worm. One of the lateral chords is near the intestine; it is compressed and barely recognizable (dart) (H&E, 200x).

Image 5

One of the most characteristic findings in human *A. costaricensis* infections is the presence of thin-shelled eggs (darts) within the wall of the intestine or appendix. In this instance, the shells cannot be distinguished, but the unsegmented ova are surrounded by clear spaces (H&E, 250x).

Image 6

At higher magnification, the undeveloped eggs are more clearly seen. A considerable number of eosinophils are present in the surrounding tissue (H&E, 500x).

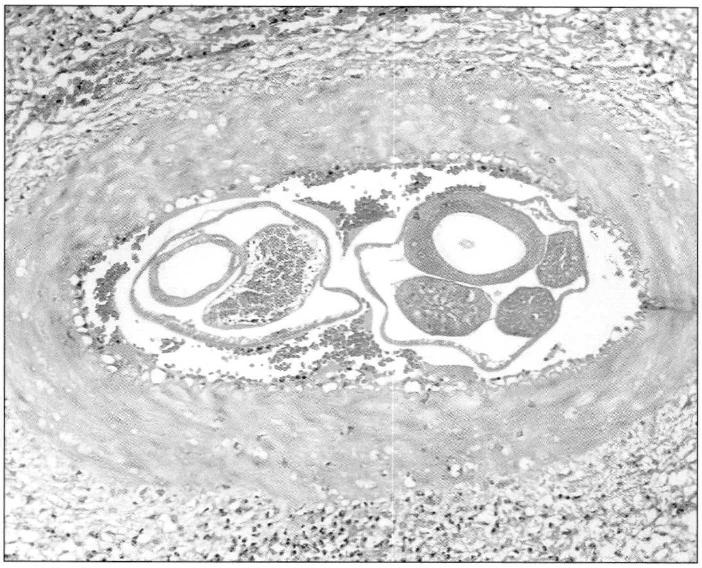

1

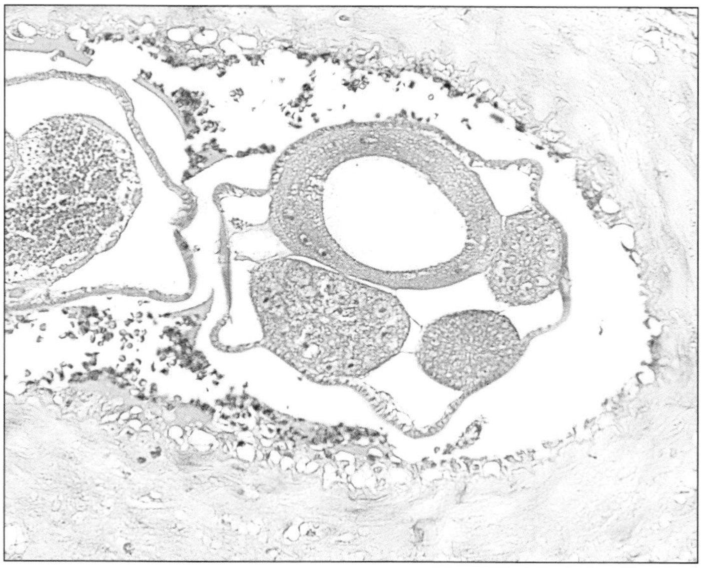

2

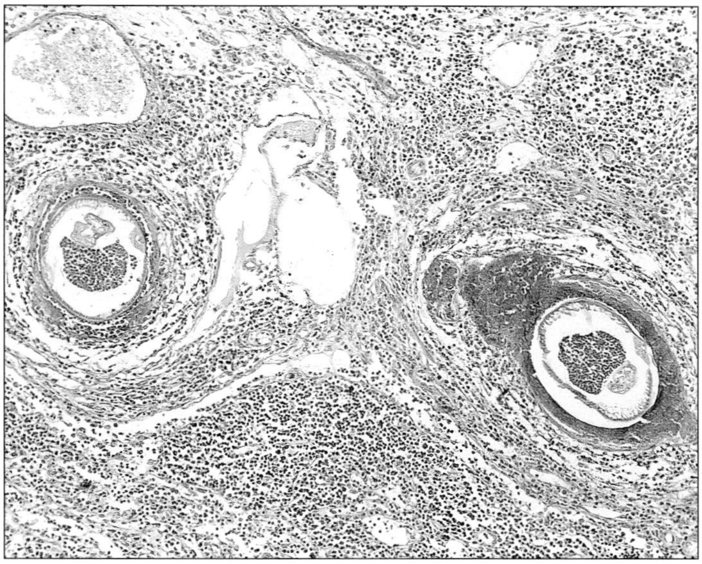

3

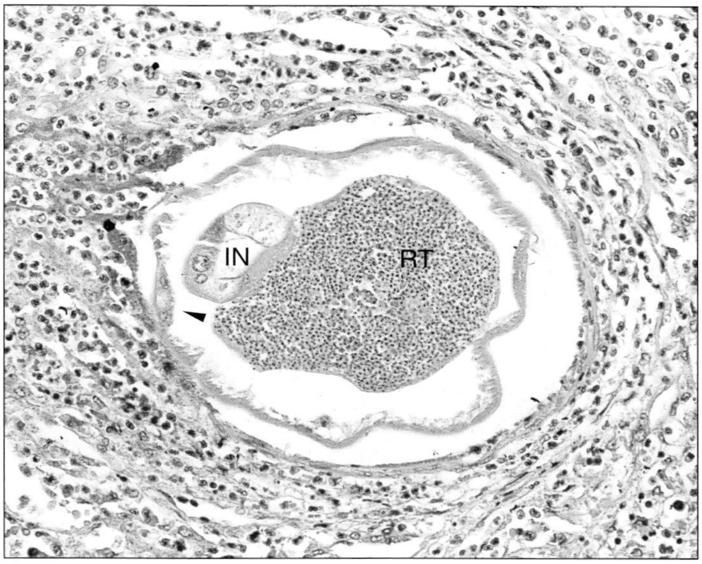

4

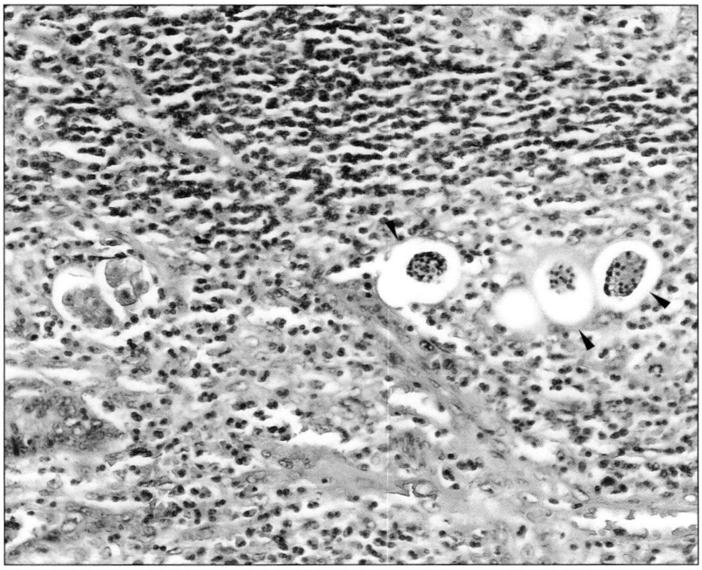

5

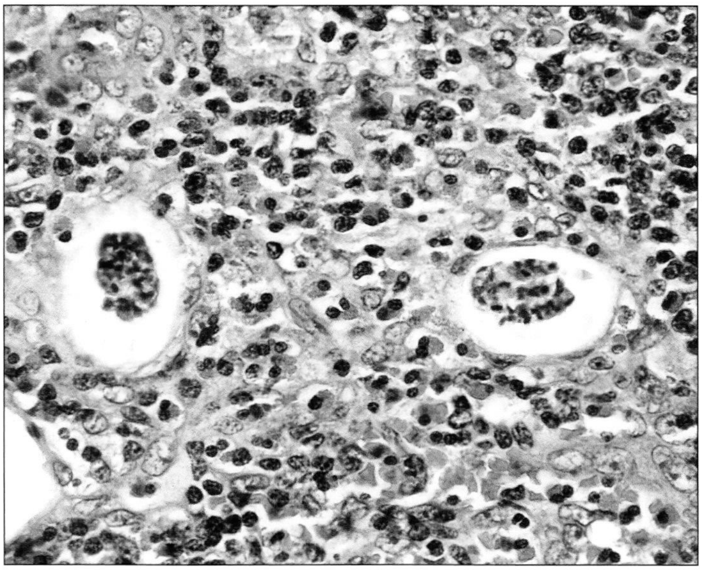

6

Gnathostoma species

The gnathostomes are spiruroid nematodes that parasitize a wide range of carnivorous and other mammals, including dogs, cats, and swine, and especially animals that feed on fish and cold-blooded vertebrates, including raccoons, opossums, and otters. Human infections with *Gnathostoma* species invariably involve larval stages of the parasite, which undergo extraintestinal migrations and produce a visceral larva migrans. Human infections are especially common in Southeast Asia and Japan, but cases have been reported from the Western Hemisphere as well, particularly in Mexico and Ecuador.

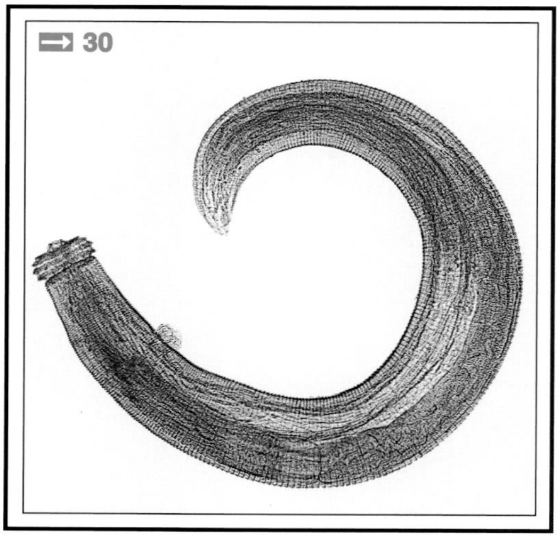

Biology and Life Cycle

In their natural hosts the adult worms are typically embedded in the gastric mucosa, where they produce a nodular tumor. Females produce a characteristic egg, which has a pluglike cap at one or both poles, depending on the species. The eggs have a roughened brown shell and contain an unsegmented ovum. They are elliptical and measure up to 80 µm in length depending on the species. Eggs discharged in feces embryonate in water and develop to the first larval stage. After hatching, the larvae are ingested by a first intermediate host, a copepod, in which they develop in the hemocoel to the third (infective) stage. Thereafter, the larvae in the infected copepod may be ingested by a variety of fish or amphibians, which serve as second intermediate hosts, and subsequently by reptiles, birds, and mammals, which become paratenic hosts. In definitive hosts other than natural ones, the larvae are unable to develop to maturity and simply wander through the tissues, where they may encyst and remain alive and infective (Plate 39:1).

Humans are infected by ingesting the raw or inadequately cooked flesh of one of the intermediate or paratenic hosts or even a copepod. The ingested larvae then migrate through the tissues, usually superficially, and invade the orbit, the eye itself, or the central nervous system. Four species, *G. spinigerum, G. hispidum, G. doloresi,* and *G. nipponicum,* have been recovered from human tissues, usually as advanced third-stage larvae. *Gnathostoma spinigerum,* which matures in cats and dogs, is the most important species causing human disease. On rare occasions, adult *G. spinigerum* worms have been recovered from humans but never from the stomach.

Pathology and Clinical Manifestations

After ingestion by the human host, larvae migrate from the intestine to the liver and on to muscular and subcutaneous tissues. The brief sojourn in the liver often causes anorexia, vomiting, abdominal pain and discomfort, and fever. Migration through the deep tissues may cause brief, sharp pains. Symptoms often mimic appendicitis, cholecystitis, cystitis, etc. Larvae reach the muscles and subcutaneous tissues after two to four weeks. During this chronic phase, which can last for many months, periodic migratory, subcutaneous swellings may occur. Pruritic but otherwise painless reddened swellings are typical. The stationary parasite, on the other hand, provokes an intense inflammatory reaction. Invasion of the central nervous system, which is extremely serious, is common, particularly in Thailand. It may produce neuritis, meningitis, or encephalitis with bizarre symptomatology and is often fatal.

The larvae and attendant symptoms may persist for many months. Diagnosis is frequently based on clinical presentation (ie, history of eating raw fish with subsequent subcutaneous migratory swellings in geographic areas where the parasitosis is endemic). Successfully removing the worm from the tissues is therapeutic and also allows for specific identification of the parasite.

Parasite Morphology

Although worms are not usually recovered from human tissues, they are robust. Females measure up to 4.0 cm in length; males are somewhat smaller. Their head bulb is set off from the rest of the body and is covered with 10 to 12 rows of recurved hooklets. Leaflike spines also cover all or part of the body depending on the species. The head bulb and spination as well as the size of this parasite make it readily distinguishable from other parasites that inhabit human tissues.

Advanced third-stage larvae from human tissues resemble the adult parasite in their gross morphologic features (⇨ 30). They measure up to 5.0 mm in length, on average, but lengths up to 12.5 mm have been reported. In addition to the head bulb, which usually has four rows of hooklets, the long, club-shaped esophagus and thick, tubular intestine with its irregular lumen can be seen through the semitransparent body wall of the intact larva (⇨ 30). Four cervical sacs in the anterior end control inflation of the head bulb, but these are not readily discernible through the body wall. The reproductive system has not yet begun its development.

In transverse sections, the body wall is relatively thin. Depending on the level of the body, the cuticle bears rows of spines (Plate 39:3). The hypodermis is thin and hardly discernible, except for the voluminous lateral chords that tend to fill the available space in the pseudocoelom (Plate 40:1–5). Few hypodermal nuclei are seen in most sections, and they appear to be randomly distributed in the cytoplasm of the chords. Because of the inapparent dorsal and ventral chords, the muscles appear to be divided into two bands rather than quadrants. The individual muscle cell is of the coelomyarian type, with the cytoplasmic portion of the cell typically taller than the contractile portion (Plate 40:4–6). Between 22 and 30 muscle cells are in each hemisphere. The esophagus is fairly round in cross-section, has a triradiate lumen, and is divided into a shorter, muscular, anterior portion (Plate 39:2) and a longer, glandular, posterior portion, which is of greater diameter (Plate 40:4). The intestine and its lumen vary in shape (Plate 40:5 & 6). The intestinal epithelium is made up of approximately 18 to 31 cells, which are more or less cuboidal and have a luminal border covered with microvilli. The number of nuclei varies according to the species (Plate 40:5 & 6). In the species recovered from humans, *G. spinigerum* has in transverse sections an average of 3 to 7 nuclei per intestinal cell; *G. hispidum* usually 1; *G. doloresi* usually 2; and *G. nipponicum* usually 1 (Plate 40:2, 3, 5, & 6). In fourth-stage larvae and in immature and mature adults, the intestinal lumen may vary in shape. The epithelial cells range from cuboidal to tall columnar cells, producing the irregular shape of the lumen. Pigmented granules are found in the cytoplasm (Plate 39:5 & 6).

The size of the gnathostomes, their tissue preferences, migratory behavior, and morphologic features, which include the head bulb, spination, and intestinal architecture, make identification and speciation straightforward. It is unlikely that the gnathostomes would be confused with any other parasites found in human tissues.

References

Akahane H, Lamothe-Argumendo R, Martinez-Cruz JM, et al. A morphological observation of the advanced third-stage larvae of Mexican *Gnathostoma*. *Jpn J Parasitol.* 1994;43:18-22.

Akahane H, Sano M, Mako T. Morphological differences in cross-sections of the advanced third-stage larvae of *Gnathostoma spinigerum*, *G. hispidum* and *G. doloresi*. *Jpn J Parasitol.* 1986;35:465-467.

Kagei N. Morphological identification of parasites in biopsied specimens from creeping disease lesions. *Jpn J Parasitol.* 1991;40:437-445.

Rusnak JM, Lucy DR. Clinical gnathostomiasis: case report and review of English-language literature. *Clin Infect Dis.* 1993;16:33-50.

Gnathostoma species

Image 1

A low-power view of a subcutaneous lesion removed from the abdominal wall of a 13-year-old Mexican boy living in southern California. The boy presented with a history of migratory lesions on the right arm, shoulder, and abdomen, and, ultimately, a nodule on the abdominal wall. Four sections are seen through a nematode parasite (H&E, 125x).

Image 2

High magnification of one of the sections of parasite, which is cut through the muscular esophagus (ES). The most conspicuous structures are the large lateral chords (LC) and the four tubes that represent the ballonets/cervical sacs (CS), which are characteristic of *Gnathostoma* species. Small spines on the surface of the cuticle are also visible (H&E, 500x).

Image 3

Higher magnification of the section cut at the level of the glandular esophagus (ES), shows spines on the surface of the cuticle (darts) (H&E, 750x).

Image 4

Transverse section through the body at the level of the intestine (IN). Note the structure of the intestinal epithelium, which has a few to several nuclei per cell, and the microvillus border of the cells (H&E, 750x).

Image 5

Transverse section through the midbody of a *Gnathostoma*. Tissue was resected from the colon wall of a Laotian. The worm is immature (H&E, 55x).

Image 6

A high-power view of the same parasite shows the thick cuticle, the moderately large lateral chords with numerous nuclei (LC), and the coelomyarian muscles. The intestine has epithelial cells of different heights, which contributes to the irregular shape of the lumen. The intestinal cells also contain significant amounts of pigmented granular material. Note the genital tubes (darts), shown here in an early stage of development. (H&E, 130x).

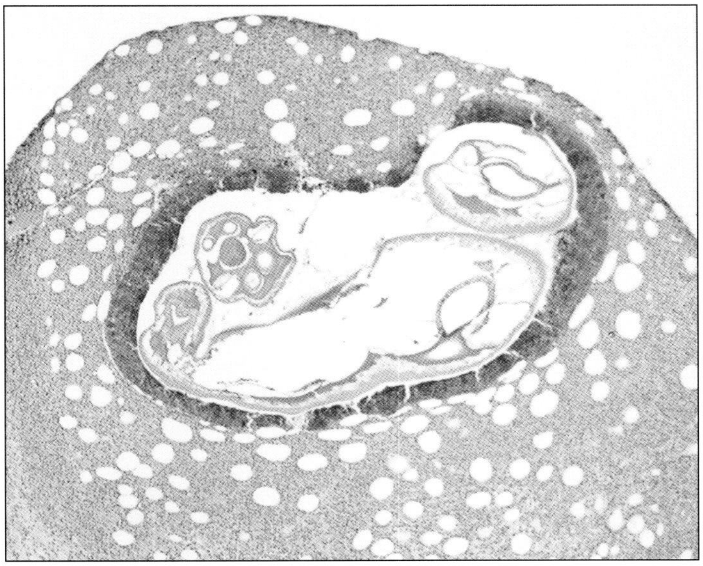

1

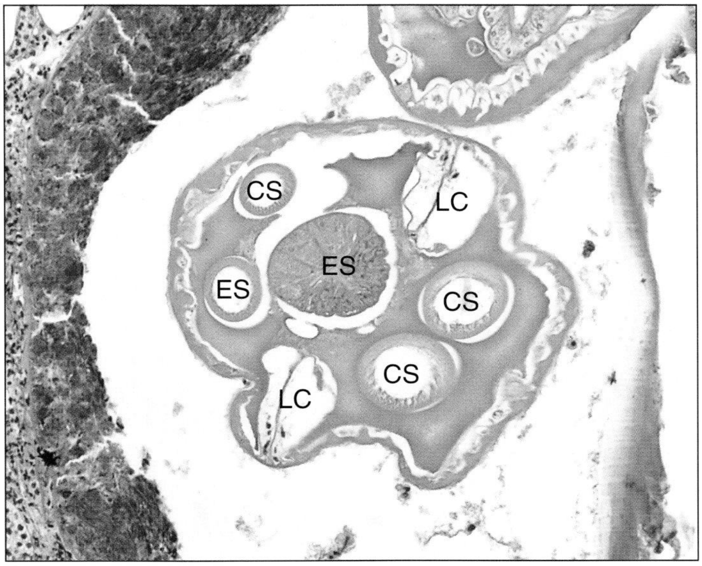

2

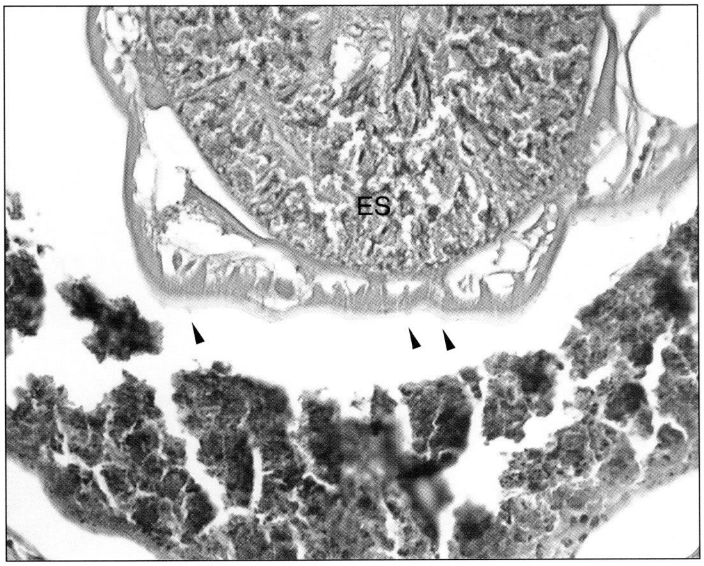

3

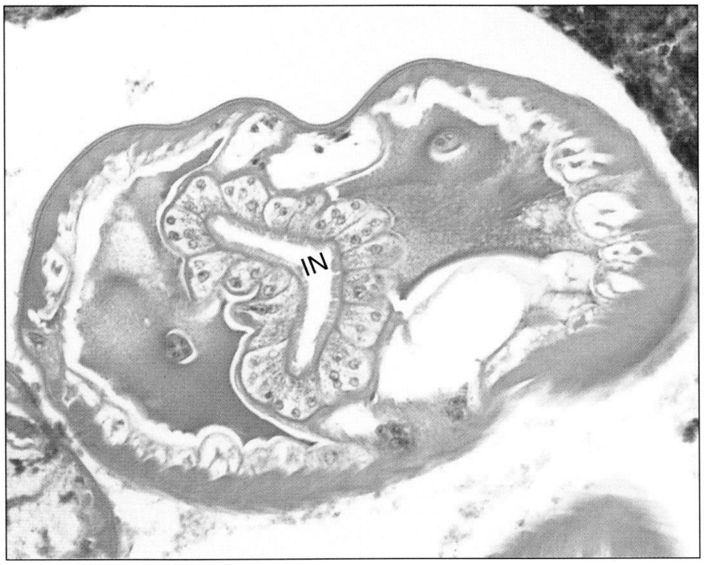

4

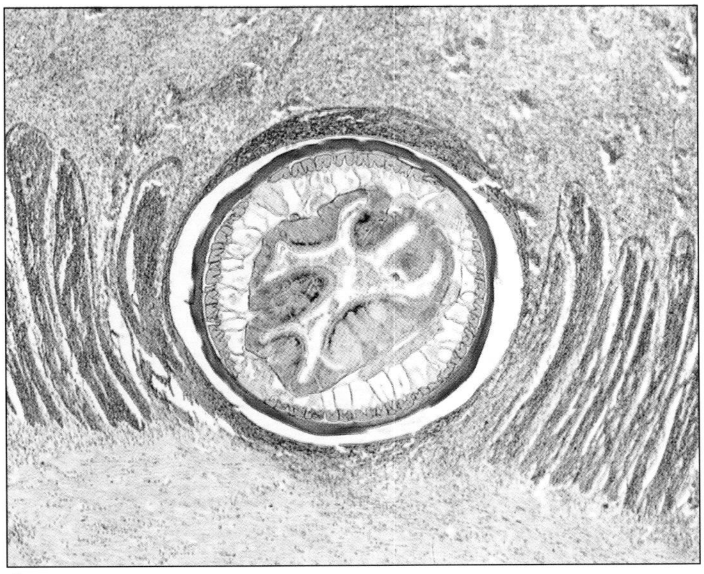

5

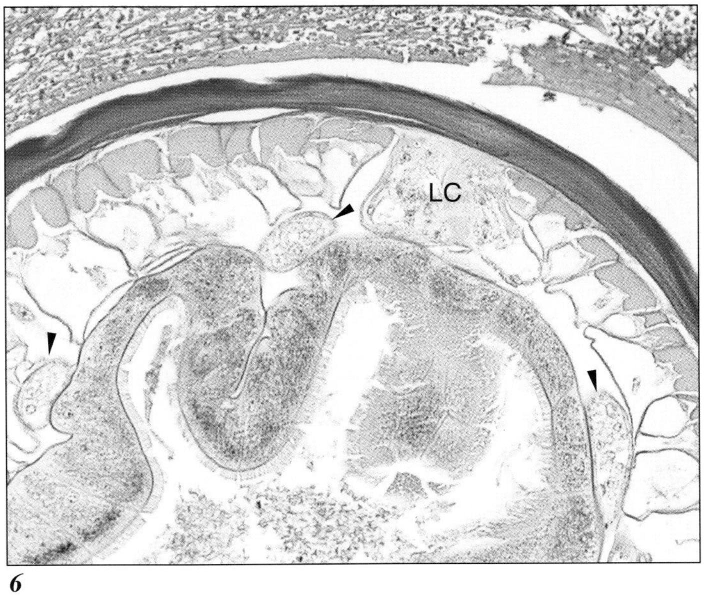

6

Plate 40

***Gnathostoma* species**

Image 1

Transverse sections of a larval *Gnathostoma spinigerum* encysted in the muscles of an intermediate host, a freshwater eel (H&E, 100x).

Image 2

At higher magnification, the esophagus (ES) and the four cervical sacs (darts) are seen. The cervical sacs are diagnostic for *Gnathostoma* species. In the other section, the voluminous lateral chords (LC) stand out. The intestinal wall is made up of cuboidal cells with microvilli on the luminal borders; the individual cells contain a few to several nuclei each (H&E, 200x).

Image 3

Note the large lateral chords (LC) in transverse sections of a larval *G. hispidum* encysted in the muscles of an intermediate host (H&E, 100x).

Image 4

At high magnification, note the glandular region of the esophagus (ES) with its triradiate lumen and the voluminous lateral chords (LC) in which hypodermal nuclei are dispersed throughout the cytoplasm (H&E, 200x).

Image 5

Transverse section through the intestinal region of *G. hispidum* shows the intestinal epithelium and the small number of nuclei (1 or 2) visible within each cell. This feature assists in the specific identification of the parasite (H&E, 200x).

Image 6

Transverse section through larval *G. doloresi* shows the intestinal epithelium. Note the lateral chords and the presence of 0 to 2 nuclei per intestinal cell (H&E, 200x).

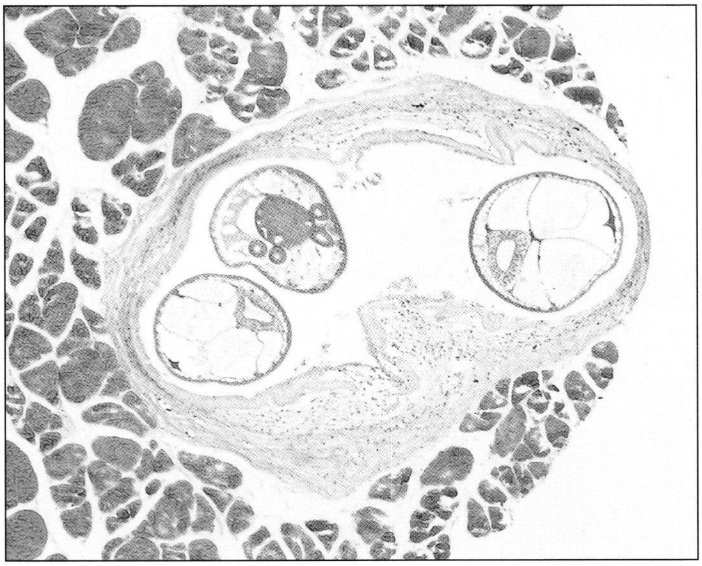

1

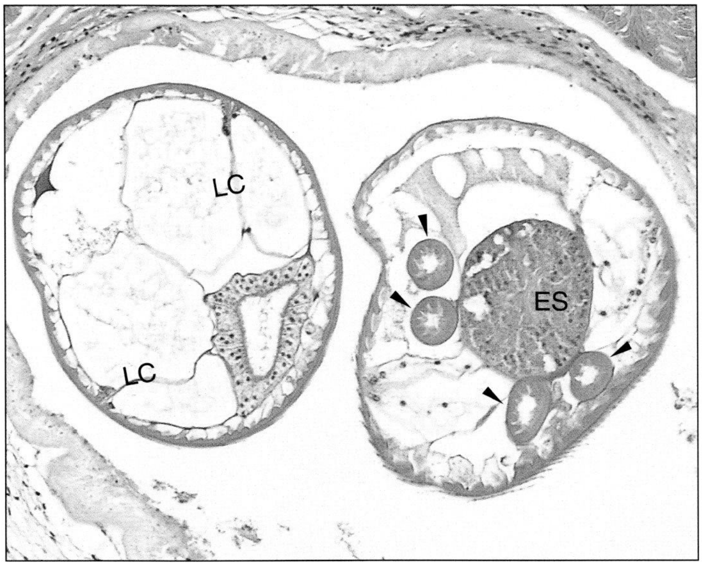

2

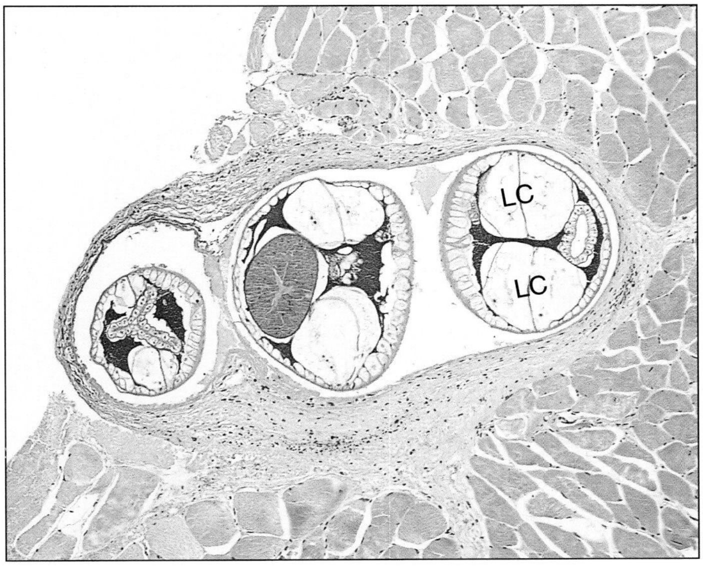

3

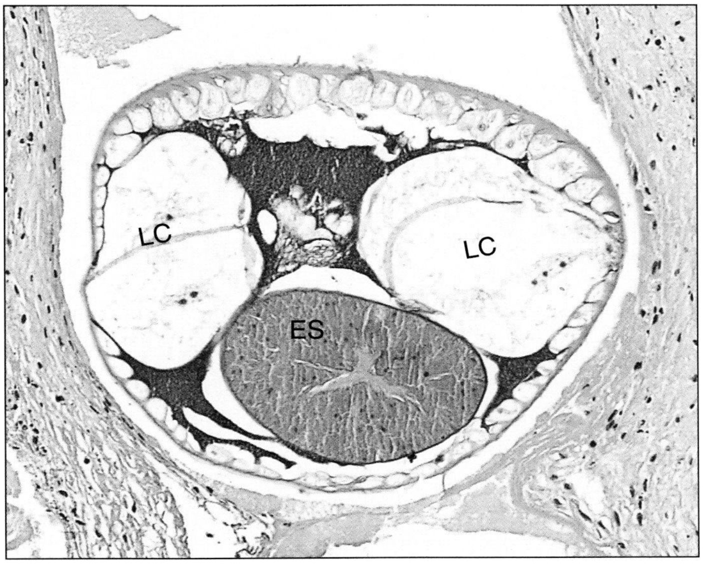

4

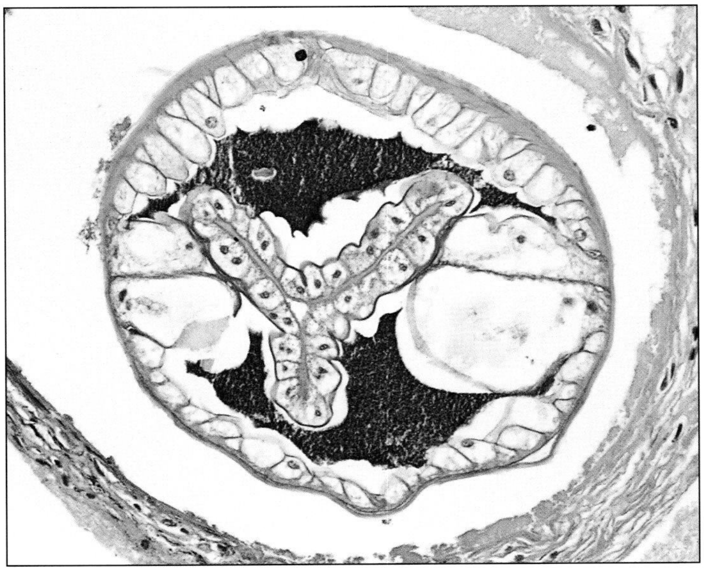

5

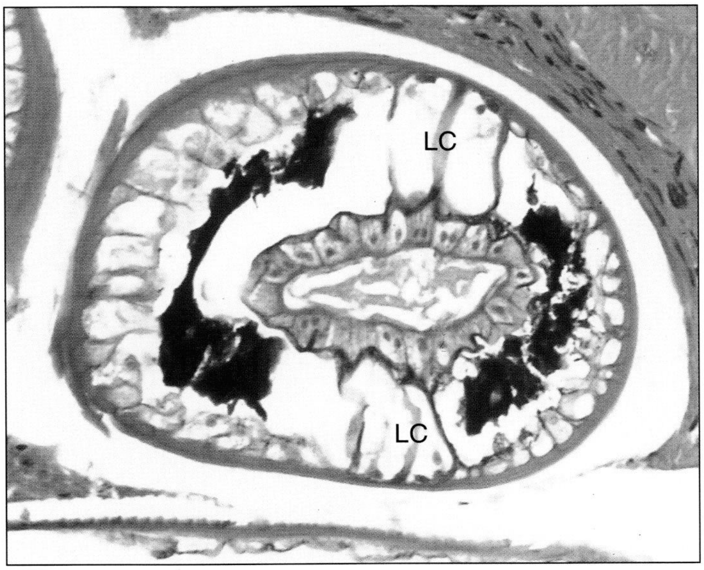

6

Gongylonema species

Species of *Gongylonema* are natural parasites of birds and mammals worldwide. More than 30 species have been described, the majority from ruminants, pigs, horses, and monkeys, as well as other animals and occasionally humans.

Biology and Life Cycle

In their natural hosts the adult worms are found in burrows in the mucosal lining of the esophagus and rumen. The female worm discharges eggs into these burrows. The eggs are eventually carried into the fecal stream as the superficial mucosal layers are sloughed, broken down in the digestive process, and ultimately discharged in feces. The eggs have a thick, transparent shell, measure about 60 by 40 µm, and contain a larva (➡ 31). Coprophagous insects such as dung beetles and cockroaches serve as intermediate hosts. Natural definitive hosts and accidental human hosts become infected by ingesting these insects. The infective larvae, encapsulated in insect tissues, are freed in the digestive process and migrate to their final destination, probably via the mucosal lining of stomach and esophagus. In humans, the worms are usually found in the mucosa and submucosa of the oral cavity. Although only about 40 human cases have been described, they have been reported from all parts of the world.

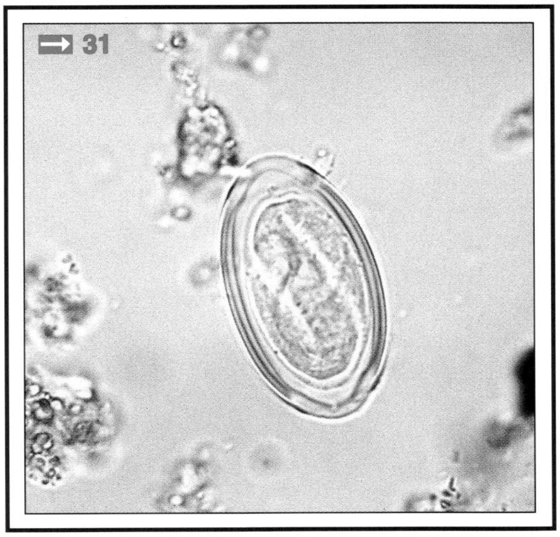

Pathology and Clinical Manifestations

Symptoms in human infections range from local irritation of tissues to a more severe stomatitis and pharyngitis caused by the active migration of the worms through the burrows in the mucosa. Patients sometimes indicate an awareness of something present and moving in the mucosa. In at least one instance, esophagostomy revealed some erosion of esophageal mucosa with oozing of blood from the lesion. Most human infections involve the lip, gums, palate, tonsils, and, rarely, the esophagus. Worms have been removed intact or have been identified along with eggs in tissue biopsy specimens.

Parasite Morphology

Gongylonema pulchrum, a common parasite in ruminants, pigs, and other animals, is generally regarded as the species most frequently seen in human infections, although this is not a certainty. The adult worms are long and slender. Females reach almost 15 cm in length (in natural hosts) with a diameter of up to 0.5 mm; males are less than one half that size (6.2 x 0.3 mm). Worms recovered from humans have been much smaller. In the male, large asymmetrical caudal alae are supported by large, paired papillae. The male also possesses long, paired dissimilar spicules. In the female, the vulva is postequatorial, usually positioned slightly anterior to the anus. In the gravid female, the reproductive tubes are filled with the typical, thick-shelled eggs that contain developing larvae. The esophagus in both sexes is long and typically divided into a short, muscular, anterior portion and a longer, glandular, posterior region. All of these features are easily recognized in transverse sections of the parasite.

In infected tissues, the burrows in the mucosa often contain typical eggs (Plate 41:1). Transverse sections through the anterior end of the worm show the conspicuous plaques (bosses) and the large cervical alae (Plate 41:2). The body is covered by a thick cuticle. Asymmetrical lateral chords are large (Plate 41:3); dorsal and ventral chords are typically inconspicuous. The muscle layer is polymyarian and coelomyarian (Plate 41:3 & 4). The esophagus shows either its muscular (Plate 41:2) or its glandular structure (Plate 41:3), depending on the level of the worm being sectioned. The intestine is a relatively simple tube in both sexes (Plate 41:4–6). In female worms, a single uterine branch is usually visible in any one section (Plate 41:4). Male worms are of smaller diameter and possess a single reproductive tube that contains developing spermatozoa (Plate 41:5 & 6). In the most posterior levels, sections may be cut through the paired spicules (Plate 41:6).

Gongylonema is readily recognized in transverse sections in tissue by its habitat preference and typical spiruroid morphologic features (ie, cuticular plaques, or bosses; cervical and lateral alae; structure of the esophagus; features of the lateral chords; and muscle layer). The presence of thick-shelled, embryonated eggs in utero is another important feature.

Reference

Illescas-Gomez MP, Osorio MR, Garcia VG, Gomez Morales MA. Human *Gongylonema* infection in Spain. *Am J Trop Med Hyg*. 1988;38:363-365.

Plate 41

Gongylonema species

Image 1

Section through esophageal mucosa shows typical burrows or tunnels containing embryonated eggs (darts) of *Gongylonema* species (H&E, 200x).

Image 2

Transverse section through the anterior extremity shows bosses (darts), cervical alae (arrows), and muscular esophagus (ES) (H&E, 250x).

Image 3

Transverse section through anterior extremity at the level of the glandular esophagus (ES) with its triradiate lumen. Note also the thick cuticle, lateral alae (darts), the large, asymmetrical lateral chords (LC), and characteristic coelomyarian muscles (H&E, 250x).

Image 4

Transverse section through the female worm illustrates the eggs in the uterine tube and the tubular intestine (IN) (H&E, 220x).

Images 5 and 6

Sections of a male worm show the reproductive tube (RT) at different levels as well as the paired spicules (dart) (H&E, 300x).

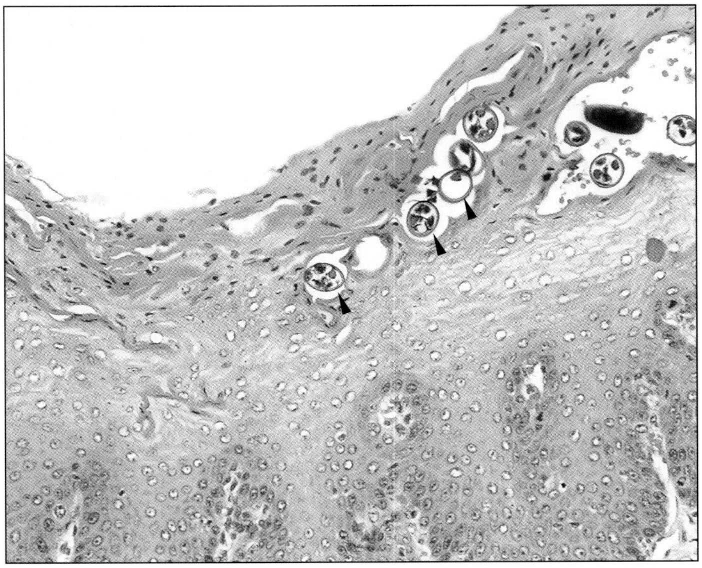

1

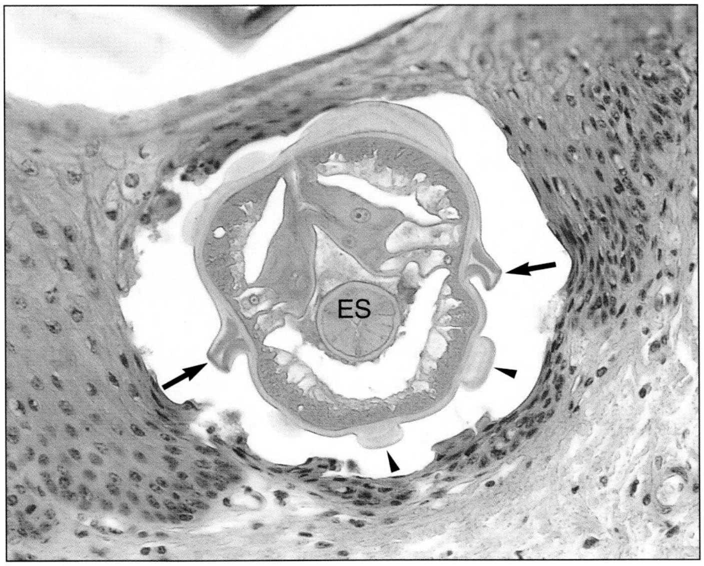

2

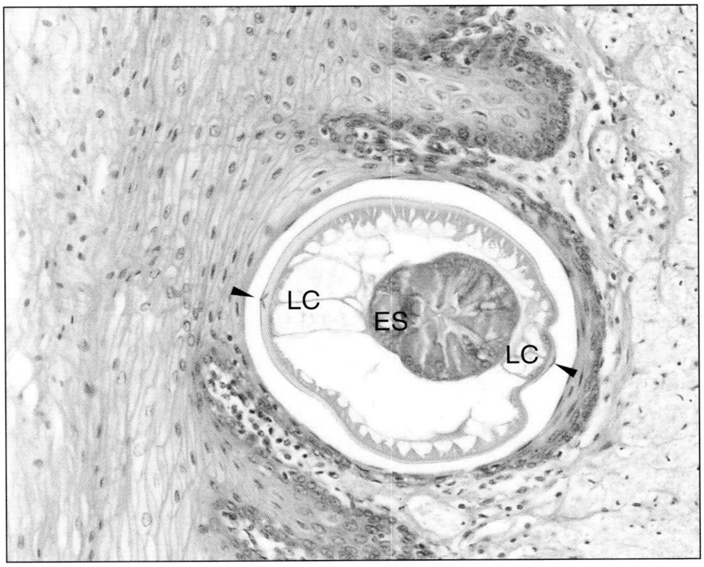

3

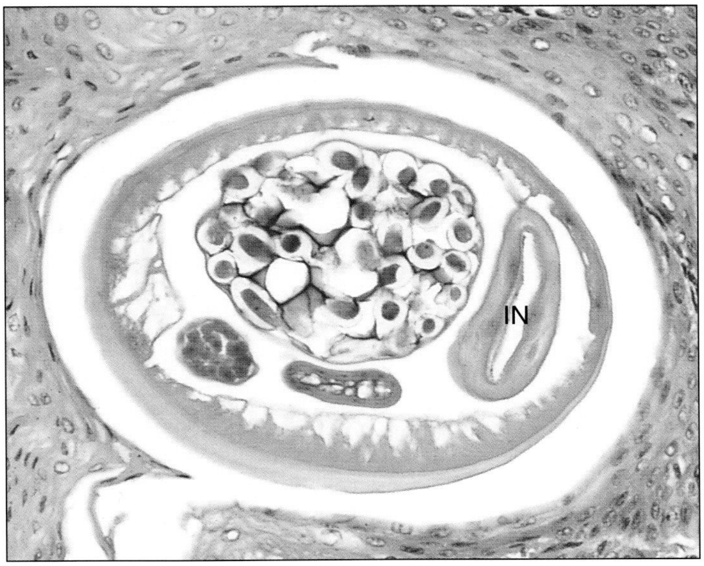

4

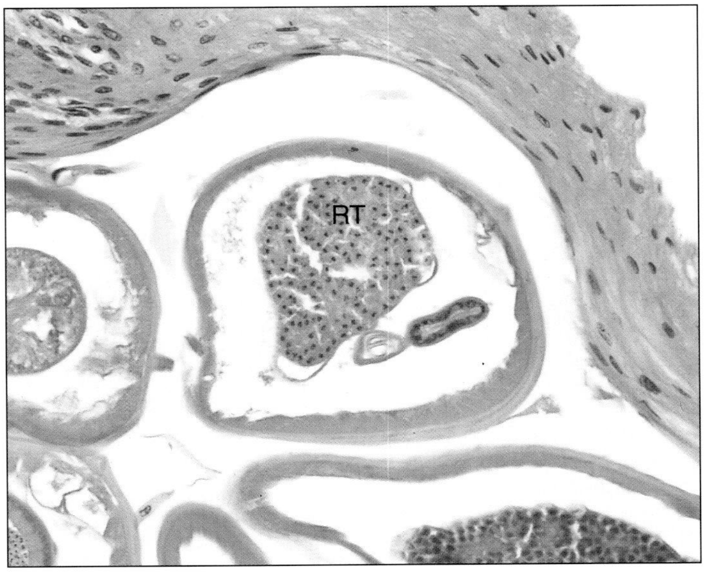

5

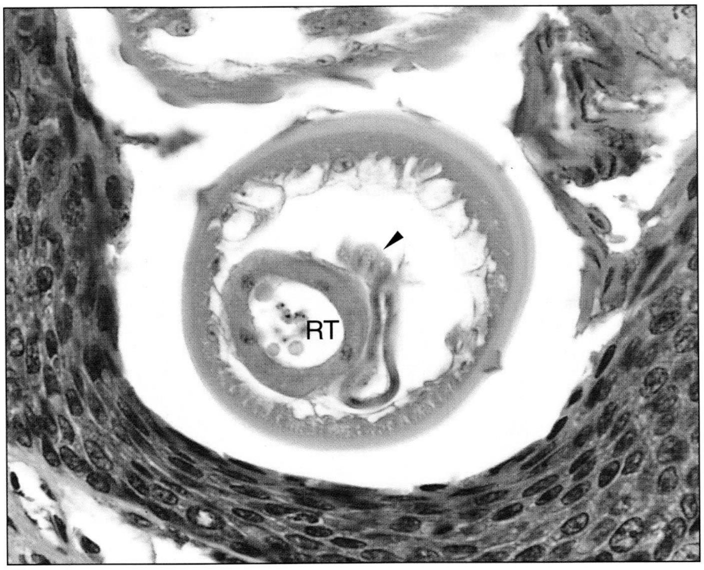

6

Uncommon Spiruroids

Some spiruroid parasites, such as *Gnathostoma* and *Gongylonema,* are frequently encountered in human tissues and can be identified in histopathologic specimens. Others, such as *Physaloptera* and *Thelazia,* occur with some frequency in humans but because of their habitats and relationships to host tissues are infrequently encountered in tissues subjected to pathologic examination. They are typically recovered intact from their human host. Despite the frequency of infection, little information is available regarding their microanatomic structure. Other spiruroids are extremely rare parasites of humans: *Rictularia* species and *Spirocerca lupi* have both been recovered only once. However, we have been able to include them in our discussion because of the availability of material from natural hosts. Another parasite, *Cheilospirura,* an acuariid, has been reported once in humans. We have no specimens from either the human case or from natural hosts, but the material we present gives some idea of the morphologic similarity of these spiruroid worms as well as some distinguishing features based on present knowledge.

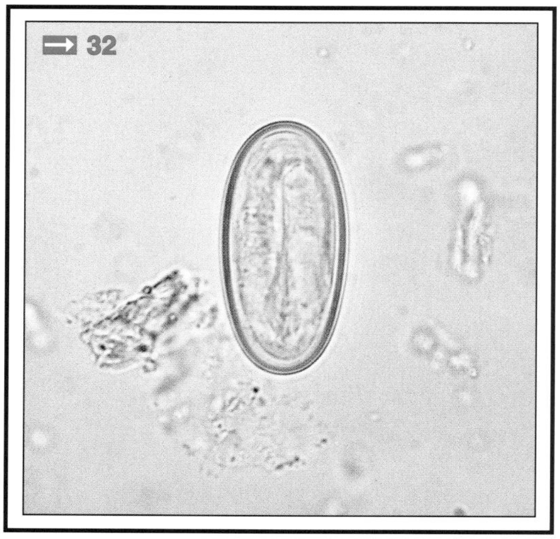

Rictularia

A gravid female worm identified as *Rictularia* species was found in a section of appendix taken in the course of a routine autopsy of a 90-year-old man in New York City.

The rictularids are natural intestinal parasites of a variety of carnivores, rodents, and bats, and they are transmitted by insect intermediate hosts. Presumably, humans may acquire infection by ingesting the intermediate host.

The adult worms are typically small. They have a well-developed buccal capsule surrounded by a row of denticles with teeth and spines at its base. The cuticle bears lateroventral rows of cuticular combs or spines along most of the body length. The male tail bears preanal and postanal pedunculated papillae and may have alae. The paired spicules are small. In the female, the vulva is near the base of the esophagus. The female produces typical thick-shelled, elongate eggs, which contain a larva.

The parasite is readily identifiable in sections of tissue. The cuticle and hypodermis are relatively thin. Dorsal and ventral chords are inconspicuous; lateral chords are tall and narrow. The muscles are well developed and are polymyarian and coelomyarian (Plate 42:1 & 2). The esophagus is muscular anteriorly and probably glandular posteriorly (although not seen) with a triradiate lumen (Plate 42:1). The intestine is tubular, and the epithelium composed of numerous columnar cells with nuclei lying near the base. The uterine branches contain typical spirurid eggs (Plate 42:2). The most useful diagnostic features are the rows of combs and spines along the length of the body (Plate 42:1 & 2). These cuticular ornamentations are equally useful in identifying intact specimens.

Physaloptera

This nematode parasitizes a wide range of animals, including amphibians, reptiles, birds, and especially mammals. Human infections with the adult stages of *Physaloptera* species have been reported from many parts of the world, especially Africa and less commonly from the Americas and parts of Asia. Most infections are diagnosed by recovery of eggs or adult parasites in feces.

The worms are large and robust and are often mistaken for immature ascarids. Females may reach 10 cm in length; males are smaller. They are typically found with the anterior end of the body buried in the mucosa of the stomach and/or intestine. The anterior extremity possesses a collarette, with the cuticle reflected anteriorly over and around the oral opening. The male has long pedunculated papillae embedded in large caudal alae, giving the impression of a well-developed bursa. In the female, the vulva is situated near or anterior to the midbody. The female produces typical spirurid eggs that measure 44 to 65 µm by 32 to 45 µm (⇨ 32).

Various insects have been implicated in the transmission of physalopterid species, and in several instances paratenic hosts have been utilized as well. Humans probably become infected by accidentally ingesting these insects.

Most often, *Physaloptera* is recovered intact from the human host. However, the nematode may also be seen in sections of the intestine. The parasite's unique morphologic features facilitate identification. The worms are large, with females reaching about 1.0 mm in diameter. The cuticle is thick. The hypodermis is thin in the submuscular areas, but the lateral chords are conspicuous. They have a narrow base but expand into the pseudocoelom and tend to occupy available space (Plate 42:3 & 4). Dorsal and ventral chords are inconspicuous by comparison. The numerous muscles are polymyarian and coelomyarian. Compared to the diameter, the muscle layer is not tall, but it is nevertheless well developed. The esophagus is divided into anterior muscular (Plate 42:3) and posterior glandular parts. The intestine is tubular with an irregular lumen due to the nature of the epithelial lining. The epithelial cells are columnar in type but irregular in height. The nucleus lies near the base of the cell. The luminal border has well-developed microvilli (Plate 42:4). The uterine tubes in the female tend to fill available space in the pseudocoelom and contain many typical spirurid eggs (Plate 42:4; ➡ 32).

Thelazia

Species of the genus *Thelazia* parasitize the conjunctival sac of a variety of mammals in many parts of the world. Human infections with *T. callipaeda*, a natural parasite of dogs and cats, are widely reported in Asia, including China, Russia, India, Japan, and Thailand. Infections have been documented in the United States, primarily *T. californiensis* in California, a parasite found in various wild animals. Infections are most frequently seen in young children. The worms measure up to 2.0 cm in length, localize in the conjunctival sac, and cause considerable inflammation and lacrimation. Gravid female worms discharge typical spirurid eggs, which are ingested along with lacrimal secretions by various species of flies. Larvae develop in the fly to the infective (third) stage and migrate to the mouthparts, which enables them to escape from the vector and to infect a new host when the fly feeds on ocular secretions of another host.

Flies belonging to *Fannia* and *Musca* have been implicated in transmission in the United States and Asia. Adult worms are usually removed intact from infected humans with forceps, so that it is unusual to see sections of the worms in conjunctival tissues. Consequently, no detailed information is available regarding the microscopic morphology of *Thelazia* species. However, (Plate 42:5) shows a transverse section of a female *Thelazia,* illustrating some features of the body. The body wall is similar to that of *Spirocerca* (Plate 42:6), *Gnathostoma* (Plate 39:5), and other spiruroids. The uterine tubes contain thick-shelled eggs, each with a first-stage larva. The position of the worm in the eye might initially suggest the possibility that the parasite might be *Loa* or *Dirofilaria.* However, knowledge of the relative sizes of the worms and details of internal anatomy eliminate *Loa* and *Dirofilaria* from consideration.

Spirocerca

Only a few species of *Spirocerca* exist. The best known is *S. lupi,* the esophageal worm of dogs. It is most common in the southeastern United States but has been reported from Central America, Africa, the Middle East, and southern Europe. The parasite has been recovered from a human host on only one occasion: from the ileum of a newborn child in Italy. Infection was apparently transmitted by transplacental migration of infective larvae from mother to fetus.

This spiruroid is large. Males measure up to 4 cm in length; females are as long as 7 cm. They are pink to bright red and typically are found in nodular masses in the thoracic region of the esophagus of the natural host. The female worm produces a typical spirurid egg, which is discharged in feces. Dung beetles serve as the intermediate host, and apparently a variety of animals, including birds, lizards, mice, and rabbits, are paratenic or transport hosts. Humans become infected by ingesting infective larvae from either the intermediate or transport hosts.

Anatomic features of the adult worm are best illustrated in a transverse section of a female worm in the canine host (Plate 42:6). The worm may measure up to 1.2 mm in diameter. The cuticle is smooth and relatively thick. The underlying hypodermis is thin in submuscular areas. The dorsal and ventral chords are usually evident, and the lateral chords are large and sometimes uneven. The hypodermal nuclei are dispersed at random in the syncytial cytoplasm. The muscles, divided by the chords into four bands, are well developed and of the polymyarian and coelomyarian type. The cytoplasmic portions of the cells are as tall or taller than the contractile portions. The esophagus is divided into muscular and glandular portions. The intestine is tubular. The nature of the epithelial lining is helpful in diagnosis. Epithelial cells are columnar and slender. The microvillus border is conspicuous, and the nuclei of the cells lie uniformly close to the luminal border. The eggs in the uterine tube are small, have a thick shell, contain a larva, and measure 30 to 38 μm by 11 to 15 μm.

References

Biocca E. Infestazione umana prenatale da *Spirocerca lupi* (Rud., 1809). *Parasitologia.* 1959;1:137-142.

Kenny M, Eveland LK, Vermalov V, Kassouny DY. A case of *Rictularia* infection of man in New York. *Am J Trop Med Hyg.* 1975;24:596-598.

Kirschner BI, Dunn JP, Ostler HB. Conjunctivitis caused by *Thelazia californiensis. Am J Ophthalmol.* 1990;110:573-574.

Hira PR. Observations on helminth zoonoses in Zambia. *E Afr Med J.* 1976;53:278-286.

Shi YE, Han JJ, Yang WY, Wei DX. *Thelazia callipaeda* (Nematoda: Spirurida): transmission by flies from dogs to children in Hubei, China. *Trans R Soc Trop Med Hyg.* 1988;82:627.

Uncommon Spiruroids

Image 1

Rictularia lucifugus. Transverse section of a female worm cut at the esophageal level shows the subventral cuticular combs (darts) (H&E, 120x). (Case courtesy of R. Lichtenfels.)

Image 2

The same parasite cut at the midbody level shows the structure of the body wall, a cuticular comb (dart), the uterine tubes (UT) containing embryonated eggs, and the tubular intestine (IN) with its tall, columnar epithelium, microvillus luminal border, and nuclei positioned near the base of each cell (H&E, 120x).

Image 3

Physaloptera species from the stomach of a raccoon. The section is through the level of the esophagus (ES) in the glandular part. Note the triradiate lumen. The cuticle is smooth and thick; the hypodermis is evident only from the large lateral chords (LC) with their narrow base, expanding into the pseudocoelom. The muscles are well developed, and the contractile and cytoplasmic portions of each are well defined (H&E, 10x).

Image 4

The worm shown in Image 3 is seen here at a more posterior level. Note again the thick cuticle, well-developed muscles, and the pale voluminous lateral chords (LC). These chords and the uterine branches (UT) contain large numbers of eggs that literally fill the body cavity. The intestine (dart) is tubular with an irregular lumen due to the different heights of the lining epithelium. (H&E, 8x).

Image 5

Thelazia californiensis from the conjunctival sac of a dog. Note the spiruroid features of the body wall and the presence of embryonating eggs in the uterine tubes (H&E, 100x).

Image 6

Spirocerca lupi. Transverse section of female worm in an esophageal tumor in a dog. Note the typical spiruroid features of the body wall. The cuticle is thick, muscles are well developed, and the lateral chords (LC) are large. The uterine tube (UT) contains many eggs, each in some stage of embryonation. The intestine (IN) is lined by a low columnar epithelium in which the luminal border has tall microvilli, and the cell nucleus in each lies near to the luminal edge (H&E, 70x).

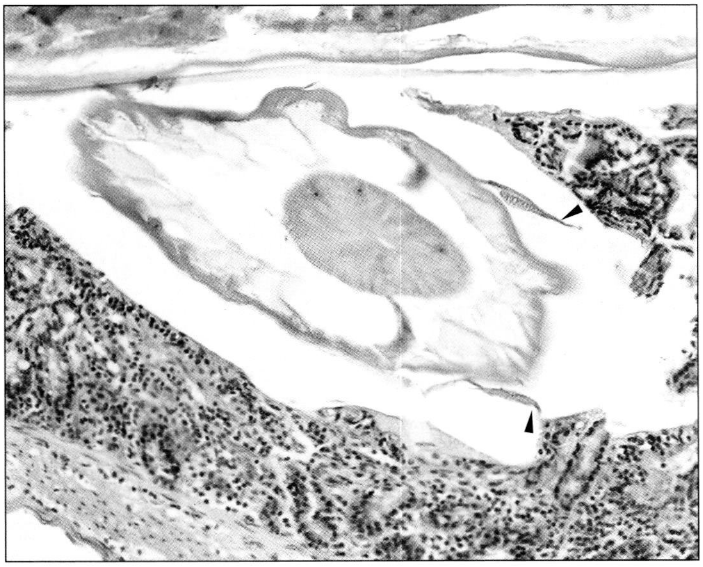

1

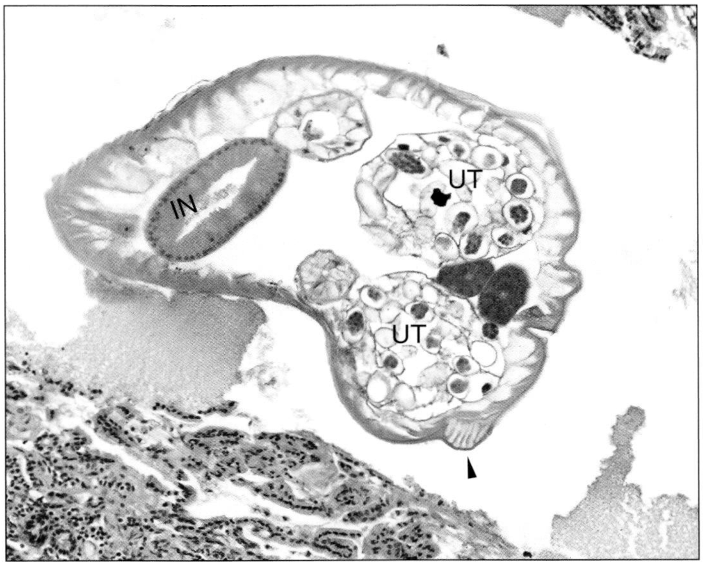

2

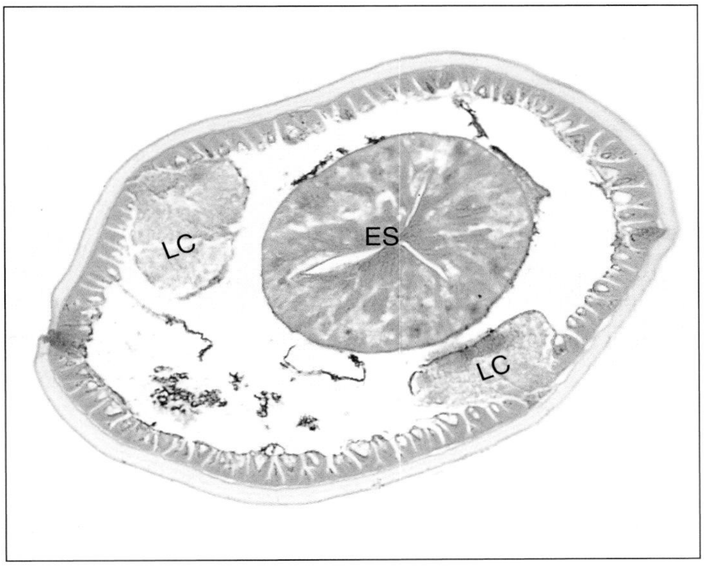

3

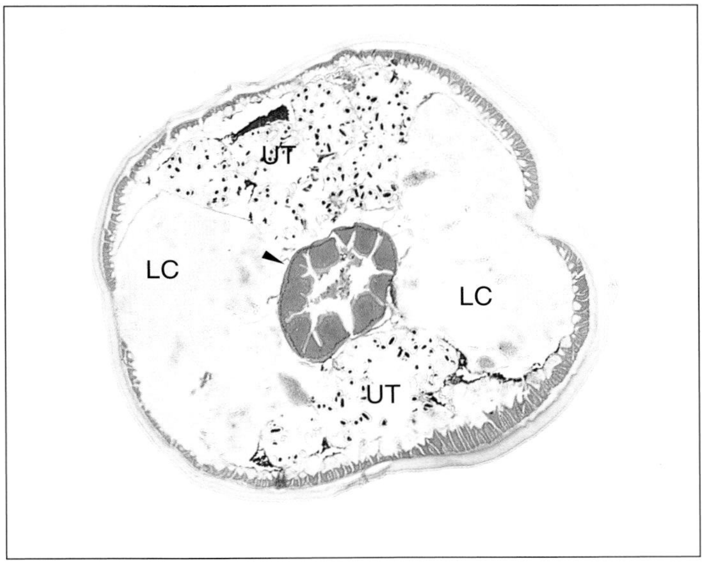

4

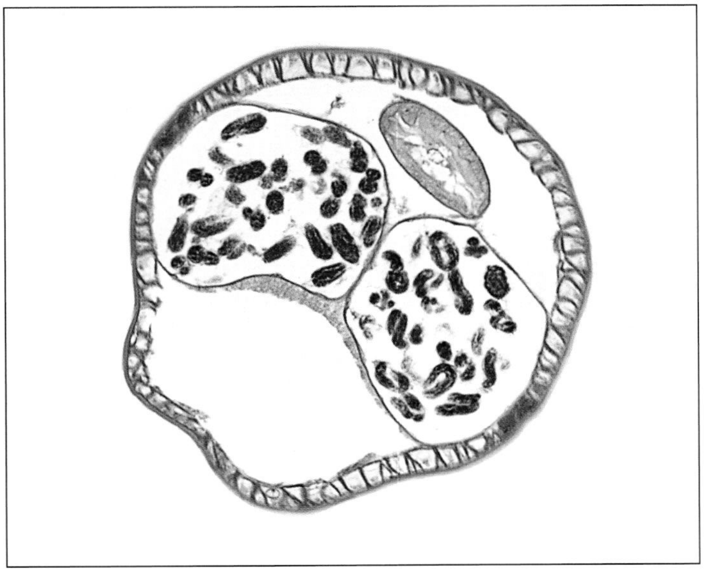

5

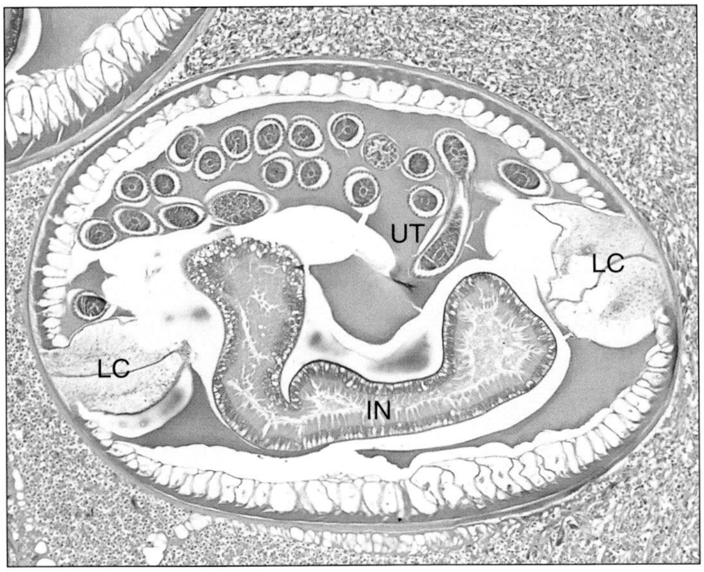

6

Filarioidea

The filariae are nematode parasites transmitted by blood-sucking arthropods, including mosquitoes, tabanid flies, gnats, and blackflies, among others. The adults are long, slender, delicate worms that live in the lymphatics, subcutaneous tissues, and connective tissues associated with the liver, gall bladder, adrenal glands, etc. A few species are found in the body cavities and in the vascular system. Because of their tissue habitats, the adults of most species are rarely seen and usually only in sectioned tissues. Infections are typically diagnosed by the presence of the microfilariae (➡ 33), which are produced by the female and found circulating in the peripheral blood or in the dermis of the host.

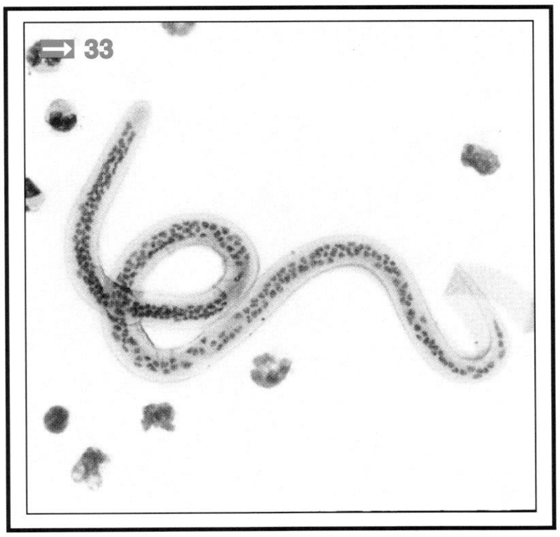

When microfilariae are ingested by an appropriate vector in the course of taking a blood meal from an infected host, they migrate from the midgut of the arthropod to certain tissues—eg, flight muscles, fat body, etc—and there develop as intracellular parasites to the infective, third stage over a period of several days to two weeks or longer. Upon reaching the infective stage, the larvae emerge from the tissues and make their way to the head and mouthparts of the vector. When the vector takes its next blood meal (➡ 34), the larvae escape and may invade the tissues of the definitive host (man or animal) by entering the bite site, migrating to specific tissues in the body, and developing to sexual maturity, which completes the life cycle. Development from infective larva to the adult stage requires a few to several months, depending on the species. Although certain species of filariae cause significant disease in humans, others are relatively innocuous. Diseases attributed to filariae are not life threatening, but they may have a significant impact on quality of life and productivity at the personal and community levels.

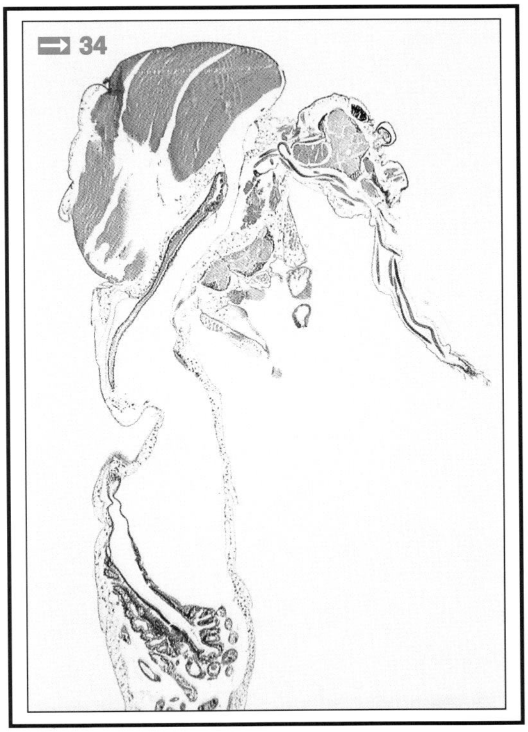

Several species of filariae are common parasites of humans and typically inhabit specific organs or tissues of the body. These include *Wuchereria bancrofti*, *Brugia malayi*, and *B. timori*, which are all found in the lymphatics; *Loa loa*, which inhabits the subcutaneous tissues; *Onchocerca volvulus*, which is found in fibrous nodules in the subcutaneous tissues; and three species of *Mansonella*—*M. ozzardi*, *M. perstans*, and *M. streptocerca*—all of which typically reside in subcutaneous or connective tissues and possibly the body cavities.

In addition to these "natural" filarial parasites of humans, several species naturally infect domestic and wild animals and may accidentally infect people and produce cryptic (nonpatent) infections. Infections in humans attributed to filariae of animals are categorized as zoonotic infections. These are among the most common zoonotic parasites encountered in human tissues, especially in the United States, and are usually caused by species of *Dirofilaria*, *Brugia*, *Dipetalonema*, and *Onchocerca*. Other more rarely encountered filariae include *Meningonema* and *Loaina*.

Wuchereria bancrofti

Bancroftian Filariasis

Wuchereria bancrofti is the most common and widely distributed filaria infecting humans. According to the World Health Organization, approximately 90 million people are infected and nearly one billion are at risk for infection. The parasite is most common in tropical and subtropical areas of the world, with the majority of infections occurring in India, Indonesia, and several other Asian countries. It is also endemic in parts of Africa, northern South America, some Caribbean Islands, and certain islands in the Western Pacific. It is most commonly associated with elephantiasis, the disease it produces in chronically infected individuals.

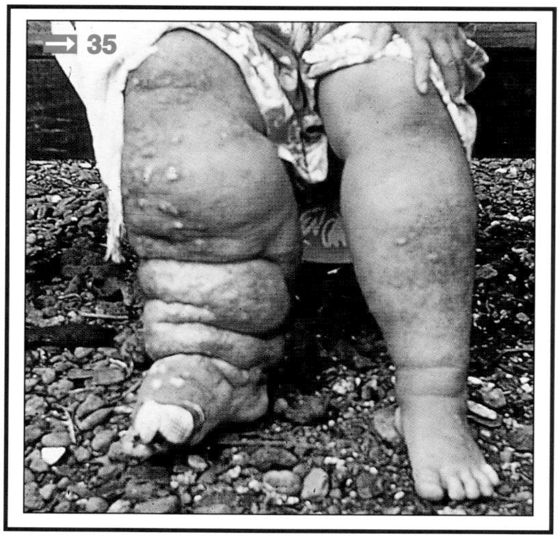

Biology and Life Cycle

The adult worms live in lymph nodes and lymph vessels, often associated with the testes, epididymis, and spermatic chord in men, and apparently, although not adequately documented, in the lateral ovarian ligaments in women. Inguinal lymph nodes have been reported to be an important site for adult worms in both sexes. On rare occasions, worms have been found in blood vessels. The female produces sheathed microfilariae, which circulate in the peripheral blood with well-defined periodicity—nocturnal in most regions of the world but diurnally subperiodic in the Western Pacific.

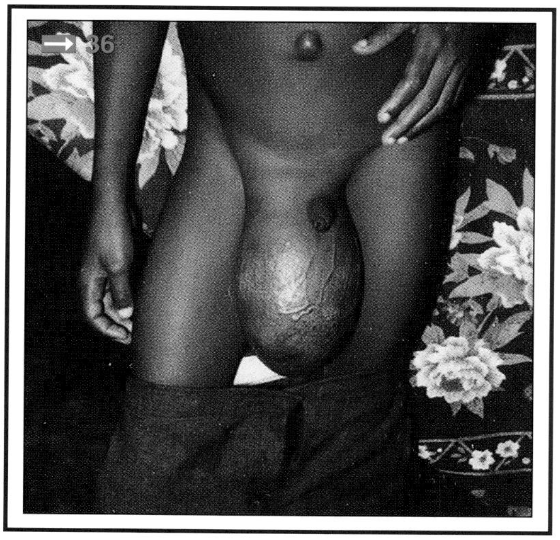

Female mosquitoes are natural vectors of this filaria. The mosquito is infected by ingesting microfilariae present in the blood of the human host at the time it takes a blood meal. The microfilariae then migrate from the mosquito's midgut to the flight muscles in the thorax, where they develop to the infective stage over a period of approximately 12 to 14 days. Thereafter, they migrate to the head and mouthparts of the mosquito and escape when it takes its next blood meal. Infective larvae can enter the bite site and infect the new host. Development from the infective stage to sexual maturity requires several months.

Pathology and Clinical Manifestations

Individuals suspected of having bancroftian filariasis must have a history of residence in or travel to an endemic area and must have been exposed to mosquitoes, the parasite's natural vector. In the early (acute) stage of patent, bancroftian filariasis, an individual may be completely asymptomatic, so that infection is noted only upon the discovery of microfilariae in the peripheral blood. This condition may persist for the duration of infection in some individuals, although in other individuals infection produces recurrent fever and malaise accompanied by bouts of lymphangitis and lymphadenitis. A transient lymphedema is not uncommon, and in long-term, chronic infections the lymphedema may progress to an irreversible state with attendant and extensive lymphatic pathology. The lymph nodes of the lower extremities and the genitalia are most frequently affected. Hydrocele is an especially common pathologic manifestation of infection in males (➡ 36). Elephantiasis or exaggerated swelling of the affected limbs or genitalia occurs in only a small percentage of infected individuals and typically results from prolonged reexposure and chronic infection (➡ 35). Characteristically, in this stage of disease microfilariae are no longer found in the peripheral blood.

Cryptic or occult forms of bancroftian filariasis occur as well. In some individuals, infections with *W. bancrofti* may cause a nocturnal, paroxysmal cough; wheezing; hypereosinophilia; and high levels of antifilarial antibodies. Microfilariae are absent from the peripheral blood but may be found trapped in lung tissues and in lymph nodes. The syndrome is referred to as tropical pulmonary eosinophilia and is usually diagnosed on clinical presentation alone. Diethylcarbamazine alleviates symptoms.

Another cryptic form of bancroftian filariasis is seen in migrant populations and new arrivals to areas where the parasite is endemic. Individuals exposed to infection develop lymphangitis, lymphadenitis, lymphedema, and eosinophilia. Adult worms are found in biopsy specimens of lymph nodes and vessels, but microfilariae are absent from the peripheral blood. This type of presentation was seen in American soldiers stationed on some of the Pacific Islands during World War II, in French soldiers in North Vietnam in the 1950s, and allegedly in American military personnel in South Vietnam in the 1960s. One might expect to see similar clinical presentations in individuals such as tourists, health workers, or any visitors to endemic areas who have been significantly exposed to infection, especially over an extended time.

Parasite Morphology

The adult worms are invariably found in lymph nodes or lymph vessels. Worms may be alive or dead and in various stages of degeneration. They lie coiled in the lymph vessel, and their presence in many transverse sections attests to their length. Typically, all levels of the filaria are encountered, and the various internal organs are easily recognized. The features of the body wall are most important for identification.

Depending on its age, the female worm may measure up to 10 cm in length, with a maximum diameter of 300 µm. Size varies somewhat with the body level. The cuticle appears smooth, although fine transverse striations are present, and is uniformly 1 to 2 µm thick except in the lateral fields, where it is thickened (Plate 43:2). The hypodermis is thin in the submuscular areas. Dorsal and ventral chords are inconspicuous. However, the lateral chords occupy as much as two fifths of the body circumference and, although relatively short, are conspicuous (Plate 43:2). Hypodermal nuclei are evident in most sections and are typically seen near the base and toward the periphery of the lateral chords. Usually only three to four muscle cells are present per quadrant. They are of the coelomyarian type and have a voluminous cytoplasmic portion (Plate 43:4; Plate 45:6). The cell nucleus may be seen in some. The height of the muscle cells varies with the contents of the pseudocoelom—that is, the muscle cells are shorter when the pseudocoelom is filled with uterine tubes or several sections of ovaries and taller when the cavity is less filled.

The morphologic structure of the reproductive system provides no clue to species identification as far as we can tell. However, the contents of the reproductive system do indicate the worm's stage of maturity, its reproductive state, and whether the female has been inseminated or is infertile. At most levels, transverse sections through the female worm contain paired uterine tubes filled with eggs developing to microfilariae (Plate 43:2). In the posterior end are several tubes, which constitute the coiled ovaries (Plate 43:4). The presence of developing eggs indicates that the ovaries are functional. If the female has been fertilized, sections cut through the distal portions of the uterine tubes show accumulations of spermatozoa. The digestive tube consists of an esophagus divided into anterior muscular and posterior glandular portions. The intestine, a simple cylindrical tube with a low epithelium, has no diagnostic value.

The male worm is much smaller than the female, usually about 4 cm in length and not more than 150 µm in diameter. The structure of the body wall is the same as in the female. The muscle cells are of approximately the same number but tend to be taller, especially the cytoplasmic portion. In the coiled tail of the male, the muscles tend to be strongly fibrillar with little evidence of the cytoplasmic portion of the individual cell (Plate 43:6). The reproductive tube is the testis, which lies in the anterior end of the worm. The remainder of the tube is straight and cylindrical and contains developing spermatozoa. Posteriorly, the ejaculatory duct joins the rectum to form the cloaca. Cuts through the paired spicules are frequently seen in this region. Fortuitous sections through the tail at the level of the cloaca may reveal the pericloacal papillae.

Worms that die in situ begin to degenerate quickly (Plate 44) and soon calcify (Plate 45:1 & 2). Depending on the state of degeneration, some of the normal architecture of the body wall may remain, so that the normal structure of the living worm can frequently be discerned (ie, thickness of cuticle, type of chords, and number of muscle cells).

References

Beaver PC. Filariasis without microfilaremia. *Am J Trop Med Hyg*. 1970;19:181-189.

Beaver PC. *Wuchereria*-like filaria in an artery associated with pulmonary infarction. *Am J Trop Med Hyg*. 1974;23:869-876.

Jungermann PJ, Figueredo-Silva J, Dreyer G. Bancroftian lymphadenopathy: a histopathologic study of fifty-eight cases from Northeastern Brazil. *Am J Trop Med Hyg*. 1991;45:325-331.

World Health Organization. *Lymphatic Filariasis: The Disease and Its Control*. Fifth Report of the WHO Expert Committee on Filariasis. Geneva, Switzerland: World Health Organization; 1992. WHO Technical Report Series 821.

Plate 43

Wuchereria bancrofti

Image 1

A characteristic presentation of a gravid adult female worm in a lymphatic vessel. The worm is coiled; hence, it is cut at several levels of the body. Eggs and developing microfilariae can be seen in the reproductive tubes (uteri) (H&E, 45x).

Image 2

Transverse section through a gravid female worm somewhat anterior to the midbody illustrates the characteristic morphologic features of the adult female. Note the thin cuticle that is slightly thickened in the lateral fields (dart), the long, low, lateral chords (LC), and the few well-developed muscle cells (MU). Paired uterine tubes (UT) virtually fill the body cavity (pseudocoelom) and contain sections through large numbers of microfilariae. The intestine (IN) is beneath and between the uterine tubes (H&E, 250x).

Image 3

Transverse section through the posterior one third of the body of a female worm. Note the characteristic features of the body wall. Within the pseudocoelom are a small tubular intestine (IN) and three sections through ovaries, all of which contain large numbers of single-cell eggs (H&E, 220x).

Image 4

Transverse section through the posterior end of a female worm. Because the ovaries are paired structures and are characteristically coiled in the pseudocoelom, several sections through the ovaries can be seen. Within the ovaries, primary oocytes and nearly mature eggs are present (H&E, 220x).

Image 5

Three transverse sections through a male worm. Note that at most levels the muscle cells, though few, are tall, with large cytoplasmic portions. The intestine is small, tubular, and sometimes inconspicuous (dart), whereas the reproductive tube (RT) is large at all levels and usually contains spermatozoa in various stages of maturation (H&E, 200x).

Image 6

Transverse section through the coiled tail of a male worm. At this level of the body, the muscle cell has a large contractile component and shows little evidence of a cytoplasmic portion (H&E, 300x).

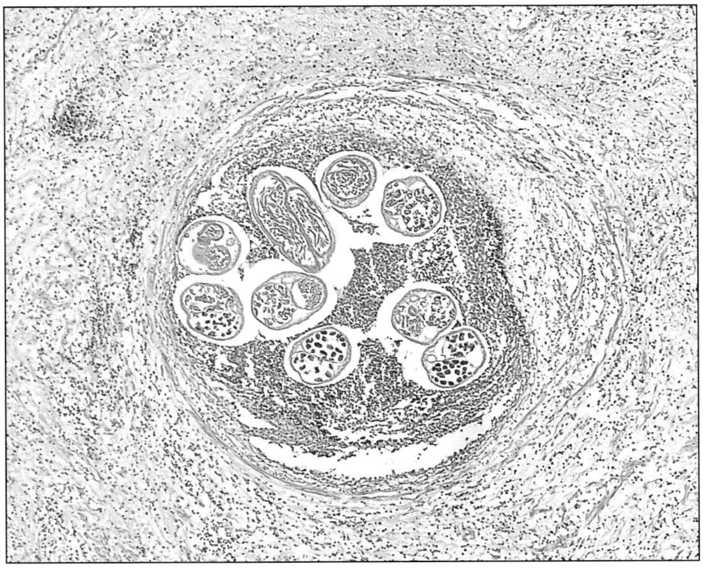

1

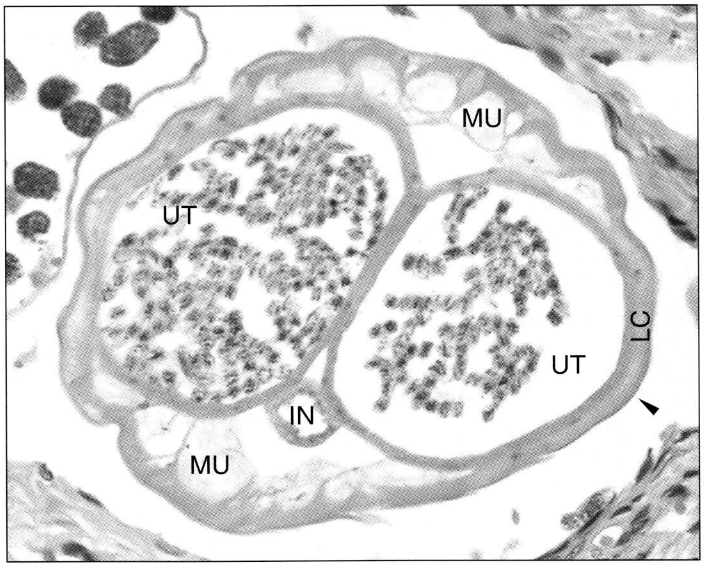

2

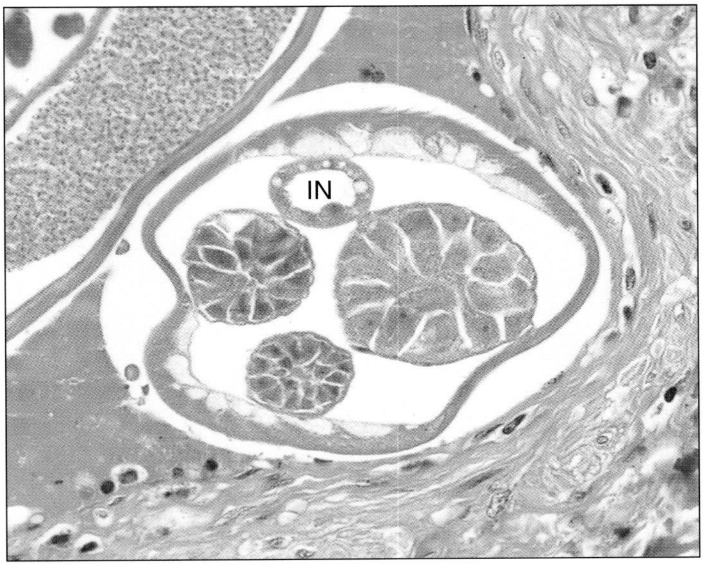

3

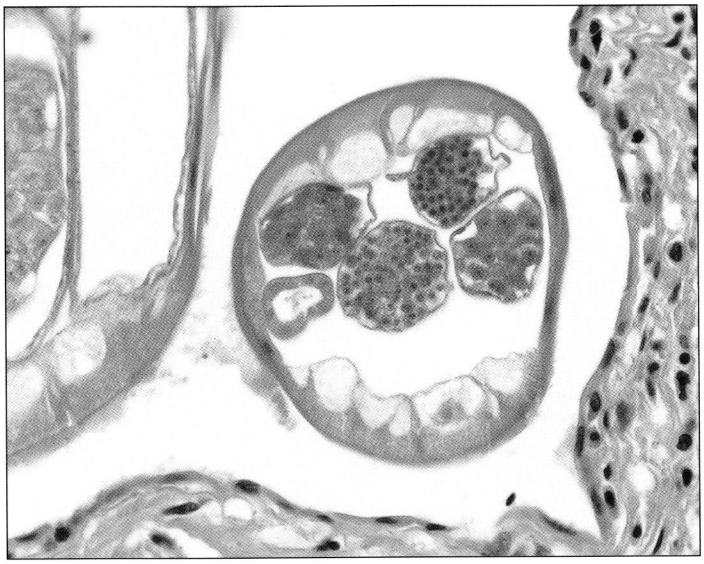

4

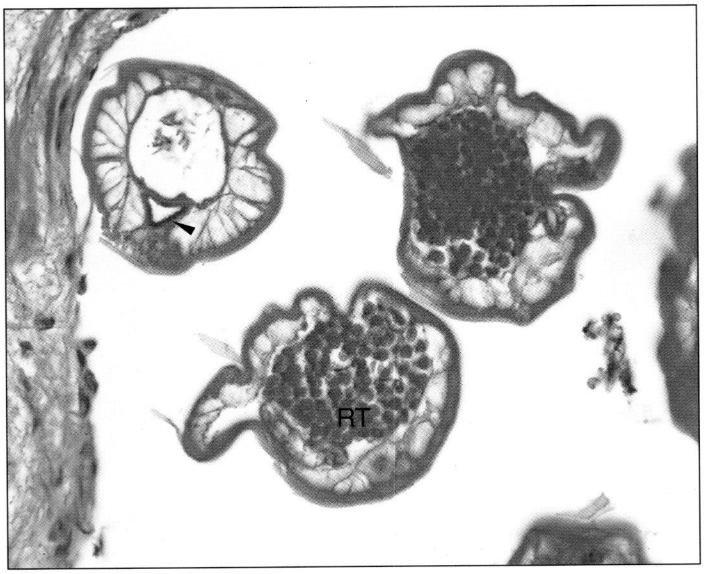

5

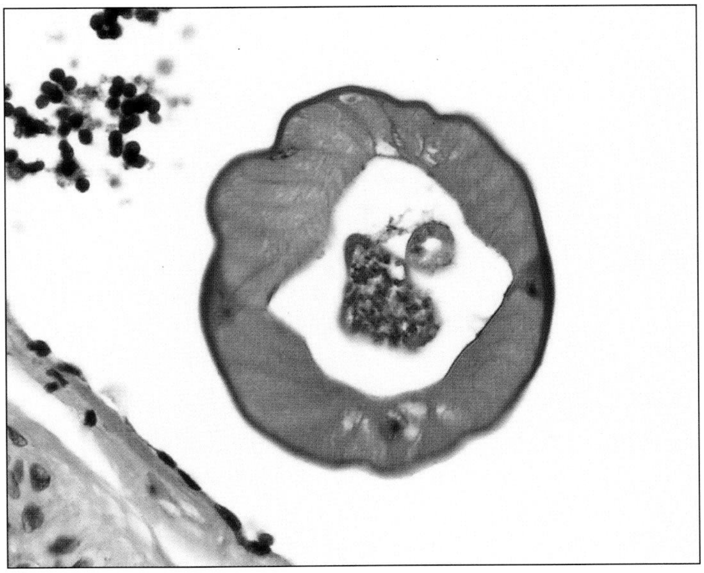

6

Plate 44

Wuchereria bancrofti

Image 1

Section through a granuloma in a lymph node contains a dead, degenerated female worm (H&E, 100x).

Image 2

High-magnification transverse section through the worm in the previous image. It is immediately evident that the worm is a gravid female, because paired uterine tubes are present and they contain elements that represent disintegrating microfilariae. The intestine is inconspicuous, but its tubular structure is evident (dart). Note that the elements of the body wall (ie, thin cuticle, lateral chords, and muscle cells) still show traces of their normal architecture (H&E, 370x).

Image 3

Another section through a dead female worm in which the features of the body wall can still be discerned. The uterine tubes (UT) are empty, suggesting that the worm may have been infertile or immature (H&E, 310x).

Image 4

Transverse section through another degenerated female worm. In spite of the degeneration, the large, compressed lateral chords and a few muscle cells are visible. The paired uterine tubes (UT) contain amorphous masses of degenerated reproductive products (eg, eggs or microfilariae). The simple, tubular intestine (IN) is easily recognized (H&E, 370x).

Image 5

Transverse sections through a dead male worm in a lymph vessel. Most of the normal architecture of the worm has been lost (Movat, 360x).

Image 6

At higher magnification, it is evident that the cuticle is swollen. One of the lateral chords is clear (darts). The number of muscle cells present is within the range seen in *W. bancrofti*. The single reproductive tube (RT) indicates that the worm is male. The smaller tube is the intestine (Movat, 700x).

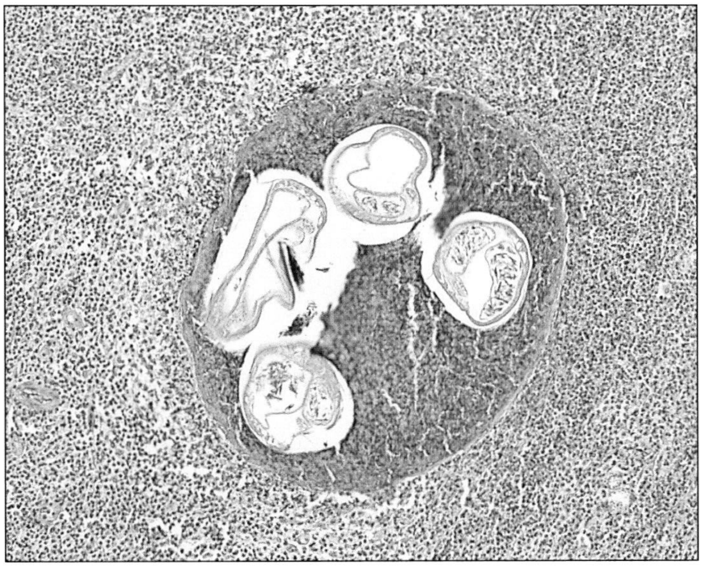

1

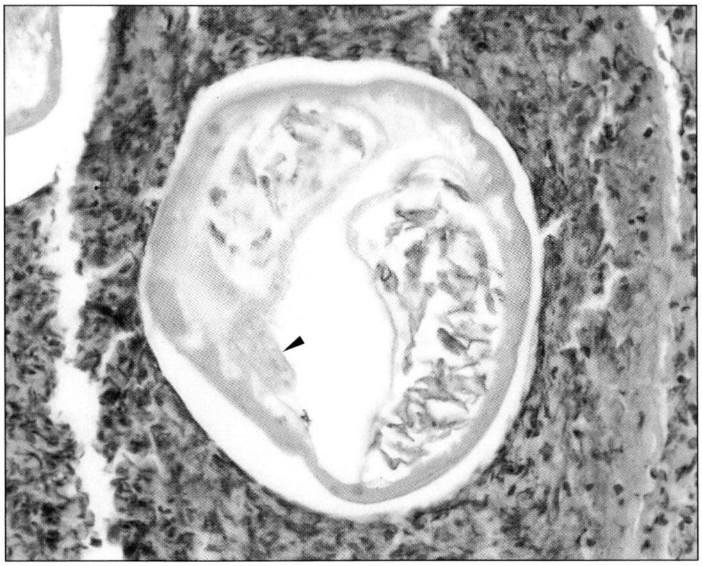

2

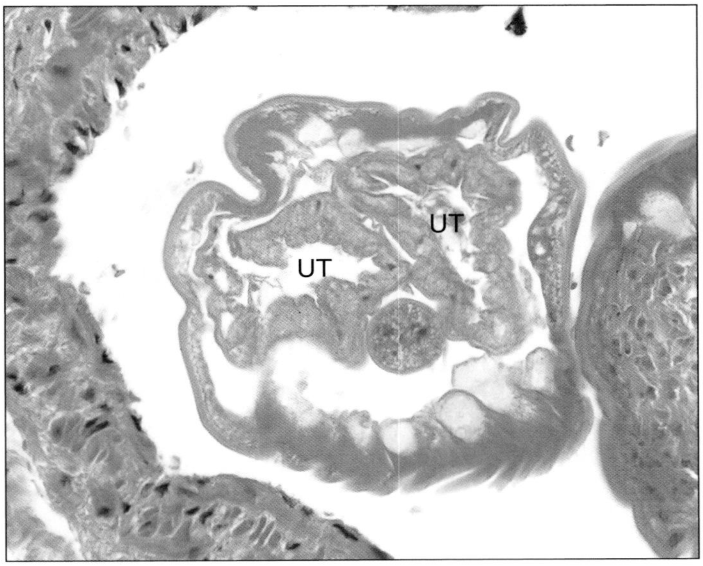

3

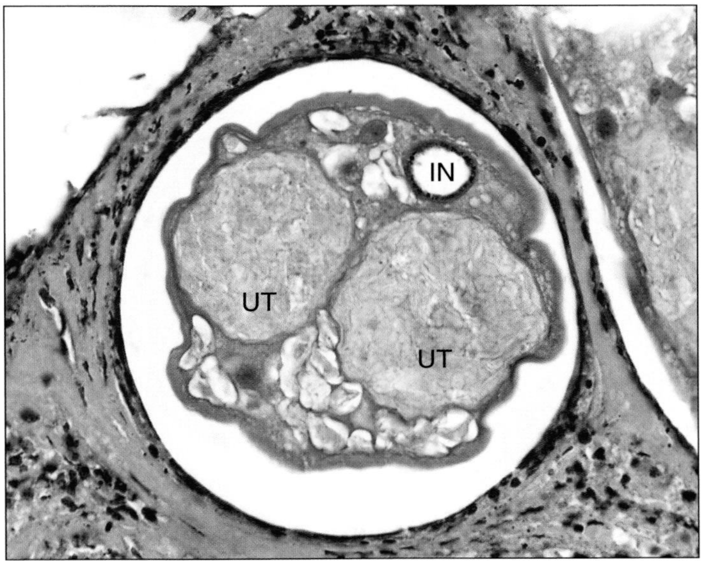

4

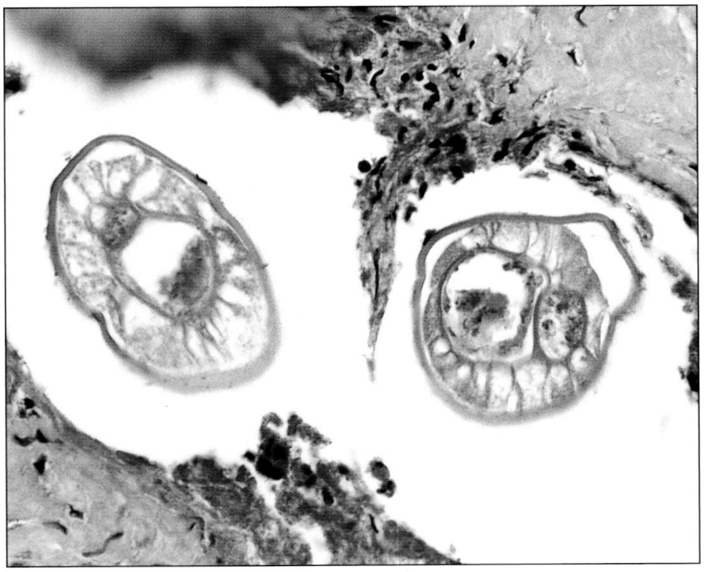

5

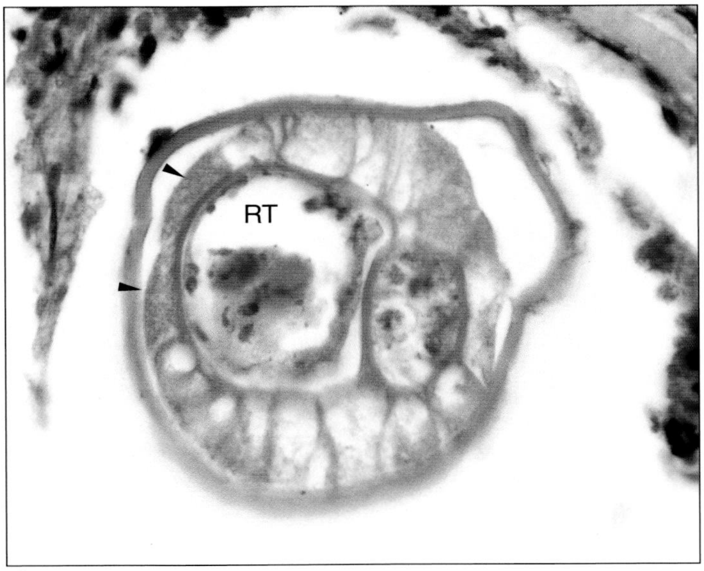

6

Plate 45

Wuchereria bancrofti

Image 1

Sections through a dead worm that has undergone calcification in situ. Note the concentric layers of fibrous connective tissue around the worm (H&E, 25x).

Image 2

At high magnification, the parasite can be clearly identified as a filarial worm. Despite the advanced degeneration and mineralization, some of the normal architecture of the worm is still apparent. Both the body wall of the filaria and the paired uterine tubes (UT) are identifiable (H&E, 170x).

Image 3

A so-called "tumor" removed from the breast of a Singapore woman was thought to contain remnants of a female *W. bancrofti* containing numerous recognizable microfilariae (H&E, 33x).

Image 4

At high magnification, numerous remnants of microfilariae are identifiable in the tissues (H&E, 300x).

Image 5

A filaria lodged in a small pulmonary artery in an infarcted area of lung was identified as *W. bancrofti.* The patient had resided in Singapore for 30 months. It is evident in this section of tissue that the worm was an infertile female, based on the absence of developing eggs or microfilariae in the reproductive tubes. The worm had a maximum diameter of 160 µm (Masson's trichrome, 140x).

Image 6

High-power view of the same worm at the level of the vagina (dart). The morphologic features of the body wall—ie, thin cuticle thickened in the lateral fields (arrow), large lateral chords, and well-developed but few muscle cells per quadrant—are consistent with a diagnosis of *W. bancrofti* (Masson's trichrome, 275x).

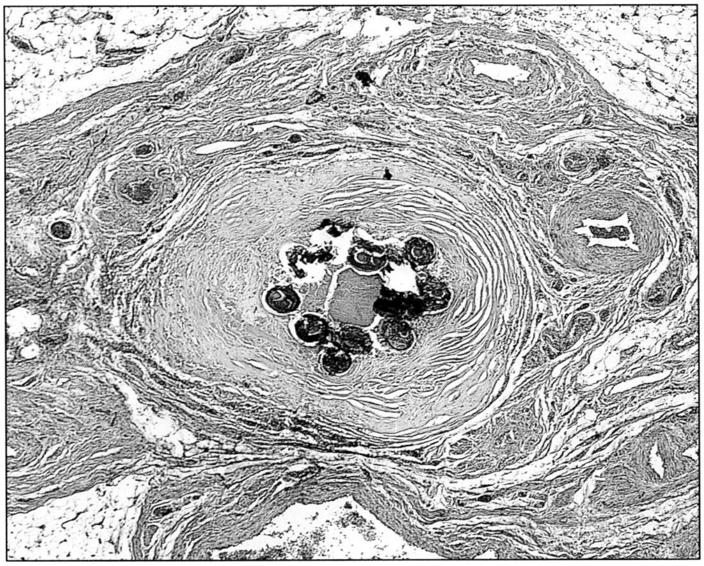

1

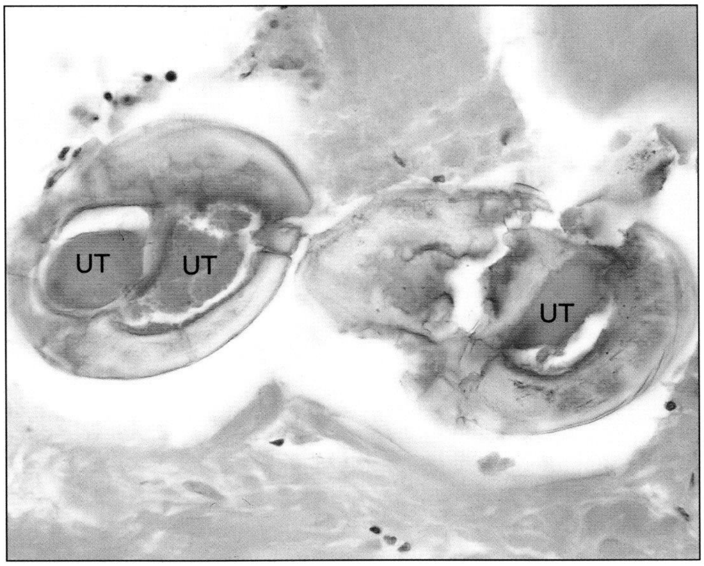

2

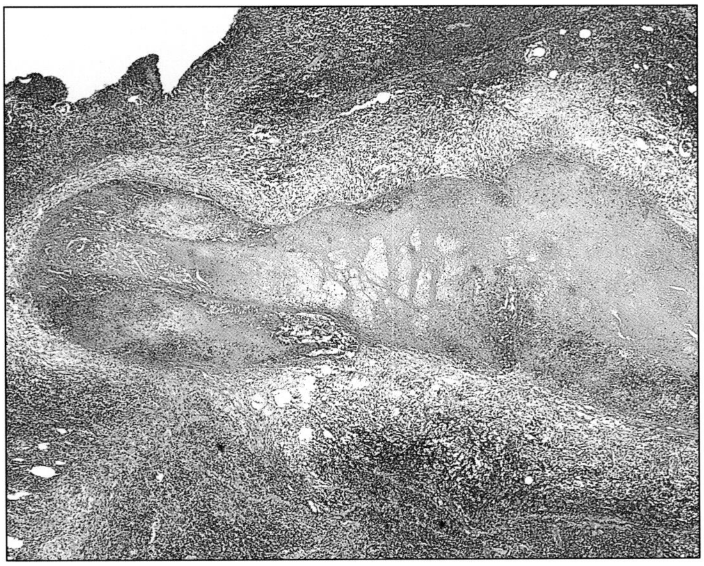

3

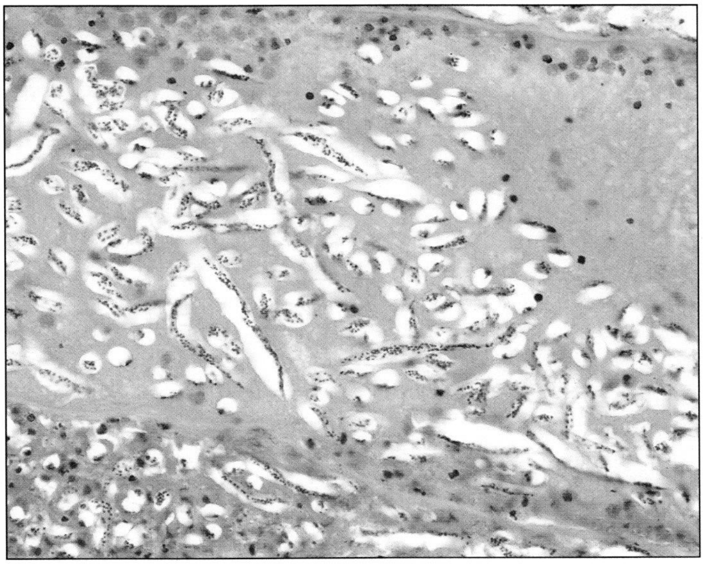

4

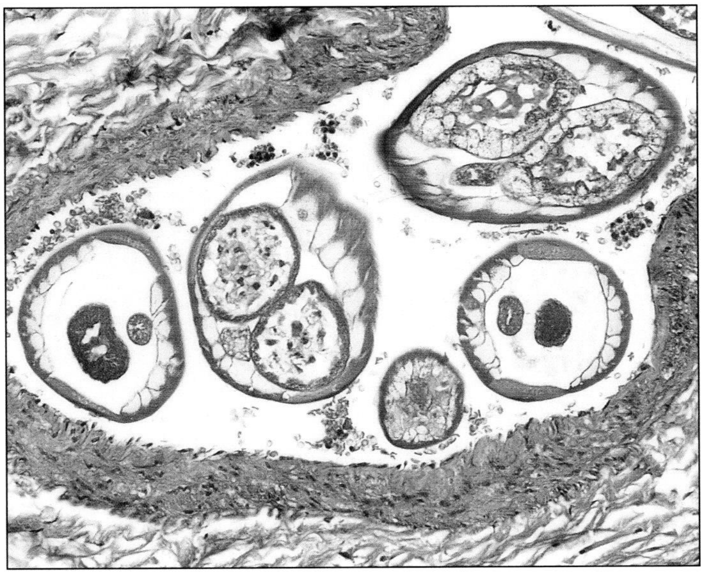

5

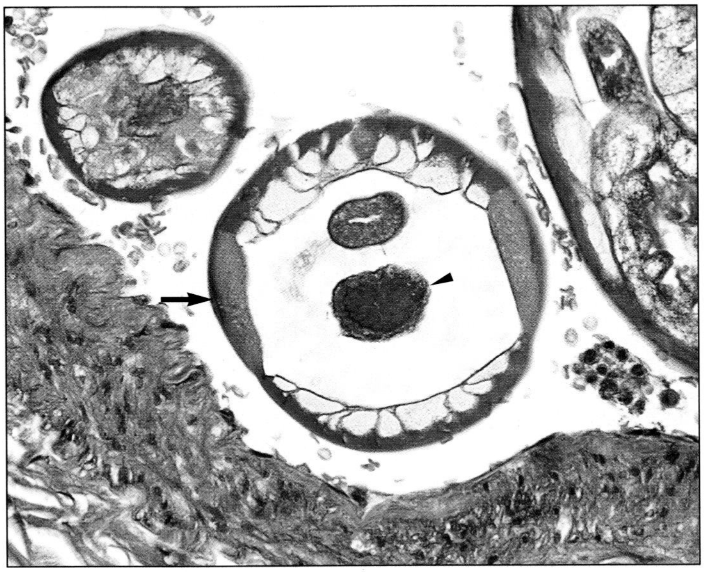

6

Brugia malayi

Brugia species

The genus *Brugia* includes an assemblage of species that are morphologically and biologically similar to *Wuchereria bancrofti*. At one time the early known species were included in the genus *Wuchereria*. In addition to the species found in humans (*B. malayi* and *B. timori*), at least eight other species of *Brugia* are natural parasites of a wide variety of animals. All or most are parasites in the lymphatic systems of their hosts and all are transmitted by mosquitoes.

An interesting aspect of brugian filariasis is their zoonotic potential. In recent years, many cases of human infections with *Brugia* parasites have been reported in areas where human brugian filariasis is nonendemic, including both North and South America. The majority of infections have been reported from the eastern and northeastern United States (Orihel and Beaver, 1989). The species responsible for these infections remain a matter of speculation.

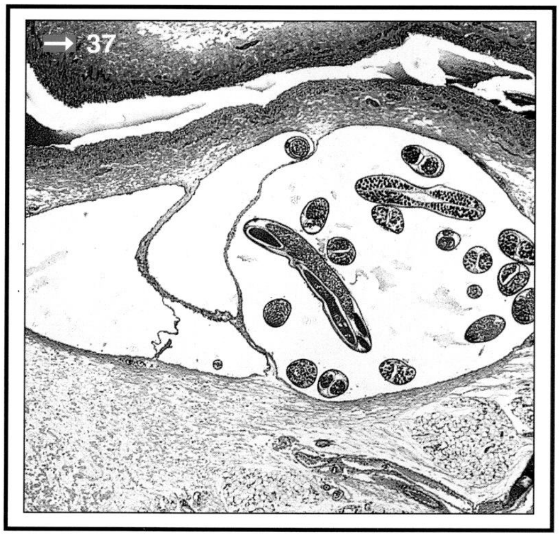

Approximately six million people worldwide are infected with *B. malayi* and *B. timori*, the majority with the former. *Brugia malayi* is limited to but widely distributed in Southeast Asia and parts of the Western Pacific. *Brugia timori* is found only in the southeastern Indonesian archipelago. Both parasites are typically found in rural populations.

Biology and Life Cycle

The sheathed microfilaria produced by the female measures about 270 µm and has a distinct tail with a terminal and a subterminal nucleus. This feature distinguishes it from microfilariae of other generic groups. The parasite is transmitted by *Mansonia*, *Anopheles*, and *Aedes* mosquitoes. When ingested by an appropriate mosquito vector, microfilariae circulating in the peripheral blood develop in the flight muscles to the infective stage in 12 to 14 days. Infective larvae that invade the human tissues via the bite site develop to adults and produce patent infections in about three months. Adult worms have an estimated lifespan of up to 10 years, while microfilariae are believed to live for about one year.

Pathology and Clinical Manifestations

Clinical presentations and pathology are similar for all of the lymphatic filariae. Although some individuals infected with *B. malayi* may have no associated symptoms, others complain of recurrent fever and malaise accompanied by bouts of lymphangitis and lymphadenitis. Lymphatic inflammation may be so intense that an abscess will form along the affected lymphatic vessel, with subsequent ulceration and scarring. This scarring has been used epidemiologically as an indicator of clinical disease in patients living in areas where brugian filariasis is endemic. Elephantiasis of the limbs is a common feature of chronic infection, but in contrast to bancroftian filariasis, the genitalia and genitourinary tract (eg, chyluria, hydrocele) are not involved. Unlike *W. bancrofti*, elephantiasis or swellings typically occur below the knee. Immigrants from nonendemic areas who become infected may have clinical symptoms (eg, lymphangitis, lymphadenitis) that are much more intense than symptoms seen in the indigenous population, and they may develop elephantiasis with greater frequency and much earlier in life. Tropical pulmonary eosinophilia occurs in areas where *W. bancrofti* and *B. malayi* overlap.

Parasite Morphology

Because *B. malayi* adults can be obtained from natural animal hosts and from experimentally infected laboratory rodents, it has not been necessary to search diligently in scarce or virtually unavailable human tissues for adult worms. Consequently, much of our knowledge of the filaria's morphology derives from examinations of animal materials collected under optimal conditions, which precludes the identification of uncertain species.

Although an individual's history of residence and travel is always useful in reaching a proper diagnosis, the potential for infections of zoonotic origin may complicate the diagnosis. Worms may be alive, dead, or in various stages of degeneration. On at least one occasion an adult worm has been found in a pulmonary artery, but it is not clear whether the parasite was *B. malayi* or of zoonotic origin.

The adult worms are morphologically similar to those of *W. bancrofti* but are smaller. Females reach lengths of approximately 55 mm with diameters of up to 180 µm; males are much smaller, with a maximum length of about 25 mm and a diameter that may reach 90 µm. Because they are usually coiled within a lymph node sinus or vessel, the worms are cut through many levels of the body (➡ 37). It is helpful to have an idea of the gross morphology of the adult worms to better interpret microscopic morphology in sectioned tissues.

The adult worms are uniform in diameter through most of the length of the body, with females being much larger than males. Both extremities taper to a smaller diameter. Both sexes have a head bulb. The esophagus is long and divided into an anterior muscular portion and a longer posterior glandular region. The intestine is a small, simple tube in both sexes. The anus (in the female) and cloaca (in the male) are near the posterior end of the body. In the female, the vulva lies in the esophageal region and opens into a muscularized, pear-shaped ovejector. The vagina is moderately long and usually coiled. It divides into paired uterine tubes that lie parallel to each other and course posteriorly through most of the length of the body, eventually terminating as seminal receptacles and leading directly into short, muscular, coiled oviducts. The latter are continuous with the long, highly coiled ovaries that fill the posterior end just anterior to the anus. In the much smaller male worm, the testis is situated in the anterior end of the body. The single genital tube courses posteriorly and ultimately joins the rectum to form the cloaca. There are paired but unequal spicules that also enter the cloaca in the dorsal aspect and may protrude from the cloaca to the exterior. The tail bears several pairs of papillae, which lie anterior and posterior to as well as around the cloaca. The worm has no alae.

In microscopic sections, the female worm may reach 180 µm in diameter, depending on its age and the level of the body. The appearance of the body wall is similar to that of *W. bancrofti*. The cuticle is relatively thin, measuring up to 2 µm in thickness over most of the body surface but twice that in the lateral fields (Plate 46:2 & 4) and often thicker still at the extremities (Plate 46:5 & 6). The hypodermis is extremely thin and difficult to discern in the submuscular regions of the body. In contrast, it expands in the lateral field to form conspicuous lateral chords that also vary in their appearance at different levels of the body. The lateral chords tend to be tall and conspicuous in the extremities (Plate 46:2 & 6) but flatter in the rest of the body (Plate 46:3 & 4). They occupy about one-third of the circumference of the body in its middle two-thirds. Dorsal and ventral chords are inapparent at most levels, but when seen they are typically tall and slender.

Musculature is well defined in both sexes. Individual muscle cells are of the coelomyarian type, with distinct contractile and cytoplasmic portions. They are tallest at the extremities (Plate 46:1 & 6; Plate 47:2) and have lower profiles at levels where the pseudocoelom is filled with organs. Usually four to five muscle cells are present per body quadrant. Muscles in the tail of the male are unusual in that the contractile portion of the cell is strong and the cytoplasmic portion seems almost nonexistent (Plate 47:5).

With regard to the female reproductive system, the structures seen depend on the level of the body. In the anterior extremity is the coiled vagina, with possibly up to several sections through the organ (Plate 46:2). In the posterior end are sections through the ovaries and oviducts (Plate 46:4 & 5). The paired uterine tubes are typically filled with developing eggs and microfilariae through most of the remainder of the body. The presence of only unsegmented eggs indicates that the female worm has not been inseminated and is infertile.

The male reproductive system is represented at all levels by a single genital tube that contains developing spermatozoa (Plate 47:1–5). In the posterior extremity, one or both spicules may be evident (Plate 47:6). The remaining tube present in male worms is the intestine, which is characteristically empty and sometimes may be difficult to find (Plate 47:4 & 5). In both sexes, the muscular esophagus has the same appearance (Plate 46:1). The glandular region is of greater diameter than it is in the female and has a distinctly granular and dark-staining appearance. Its triradiate lumen is always evident. The intestine in both sexes is a simple tube with a low, cuboidal epithelium, usually devoid of any contents and often pushed against the body wall by other organs in the pseudocoelom (Plate 46:3; Plate 47:4 & 5).

Brugia malayi may be distinguished from its close relative, *W. bancrofti*, by its smaller size, thicker cuticle, and the prominent thickening of the cuticle in the lateral fields.

References

Franz M, Buttner DW. Histology of adult *Brugia malayi*. *Trop Med Parasitol*. 1986;37:282-285.

World Health Organization. *Lymphatic Filariasis: The Disease and Its Control*. Fifth Report of the WHO Expert Committee on Filariasis. Geneva, Switzerland: World Health Organization; 1992. WHO Technical Report Series 821.

Plate 46

Brugia malayi, Female

Image 1

Transverse section through the muscular portion of the esophagus near the level of the nerve ring. This section illustrates the triradiate lumen of the esophagus, the hypodermis, and the few muscle cells (four to five) in each quadrant of the circumference of the body wall. The hypodermis is virtually impossible to define except as the lateral chords (LC) (Masson's trichrome, 360x).

Image 2

Transverse section through the anterior extremity at a level just posterior to the esophageal-intestinal junction. Note the thin cuticle, which is thickened in the lateral fields (dart), the large lateral chords (LC), and the tall coelomyarian muscle cells. The intestine (IN) has a thick lining. The other three tubes represent the coiled vagina, and one of these (uppermost) contains microfilariae in position to be discharged from the body (Masson's trichrome, 360x).

Image 3

This section of worm is through the midbody and is quite typical. At this level, female worms may measure as much as 180 µm in diameter. The paired uterine tubes characteristically contain developing eggs or microfilariae, as seen here. The intestine is represented by the small tube and is usually squeezed between the uterine branches in the midline of the body. Note the structure of the body wall, including the thin cuticle, large, low, lateral chords, and few muscle cells (Masson's trichrome, 125x).

Image 4

This section is through the posterior third of the worm. The paired, large-diameter tubes are ovaries (OV) at the level of growth zone. The unsegmented eggs are spindle shaped. The two small-diameter tubes are oviducts with their thick muscular coat. The intestine (arrow) is the small irregular tube with a low epithelial lining of cells (Masson's trichrome, 125x).

Image 5

Because the ovaries may be coiled or looped in the posterior end of the female, several sections may fill the pseudocoelom. In this section, four portions of the germinal zone of the ovaries are seen. Each contains oogonia arranged around a central rachis. The intestine has been pushed to one side of the cavity (Masson's trichrome, 825x).

Image 6

The posterior extremity is tapered and has a smaller diameter than the remainder of the body. In this transverse section, the thickening of the cuticle in the lateral fields is evident. The lateral chords are tall and conspicuous, as are the muscle cells. The rectum has a large lumen with low epithelium (Masson's trichrome, 360x).

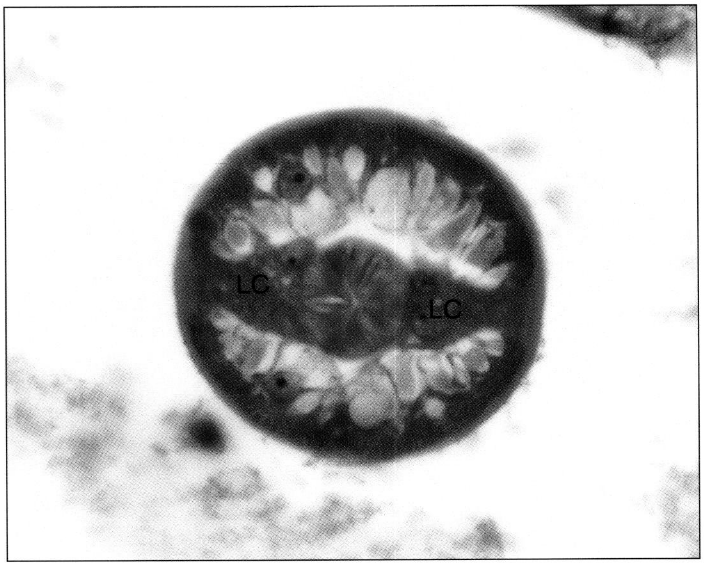

1

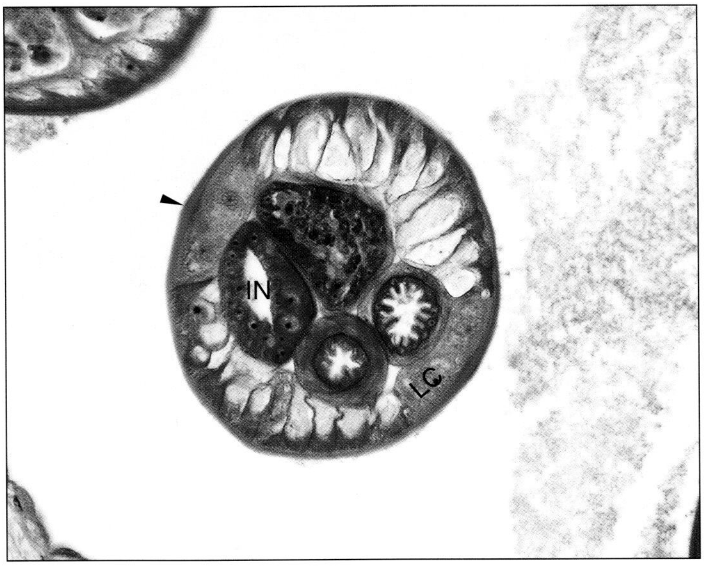

2

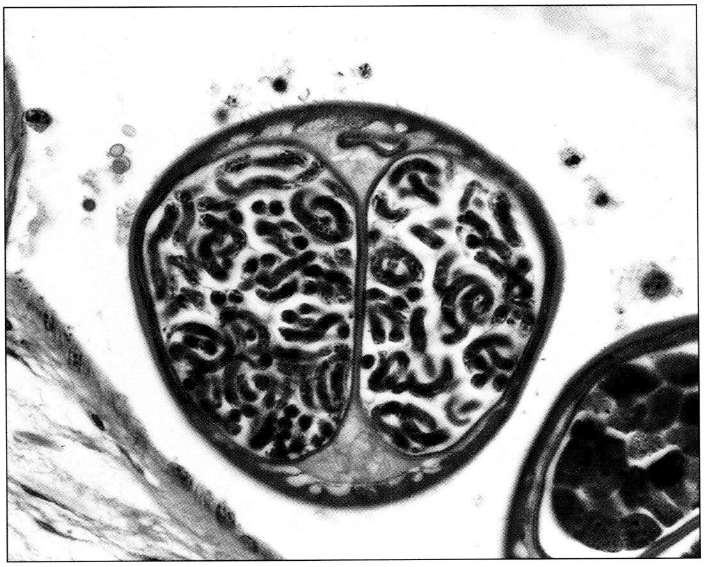

3

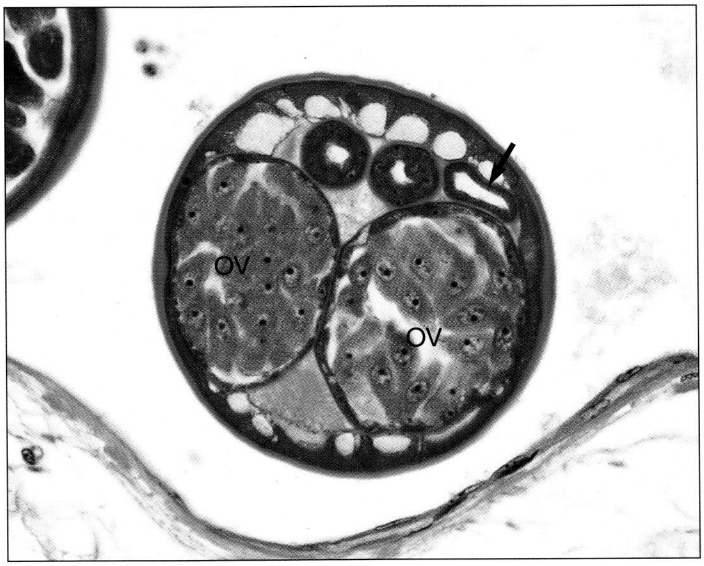

4

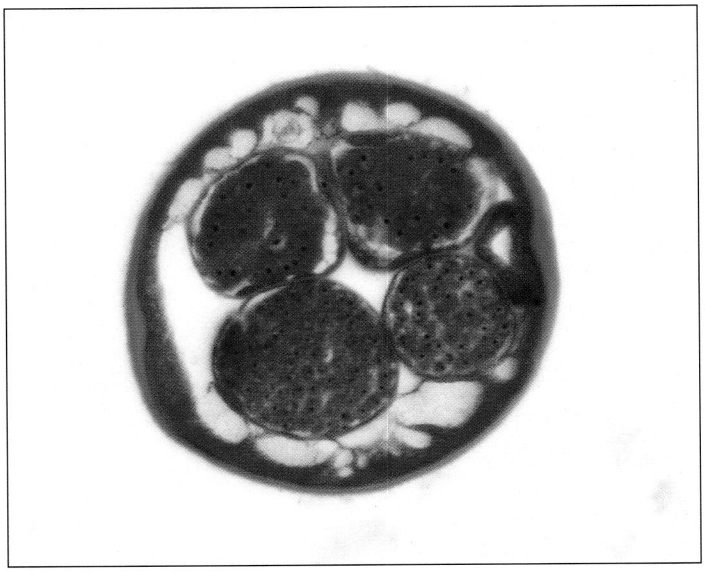

5

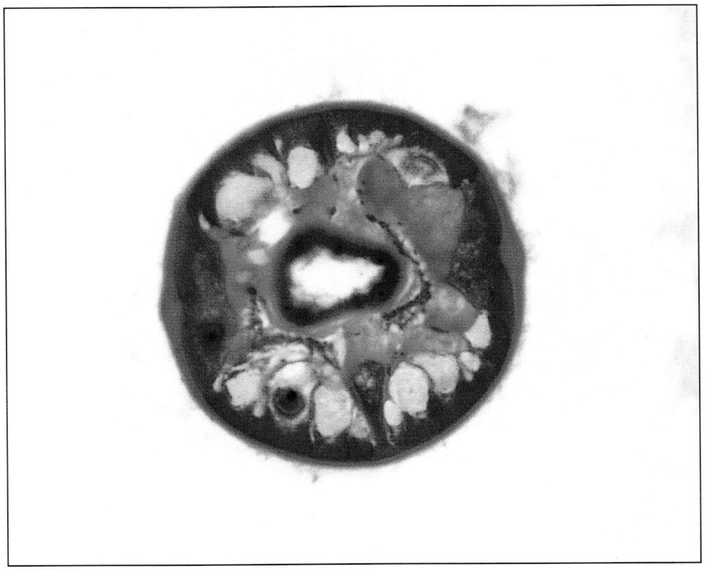

6

Plate 47

Brugia malayi, Male

Image 1

Transverse section through the anterior extremity of the worm shows intestine and the testis (dart). The structure of the body wall of the male does not differ from that of the female (Masson's trichrome, 800x).

Image 2

At virtually all levels, the male worm in transverse section contains only two tubes: the thin-walled intestine and a reproductive tube containing developing spermatozoa. The reproductive tube varies in its size and contents (Masson's trichrome, 500x).

Image 3

At high magnification, this transverse section demonstrates the typical morphologic features of a male worm. Note the thickening of the cuticle in the lateral fields. The male worm has a maximum diameter of 70 µm (Masson's trichrome, 800x).

Image 4

At a more posterior level, significant changes in the maturation of the spermatozoa can be seen. Each is small and spindle shaped. In this transverse section, the intestine has been pushed to the lateral margin of the pseudocoelom (IN) (Masson's trichrome, 500x).

Image 5

At the level of the coiled tail, the body wall changes considerably in its gross appearance. The lateral chords (dart) appear squeezed by the muscle cells and are conoid. The individual muscle cells show almost no cytoplasm (Masson's trichrome, 500x).

Image 6

Near the cloacal opening, sections through one or both spicules can generally be seen. A segment of the longer left spicule is illustrated (arrow). Note also the intestine (IN) and ejaculatory duct (EJ) (Masson's trichrome, 500x).

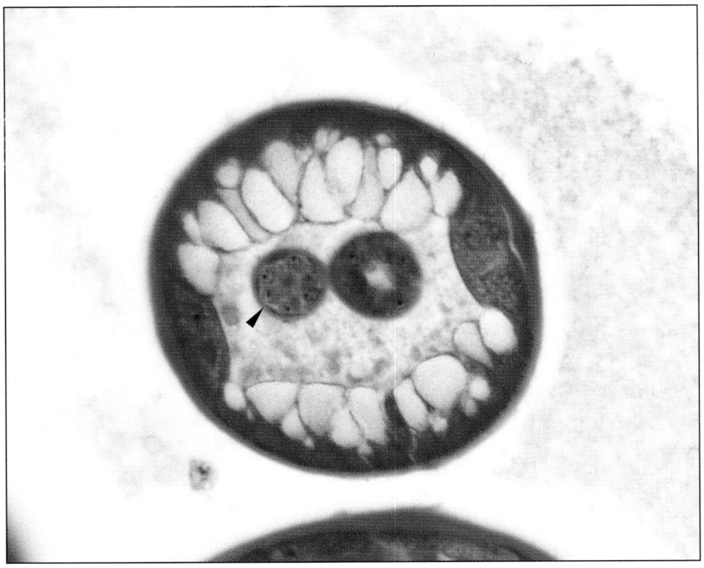

1

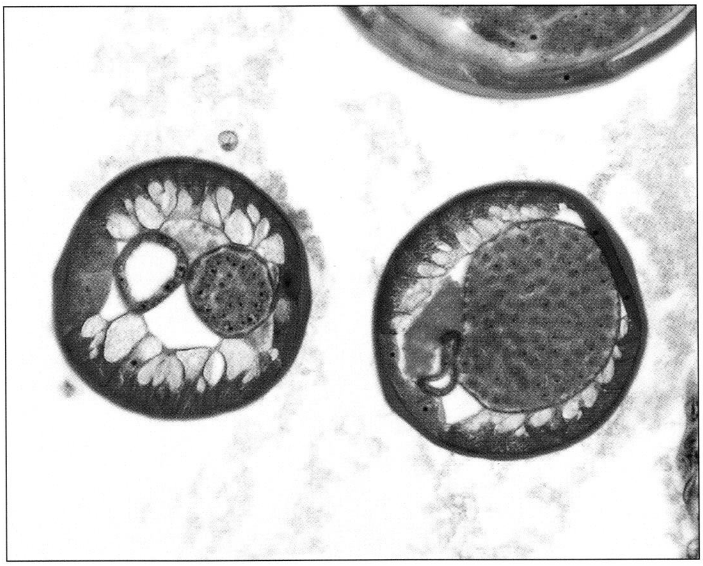

2

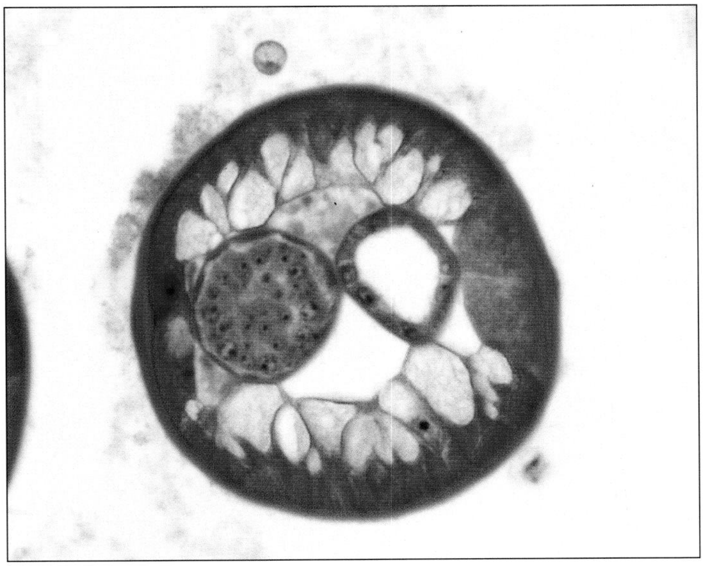

3

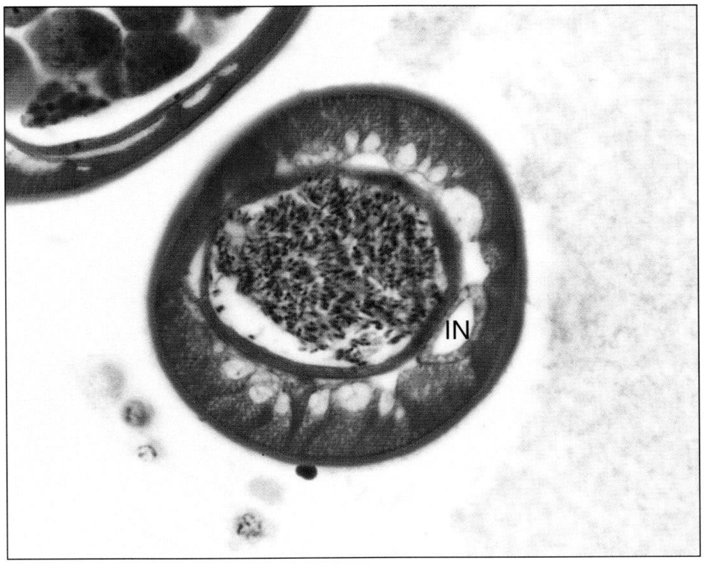

4

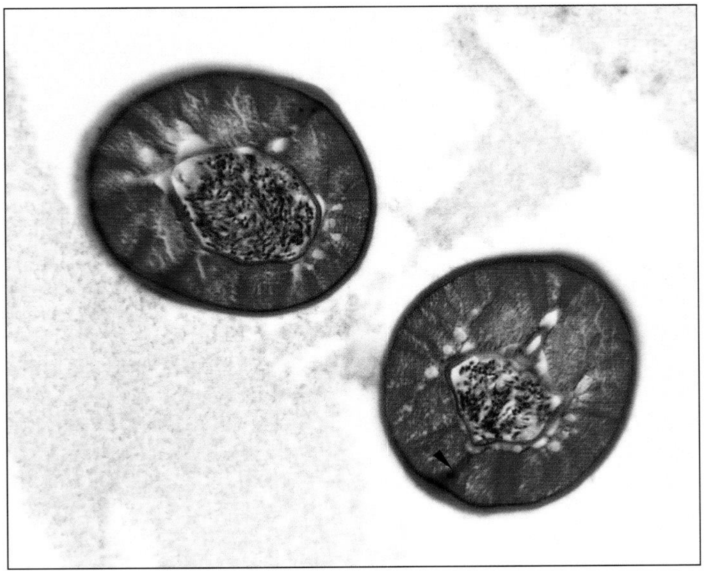

5

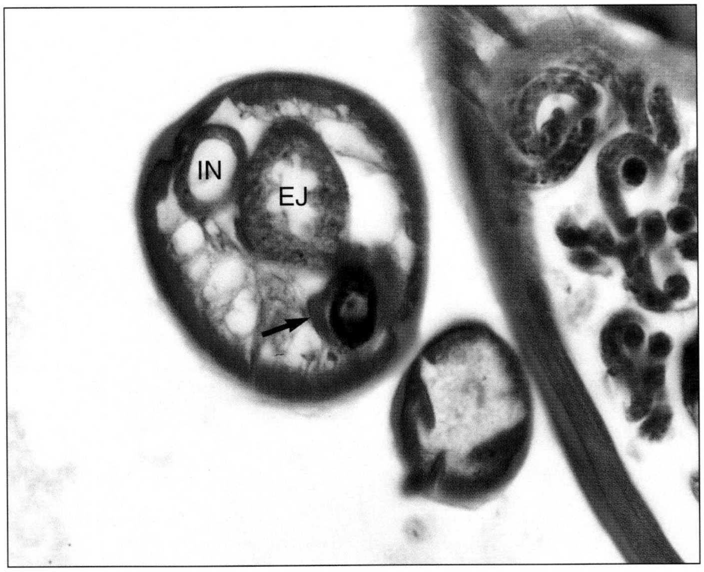

6

Brugia species

Zoonotic *Brugia* species

Several species of *Brugia* are natural parasites of animals worldwide. These species dwell essentially in the lymphatic system, produce microfilariae that circulate in the blood, and use mosquitoes as natural vectors. They do not appear to produce lymphedema in their animal hosts. Some of these species are found in domestic animals such as dogs and cats; others infect animals that live close to or in the human environment such as rabbits and raccoons. Zooanthropophilic mosquito species may accidentally transmit the infective stages by feeding first on an infected animal and then on a human approximately two weeks later.

These infections are relatively rare: only 32 cases have been published thus far. The first case was reported in the United States in 1962, but all of the others have been documented after 1977. Most infections have been found in the northeastern United States. A few have been reported in South America, specifically in Colombia, Brazil, Ecuador, and Peru.

Pathology and Clinical Manifestations

Individuals who are usually in good health present most frequently with a possibly tender mass in the cervical, axillary, or inguinal regions of two to several weeks' duration. Preoperative diagnoses may include enlarged lymph node, lymphoma, lipoma, and papilloma. Microscopic examination usually reveals a lymph node with a nonspecific lymphadenitis and preservation of the node's normal architecture, along with follicular hyperplasia and moderate eosinophilia. A nematode worm is usually found lodged in a dilated lymphatic vessel in the capsule or cortex or near the hilus of the node. The worm may be alive, with most of its normal architecture well preserved, or dead and surrounded by a granulomatous reaction. Removing the nodes eliminates further patient complaints.

These infections typically are cryptic (ie, no microfilaremia). On rare occasions, however, gravid female worms have been found in the tissues of patients who had no microfilariae in their blood after repeated follow-up examinations. In one report, a diagnosis of zoonotic *Brugia* infection in an immunosuppressed infant was based on microfilariae circulating in the peripheral blood; in another report, microfilariae, clearly *Brugia* species, were found in a patient from Ethiopia who had never resided in an area where human brugian filariasis is endemic.

Although almost all of the zoonotic *Brugia* have been found in the lymphatic system, one report involved an adult worm lodged in a pulmonary artery (Plate 49:5). Such a location is unusual but not completely unexpected; experimental inoculation of gerbils with infective larvae of *Brugia* species results in adult worms lodging in pulmonary arteries.

Parasite Morphology

Specific identification of the *Brugia* species found in human tissues is not possible because so little work has been done at the microanatomic level with existing species. Besides *B. malayi*, only *B. beaveri* has been studied to any degree. Infections have been reported from a number of different geographical areas, which suggests that several species of *Brugia* are involved. This may even be true in the United States, but data on *Brugia* species and distribution are scanty. The characteristics of the zoonotic *Brugia* species that are described in the following paragraphs are based on existing knowledge and new information gathered from the cases.

Female worms range from 50 to 120 µm in diameter with an average of about 100 µm. The cuticle is thin (about 1 to 2 µm thick) but becomes thicker in the lateral fields, just as it does in *B. malayi* (Plate 49:6). No distinct layers are visible in the cuticle. The surface bears fine transverse striations, which are evident only with appropriate orientation. Lateral chords are large and conspicuous and may occupy up to 30% of the total circumference. Dorsal and ventral chords may be evident but often are inconspicuous. Muscles are coelomyarian and range between three and five per quadrant; both contractile and cytoplasmic portions are distinct (Plate 49:3 & 6).

Uterine tubes are large and whether full or empty they usually fill the pseudocoelom. Their contents are usually unsegmented ova, which are alive or degenerated (Plate 49:3 & 6; Plate 50:4). The intestine is a small tube with a relatively thin wall; one must be careful not to confuse it with the uterine branches (Plate 49:3; Plate 49:6). Even in the degenerated state, the female worm can be identified in part by its size and by the contents of the pseudocoelom (Plate 50:6).

The male worm is much smaller than the female, with a diameter of 35 to 55 µm. Only one reproductive tube is present at all levels (except at the esophageal level, which usually has no reproductive structures) (Plate 50:2). Sections through the posterior end of the worm usually show one or both spicules (Plate 50:2). Muscles and lateral chords appear as they do in the female, except that in the tail region the appearance of the muscle cells is as described for *B. malayi*—that is, the cytoplasmic portion of the individual cell is virtually nonexistent (Plate 48:6).

Plate 48 shows typical morphologic features of *B. beaveri* from a raccoon. The male and female worms in these specimens were alive when fixed, and as a result, their normal architecture under optimal conditions was preserved. Because our knowledge of the animal species currently is limited to *B. beaveri,* species identifications are unlikely. Generic identification should not be a problem, however.

References

Baird JK, Neafie RC. South American brugian filariasis: report of a human infection acquired in Peru. *Am J Trop Med Hyg*. 1988;39:185-188.

Orihel TC, Beaver PC. Zoonotic *Brugia* infection in North and South America. *Am J Trop Med Hyg*. 1989;40:638-647.

Simmons CF Jr, Winter HS, Berde C, et al. Zoonotic filariasis with lymphedema in an immunodeficient infant. *N Engl J Med*. 1984;310:1243-1245.

Plate 48

Brugia beaveri

Image 1

Transverse section through the anterior extremity frequently reveals the well-developed muscular portion of the esophagus. Note the cuticularized triradiate lumen. At this level, the lateral chords are usually large and conspicuous. Note the typical *Brugia* features of the body wall (Masson's trichrome, 740x).

Image 2

Female worm at the midbody level. The pseudocoelom is filled with the paired uterine tubes, which may contain microfilariae, as shown here, or eggs in various stages of development. The intestine is invariably small and tubular. At this level, a female worm measures about 100 µm in diameter (Masson's trichrome, 380x).

Image 3

In the posterior third of the body, a variety of reproductive tubes can be seen. In this section, the terminal portion of one uterine tube (seminal receptacle) is filled with sperm; and an egg (arrow) is present as well. Note also the two sections of ovary (germinal zone) (OV), the two sections of thick-walled, muscular oviducts, and the intestine (IN). Features of the body wall are sometimes not clearly evident, as seen here (Masson's trichrome, 330x).

Image 4

Normal appearance of the male worm at most levels. Typically, the pseudocoelom contains only two tubes: the intestine and the reproductive tube, which is filled with developing spermatozoa. This section illustrates the typical features of the cuticle, including its thickened portion in the lateral fields (dart), the large lateral chords, and the few well-developed muscle cells. At the midbody level, the male worm has an average diameter of 70 µm (Masson's trichrome, 740x).

Image 5

At more posterior levels, the male reproductive tube contains nearly mature spermatozoa (Masson's trichrome, 740x).

Image 6

In the region of the coiled tail, the body has a characteristic appearance, ie, the fibrillar or contractile portion of the muscle cell is expanded and the cytoplasm is not evident. The lateral chords (arrow) are reduced in size and volume. The intestine is small and somewhat obscure (dart), whereas the reproductive tube is much larger and contains spermatozoa (Masson's trichrome, 740x).

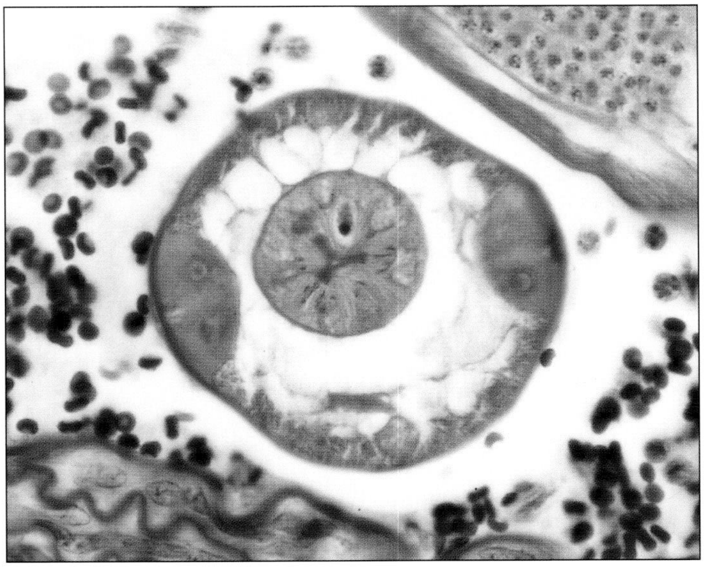

1

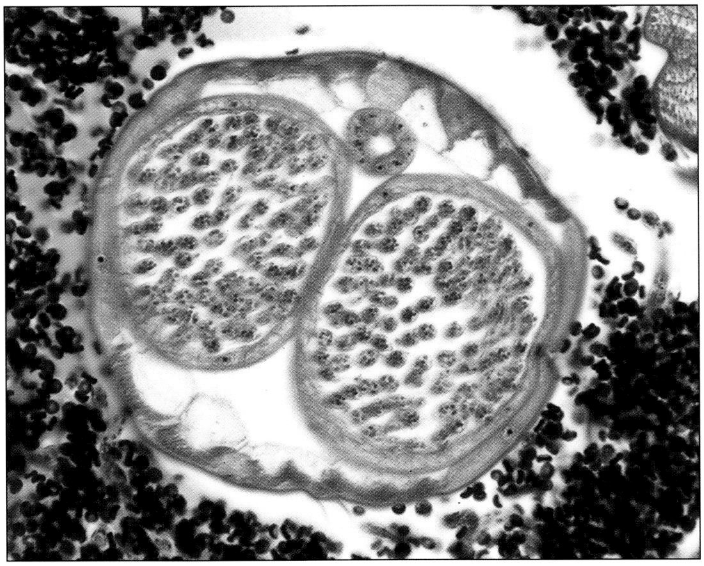

2

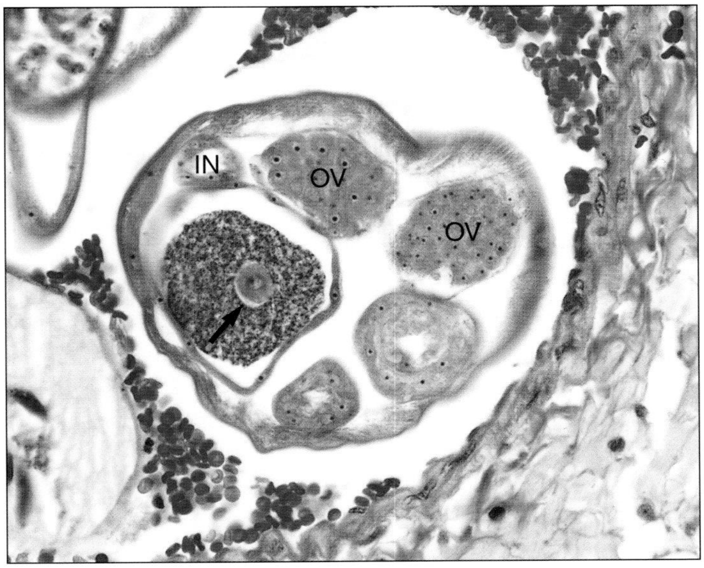

3

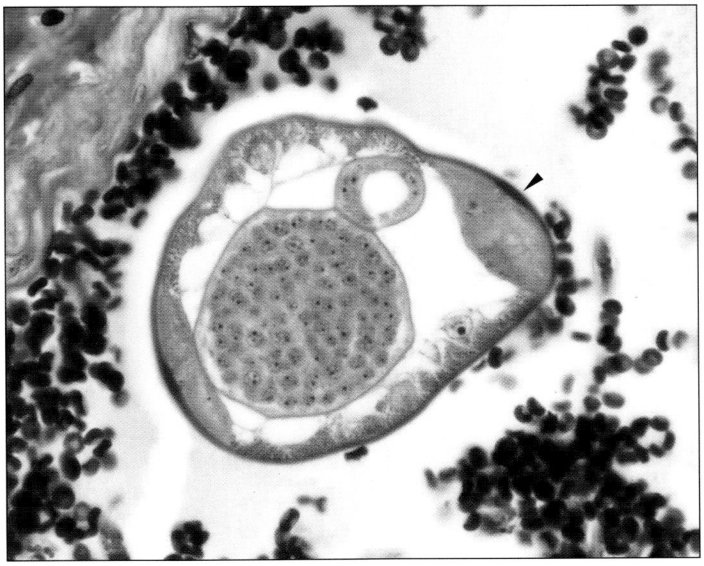

4

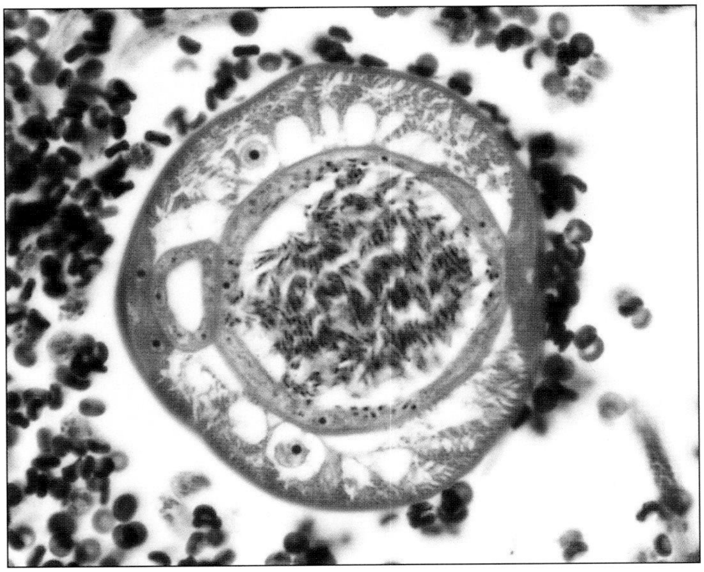

5

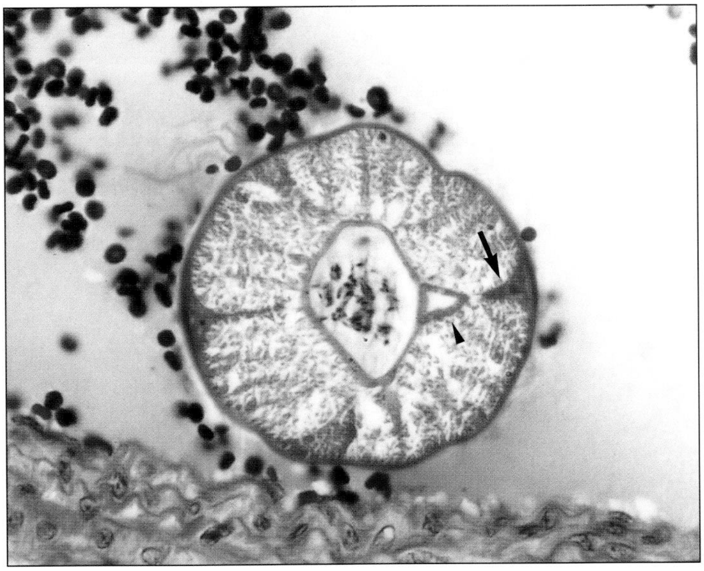

6

Plate 49

Zoonotic *Brugia*

Image 1

Section through a lymph node removed from an Ohioan. A nematode parasite is coiled in a dilated, subcapsular lymph vessel (H&E, 40x). (Case courtesy of Y. Gutierrez.)

Image 2

At higher magnification, transverse and longitudinal sections through a sexually mature female filaria (H&E, 180x). (Case courtesy of Y. Gutierrez.)

Image 3

At still higher magnification, the morphologic features of the parasite indicate that it is a species of *Brugia*. The worm has a maximum diameter of 48 μm. The degenerating eggs in the uterine tubes (UT) indicate that although the worm is sexually mature, it is infertile (H&E, 900x). (Case courtesy of Y. Gutierrez.)

Image 4

This female worm found in a lymph node in the breast of a woman from New York measured 56 μm in diameter. The worm is in good condition, and the morphologic features that aid in its identification as a *Brugia* species are evident. The eggs in the uterine tubes indicate that the worm is sexually mature (H&E, 360x).

Image 5

Transverse section through a small artery in the lung of an individual who had worked in India. Lodged in the vessel are two intact sections of a filarial parasite (H&E, 100x).

Image 6

At much higher magnification, the morphologic features of the parasite—ie, the thin, smooth cuticle, large lateral chords, and few muscle cells—indicate that it is a species of *Brugia*. The paired uterine tubes, one of which contains degenerating, unsegmented eggs, indicates that the worm is sexually mature but infertile. Note the small tubular intestine (dart). The worm measures 110 μm at midbody (H&E, 320x).

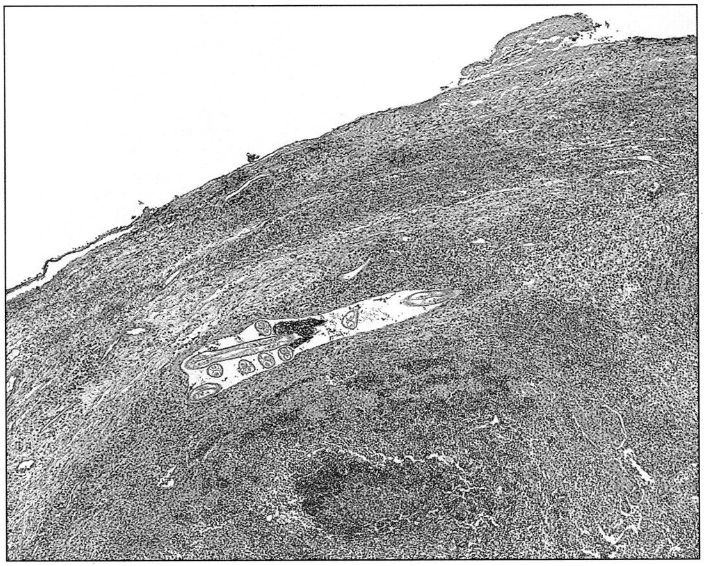

1

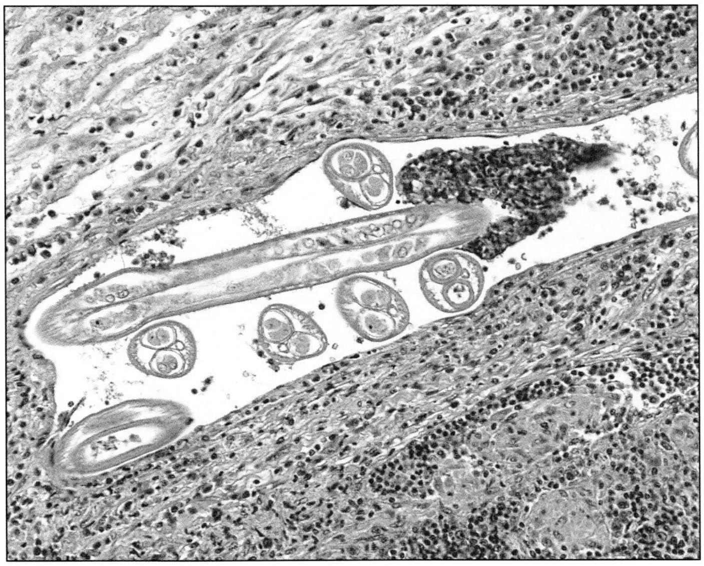

2

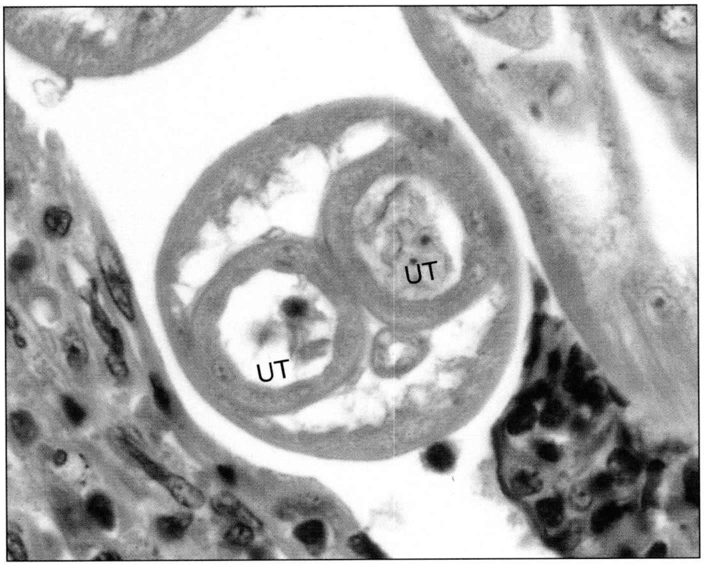

3

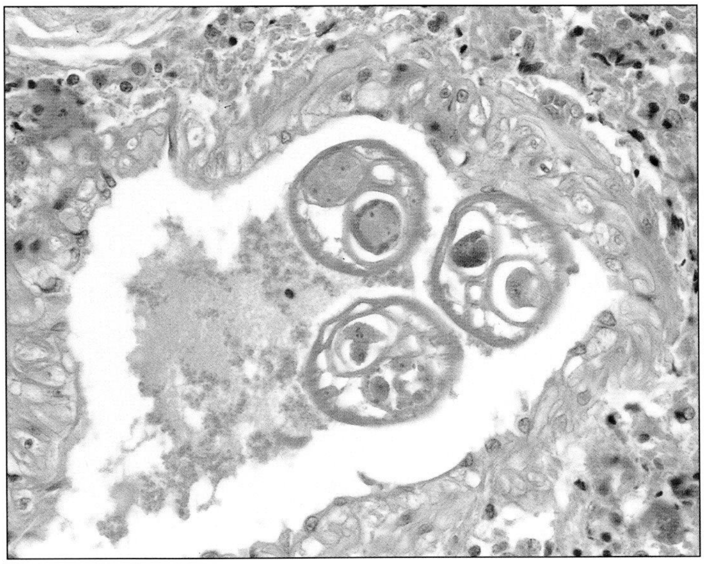

4

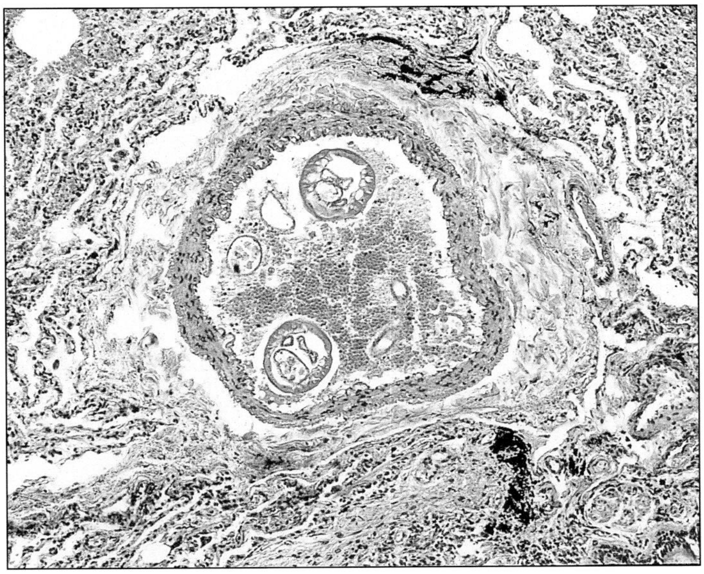

5

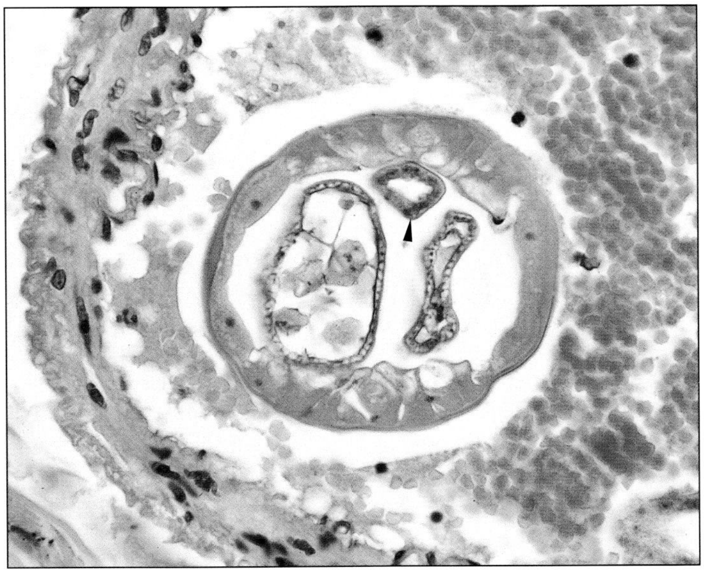

6

Plate 50

Zoonotic *Brugia*

Image 1

Section through an inflamed cervical lymph node shows a lymph vessel containing a highly coiled nematode parasite. The node was removed from an individual who six months previously had visited the Amazon rain forest in Peru (H&E, 45x). (Case courtesy of AFIP.)

Image 2

At higher magnification, the several sections of worm reveal that it is a male with features characteristic of *Brugia.* Some of the sections are cut through the posterior end of the worm at the level of the spicules (arrows). This worm measured approximately 50 μm in diameter (H&E, 300x). (Case courtesy of AFIP.)

Image 3

Another lymph vessel in the node shown in the two previous images contains a gravid female worm. The paired uterine tubes in all of the sections contain eggs in various stages of development to microfilariae. One section is cut through the seminal receptacle (arrow), which is packed with sperm and two eggs (H&E, 200x). (Case courtesy of AFIP.)

Image 4

At much higher magnification, this female worm has all of the morphologic features of *Brugia.* The paired uteri contain eggs in various stages of segmentation. It is most unusual to see gravid female worms in these zoonotic infections (H&E, 800x). (Case courtesy of AFIP.)

Image 5

A section of a nodule removed from the arm of a Louisianan. The dead female worm had undergone appreciable degenerative changes (H&E, 100x).

Image 6

At higher magnification, the female worm, which measures approximately 120 μm in maximum diameter, has morphologic features of *Brugia* species. The cuticle is thin and appears thickened in the lateral field (arrow). The lateral chords occupy a significant portion of the circumference of the body, and the muscle cells are relatively few. The presence of degenerating eggs in some of the uterine tubes indicates that the worm was sexually mature but infertile (H&E, 400x).

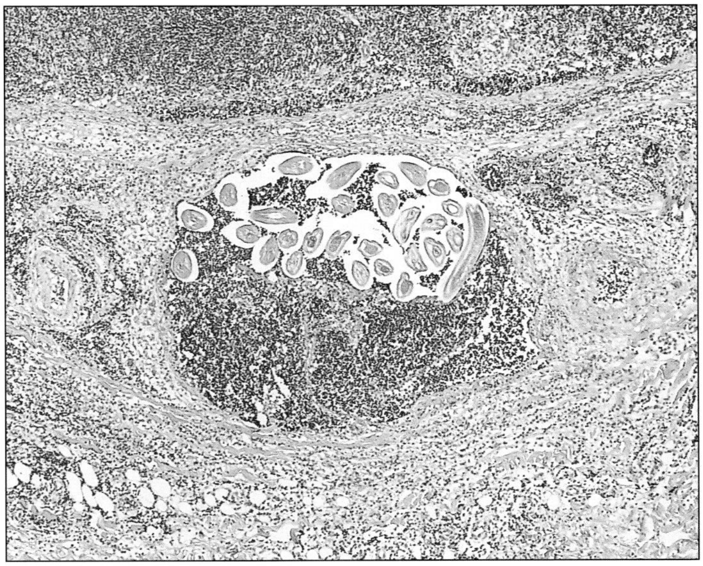

1

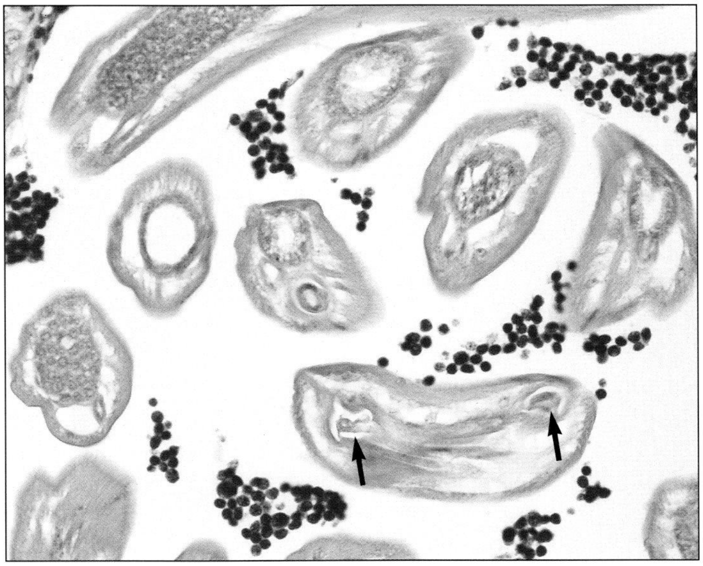

2

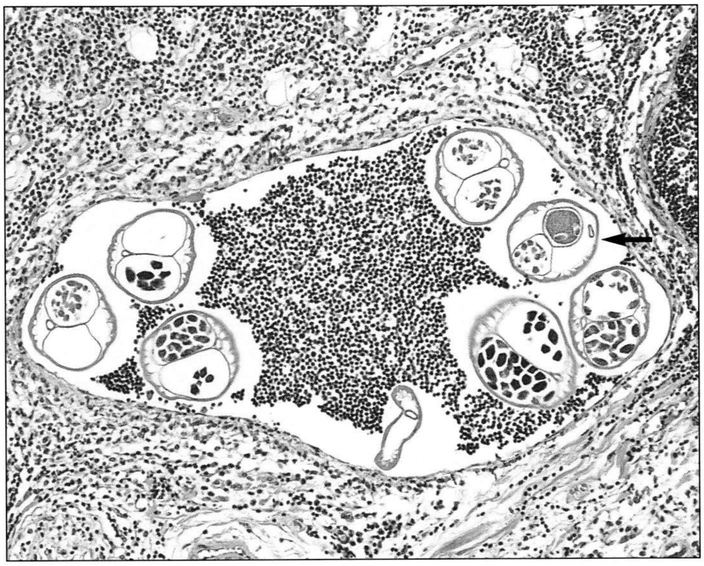

3

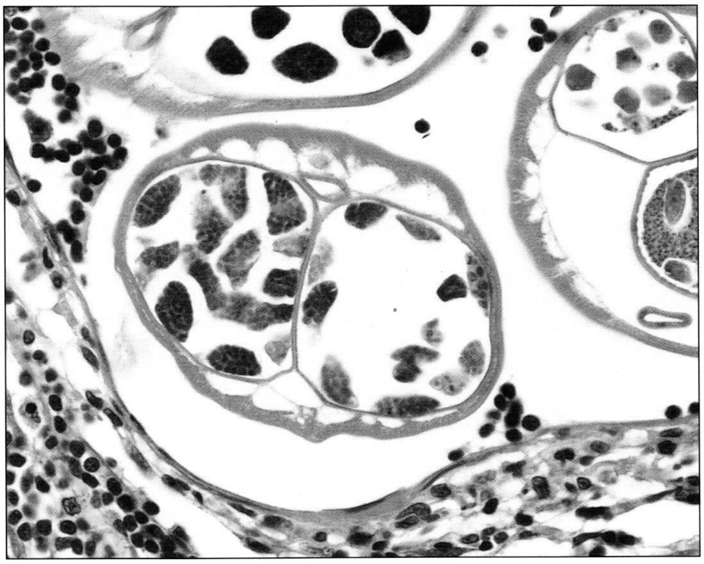

4

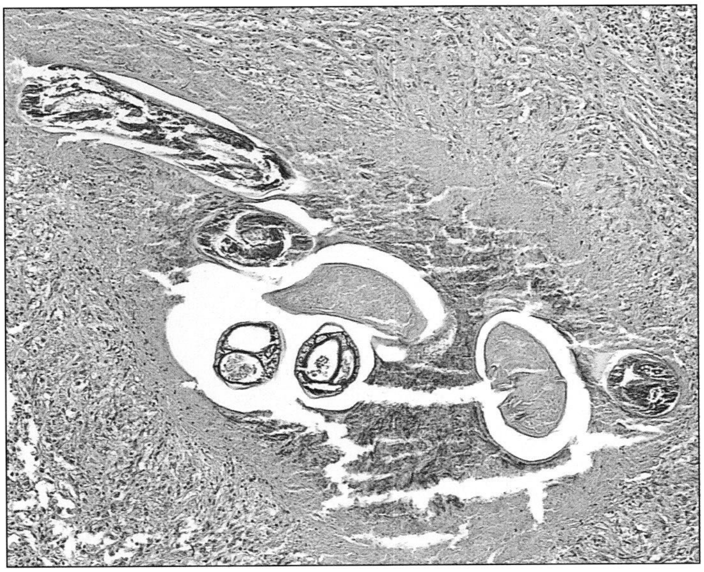

5

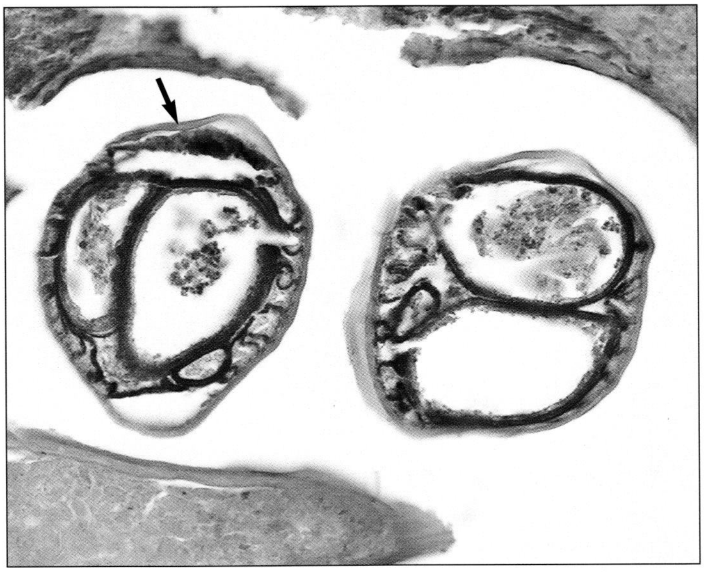

6

Onchocerca volvulus and *Onchocerca* species

Human onchocerciasis is an important medical, public health, and socioeconomic problem in parts of tropical Africa and, to a lesser extent, in Latin America, where *Onchocerca volvulus* is endemic. The parasite resides in the subcutaneous tissues and causes severe itching, disfiguring skin lesions, and potentially severe ocular lesions, which may lead to blindness. Onchocerciasis is frequently referred to as "river blindness," because of the close association between the disease and fast-moving rivers and streams where the vector breeds and humans are infected. More than 17 million people worldwide, the majority of them in Africa, are infected with the parasite.

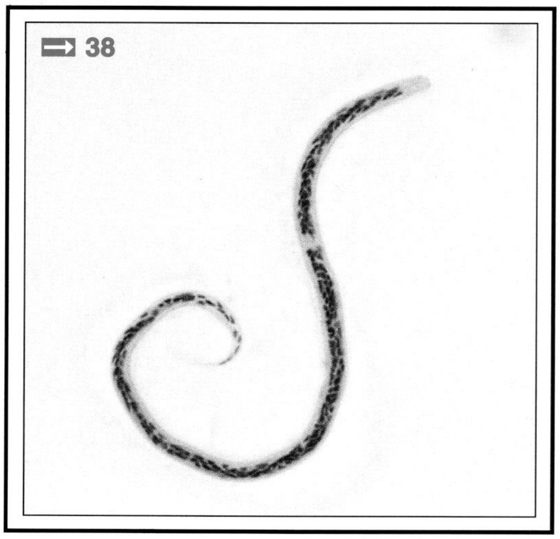

Biology and Life Cycle

The adult worms live in the subcutaneous tissues enmeshed in fibrous connective tissue nodules that, if superficial, are easily palpable and may be widely distributed over the body. The distribution of nodules on the body varies with the geographic region. Nodules may be in deeper tissues and therefore impalpable, but this is less common. The average nodule measures 2 cm in diameter, but smaller and larger ones frequently occur. Each nodule contains between 1 and 10 worms, with a male to female ratio of 1.1 to 1.2. The female worm produces unsheathed microfilariae (➡ 38), which measure approximately 309 µm in length, have diameters of 5 to 9 µm, and reside in the dermal layers of the skin. Diagnosis is made by examining skin snips for microfilariae. Blackflies of the genus *Simulium* are natural vectors of *O. volvulus*. Development from microfilaria to infective larva in the vector requires about 5 to 7 days, depending on the environmental temperature. Prepatent development in the human host varies considerably but usually requires 12 to 15 months.

Pathology and Clinical Manifestations

A huge body of literature is devoted to the clinical and pathologic aspects of human onchocerciasis. Briefly, onchocerciasis is associated with a wide spectrum of clinical diseases—dermal, lymphatic, and ocular. Skin lesions result from host inflammatory response to dead or dying microfilariae, which are widely dispersed in the dermis. The most common is an intensely pruritic dermatitis. Skin changes of a chronic nature include atrophy, hypertrophy, and abnormal pigmentation. Lymph nodes draining the areas of dermatitis, typically inguinal and femoral nodes, may become enlarged and fibrosed. Along with skin atrophy, the condition of hanging groin develops. In Yemen and occasionally in Africa, a chronic, hyperreactive, localized dermatitis may be seen, with intense itching, papules, pustules, edema, darkening of the skin, and enlarged regional lymph nodes. This condition, called "Sowda," predominates in young, adult males and is usually localized to a lower limb.

Live microfilariae invade the ocular tissues and stimulate little inflammatory response. They may be found in the conjunctiva, cornea, sclera, anterior and posterior chambers, vitreous, retina, optic nerve, etc. Each dead microfilaria stimulates a limited inflammatory response, and in chronic infection the cumulative effect of dying microfilariae produces considerable inflammation and scarring. Because the eye depends on clarity for normal function, even minor scarring causes visual impairment.

Individuals with demonstrable microfiladermia often have no palpable nodules. Occasionally, individuals have nodules but no microfilariae. Other growths or tumors, such as lipomas, sebaceous and dermoid cysts, foreign body granulomas, or even enlarged lymph nodes, must not be confused with true onchocercal nodules. A diagnosis can be confirmed by needle aspiration and demonstration of filarial tissues in the aspirate or by removal and histopathologic examination of the nodules.

Parasite Morphology

The adult female worm is large, up to 70 cm in length with a maximum diameter of about 0.4 mm, and lies tightly coiled in the nodule. Males are much smaller, reaching only about 42 mm in length with a diameter of approximately 0.2 mm. Because adult worms are tightly coiled within a nodule, almost every level of the worm can be seen in a few sections (Plate 51:1). It is possible to identify the sex of the worm, assess its reproductive state, and determine whether it is live or dead. Microfilariae are typically distributed throughout the dermis (Plate 51:2).

The body wall has characteristic features that aid in identification. In the female, the multilayered cuticle is 5 to 7 µm thick, and its cortical surface bears conspicuous transverse thickenings, or ridges, spaced between 50 and 70 µm apart. These are seen in longitudinal views of the body (Plate 52:3 & 4). The ridges increase the thickness of the cuticle substantially. The middle layer is divided transversely into striae, usually two for each external ridge. The number of striae between consecutive external ridges has been suggested as a means of identifying species of *Onchocerca* (Plate 52:4). However, this number may vary with the level of the body. A thin, fibrous, basal lamella interfaces with the hypodermis. A striking feature in the female is the highly developed hypodermis and significant reduction in the musculature. At most levels of the body, only a few muscle cells are visible in each body quadrant. These are often much reduced and vestigial in appearance (Plate 51:4 & 5). At the extremities, the muscles may be somewhat better developed (Plate 51:6). The pseudocoelom is usually filled with reproductive organs, and at most levels the paired uteri contain developing or fully mature microfilariae (Plate 51:4 & 5). Other structures, such as ovaries and oviducts, are visible in cuts through the posterior end of the body (Plate 51:6). The esophagus is short and muscular, has a triradiate lumen, and is seen only in the anterior end of the body. The intestine is a small, simple tube and often has an irregular lumen. In some worms, the intestinal cells may be filled with spherogranules.

The male cuticle differs in its appearance from the female cuticle. Deep striations give the male cuticle an annulated appearance, which is best seen in longitudinal and oblique sections of the worm (Plate 52:1). In transverse sections, the body wall of the male worm looks more like that of a typical filaria. The cuticle is moderately thin. The hypodermis is also thin in the submuscular areas. Lateral chords are conspicuous but not as highly developed as in females. Muscle cells are much better developed and are strong at all body levels, with usually three or four cells per quadrant (Plate 52:2). The reproductive system is represented by a single tube that contains developing spermatozoa (Plate 52:1 & 2). As in females, the intestine is a simple tube. The lumen may be irregular, and spherogranules may be seen.

Onchocerca volvulus can be easily recognized in tissues by several features. To be infected with *O. volvulus*, an individual must have a history of travel to or residence in an endemic area either in Africa or Central or South America. Adult worms are encased either in discrete nodules or in loose connective tissues from deeper parts of the body. Key characteristics of the female worm are size and morphology of the body wall (ie, cuticular ridges, striae, highly developed hypodermis, and reduced muscle development). Male worms display the characteristic cuticular annulations and can be found in association with female worms. Both males and females differ from species of *Dirofilaria* in subcutaneous tissues, especially in structure of the cuticle and other elements of the body wall.

Zoonotic *Onchocerciasis*

Several species of *Onchocerca* are parasites of cattle, horses, and related ungulates throughout the world, including the United States. Despite our knowledge of their existence, details of their geographic distribution, prevalence, life cycles, and vector requirements have not been determined in most instances.

On rare occasions, animal *Onchocerca* species accidentally infect humans. Cases have been reported in the United States, Canada, Japan, and Russia. In no instance had the patient traveled to or resided in areas where human onchocerciasis is endemic. Worms are most easily identified if segments or intact worms can be removed from the tissues. When material is limited to microsections, the morphologic features of the body wall, particularly the cuticle, are crucial factors for diagnosis (Plate 52:5). The transverse ridges are conspicuous, and even the striae in the middle layer of the cuticle can be seen and counted (Plate 52:6). The worm shown in (Plate 52:5 & 6) was found in the tissue of an Illinois resident who had not left the United States and had never traveled to any state beyond the states contiguous with Illinois.

References

Beaver PC, Horner GS, Bilos JZ. Zoonotic onchocerciasis in a resident of Illinois and observations on the identification of *Onchocerca* species. *Am J Trop Med Hyg*. 1974;23:595-607.

Murdoch ME, Hay RJ, Mackenzie CD, et al. A clinical classification and grading system of the cutaneous changes in onchocerciasis. *Brit J Dermatol.* 1993;129:260-269.

Schulz-Key H, Ginger CD, Duke BOL, Büttner DW. The *Onchocerca* nodule and the adult filariae: normal structure, changes during chemotherapy and optimal recovery of worm material. *Trop Med Parasitol.* 1988;39(suppl IV):329-486.

World Health Organization. Third Report of the WHO Expert Committee on Onchocerciasis. Geneva, Switzerland: World Health Organization; 1987. WHO Technical Report Series 752.

Plate 51

Onchocerca volvulus

Image 1

A scanning view through an *Onchocerca* nodule illustrates many transverse and longitudinal sections through what appears to be both male and female adult worms (H&E, 8x).

Image 2

Microfilariae are easily recognized in the dermis of the skin. One must be careful in making a diagnosis of *O. volvulus* solely on the presence of a microfilaria in the skin, however, because microfilariae of *M. streptocerca* occupy the same tissues, and the geographic distribution of these two parasites frequently overlaps (H&E, 325x).

Image 3

Sections through male (arrows) and female worms in same nodule. Note the smaller diameter of the male worm and the presence of only one reproductive tube. Two tubes are seen in sections of the female (H&E, 80x).

Images 4 and 5

Female worms in transverse section show typical morphologic features, ie, moderately thick cuticle, well-developed hypodermis, and weak musculature (MU). The paired uterine branches contain developing microfilariae. Note also the small intestinal tube (IN) (H&E, 160x).

Image 6

Transverse section through the posterior end of a female worm contains sections of ovaries in addition to the intestine (IN) (H&E, 160x).

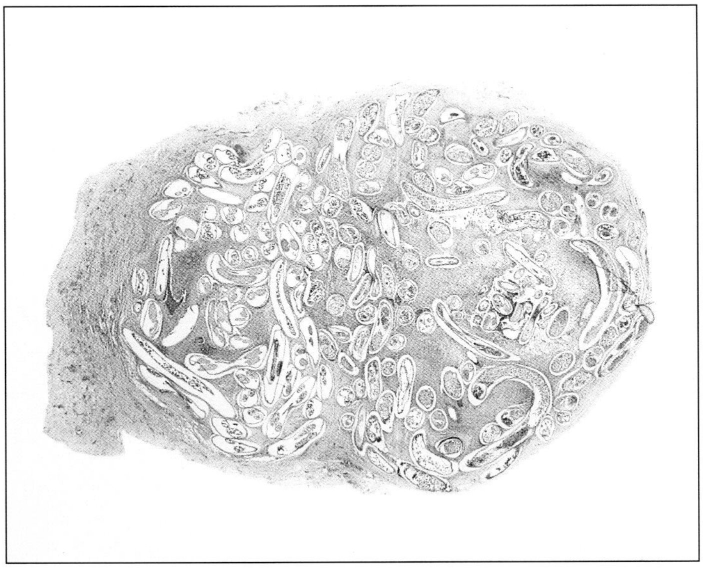

1

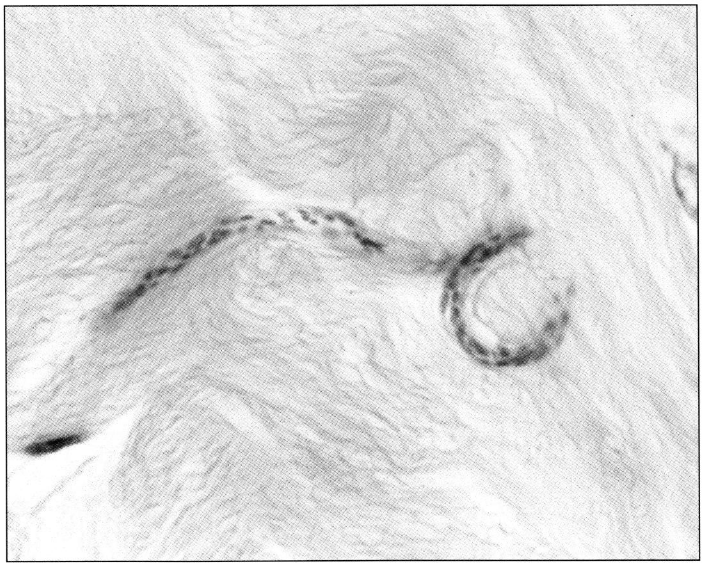

2

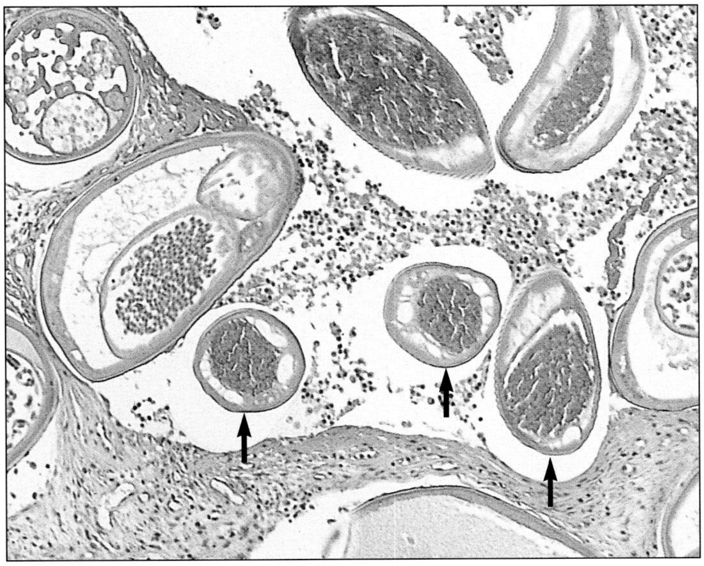

3

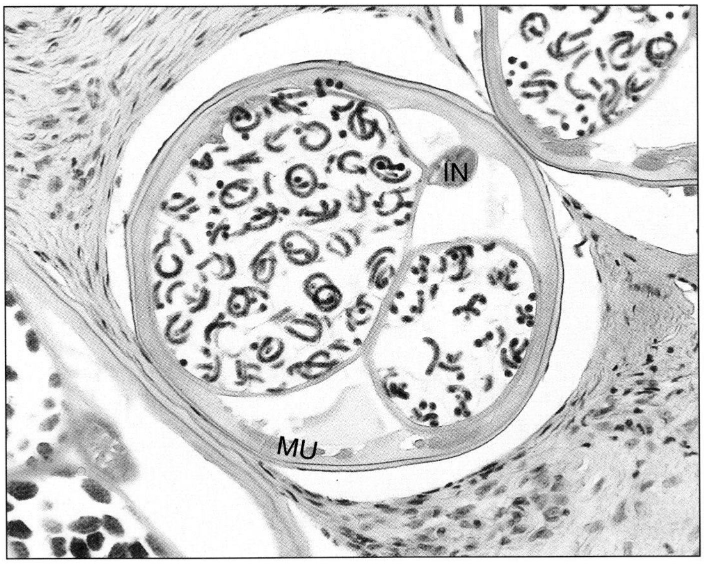

4

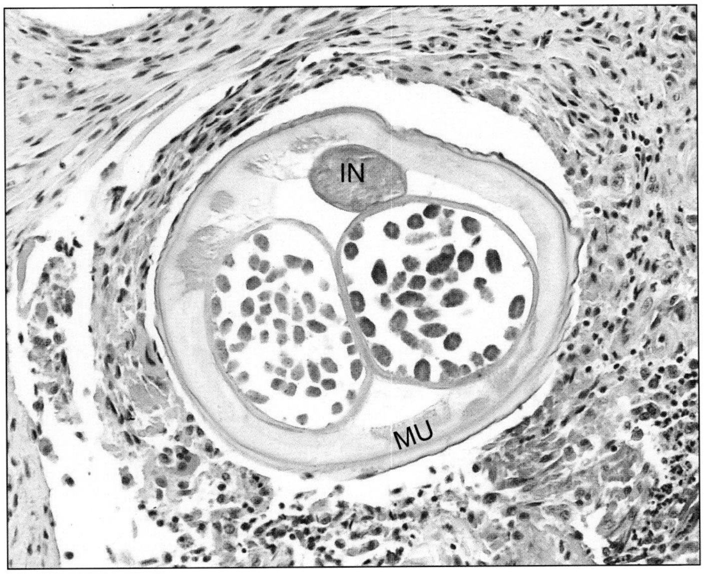

5

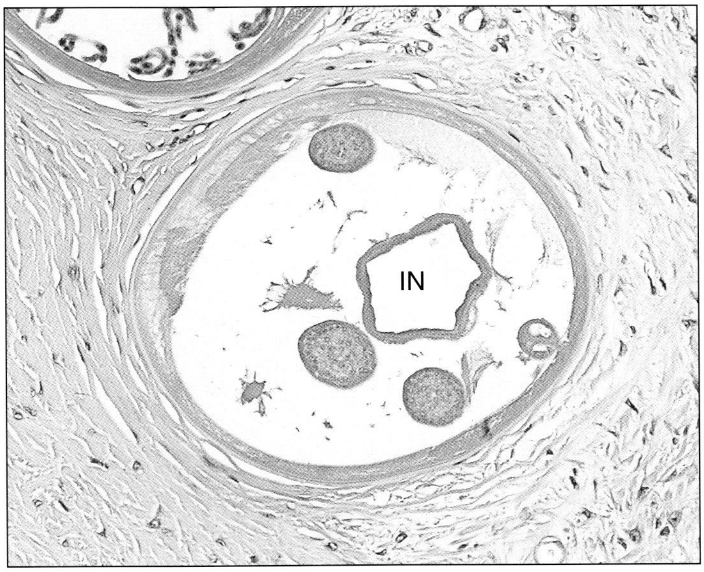

6

Plate 52

Onchocerca volvulus and *Onchocerca* species

Image 1

Multiple sections of a male *O. volvulus* worm in a nodule (H&E, 40x).

Image 2

Transverse section through the same male worm shows the typical body wall architecture. Note the relatively thin cuticle, the conspicuous but not overdeveloped hypodermal (lateral) chords (keyline), and the well-developed coelomyarian muscles, which number three to four in each quadrant. The reproductive tube contains developing spermatozoa. The smaller tube is the intestine (H&E, 230x).

Image 3

Tangential section through a female worm illustrates the cuticular rings (darts) on the surface of the cuticle (Masson's trichrome, 200x).

Image 4

A. High magnification of an unstained section shows the cuticular rings on the surface of the cuticle and the underlying striae (ST).

B. A stained section of the worm illustrates the same features less clearly (Masson's trichrome, 120x).

Image 5

Section through an immature *Onchocerca* in an inflammatory nodule in a woman who had never traveled beyond the midwestern region of the United States. The prominent ridges in the cuticle immediately identify the worm as an *Onchocerca* species (Trichrome, 100x).

Image 6

The same worm at high magnification shows both the ridges on the surface of the cuticle and the striae in the middle layer (darts) (Trichrome, 350x).

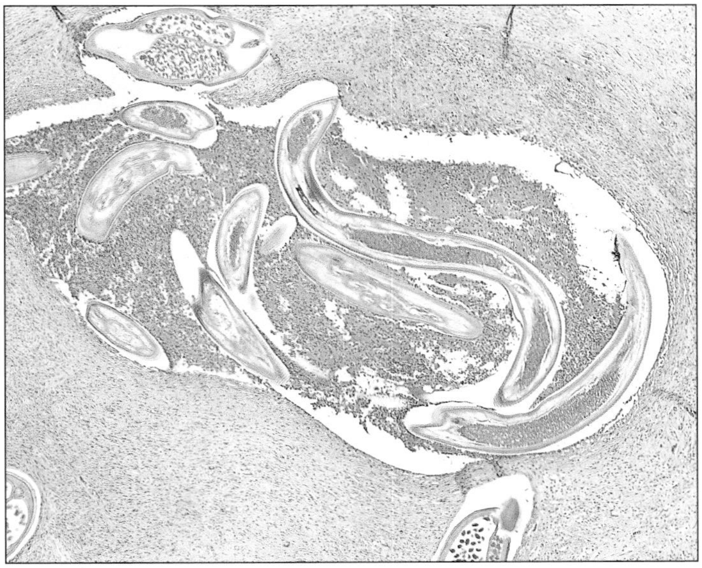

1

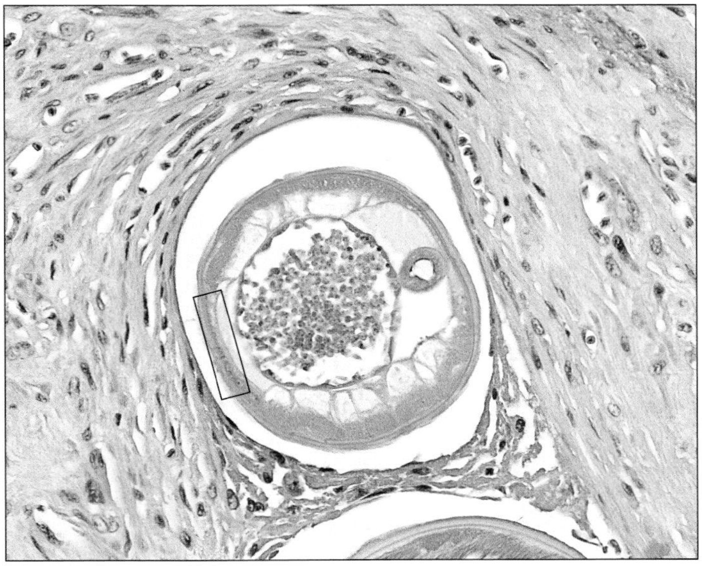

2

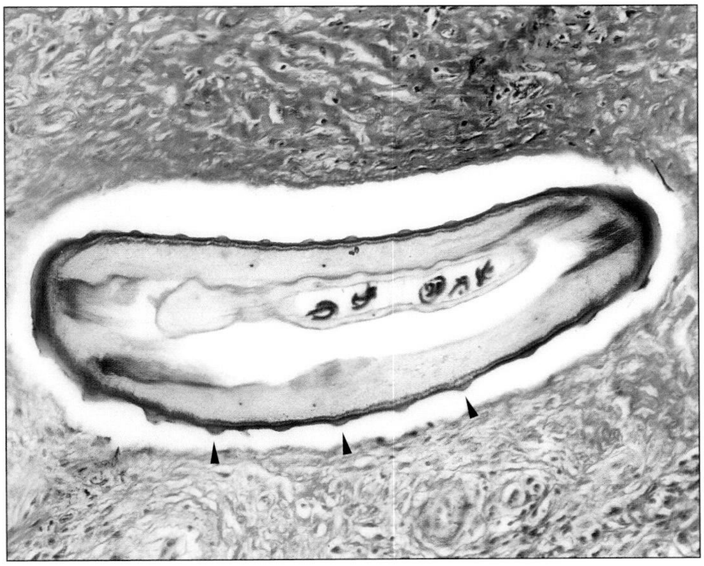

3

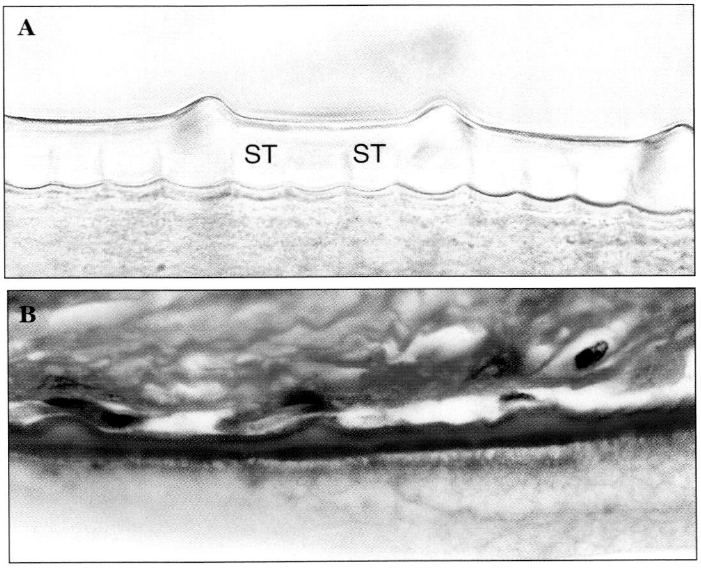

4

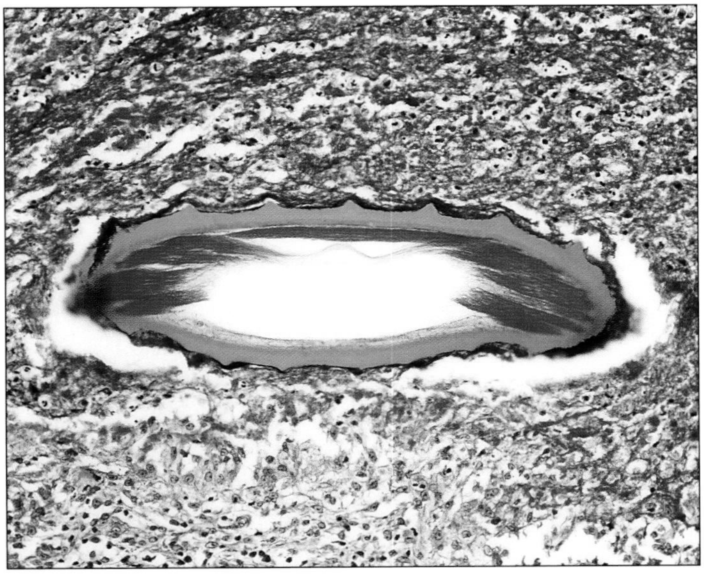

5

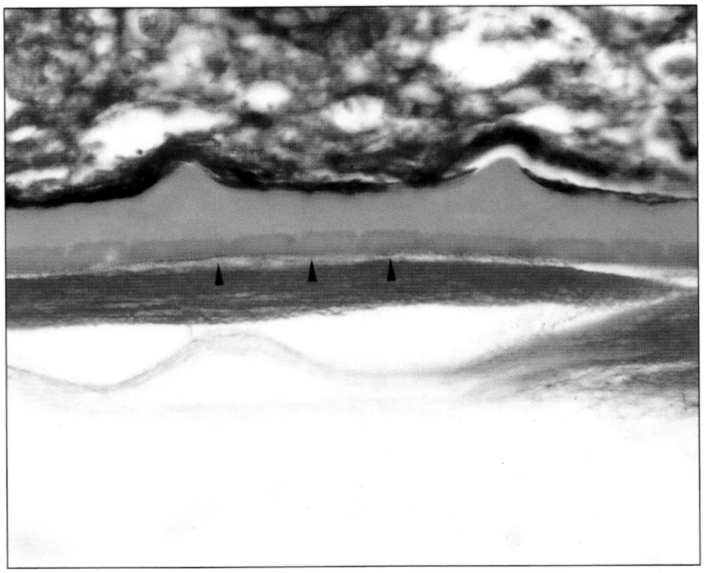

6

Loa loa

Loa loa is distributed throughout the human population in the rain forests of West and Central Africa. The filaria is often referred to as the African eye worm, because the adult parasite frequently wanders into the ocular conjunctivae, causing considerable discomfort. Visitors to endemic areas often acquire the parasite but are unaware of its presence until after they return home.

Biology and Life Cycle

The adult worm resides in and wanders freely through the subcutaneous tissues and the ocular conjunctivae (⇒ 39). Their invasion of these sensitive tissues produces considerable pain and apprehension in the affected individual. The female worm produces a distinctive, moderately large, sheathed microfilaria, which circulates in the peripheral blood with a diurnal periodicity. Species of the blood-sucking tabanid, *Chrysops* (also known as the deerfly), are natural vectors of the filaria. Microfilariae develop to the infective stage in the fat body of the fly over a period of about 7 days. Infective larvae entering human tissues reach adulthood in approximately 5 months. A related species of *Loa*, *L. papionis,* parasitizes monkeys in the forest canopy and uses other species of *Chrysops* as vectors but is not regarded as a reservoir of human infections. The parasite from humans can be easily maintained in experimentally infected monkeys.

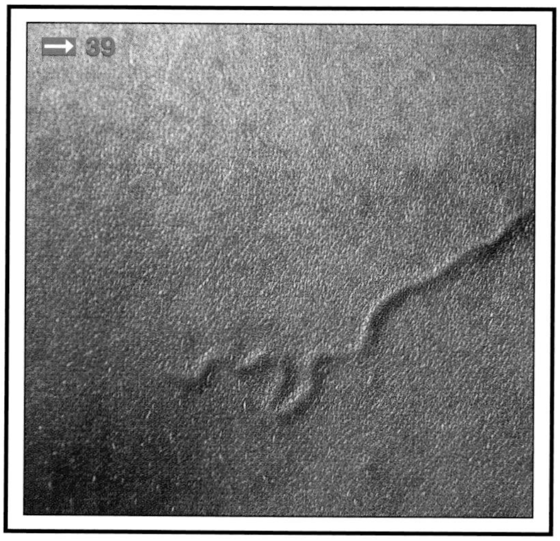

Pathology and Clinical Manifestations

Infected individuals may be essentially asymptomatic although microfilaremic. Often they become aware of their infection when adult worms move into the ocular conjunctivae. Although the worms cause considerable insult to host tissues, they do not produce any permanent damage and can be easily removed from these tissues intact. Some individuals who are amicrofilaremic may develop Calabar swellings, which are areas of erythema and angioedema as large as 5 to 10 cm that usually resolve in days but often recur intermittently. This syndrome typically involves the extremities and is regarded as the host response to the parasite or parasite antigens. Visitors to endemic areas who become infected show greater allergic or hyperreactive symptomatology than do local residents. They may also develop severe eosinophilia that reaches 30% to 60% of the total white blood cell count. Nephropathy, cardiomyopathy, and encephalopathies have been described in association with loiasis, but all of these require further study and documentation. Severe encephalitic complications that lead to coma and sometimes death after therapy with diethylcarbamazine have been reported in individuals with increased levels of microfilariae (> 50,000/mL) at the onset of treatment. Conservative treatment with diethylcarbamazine is essential for patients in these circumstances. To consider a diagnosis of loiasis, the patient must have lived in or traveled to an endemic area.

Parasite Morphology

The adults are robust worms of moderate size. Females reach lengths of 7.0 cm and have a maximum diameter of 0.5 mm. Males are smaller, measuring up to 3.5 cm by 0.35 to 0.40 mm. They have been recovered from subcutaneous tissues in most parts of the body. Living worms migrating through the tissues typically do not provoke a host inflammatory response, but dead or dying worms do (⇒ 39).

The cuticle is moderately thick, up to 10 μm over most of the body but twice as thick in the lateral fields (Plate 54:4). The surface, although smooth, bears small bosses that are dome shaped and about 3 to 8 μm high. In females, these structures are found from a level near the base of the esophagus to the end of the tail. These may be conspicuous in transverse sections (Plate 53:3 & 5; Plate 54:4). Bosses tend to be more numerous in females and sometimes appear to be in small groups.

The hypodermis is thin in submuscular areas (Plate 54:2 & 4) but expands laterally into conspicuous lateral chords, which may occupy 15% to 25% of the circumference of the worm (Plate 53:2; Plate 54:2). Dorsal and ventral chords are typically slender (Plate 53:4) and not always apparent. The musculature is strong and well developed. Muscle cells are coelomyarian, usually with 8 to 12 cells in each quadrant of the body. The contractile and cytoplasmic portions are well demarcated, with the contractile taller than the cytoplasmic at most levels but not at the extremities (Plate 53:1 & 4). Occasionally, the muscle cell nucleus is seen lying in the cytoplasmic portion of the cell (Plate 53:1; Plate 54:3). The pseudocoelom is usually filled with reproductive tubes and a single intestinal tube. In the anterior end of both sexes is the strong, muscular esophagus (Plate 53:1). Posterior to the esophagus, the intestine appears as a small, simple tube that extends to the posterior end of the body without looping or coiling and joins the rectum (female) or cloaca (male).

The arrangement of the reproductive tubes in the female helps identify the parasite. With the exception of *Loaina*, the paired reproductive tubes course posteriorly in parallel fashion in all of the filariae discussed. Typically, the two branches of the uterus, both seminal receptacles, the two oviducts, and both ovaries are seen, depending on the level of the sections, but never all of them in a single section. In contrast, in the female *Loa*, the reproductive tubes are looped and coiled, and one entire branch is displaced anteriorly, bringing one ovary to a position near midbody while the other lies further posteriorly. This results in uterine tubes and seminal receptacles in the same transverse section (Plate 53:2) or uterine tubes and ovaries in the same section (Plate 53:4). In the male worm, the single reproductive tube is apparent, along with the intestine, which fills the pseudocoelom (Plate 54:2 & 3). Sections through the posterior end of the male typically show the caudal alae, one or both spicules (Plate 54:5 & 6), and sometimes the large pedunculated caudal papillae (Plate 54:6).

References

Negesse Y, Lanoie LO, Neafie RC, Connor DH. Loiasis: "Calabar" swellings and involvement of deep organs. *Am J Trop Med Hyg*. 1985;34:537-546.

Nuttman TB, Miller KD, Mulligan M, Ottesen EA. *Loa loa* infections in temporary residents of endemic regions: recognition of a hyperresponsive syndrome with characteristic clinical manifestations. *J Infect Dis*. 1986;154:10-18.

Orihel TC, Eberhard ML. *Loa loa*: development and course of patency in experimentally infected primates. *Trop Med Parasitol*. 1985;36:215-224.

Plate 53

Loa loa

Image 1

Transverse section through the anterior extremity of a female *Loa loa* shows the muscular esophagus. Note the strong musculature of the body wall with its taller cytoplasmic portions and the occasional muscle cell nucleus (Trichrome, 110x).

Image 2

Section through the female illustrates the structure of the body wall. Note the prominent lateral chords (dart) and the simple intestine (IN). Sections of three uterine tubes containing microfilariae and the seminal receptacle (SR) are also present (Trichrome, 130x).

Image 3

Another level illustrates thickening of cuticle in lateral fields (arrow), and, in the pseudocoelom, a uterine tube containing microfilariae (UT), another with segmenting eggs (UE), ovaries (darts), oviducts (OD), and the intestine (IN) (Trichrome, 130x).

Image 4

This section shows two uterine tubes (UT) with developing microfilariae and two sections of ovary (Trichrome, 130x).

Image 5

Another level of the body contains uterine tubes (UT), ovaries (darts), and the intestine. Note bosses on the surface of the cuticle (arrows) (Trichrome, 130x).

Image 6

Sections through an ovary and the intestine (IN) are seen through the posterior end (Trichrome, 130x).

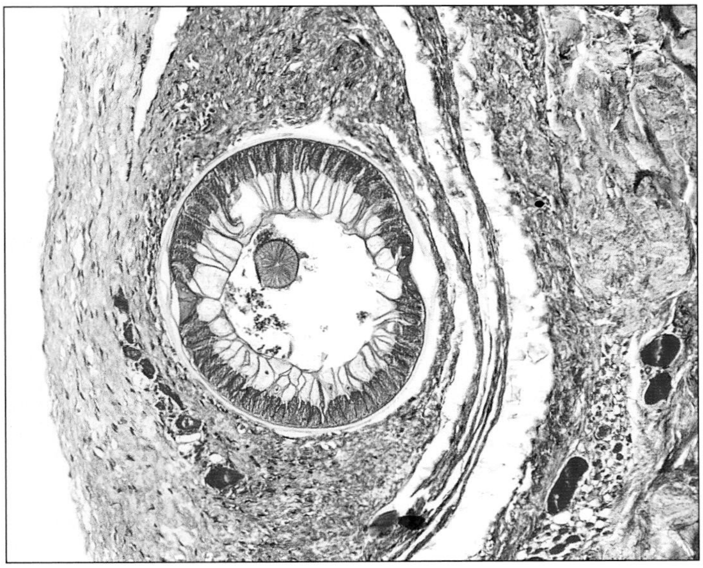

1

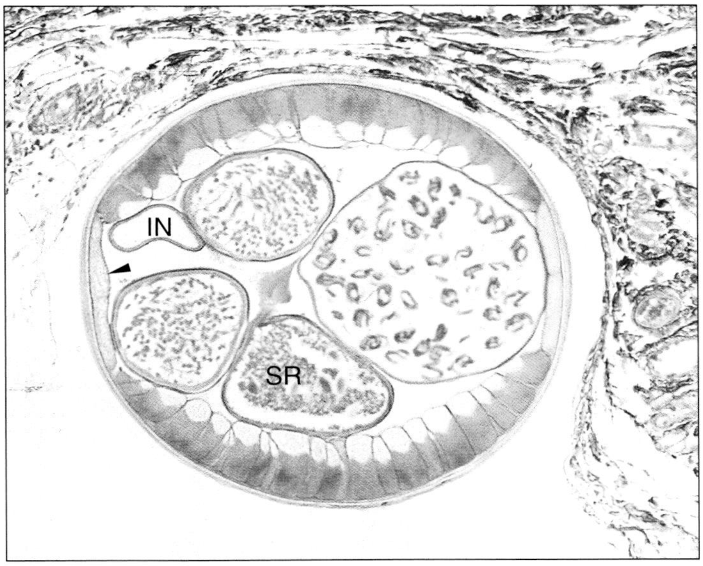

2

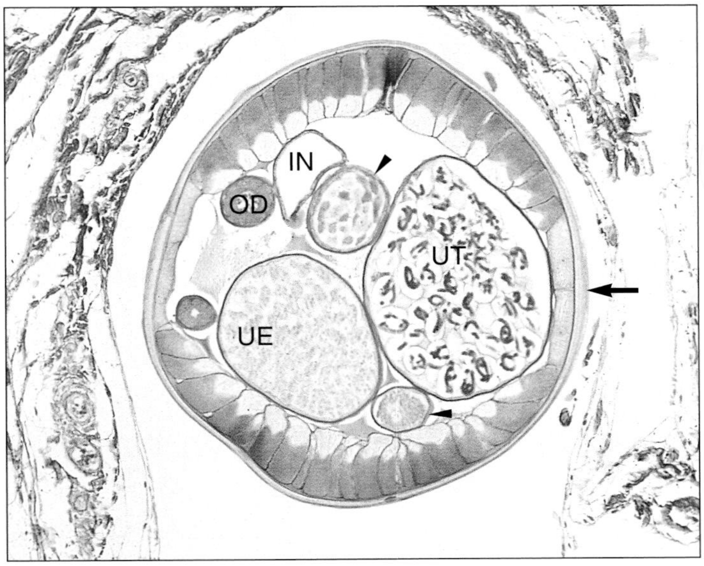

3

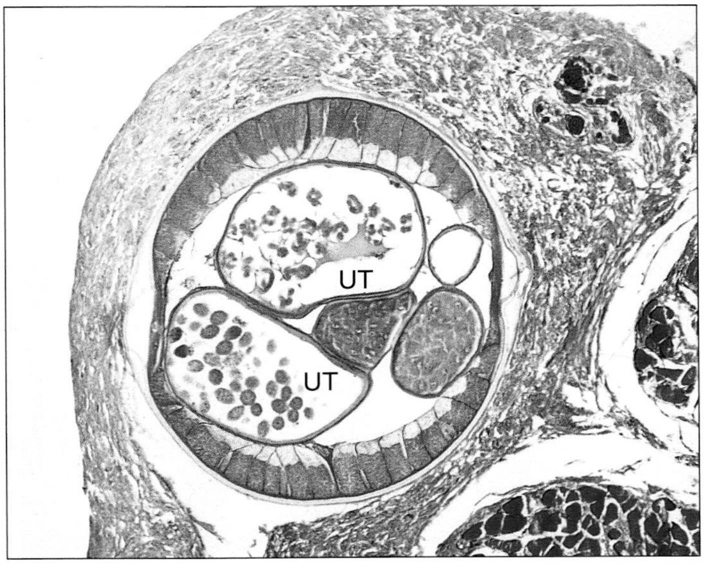

4

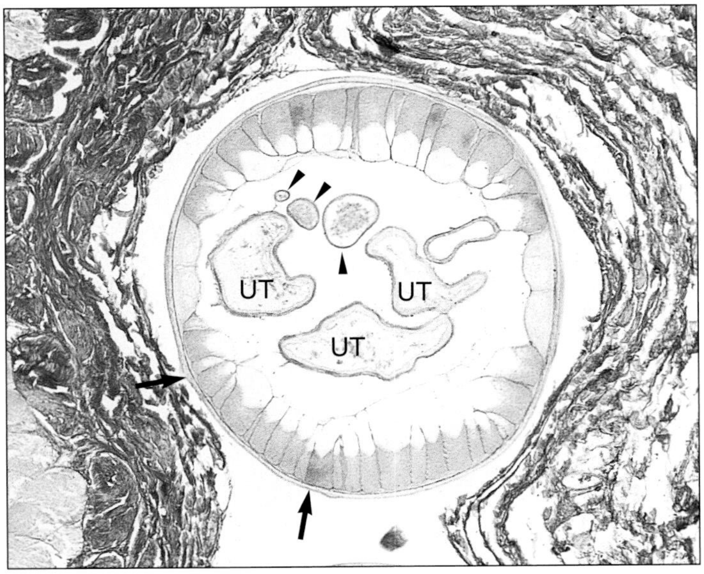

5

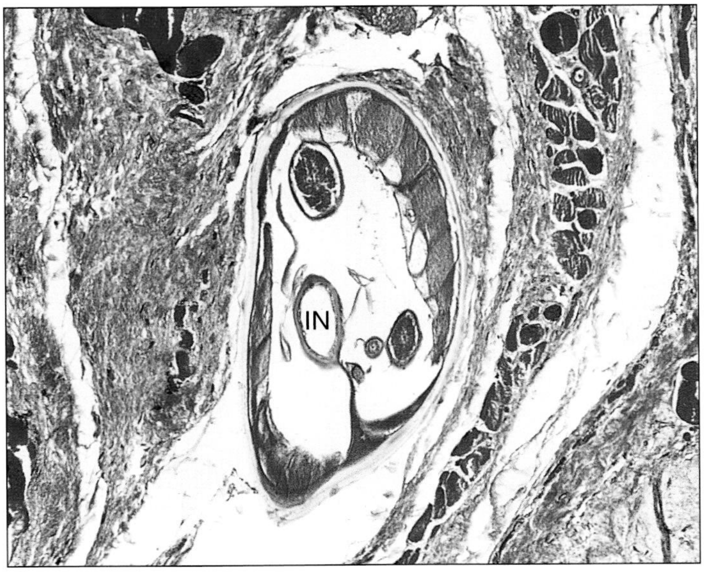

6

Plate 54

Loa loa

Image 1

Low-power view shows a male *Loa loa* in subcutaneous tissues. Worms tend to coil in the tissues, resulting in several sections of the same worm at different body levels (Trichrome, 40x).

Image 2

A typical section through a male worm illustrates the features of the body wall: the moderately thick cuticle, thin, pink-staining hypodermis, conspicuous lateral chords (arrows), and well-developed muscles. A large reproductive tube filled with developing spermatozoa is also visible. Note the small, tubular intestine (dart) (Trichrome, 110x).

Image 3

Muscle cell nuclei (dart) can be seen in this section. The male reproductive tube varies in muscularity and contents (developing spermatozoa) (Trichrome, 110x).

Image 4

High-power view of the body wall shows the thickening of the cuticle, some evidence of its layered structure, a boss (arrow), the thin, submuscular hypodermis, and the lateral chords. Note the hypodermal nucleus near the base and periphery of the chord. The structure of the individual muscle cell is well defined (Trichrome, 470x).

Image 5

At the level of the tail, the thick caudal alae are conspicuous (AL). Note the segment of spicule (dart) and the intestine (arrow) (Trichrome, 270x).

Image 6

A cut through the end of the tail shows the alae (AL), the embedded, large pedunculated papillae (PA), spicule (dart), and cloaca (CL) (Trichrome, 270x).

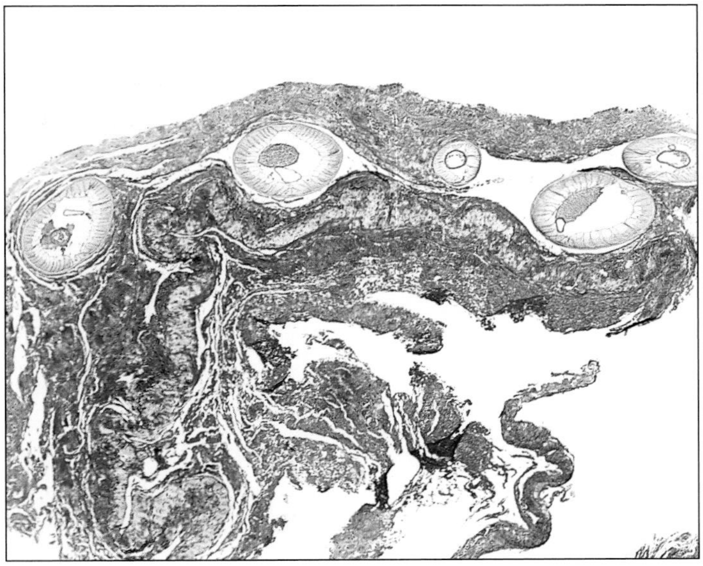

1

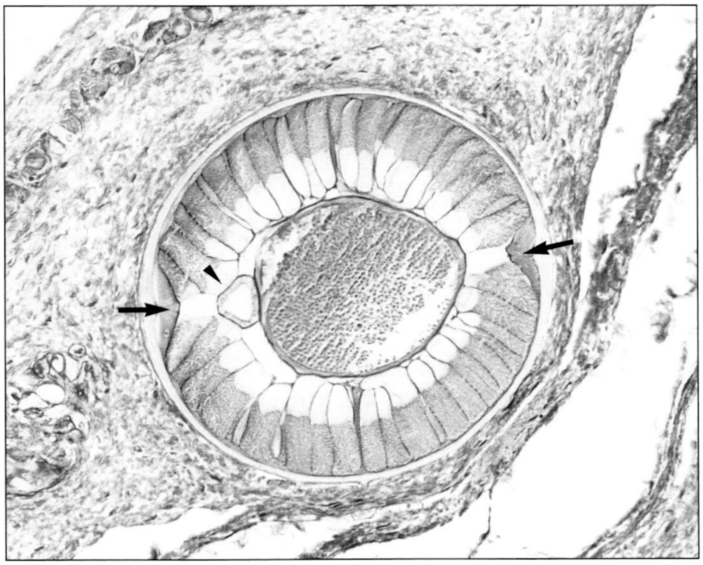

2

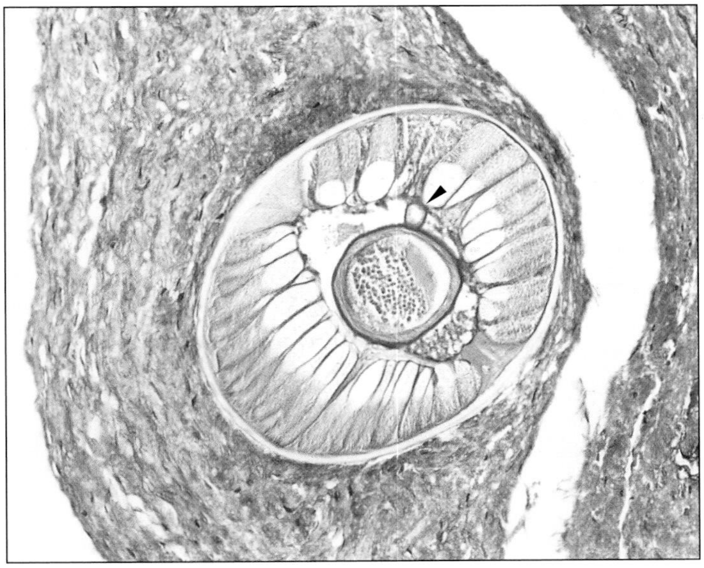

3

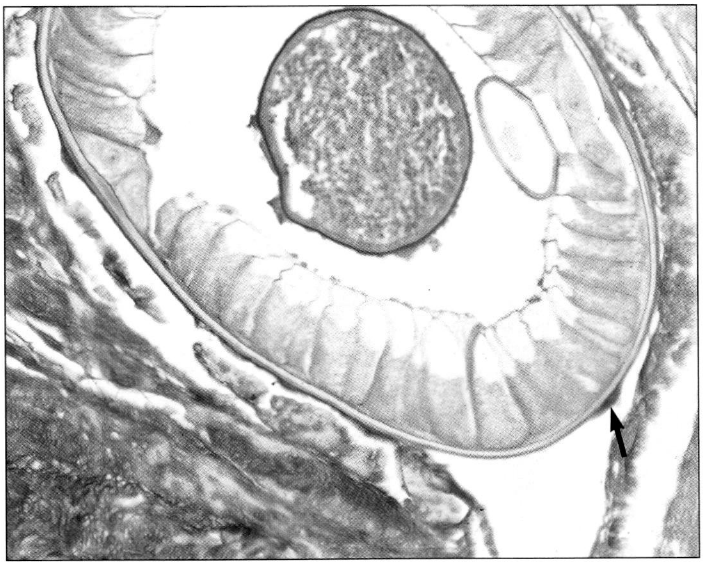

4

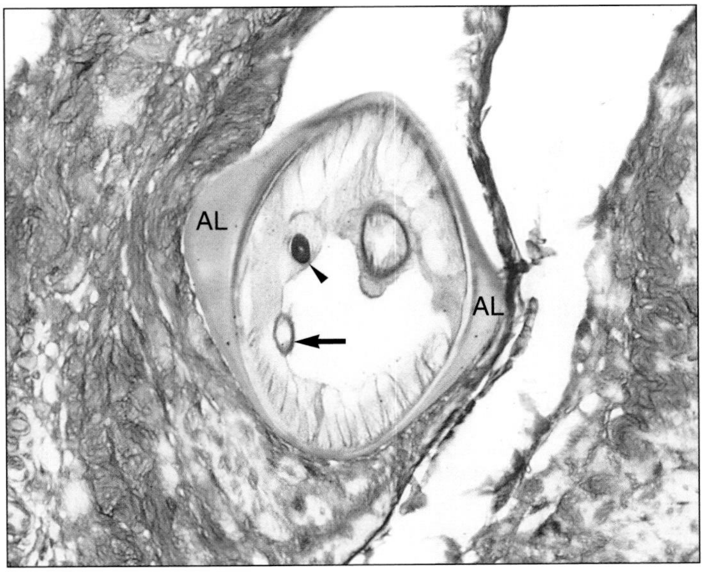

5

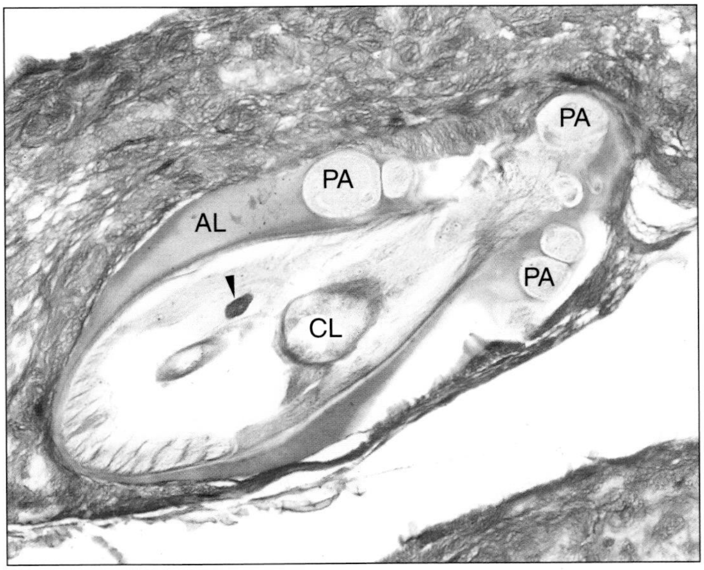

6

Mansonella perstans

Mansonella species

Three species of *Mansonella*—*M. perstans*, *M. ozzardi*, and *M. streptocerca*—are natural parasites of humans. For the most part, they cause little or no disease. Consequently, they have received little attention over the many decades since their discovery. Because they are tissue dwellers, however, they may require diagnosis in tissue specimens. *Mansonella perstans* primarily inhabits the connective tissues of abdominal organs but has been recovered frequently from hernial sacs. *Mansonella streptocerca* lives in the dermal layers of the skin, but our knowledge of the parasite is still fragmentary and sketchy. Until recently, much confusion has surrounded *Mansonella ozzardi*. Originally, it was believed to inhabit the abdominal cavity and the mesenteries. Recent studies have indicated that the parasite lives in the subcutaneous tissues of the human body. Although adult worms of *M. ozzardi* have been recovered intact from tissues of experimentally infected monkeys, worms have rarely been obtained in situ. Consequently, we are unable to provide histologic descriptions of this species in tissue. It can be assumed, with some confidence, that *M. ozzardi* shares many morphologic characteristics with the adults of *M. perstans* and *M. streptocerca*, but this is still speculation.

Mansonella perstans was discovered about 100 years ago when the microfilaria was found in the blood of a Congo native. Information collected since then indicates that the filaria is widely distributed in the tropical regions of Africa and is also present along the north coast of South America, the Amazon region, and possibly on some islands in the Caribbean.

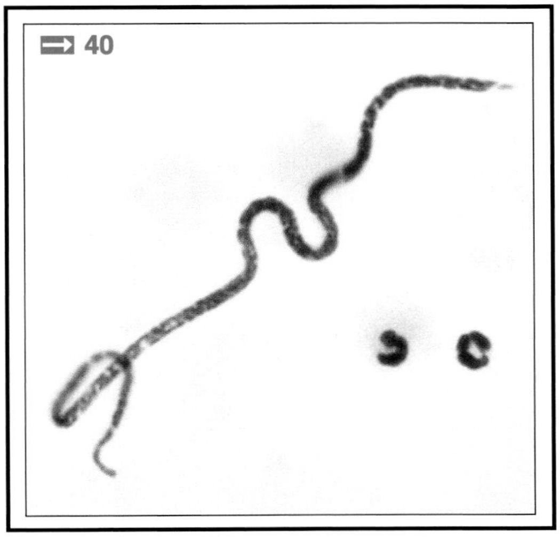

Biology and Life Cycle

The adult worms are usually found in connective tissues associated with organs in the abdominal cavity. In recent years worms have been found in hernial sacs during surgical repair. Females produce small (225 x 5 µm), unsheathed microfilariae with characteristic morphologic features (⇒ 40). Microfilariae circulate in the blood without any periodicity. *Culicoides* species are natural vectors, and microfilariae develop in the vector to the infective stage over several days. The length of prepatent development in humans has not been established but is estimated to be just a few months. Microfilariae similar to those of *M. perstans* have been seen in anthropoid apes and in some monkeys. Their precise taxonomic status and relationship to *M. perstans* have not been determined.

Pathology and Clinical Manifestations

A large percentage of people infected with *M. perstans* are asymptomatic. Others experience pruritus, angioedematous swellings similar to Calabar swellings, vague pain in serous cavities or the liver, and fever and headache. Symptoms seem more frequent and of greater intensity and duration in people from nonendemic areas. Adult worms have been found in connective tissues associated with the pancreas, kidney, liver, mesenteric lymph nodes, gall bladder, and in hernial sacs. Living worms usually do not provoke an inflammatory response, whereas dead worms do. *M. perstans* is believed to cause "bung-eye" and "bulge-eye" diseases, which are seen in people from Uganda and are characterized by swelling of the eyelid, or proptosis, as well as painless nodules (containing a filaria) in the conjunctivae.

Parasite Morphology

The adult worms are long and filamentous. Females may reach lengths up to 8.0 cm, with diameters of 0.12 mm. The males are much smaller, about 4.5 cm by 0.06 mm. A recent study at the Armed Forces Institute of Pathology offered the following criteria for identifying *M. perstans* in human tissues. Females measure 80 to 125 µm in diameter, males 45 to 60 µm. The thin, smooth cuticle measures about 1 to 2 µm, with thickenings in the lateral fields (Plate 55:6). The lateral chords are large and flattened and contain melanin granules (Plate 55:3 & 4). Dorsal and ventral chords are obscured. Eight to 12 muscle cells of the coelomyarian type are present per body quadrant. Reproductive tubes fill the pseudocoelom in females (Plate 55:2–4), less so in males (Plate 55:5). The intestine is a simple tube that is usually pushed against the body wall (Plate 55:3). Even in dead and degenerating worms, the characteristics of the cuticle and the pigment deposits in the degenerate lateral chords are retained (Plate 55:6). *Mansonella perstans* may be recognized by its tissue location, size, and the presence of melanin granules in the lateral chords.

References

Baird JK, Neafie RC, Lanoie L, Connor DH. Adult *Mansonella perstans* in the abdominal cavity in nine Africans. *Am J Trop Med Hyg*. 1987;37:578-584.

Baird JK, Neafie RC, Connor DH. Nodules in the conjunctiva, Bung-eye, and Bulge-eye in Africa caused by *Mansonella perstans*. *Am J Trop Med Hyg*. 1988;38:553-557.

Plate 55

Mansonella perstans

Image 1

Low-power view of fertile female worm in peripancreatic connective tissue (H&E, 100x) (AFIP No. 1738807).

Image 2

High-power view of previous image shows sections through paired uterine tubes (UT), the ovaries (OV), and the seminal receptacle (SR). The sections reveal the characteristic appearance of the body wall. Note the absence of any inflammatory response to the presence of the worm (H&E, 320x).

Image 3

Transverse section of female worm through uterine tubes filled with microfilariae. Note the characteristic pigment (melanin) deposits in the lateral chords (arrow). The worm lies in perilymphatic connective tissue (H&E, 430x).

Image 4

High-power view of another section better illustrates the pigment deposits (arrow) in the lateral chord (H&E, 645x).

Image 5

Sections through male worm show single genital tube (GT) and tubular intestine (dart) (H&E, 150x).

Image 6

Transverse section through a dead female worm. The thin cuticle is thickened in the lateral fields. Although muscle and lateral chords have undergone extensive degeneration, pigment can still be seen in the remnants of the lateral chords (arrows) (H&E, 430x) (AFIP No. 377599).

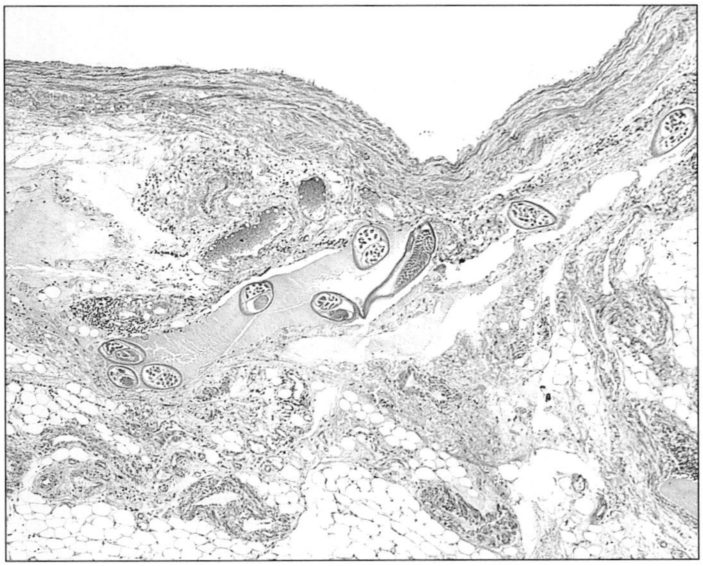

1

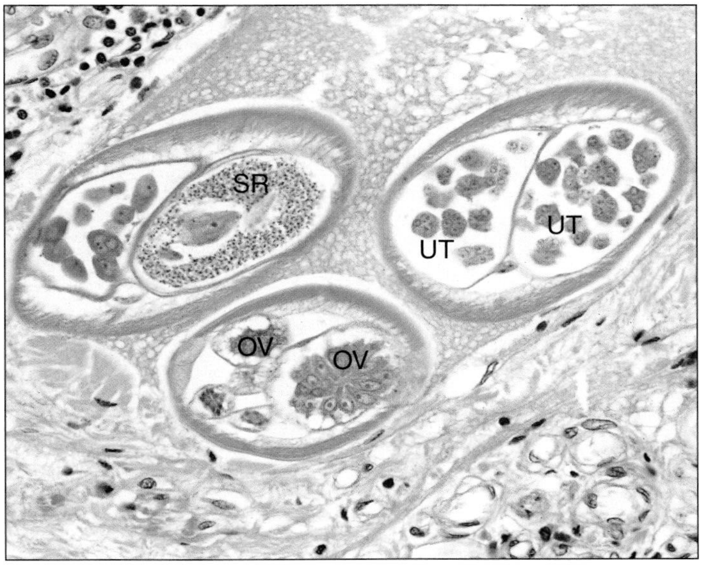

2

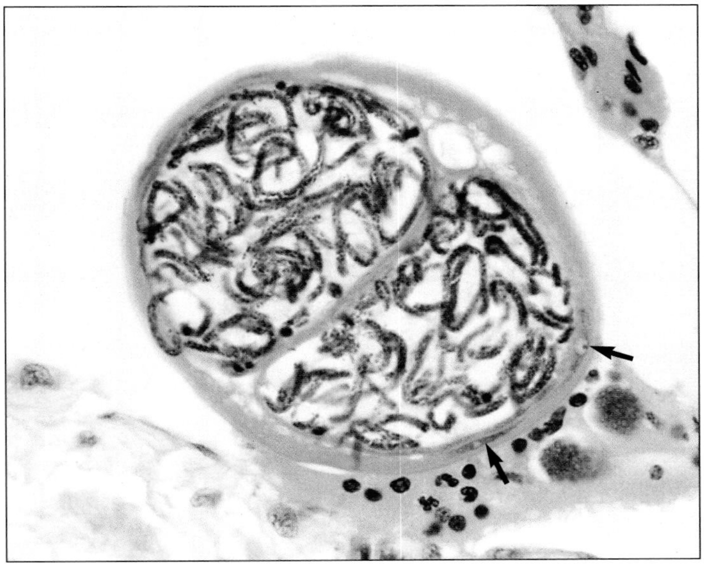

3

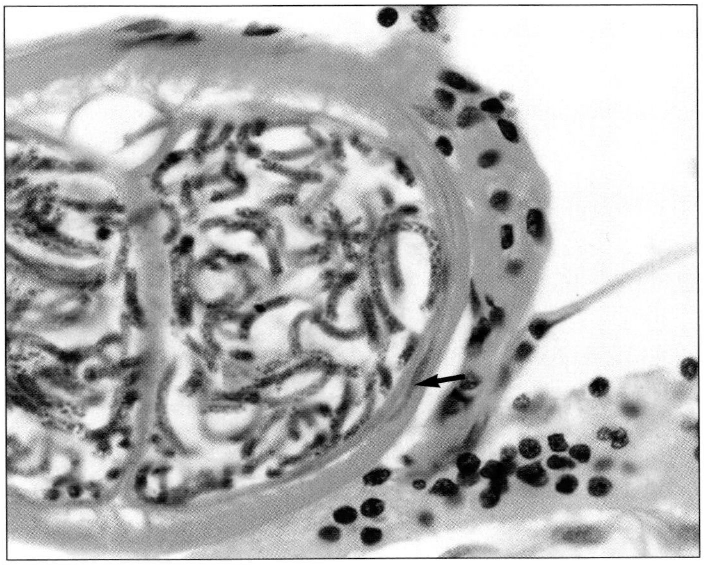

4

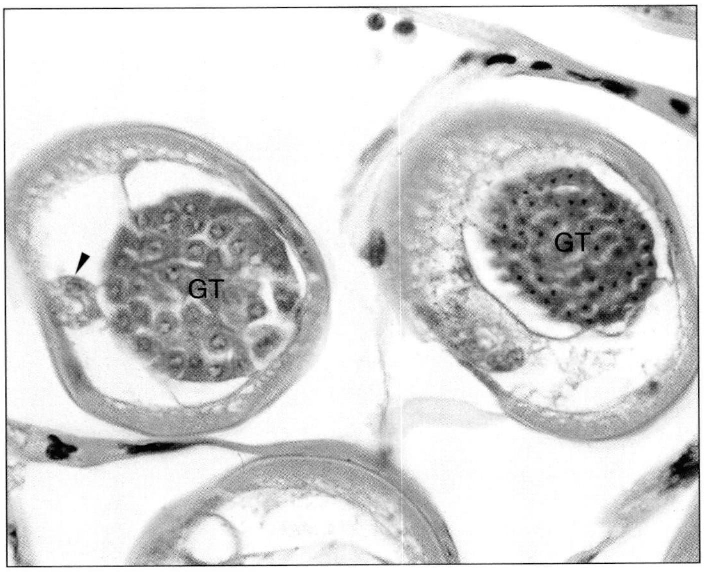

5

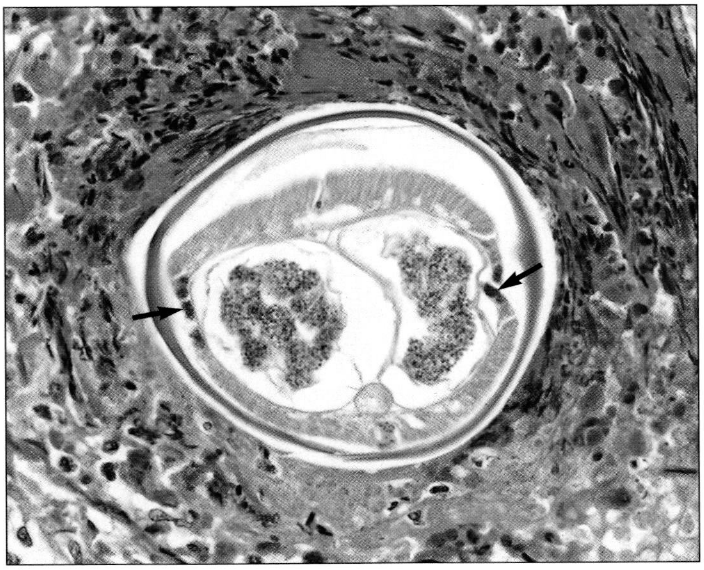

6

Mansonella streptocerca

The microfilariae of *M. streptocerca* were discovered in the skin of a patient from Ghana about 70 years ago. Microfilariae and adult worms were reported from chimpanzees and gorillas 20 years later. The adult worms were eventually collected from human tissues in 1972, some 50 years after the parasite was discovered. *Mansonella streptocerca* is restricted in its geographic distribution to the rain forests of West and Central Africa. In addition to humans, the filaria also infects anthropoid apes.

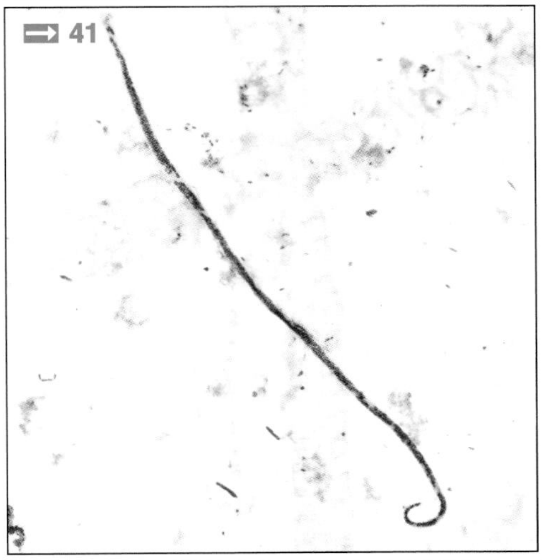

Biology and Life Cycle

The adult worms as well as the microfilariae live in the dermis. The microfilaria, with its characteristic crooked tail, measures about 240 by 5 μm and has no sheath (➡ 41). Species of blood-sucking gnats of the genus *Culicoides* are thought to be the natural vectors, but information in this regard is limited. Prepatent development in humans is estimated to be only a few months, but no firm experimental data are available to support this.

Pathology and Clinical Manifestations

Streptocerciasis does not receive much medical attention in areas where it occurs. Many regard it as an innocuous parasite. In the few studies that have been conducted, approximately one-third of infected individuals were asymptomatic. In the remainder, a dermatitis characterized by pruritus, hypopigmented macules, and papules and referred to as streptocercal dermatitis was the major clinical feature of infection. Physical examination usually reveals inguinal lymphadenopathy but no lymphedema or elephantiasis, as some have speculated. Treatment with diethylcarbamazine usually results in the death and degeneration of adult worms in the skin. Microfilariae are also destroyed in situ after administration of diethylcarbamazine.

Parasite Morphology

Our knowledge of the size and morphology of the adult stages of *M. streptocerca* remains somewhat fragmentary. Most information from human infections is based on histopathologic material obtained after treating infected individuals with diethylcarbamazine. Intact worms have been obtained only rarely from humans and occasionally from chimpanzees. The combination of these sources of information provides the following description. Adult females measure approximately 28 mm in length with a maximum diameter of 85 μm; males are much smaller, with a length of approximately 18 mm and a diameter of 50 μm. Adult worms are typically found coiled in the dermis (Plate 56:1). The cuticle in both sexes is thin, 1 to 2 μm, but is slightly thicker in the lateral fields (Plate 56:3). The lateral chords are broad and flattened, and their limits are sometimes obscured. Dorsal and ventral chords are usually not apparent. The muscles are coelomyarian, with between 8 and 12 cells in each quadrant of the body. The contractile portion of the cell is much taller than the cytoplasmic portion, apparently at all levels (Plate 56:4). The esophagus is short and not distinctly divided into muscular and glandular parts. The intestine is a simple tube with a diameter of about 10 μm in both sexes. It is lined by simple cuboidal cells (Plate 56:4).

In the female, the paired uterine tubes fill the pseudocoelom and occupy most of the length of the body (Plate 56:2–4). They are filled with developing microfilariae. The oviducts and ovaries, the latter divided into germinal and growth zones, are confined to the last 2 mm of the body. The tail is about 100 to 150 μm in length. In the male the muscles are tall, and the cytoplasmic portion of the individual cell may be well defined, particularly in the posterior end of the body (Plate 56:6). The pseudocoelom contains the single reproductive tube, which is filled with developing spermatozoa.

Individuals suspected of having streptocerciasis must have traveled to the rain forest belt of West and Central Africa. The parasite can be quickly differentiated from other filariae, such as *Dirofilaria* species, by its tissue preference, small size, and thin cuticle, which lacks both external longitudinal ridges and internal cuticular ridges in the lateral fields.

References

Gardiner CH, Meyers WM, Lanoie LO. Recovery of intact male and female *Dipetalonema streptocerca* from man. *Am J Trop Med Hyg*. 1979;28:49-52.

Meyers WM, Connor DH, Harman LE, et al. Human streptocerciasis: a clinicopathologic study of 40 Africans (Zairians) including identification of the adult filaria. *Am J Trop Med Hyg*. 1972;21:528-545.

Plate 56

Mansonella streptocerca

Image 1

Low-power view of a female worm coiled in the dermis of the skin (H&E, 100x).

Image 2

The characteristic features of the female worm are shown at higher magnification. At most levels, the paired uterine tubes are likely to be filled with developing microfilariae. The intestine is small and generally pushed against the body wall (dart) (H&E, 400x).

Image 3

A typical transverse section of a female worm. Note the large uterine tube (UT) containing microfilariae; the intestine (dart) is a simple tube (H&E, 800x).

Image 4

Another transverse section through the paired uterine tubes. Note the small tubular intestine (dart). The coelomyarian structure of the muscle cells is somewhat masked by the absence of any sizeable cytoplasmic elements (H&E, 800x).

Image 5

At lower power, several sections through a male worm are seen. Sex determination is facilitated by the presence of a single reproductive tube that fills the pseudocoelom (Movat, 150x).

Image 6

At higher magnification, the reproductive tube (darts) and the relatively obscure intestine (arrow) are seen. Note the structure of the muscle cells (Movat, 440x).

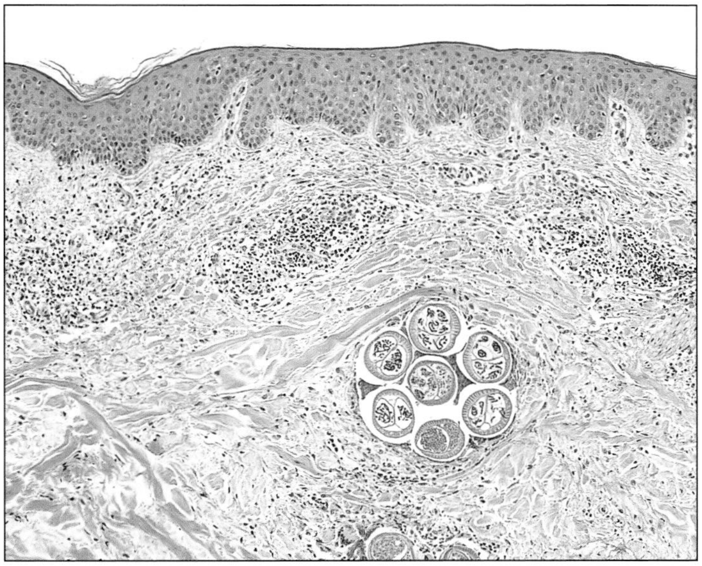

1

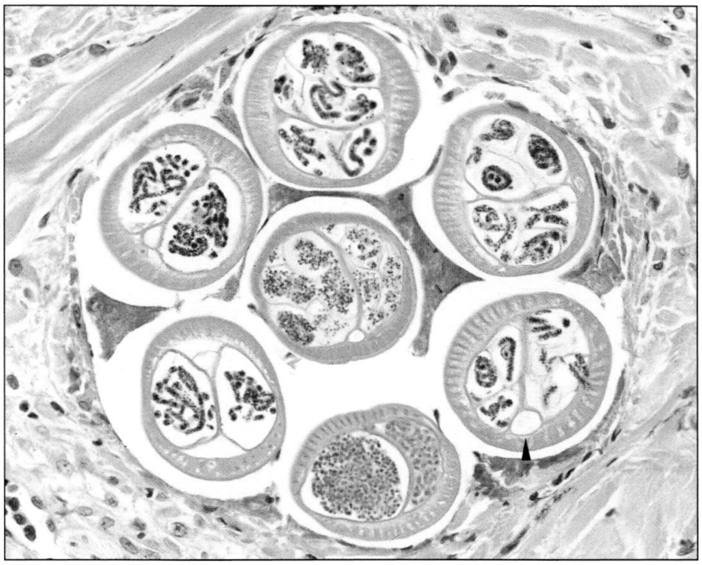

2

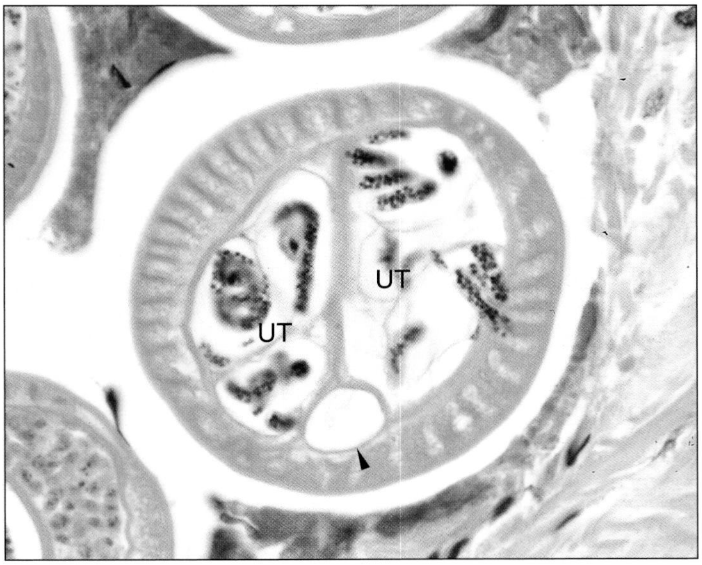

3

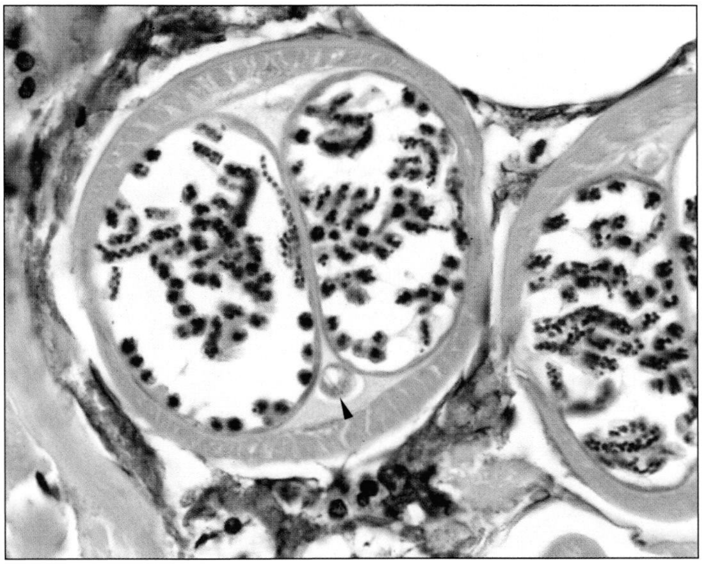

4

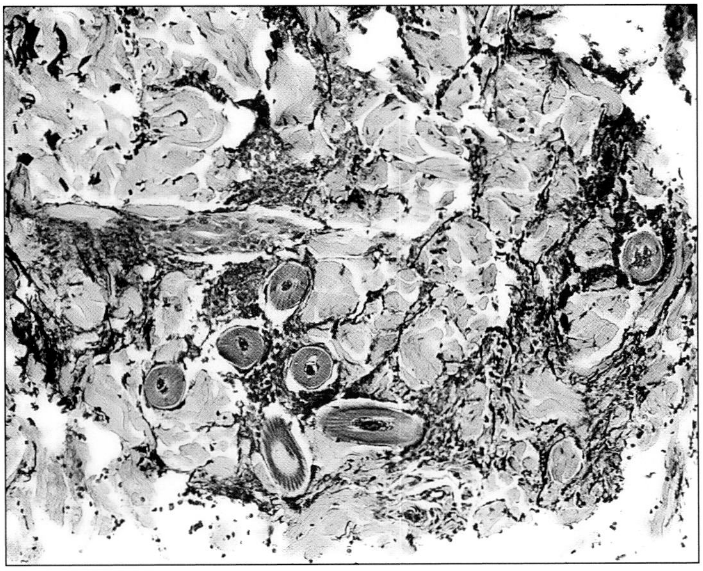

5

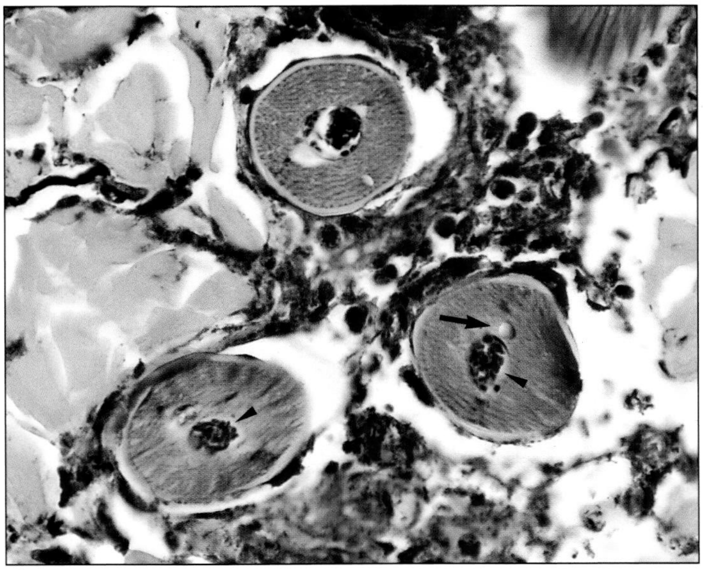

6

Dirofilaria species

The dirofilariae are natural parasites of a wide variety of animal species throughout the world. These filariae have a high zoonotic potential. Human infections have been documented from many parts of the world and occur with significant frequency in the United States, Europe, the Mediterranean region, Japan, and Australia.

Biology and Life Cycle

The genus *Dirofilaria* includes at least 24 species, which can be divided into two groups: parasites that inhabit the heart and vascular system of their hosts and those that inhabit the subcutaneous tissues.

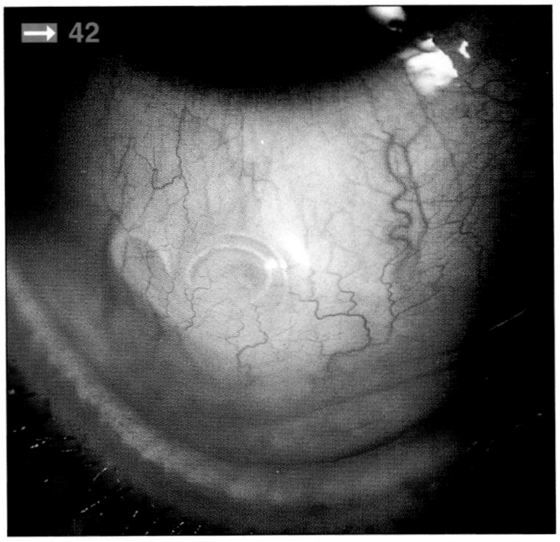

The adult female of the species produces unsheathed microfilariae that circulate in the peripheral blood of the definitive host. With few exceptions, these filariae use mosquitoes as vectors. Microfilariae typically develop to the infective stage in the malpighian tubules of the mosquito; some develop in the fat body. Development requires approximately two weeks but varies depending on the species. Infective larvae that escape from the mosquito host and enter the tissues of the definitive host, whether it is a natural or an accidental host such as a human, require several months to reach the sexually mature, adult stage.

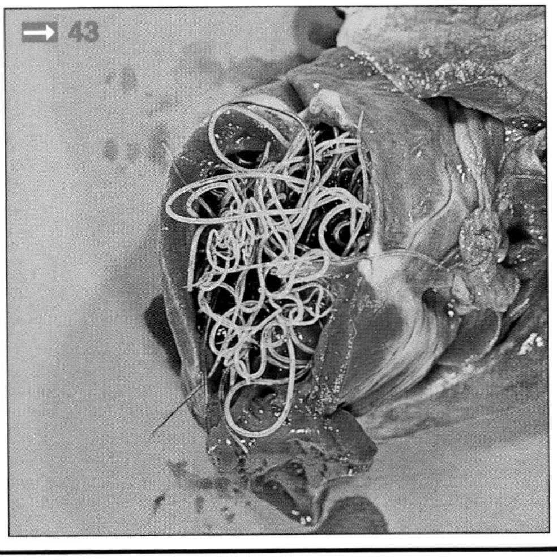

In the United States, *D. tenuis*, a parasite of raccoons, is regarded as the most common agent of subcutaneous infections, especially in the southeastern part of the country. *Dirofilaria ursi*, a subcutaneous parasite of bears in the northern United States and Canada, has also been identified as a probable source of infection in several cases. On one occasion, *Dirofilaria striata*, a filaria of the bobcat, was removed from the orbit of a boy in North Carolina. In Europe, *D. repens*, a common subcutaneous parasite of the domestic dog, is the most important agent of subcutaneous infections in humans. More than 100 human cases of *D. repens* have been reported in Italy alone. Infections involving the heart and lungs are attributed to the dog heartworm, *D. immitis*, which has nearly worldwide distribution.

Pathology and Clinical Manifestations

These infections are typically cryptic in humans, although gravid females have been recovered from tissues. Human infections are of two types: subcutaneous and pulmonary.

Subcutaneous Infections

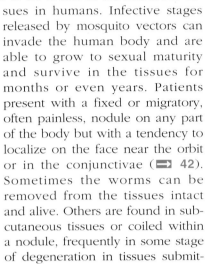

Dirofilariae that inhabit the subcutaneous tissues of their natural hosts tend to be found in subcutaneous tissues in humans. Infective stages released by mosquito vectors can invade the human body and are able to grow to sexual maturity and survive in the tissues for months or even years. Patients present with a fixed or migratory, often painless, nodule on any part of the body but with a tendency to localize on the face near the orbit or in the conjunctivae (➡ 42). Sometimes the worms can be removed from the tissues intact and alive. Others are found in subcutaneous tissues or coiled within a nodule, frequently in some stage of degeneration in tissues submitted for pathologic evaluation (Plate 58:1 & 2).

Sexually mature but infertile females and sexually mature males are found most often, females more frequently than males. Usually only one worm is present. On occasion two or more have been recovered from separate lesions. Gravid females are rarely encountered and patent infections are even rarer.

Pulmonary Dirofilariasis

Human pulmonary dirofilariasis is an important zoonosis in the United States as well as in other parts of the world. *Dirofilaria immitis*, the heartworm of dogs, is the agent of infection. The adult worms live in the right side of the heart and produce a debilitating disease in dogs (➡ 43). The infective stages of the filaria accidentally invade human tissues after a blood meal by an infected vector. Larvae develop for a time in subcutaneous tissues, then migrate to the right side of the heart. There, they either die or become moribund and are swept up into the pulmonary arteries, where they lodge in a small-caliber vessel and produce an infarct and, ultimately, a granulomatous coin lesion (Plate 60:3). Most individuals (more than 60%) are asymptomatic, while the remainder complain of cough, chest pain, or hemoptysis. In asymptomatic individuals, lesions are usually discovered incidentally during routine radiographic examination or in the course of examination for a different problem. The coin lesion measures about 1 to 3 cm in diameter and mimics a primary or metastatic lung tumor. Pathologically, the typical nodule is a spherical subpleural infarct with a central thrombosed artery containing the parasite in some stage of degeneration (Plate 60:3). Typically, a single nodule is present, but two or more nodules have occasionally been reported in the same patient.

Parasite Morphology

The morphologic features of the *Dirofilaria* species are fairly uniform. Grossly, adult worms are large. Females vary in length from several to more than 30 cm with diameters that may reach 0.6 mm, depending on the species. Males are much smaller in length and diameter. In both sexes, the anterior extremity is plain and devoid of any cuticular ornamentation. The female tail is short and without ornamentation. In contrast, the posterior end of the male is spirally coiled, and the tail is short. The tail has caudal alae supported by large, pedunculated papillae that are most frequently arranged in pairs in preanal, adanal, and postanal positions. The number and arrangement of these papillae are useful taxonomic characteristics. In the male, paired, unequal, and dissimilar spicules have structural features that are also used in taxonomy. The structure of the cuticle and its surface, the hypodermis, and the musculature (essentially the body wall) are among the features most useful in identification. The reproductive system and its contents establish the sex, the degree of maturity, and the fertility of the individual worm. Identification to the generic level poses little difficulty in most cases. However, species identifications are not always possible because knowledge of the microscopic anatomy of most of the species is limited and few morphologic features are likely to provide clues as to species identification. Frequently, species diagnosis is based on the tissue site, the size of the worm, cuticular features, and the geographic region where the infection was possibly acquired.

Subcutaneous Infections

Dirofilaria tenuis is the species most frequently encountered in human infections in the southeastern United States, where the parasite is enzootic. The appearance of the adults in transverse sections at all important levels of the body as well as some key structural features are shown in Plate 57. In general, the cuticle is relatively thick and multilayered and has longitudinal ridges on its surface (Plate 57:5). At least one species, *D. striata,* has inconspicuous lateral alae (Plate 63:1 & 2). The inner surface of the cuticle has lateral cuticular ridges (Plate 57:6). The hypodermis is thin in the submuscular region but expands into large lateral chords (Plate 57:2 & 6). Small dorsal and ventral chords are also present but they are usually inconspicuous. The muscles of the body wall are well developed and are of the coelomyarian type (Plate 57:5). Their numbers in each quadrant of the body wall vary with the species of worm.

Living, dead, and degenerating worms are encountered in the tissues, and all are recognized rather easily. Female worms typically measure 300 μm or more in diameter, depending on the species; males are smaller, about 150 to 200 μm in diameter. In dead worms, the soft tissues (muscles, hypodermis, and lining epithelium of the intestine and reproductive tubes) degenerate quickly and lose their normal architecture and appearance (Plate 59:2–4). Frequently, only the connective tissue that ensheathes the individual body organs is recognizable. Eggs and spermatozoa within the reproductive tubes also deteriorate but may still be recognized (Plate 58:5 & 6). They frequently degenerate into an amorphous mass. Muscle cells lose their individual character, boundaries are lost, and collectively they have the appearance of an amorphous band of tissue (Plate 59:3). The hypodermis and particularly the lateral chords may swell, and the chords often have a granular, frothy, or vacuolated appearance (Plate 62:3). The cuticle is most resistant to the degenerative process. It often swells significantly, which emphasizes its multilayered structure (Plate 59:1 & 6; Plate 62:4). The lateral, internal, cuticular ridges also swell and present an exaggerated appearance (Plate 59:6). Generally, the longitudinal ridges on the surface of the cuticle show minimal change.

Occasionally, dirofilariae are found that lack longitudinal ridges in the subcutaneous tissues but their specific identity has not been determined. In extremely degenerated worms, sometimes only the cuticle or remnants of it remain (Plate 59:6). Because other filariae that have been studied in microsections do not have the unique cuticular structure of dirofilariae, a diagnosis of *Dirofilaria* can be based on cuticle alone in some cases (Plate 59:6).

Close examination of the reproductive tubes in these worms can assist in determining sex, maturity, and fertility. In typical transverse sections, females have two or more reproductive tubes (paired uteri, ovaries), depending on the level through which the sections were cut (Plate 58:3 & 4). One must not confuse a single digestive tube (intestine) with reproductive structures. In sections cut at most levels, male worms have a single section of intestine and only one reproductive tube (Plate 59:2; Plate 62:3). Sexual maturity can be determined by examining the contents of the reproductive tubes. In sexually mature females, the ovaries contain developing eggs (Plate 58:6). Frequently, mature eggs can be seen in the uterine tubes (Plate 58:5). The male reproductive tube contains developing and mature spermatozoa (Plate 57:4). Unsegmented eggs indicate that the female is infertile and strongly suggest the absence of male worms in the tissues. The presence of microfilariae in utero in the female indicates that a male worm was present in the human tissues, even if it is never found (Plate 62:1 & 2).

Pulmonary Infections

A majority of the *Dirofilaria* infections involving the heart and lungs are caused by *D. immitis,* and they occur wherever this species is enzootic in the canine population. Intact worms of both sexes have been found, usually at autopsy, in the right heart or great vessels, but the majority of cases involve the pulmonary arteries. The worms are generally dead and in different stages of degeneration or disintegration (Plate 60:4; Plate 61:2 & 3). In the living *D. immitis* worm in transverse section, the cuticle is multilayered and thick, smooth on its surface, and thickened in the lateral fields by an internal cuticular ridge. Large lateral chords and numerous muscle cells of the coelomyarian type are present (Plate 60:1 & 2). In the dead or dying worm, the appearance of these structures is altered (Plate 60:4). Lateral chords often have a frothy appearance (Plate 61:2), are swollen, or may be totally unrecognizable. Depending on the state of degeneration, the muscles may show their coelomyarian structure (Plate 60:4; Plate 61:5), or they may have an amorphous, structureless appearance that provides no clue as to their normal architecture (Plate 60:6). However, even when undergoing mineralization, evidence of the body wall's normal architecture may remain (Plate 61:2). The sexes can still be differentiated on the basis of genital structures and to some extent on the basis of size. Although female worms are typically infertile, with degenerating eggs in their uterine tubes, instances of gravid females with microfilariae present in the uteri have been documented (Plate 61:4). Unfortunately, individuals have occasionally mistaken artifactual structures in the uteri for microfilariae (Plate 61:5 & 6). In a few instances, *D. repens* has been identified in nodules in the lung (Plate 60:5 & 6).

In summary, all dirofilariae can be identified at the generic level on the basis of body characteristics (ie, thick, multilayered cuticle with lateral internal ridges, large lateral chords, and coelomyarian musculature). Sexes are most reliably identified by the reproductive tubes. A study of the surface of the cuticle (ie, presence or absence of longitudinal ridges, small lateral alae, etc) assists to some extent in identifying species. In dead worms, the multilayered cuticle and its lateral internal ridges separate the dirofilariae from other zoonotic species of filariae.

A species diagnosis is not critical and is perhaps best left to experts. Generic diagnosis is sufficient and is not difficult, because morphology, epidemiology, and clinical onset of infection are similar or the same for most of the species. A question that is often raised is whether the parasites can multiply within the human host. This is not possible, however, because worm burden depends totally on the inoculum of infective stages.

References

Akaogi E, Ishibashi O, Mitsui K, et al. Pulmonary dirofilariasis cytologically mimicking lung cancer: a case report. *Acta Cytol.* 1993;37:531-534.

Cancrini G, D'Amelio S, Mattiucci S, Coluzzi M. Identification of *Dirofilaria* in man by multilocus electrophoretic analysis. *Ann Trop Med Parasitol.* 1991;85:529-532.

Gutierrez Y. Diagnostic features of zoonotic filariae in tissue sections. *Hum Pathol.* 1984;15:514-525.

Pampiglione S, Fedeli F. Dirofilariasi polmonare umana: aspetti parassitologici del secondo caso segnalato in Italia. *Parassitologia.* 1991;33:153-157.

Pampiglione S, Trotti GC, Rivasi F. La dirofilariose humaine en Italie. *Ann Parasitol Hum Comp.* 1991;66:195-203.

Ro JY, Tsakalakis PJ, White VA, et al. Pulmonary dirofilariasis: the great imitator of primary or metastatic lung tumor. A clinicopathologic analysis of seven cases and a review of the literature. *Hum Pathol.* 1989;20:69-76.

Plate 57

Dirofilaria tenuis

Image 1

Section through the anterior extremity at the level of the esophagus (ES) (H&E, 200x).

Image 2

Section at the level of the paired uterine tubes (UT), which are filled with developing microfilariae. Note the well-developed body wall with its coelomyarian muscles (MU). The intestine (IN) is the thin-walled tube devoid of any contents (H&E, 200x).

Image 3

A more posterior level of the paired uterine tubes (UT), which contain developing eggs. The uterine tubes fill the pseudocoelom, somewhat compressing the height of the muscle layer (H&E, 200x).

Image 4

Section through a male worm shows the typical single reproductive tube (RT) and the intestine (IN). Although not sharply delineated, the presence of longitudinal ridges (darts) on the surface of the cuticle is also evident (H&E, 200x).

Image 5

At high magnification, the longitudinal ridges (arrows) and the layers of the cuticle can be seen. Note the muscle cell nucleus (dart) (H&E, 400x).

Image 6

High-power view of the lateral margin of the body shows the lateral, internal cuticular ridge (dart), which is characteristic of most dirofilariae (H&E, 800x).

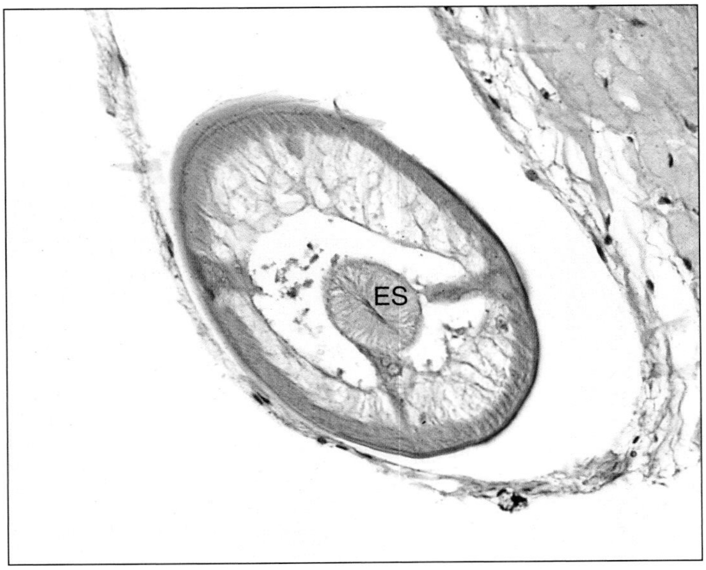

1

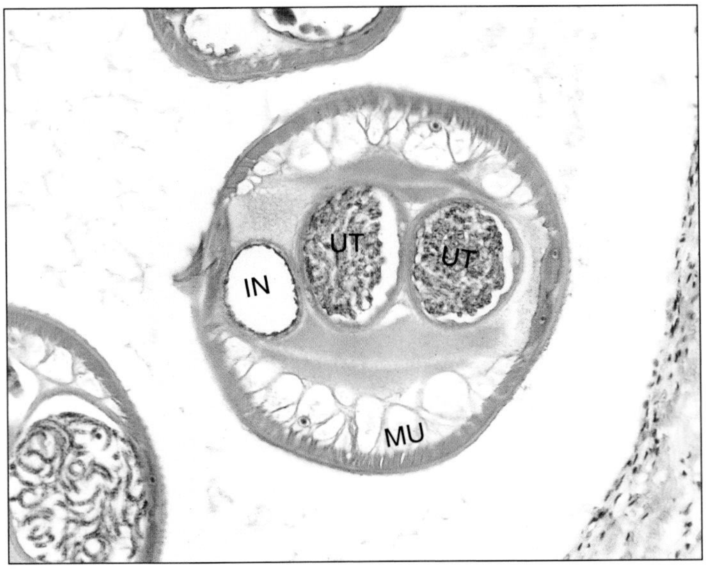

2

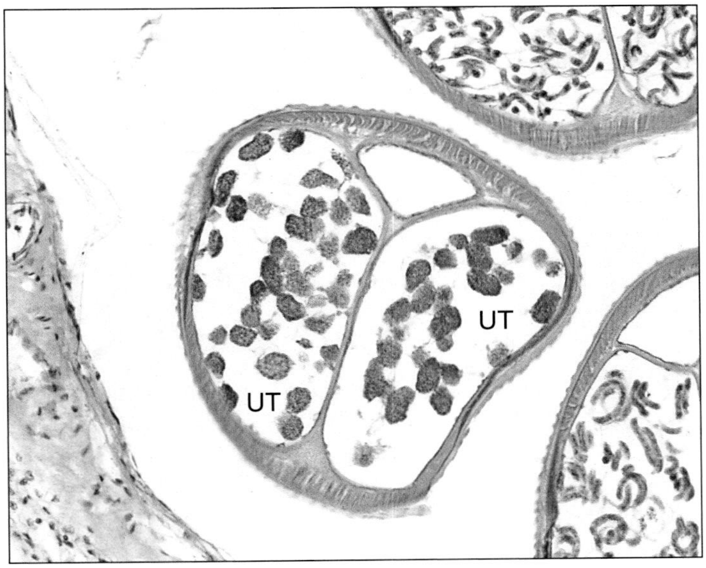

3

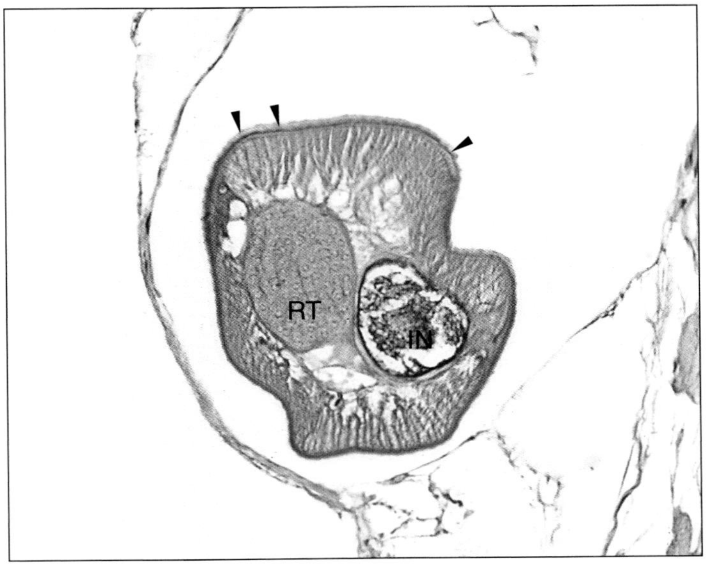

4

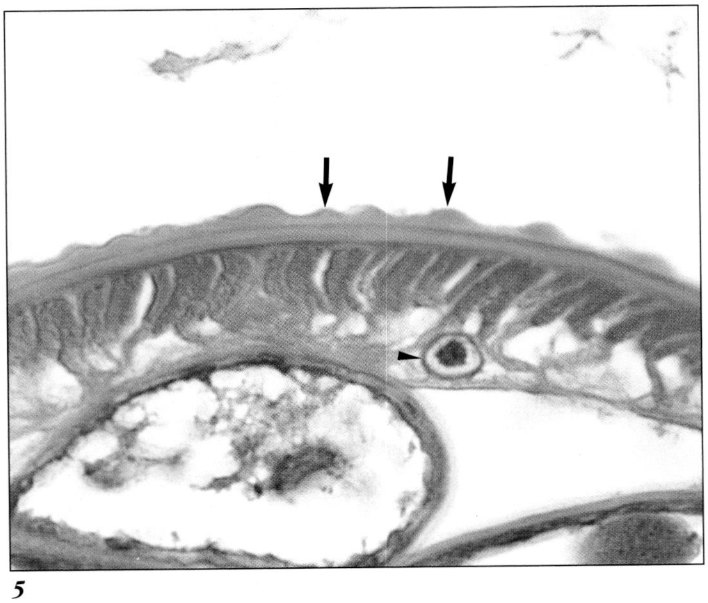

5

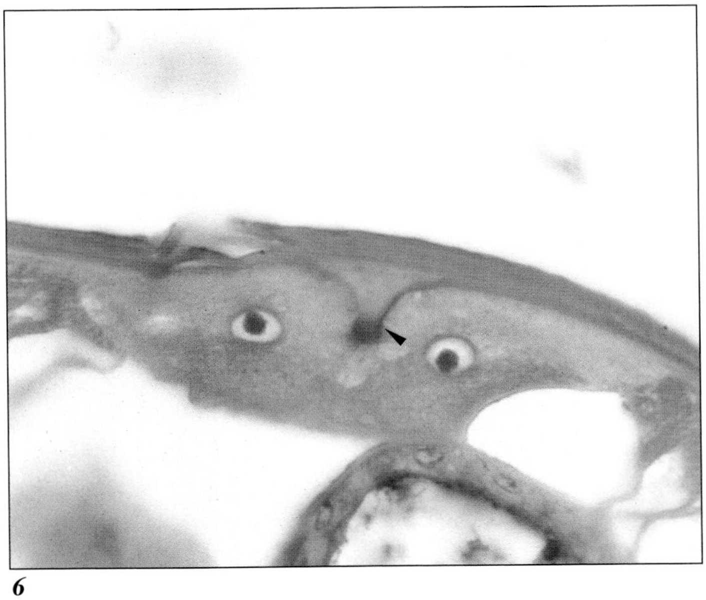

6

Plate 58

Dirofilaria species

Image 1

Section through a skin biopsy specimen from the forearm of a Louisianan shows one tangential and two transverse sections of a female *Dirofilaria.* Note the inflammation around the worm (H&E, 30x).

Image 2

Section through a subcutaneous nodule removed from the arm of a Floridian shows multiple transverse sections of a worm (darts). The nodule measures approximately 0.60 cm in diameter. The central portion of the nodule surrounding the worm is made up of an acute inflammatory infiltrate consisting of neutrophils and fibrin. Within the wall of the nodule are chronic inflammatory cells and a moderate amount of granulation tissue (H&E, 10x).

Image 3

Several transverse sections through an infertile female worm of the *D. tenuis* type from the forearm of a Floridian. All sections of the worm are through the paired uterine tubes; one section includes an oviduct (dart). The sections of worm illustrate the characteristic features of the body wall of an adult *Dirofilaria* (H&E, 75x).

Image 4

A higher magnification of the worm seen in Image 3 illustrates in greater detail the structure of the multilayered cuticle, especially the longitudinal ridges on the surface (darts). Note also the lateral internal cuticular ridge (arrow) and the large lateral chords (LC). The worm is undergoing some degeneration, so that the structure of individual muscle cells is not sharp (H&E, 260x).

Image 5

Transverse section through the female worm shown in Image 2. Note especially the pair of large uterine tubes (UT) containing degenerating eggs and the intestine (IN) (Trichrome, 180x).

Image 6

Another level of the same worm illustrated in Image 2 shows the germinal (darts) and growth zones of the ovaries (arrows). These indicate that the worm was sexually mature (Trichrome, 180x).

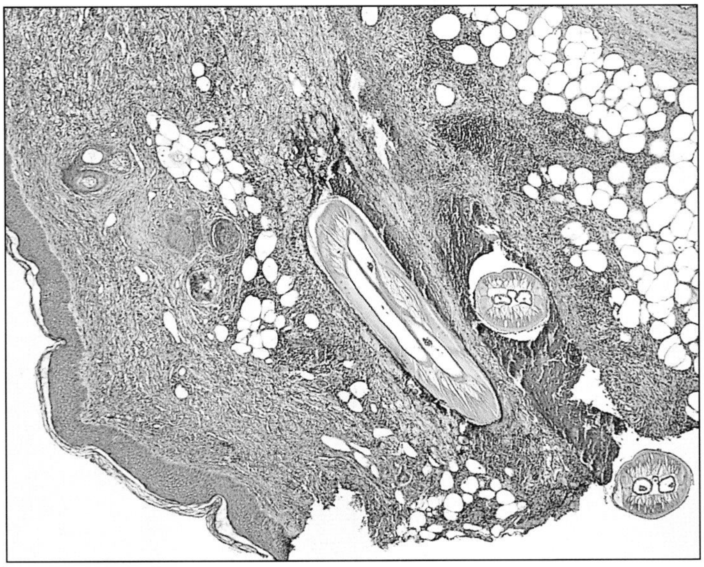

1

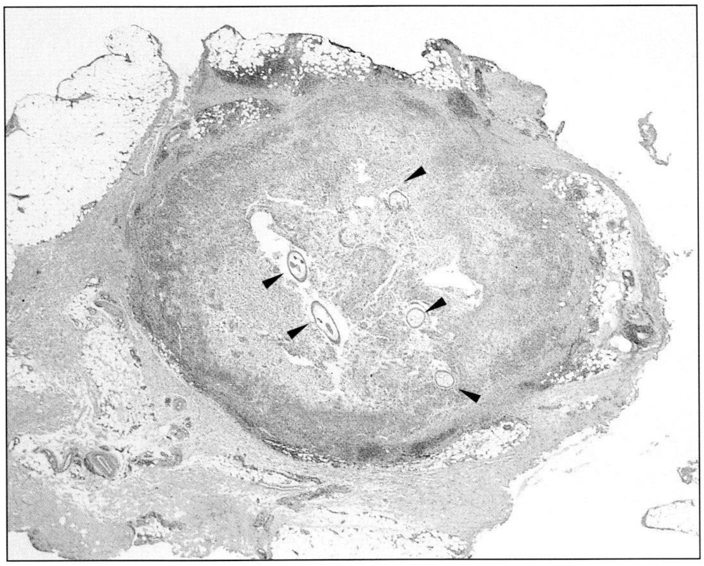

2

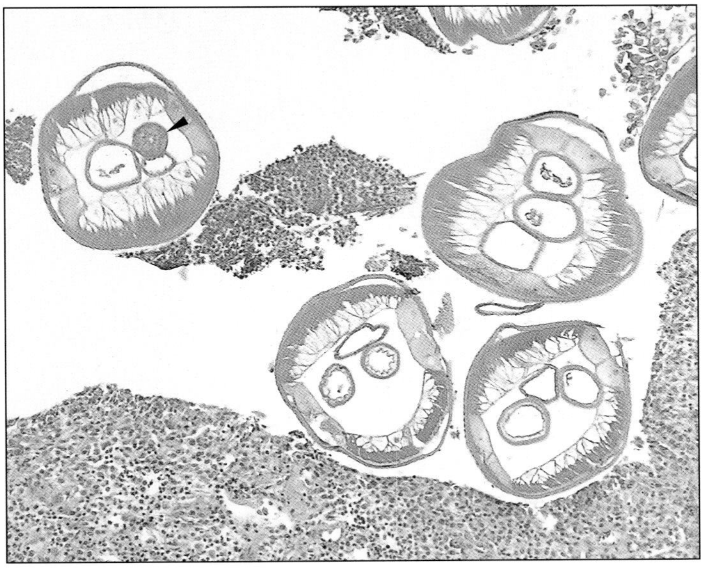

3

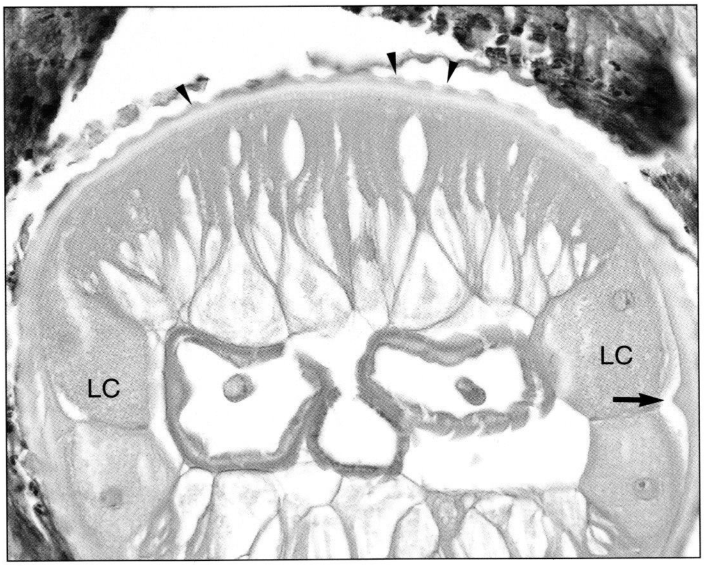

4

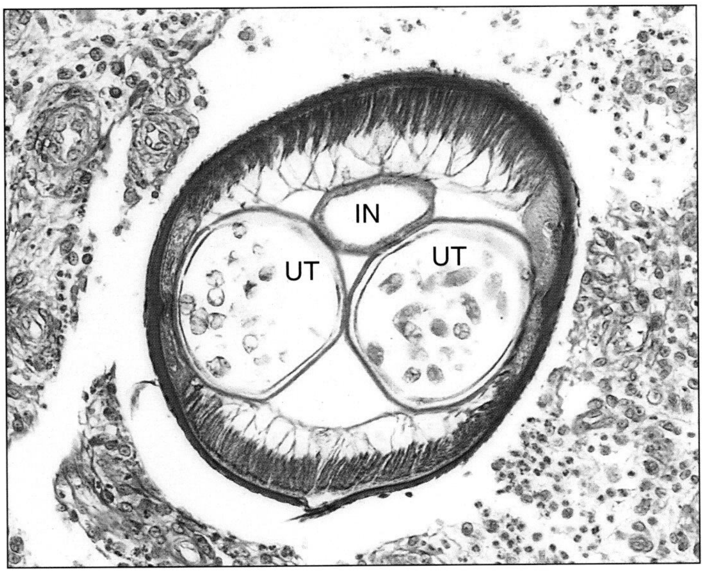

5

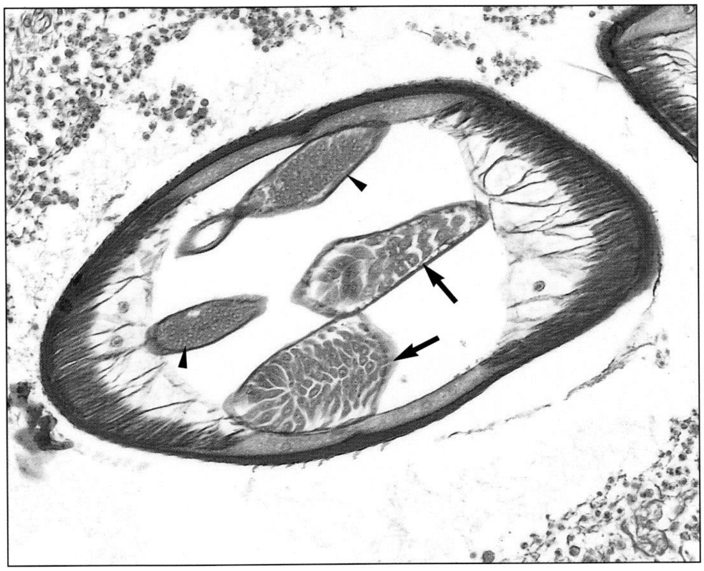

6

Dirofilaria species

Image 1

Dead and degenerate *D. tenuis,* in a subcutaneous cyst removed from near the eye of a Floridian. Transverse sections at different levels show different degrees of degeneration (H&E, 100x).

Image 2

In this section of worm, the longitudinal ridges on the thick cuticle (darts) can be seen clearly. The size of the worm (0.18 mm in diameter), the presence of only one reproductive tube (RT), and the intestine (arrow) indicate that the worm is male (H&E, 200x).

Image 3

This transverse section shows the thick cuticle; lateral internal cuticular ridges (darts); and strong musculature (MU). Only two tubes are seen in the pseudocoelom (arrows) (H&E, 200x).

Image 4

In this section, the worm is still recognizable. The layers of cuticle have separated (arrows), but the conspicuous internal cuticular ridge can still be seen (dart) (H&E, 200x).

Image 5

Only the cuticle remains of this section of worm. The three major layers have separated in the lateral fields, and the internal cuticular ridges are conspicuous (darts) (H&E, 200x).

Image 6

At another level, only the cuticle remains. It is swollen and its layers are evident. Note the internal cuticular ridges (darts). A diagnosis of *Dirofilaria* is possible based on these features of the cuticle (H&E, 200x).

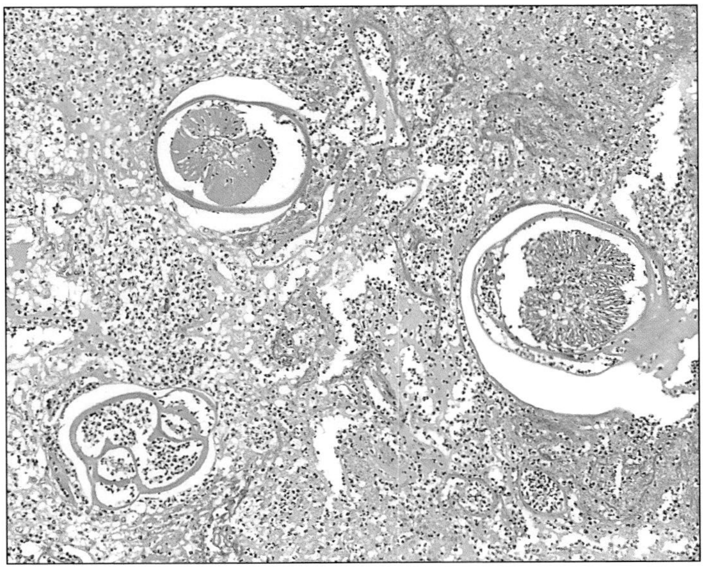

1

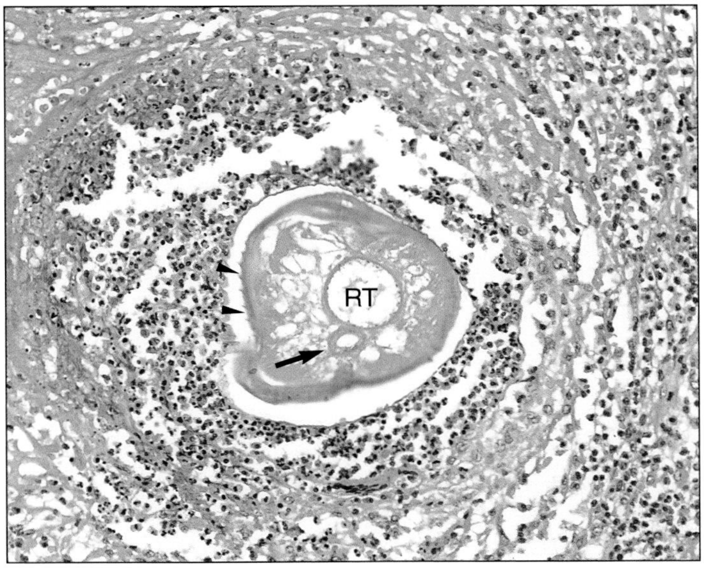

2

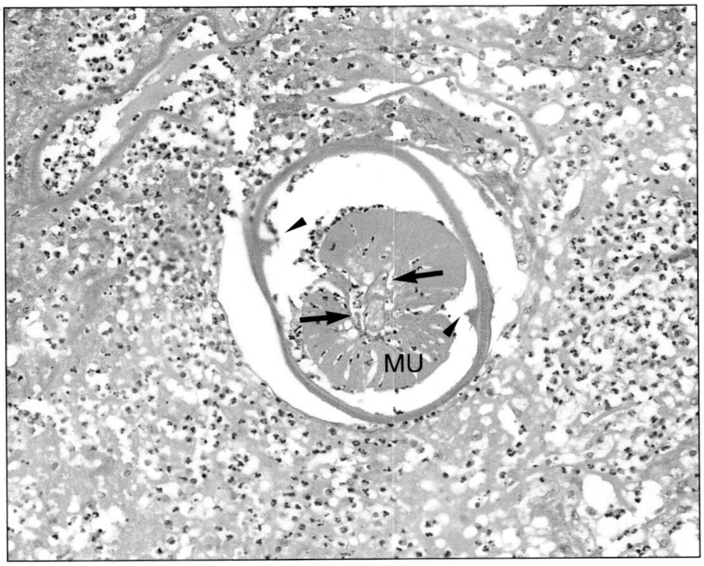

3

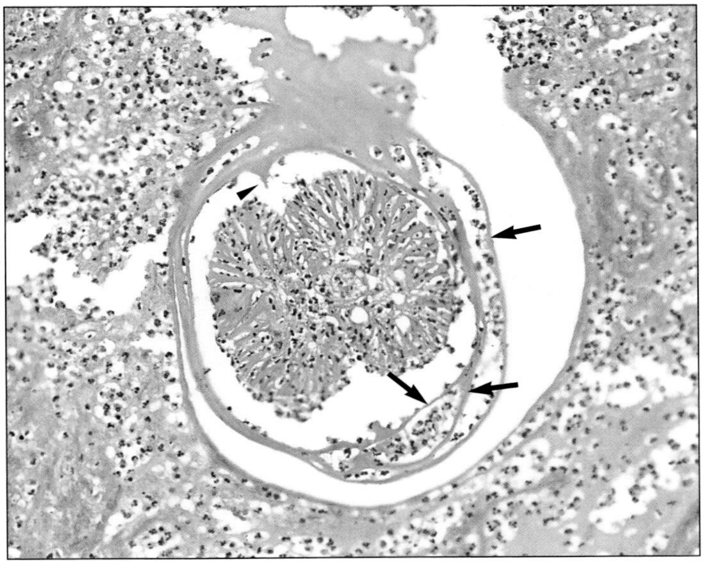

4

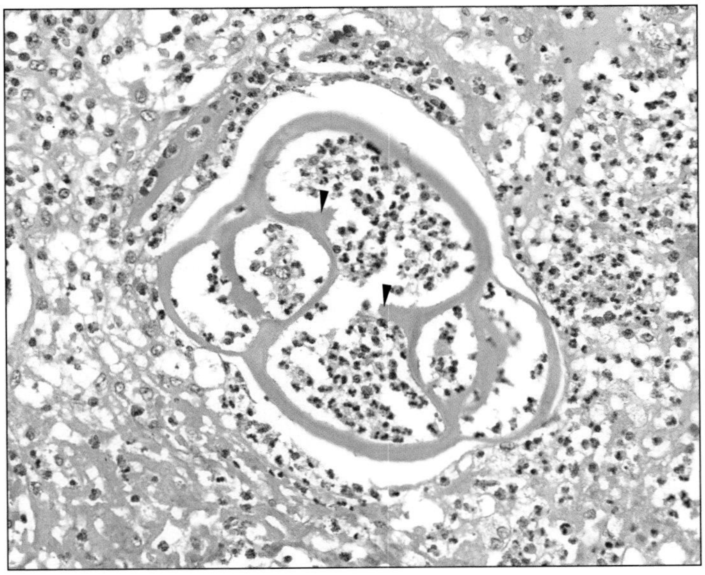

5

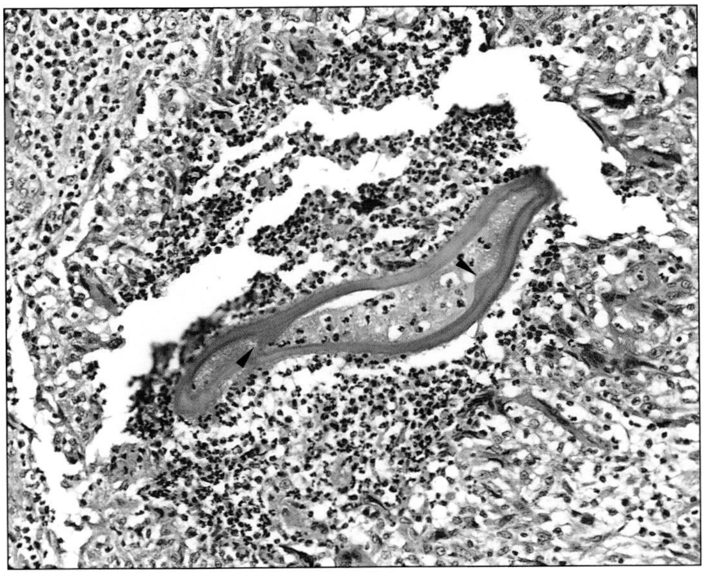

6

Dirofilaria species

Image 1

Transverse section through sexually mature adult female *D. immitis.* Note the thick, smooth cuticle, the large lateral chords (dart), and the tall, slender coelomyarian muscles. The worm measures 0.6 mm in diameter. The small tubular structure is the intestine (arrow), which shares the pseudocoelom with the paired uterine tubes (H&E, 60x).

Image 2

Transverse section through a male worm shares the same morphologic features of the body wall as seen in a previous section. Note the lateral, internal, cuticular ridges (darts). The two tubes are the intestine (IN) and the reproductive tube (H&E, 60x).

Image 3

Coin lesion measuring about 1 cm in diameter in the lung of a resident of Connecticut. The lesion involves a pulmonary artery and contains sections of a nematode (darts) in an advanced state of degeneration. The lesion and parasite are typical of *D. immitis* (H&E, 4x).

Image 4

Transverse section of a worm measuring 0.18 mm in diameter with a thick, swollen cuticle that bears a prominent internal ridge (darts) on each side. The soft parts are degenerate, but it is apparent that the muscles were well developed. Only one tube is clearly seen in this immature worm, although two are seen in most sections, indicating that the parasite is male (Trichrome, 180x).

Image 5

Sections of a filaria in a pulmonary artery in the lung of a resident of Italy (H&E, 35x).

Image 6

At high magnification, the cuticle bears longitudinal ridges, is multilayered, and has conspicuous internal ridges in the lateral fields. These features are typical of *Dirofilaria.* The size of the worm, the longitudinal ridges, and the geographic region in which the infection occurred indicates that the worm is *D. repens.* The pulmonary location of the worm is unusual and in no way typical of *D. repens* in humans (H&E, 450x).

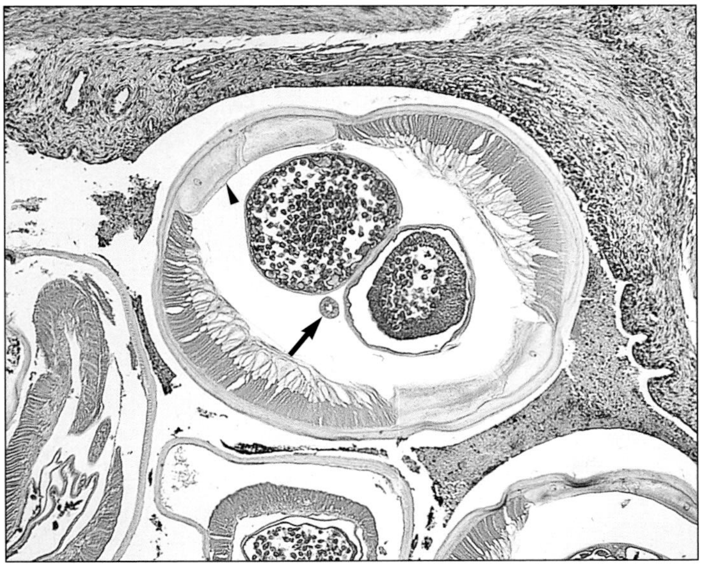

1

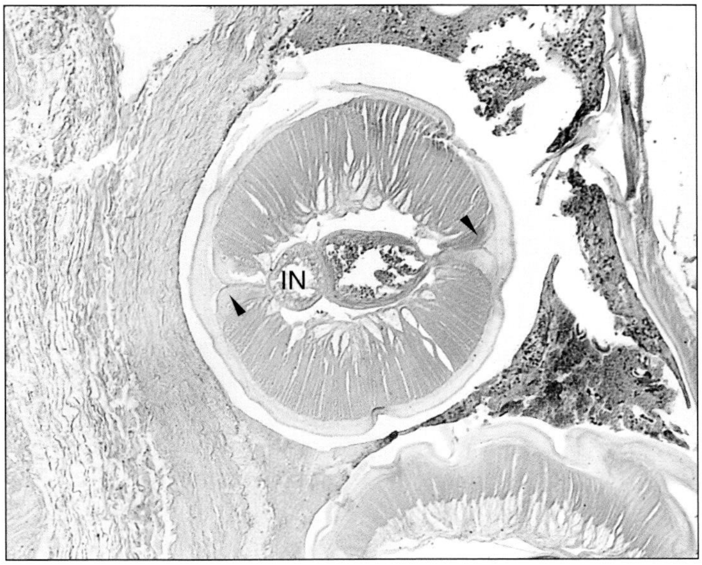

2

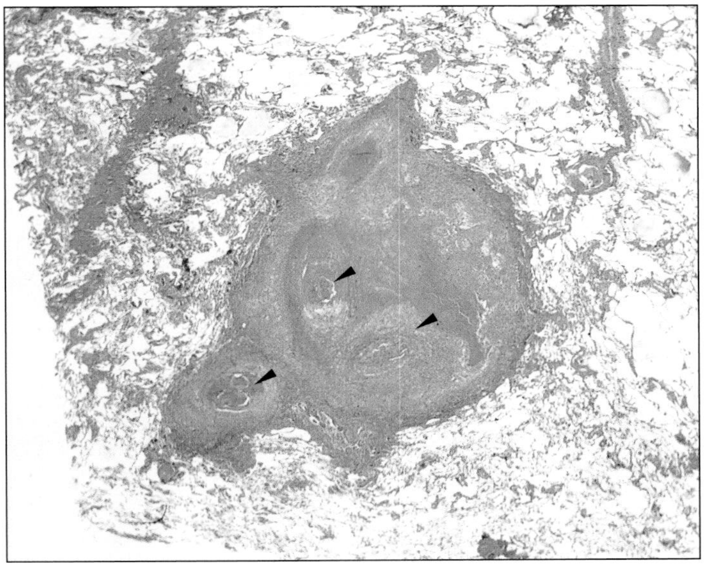

3

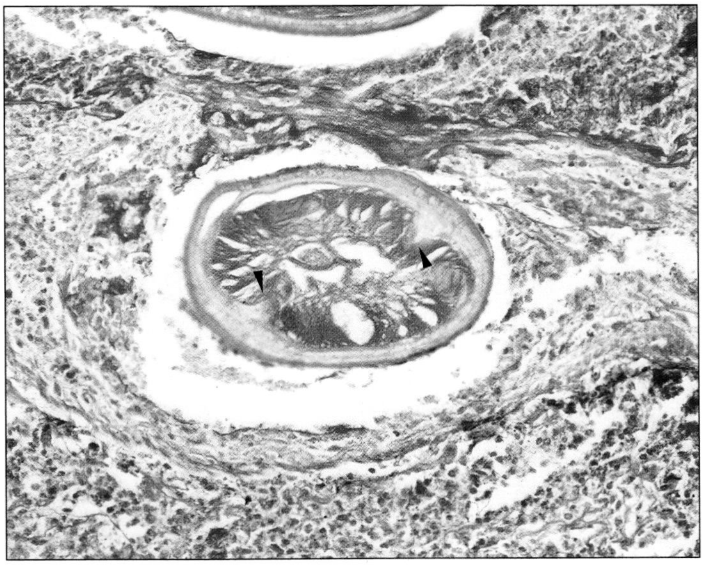

4

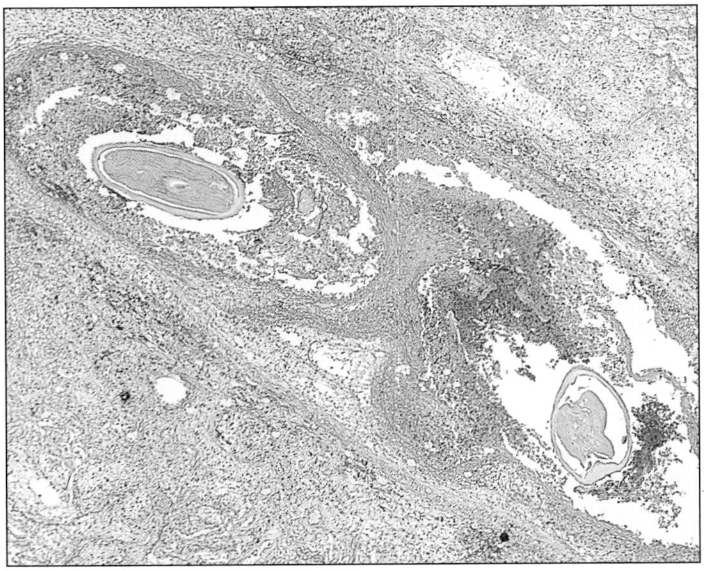

5

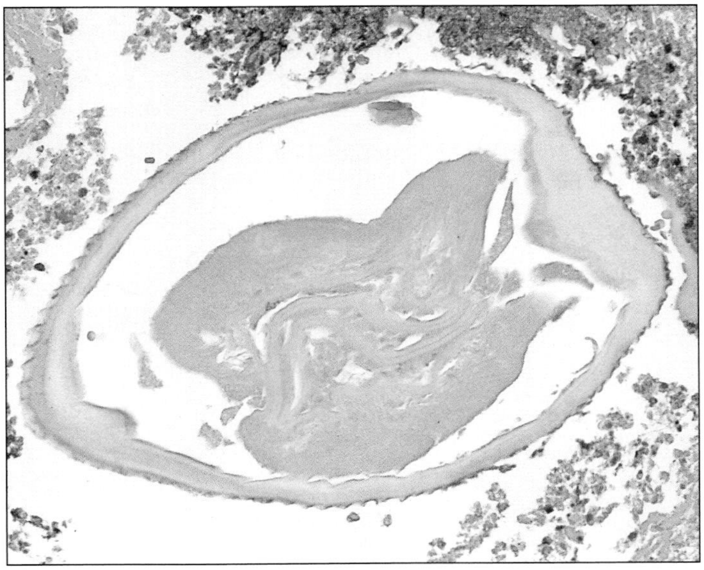

6

Plate 61

Dirofilaria species

Image 1

Section through a coin lesion shows a dead, calcifying worm in a pulmonary artery (unknown stain, 40x).

Image 2

Transverse section of the worm, which measures 0.15 mm in diameter. Although the parasite is in an advanced state of degeneration, the thickened, multilayered, smooth cuticle (CU) with much-exaggerated internal cuticular ridges (dart) can still be discerned. The hypodermis and lateral chords are recognizable, as are the muscles. At least one tube (arrow) is seen. The structures of the cuticle, hypodermis, and muscles identify the worm as *D. immitis.* Its size suggests that it is male (unknown stain, 275x).

Image 3

Another section of worm, with much-advanced degeneration, is still recognizable as a nematode. If morphologic features had to be relied upon, diagnosis would be difficult. Its tissue habitat would be highly suggestive of a *D. immitis* (H&E, 275x).

Image 4

Transverse section of a gravid female worm in a pulmonary artery of a Colombian with leukemia. One of the uterine tubes contain microfilariae. The worm, which measures about 0.30 mm in diameter, was originally identified as a *Wuchereria bancrofti.* However, the thick cuticle, internal cuticular ridges, and nature of the musculature indicate that the parasite is *D. immitis* (H&E, 200x).

Image 5

Transverse section of a female worm in a pulmonary nodule of a Japanese. The size of the worm and the structure of the multilayered cuticle with internal cuticular ridges (dart) indicate that it is a *D. immitis.* Objects (arrows) in the paired tubules were interpreted as microfilariae (H&E, 250x).

Image 6

At higher magnification, the objects shown in Image 5 (darts) are seen to be folds of degenerating tissues (H&E, 875x).

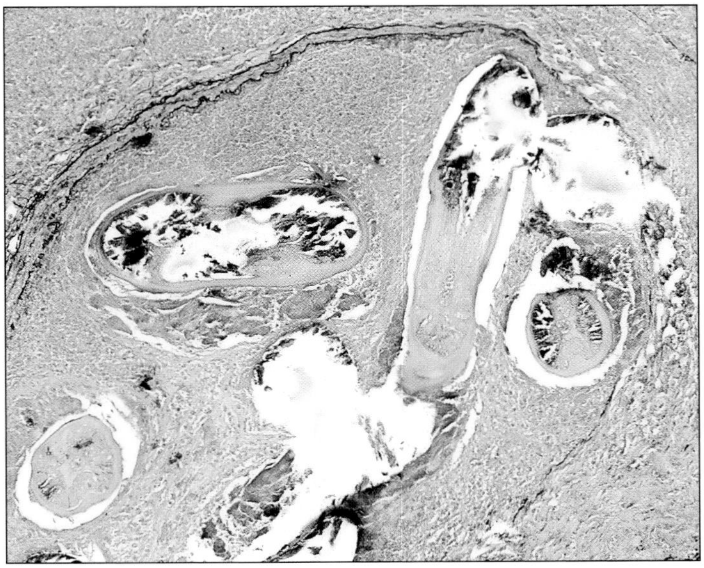

1

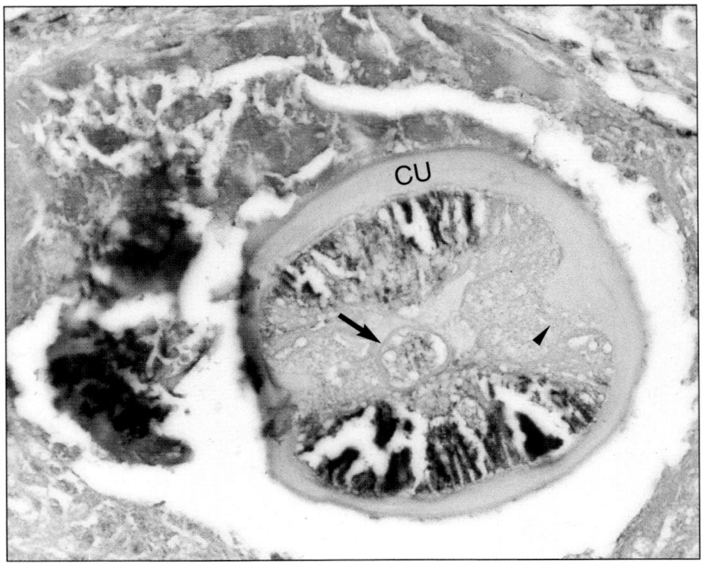

2

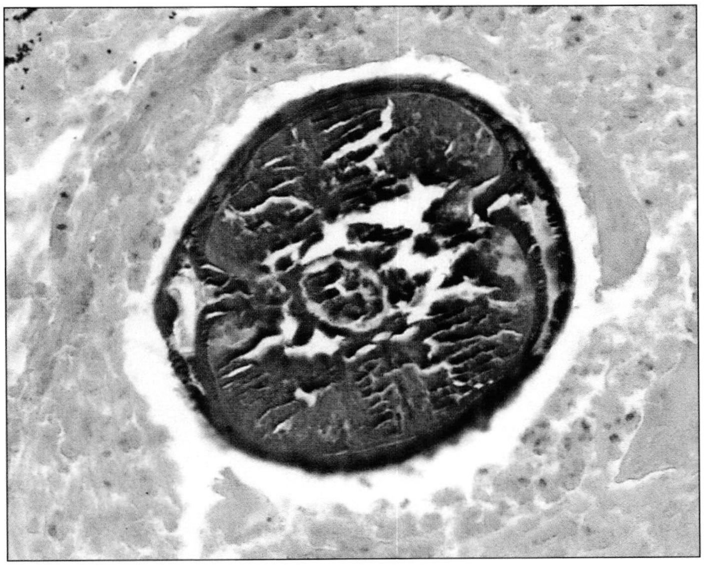

3

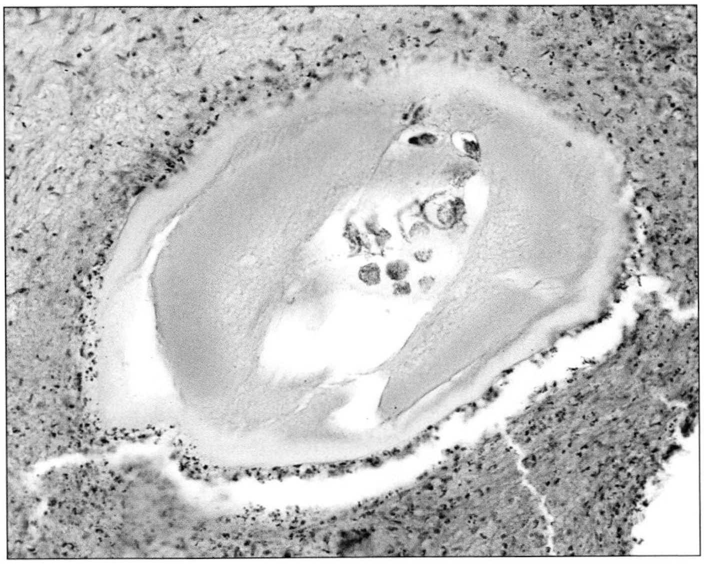

4

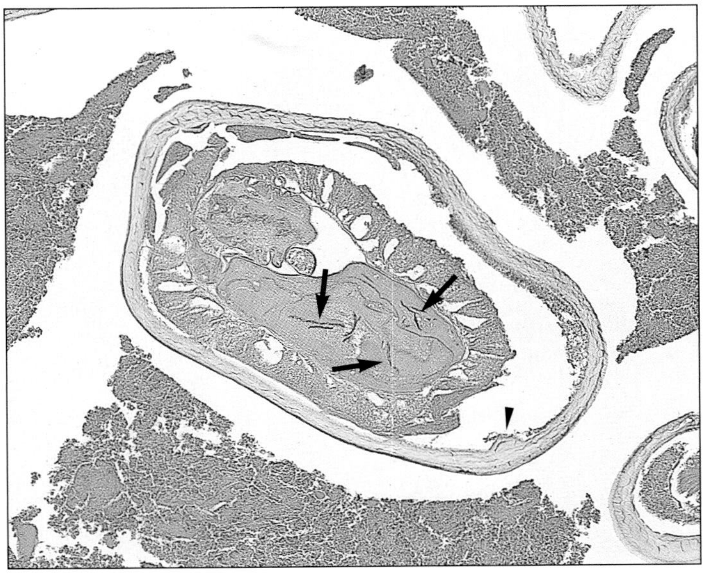

5

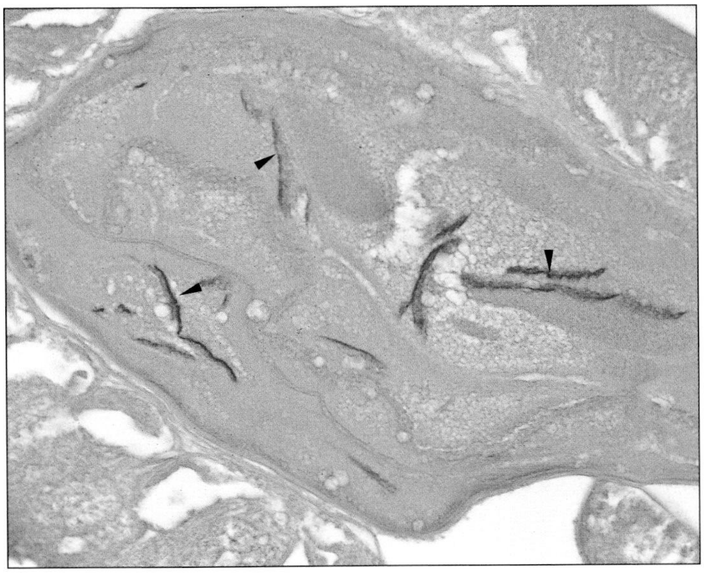

6

Plate 62

Dirofilaria species

Image 1

Section through a subcutaneous nodule removed from the thigh of a Louisianan. The worm, probably *D. tenuis*, is gravid; a branch of the uterus is filled with microfilariae (H&E, 50x).

Image 2

Transverse section through a female worm shows the uterine branches with sections of microfilariae (keyline). The worm was in a nodule removed from the abdominal wall of a Floridian. Although the worm is dead, much of the normal architecture of the body wall has been preserved. Note also the longitudinal ridges on the surface of the cuticle (darts), which help identify the worm as *D. tenuis* (H&E, 200x).

Image 3

Transverse section through a male worm in a subcutaneous nodule. Although the worm, which has a diameter of 0.23 mm, is dead, it has a thick cuticle with suggestions of longitudinal ridges, strong muscles, and large lateral chords (LC). The inner surface of the cuticle has cuticular ridges (darts). The small tube in the pseudocoelom is the intestine; the larger one is the male reproductive tube (RT) (H&E, 200x).

Image 4

A dead, degenerated male worm removed from the subcutaneous tissues of a resident of Italy. Longitudinal ridges can be seen in the cuticle. In the smaller section, the caudal alae (arrows), characteristic of *Dirofilaria*, are conspicuous. This worm is *D. repens*. Human cases are common in the Mediterranean region (H&E, 270x).

Image 5

Transverse section through a female *D. repens* in a subcutaneous nodule. Note the relatively thick cuticle with longitudinal ridges, broad lateral chords, and numerous tall coelomyarian muscle cells. The worm appears to be infertile, judging from the absence of eggs or microfilariae in the paired uterine tubes (Trichrome, 150x).

Image 6

Transverse section through an infertile female worm in a subcutaneous nodule removed from the neck of a French Canadian trapper. The body wall is typical of *Dirofilaria* species. The longitudinal ridges on the cuticle are sharp rather than rounded, which is characteristic of *D. ursi* (H&E, 200x).

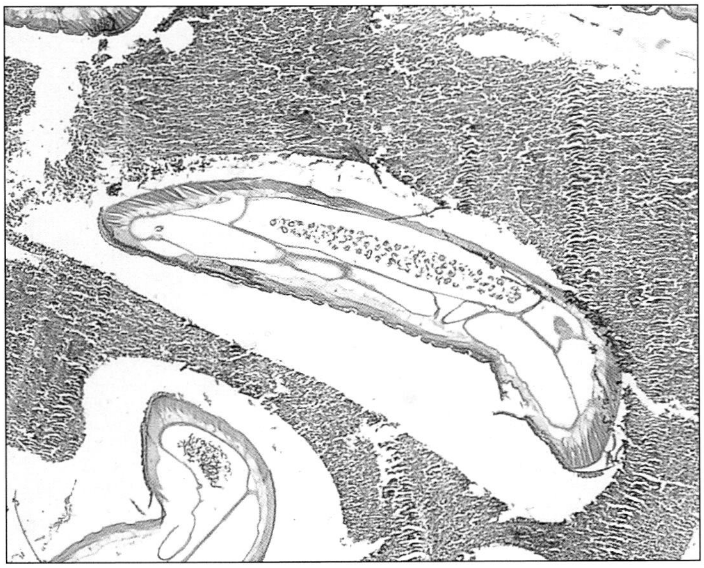

1

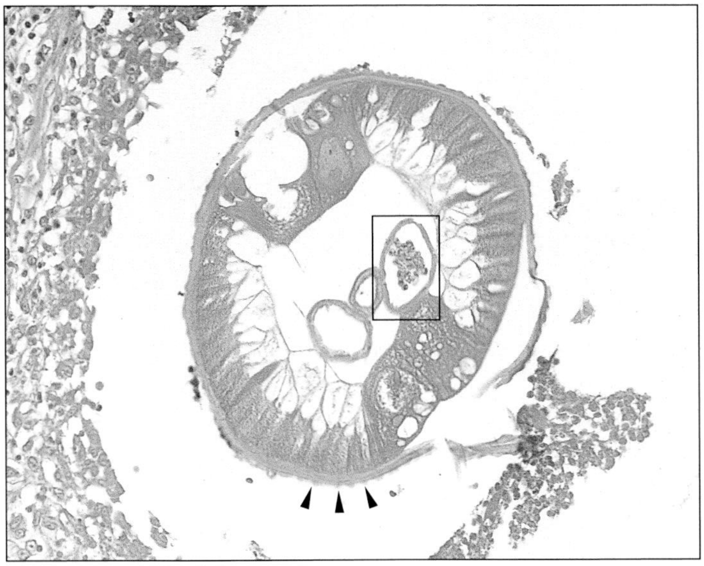

2

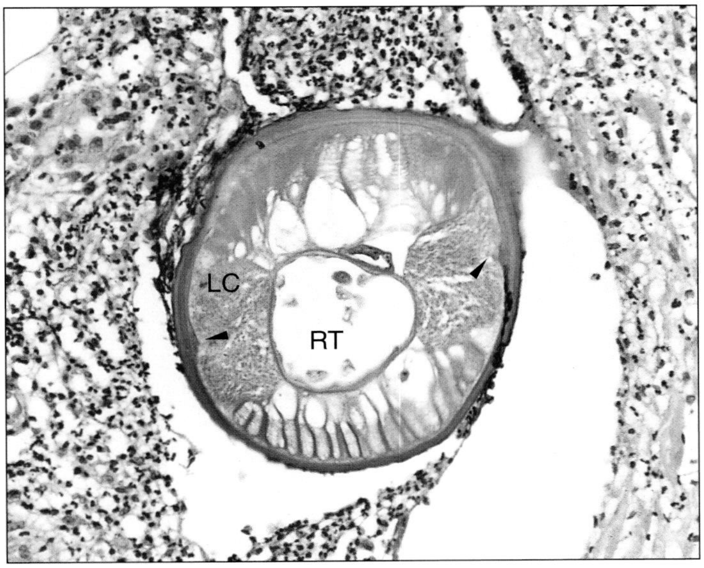

3

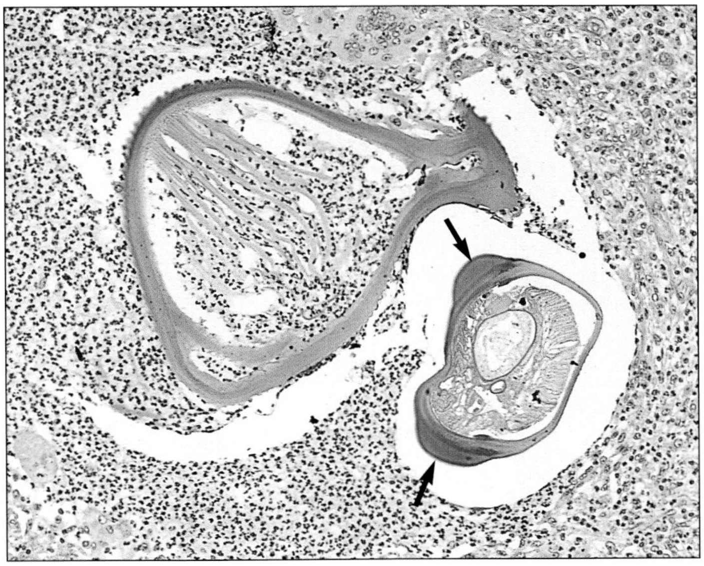

4

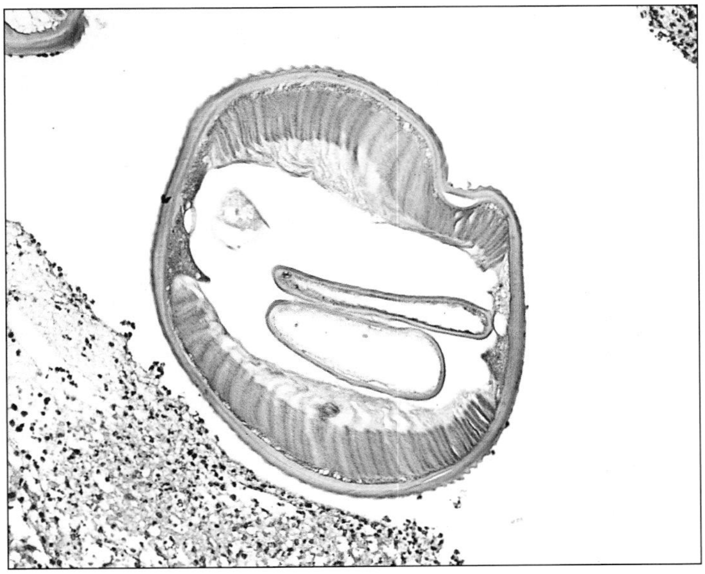

5

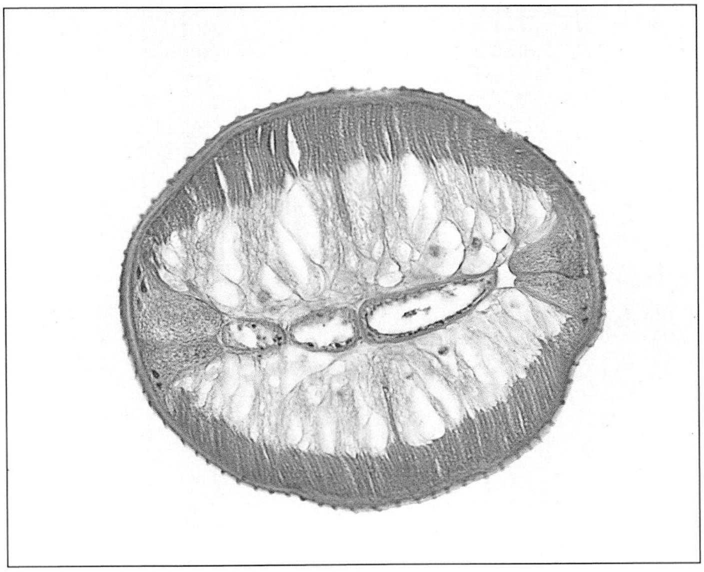

6

Uncommon Filariae

Several species of filariae have been identified in humans either by the microfilaria stage or by the immature or adult stages. Of those identified by the microfilariae, usually no matching adult is present (eg, *Microfilaria bolivarensis, Microfilaria semiclarum*). Consequently, little is known or can be said about the parasites. In other cases, the microfilaria has been matched with the adult parasite from its natural host (eg, *Meningonema peruzzii*). In still others the adult has been recovered intact from the tissues and a proper identification made (eg, *Loaina* species). *Meningonema peruzzii* and *Loaina* have on rare occasions been found in humans, and although our knowledge of them is limited, we discuss them briefly.

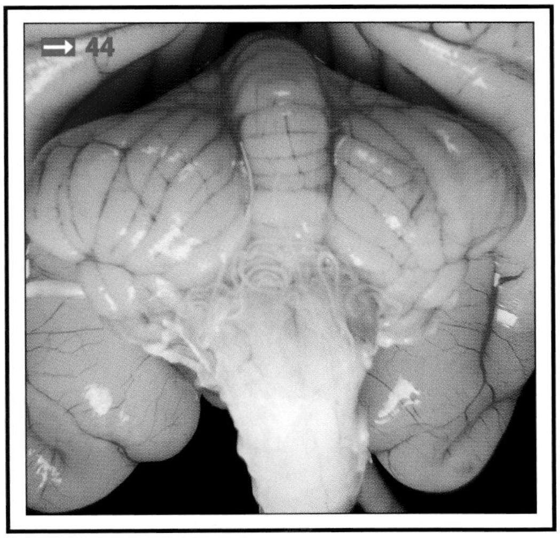

Meningonema peruzzii

Microfilariae found in the cerebrospinal fluid of two individuals in Zimbabwe who had developed neurologic disorders were mistakenly identified as *Mansonella perstans*. These microfilariae were subsequently recognized as those of *M. peruzzii*, a filaria that inhabits the meninges and subarachnoid spaces in the brain of cercopithecoid monkeys in Africa (➡ 44). Because the patients eventually recovered spontaneously or after treatment with Melarsoprol, the adult worms were never recovered. Thus, our knowledge of this filaria is limited to studies carried out on infected monkeys.

In the simian host, the small and sheathed microfilariae circulate in the peripheral blood and are found in the cerebrospinal fluid. Infected monkeys show no signs or symptoms of infection. Unfortunately, no information is available regarding the life cycle of the filaria or the vectors that transmit it.

The gross morphologic characteristics of the parasite and its microfilaria have been described by Orihel and Esslinger (1973). Adult worms are of moderate size. The female has an average length of 10 cm and a maximum average diameter of 0.47 mm; the male is less than half this size, 4.1 cm by 0.23 mm. The body wall is thin and nearly transparent. The cuticle is smooth and without apparent transverse striations. The anterior end is obovate in shape and of greater diameter than the rest of the body. The tail is long in both sexes and lacks alae, lappets, or terminal protuberances. The male has paired, unequal, dissimilar spicules. The microfilariae, unlike those of *M. perstans,* have a tight sheath that is often difficult to see. The body measures 170 by 4 µm, which is a bit smaller than that of *M. perstans*.

Only the female worm has been seen in sectioned tissues, and even this material is limited. However, the unique habitat of the filaria sets it apart from most other species (Plate 63:3). In addition, the thin and weakly developed body wall and, even more unusual, its quadridelphic female reproductive system (ie, four uterine branches, oviducts, and ovaries) are key diagnostic features of the parasite (Plate 63:4). Patients infected with the parasite have a history of travel or residence in Africa, particularly in an environment shared with primates.

Loaina species

A small, sexually mature male worm measuring 4.5 mm in length was removed from the anterior chamber of the eye of a man in Colombia. Its morphologic features indicated that it was an undescribed species of *Loaina*, a filaria normally found in the subcutaneous tissues of rabbits in the southeastern United States and probably elsewhere as well. Morphologically, *Loaina* bears a remarkable resemblance to *Loa*, a common human parasite, but the two genera are distinct in host preference, size, and cuticular ornamentation. Also, *Loaina* utilizes species of mosquitoes as vectors; *Loa* is transmitted by deerflies.

Details of the microanatomic features of *Loaina* are limited. Studies to date show a great similarity between *Loa* and *Loaina* in the structure of the body wall and the distribution of the parts of the female reproductive system at different body levels. This is immediately evident when comparing the two (Plate 53:2 vs Plate 63:5 & 6). The female *Loaina* measures about 3 cm in length and has a diameter of approximately 0.42 mm. The male is smaller, with an average length of 1.4 cm and a diameter of about 0.3 mm. The cuticle is moderately thick but lacks the bosses seen in *Loa*. The hypodermis is thin in the submuscular areas, but the lateral chords are expanded and conspicuous (Plate 63:5). The muscles are well developed and of the coelomyarian type; they number eight or fewer per body quadrant (Plate 63:5). Both contractile and cytoplasmic portions are equally developed (Plate 63:6). Dorsal and ventral hypodermal chords are easy to identify. Because one set of reproductive tubes lies in the anterior half of the body of the female and the other in the posterior part, and because they tend to be coiled and looped, all levels of each tube (ie, uterus, oviducts, and ovaries) can usually be seen in any transverse section (Plate 63:5). Features of the male have not been described in sections.

References

Botero D, Aguledo LM, Uribe FJ, et al. Intraocular filaria: a *Loaina* species from man in Colombia. *Am J Trop Med Hyg.* 1984;33:578-582.

Orihel TC. Cerebral filariasis in Rhodesia: a zoonotic infection? *Am J Trop Med Hyg.* 1973;22:596-599.

Beaver PC. Intraocular filariasis: a brief review. *Am J Trop Med Hyg.* 1989;40:40-45.

Plate 63

Uncommon Filariae

Image 1

Dirofilaria striata. Female worm within muscle sheath shows typical *Dirofilaria* morphology. This worm is in the tissues of the natural host, the bobcat (H&E, 150x).

Image 2

High-magnification image shows the ala in the lateral line of the body (dart). This feature distinguishes *D. striata* from all other known species of *Dirofilaria* in the Western Hemisphere (H&E, 400x).

Image 3

Section through the brain of a monkey shows several sections of a female *M. peruzzii* lying in the meninges. At this low magnification, the thin body wall of the worm is clear (H&E, 40x).

Image 4

At higher magnification, two transverse sections show the thin body wall. One can see the poorly developed muscles (keylines) and the broad but flattened lateral chords (between the two keylines). The four branches of the uterus contain microfilariae. The flattened tube in the same section is the intestine (dart). In the other section, six segments of uterine tubes are seen. The intestine (IN) displays its normal tubular appearance with a low cuboidal epithelium (H&E, 120x).

Image 5

Loaina species. Transverse section through a gravid female worm shows its typical appearance. The five sections of uterine tube contain developing eggs and microfilariae. The intestine (dart) is a simple tube. The structural features of the body wall are especially clear (Trichrome, 140x).

Image 6

The architecture of the body wall at higher magnification reveals the cuticle, underlying hypodermis, large lateral chords (LC), and well-developed coelomyarian muscles (MU) (Trichrome, 400x).

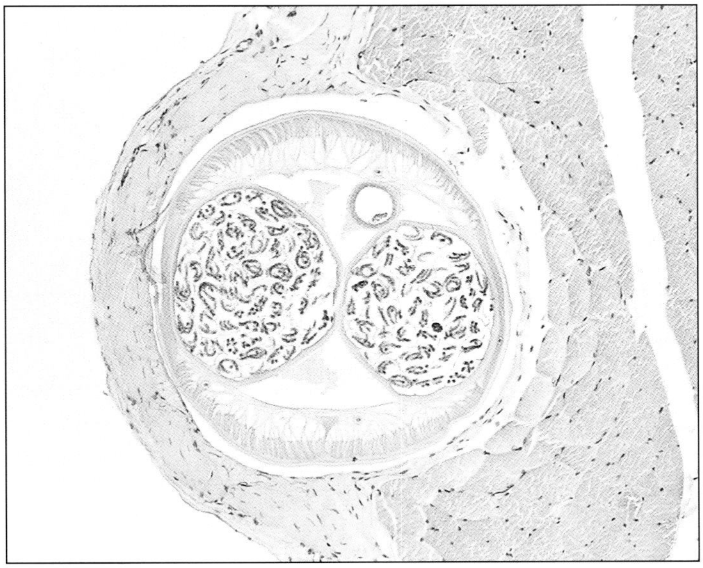

1

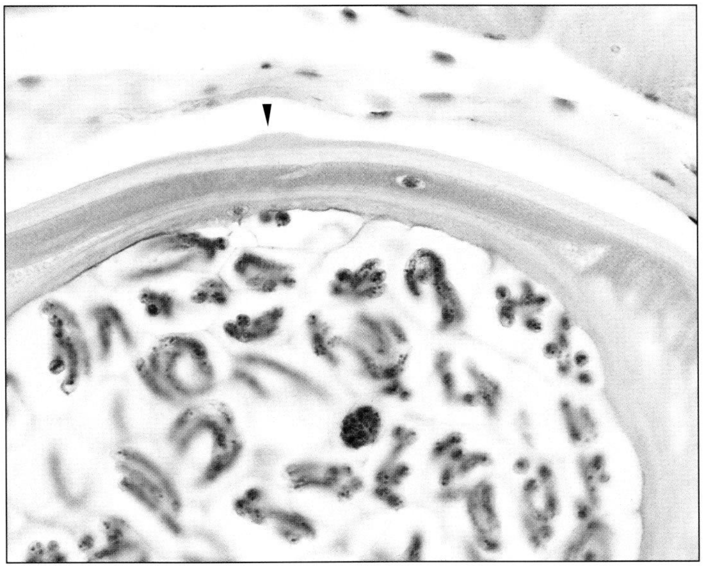

2

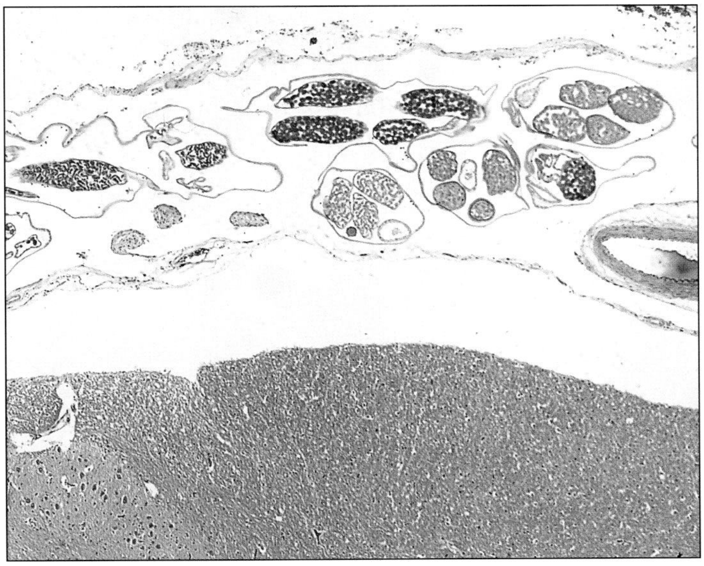

3

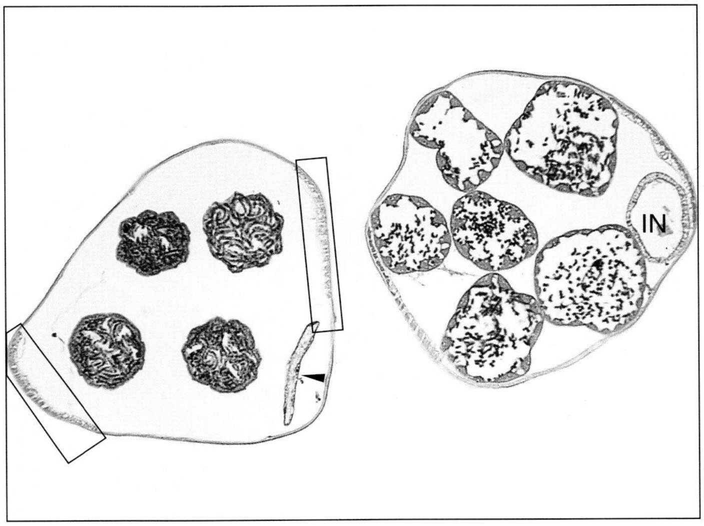

4

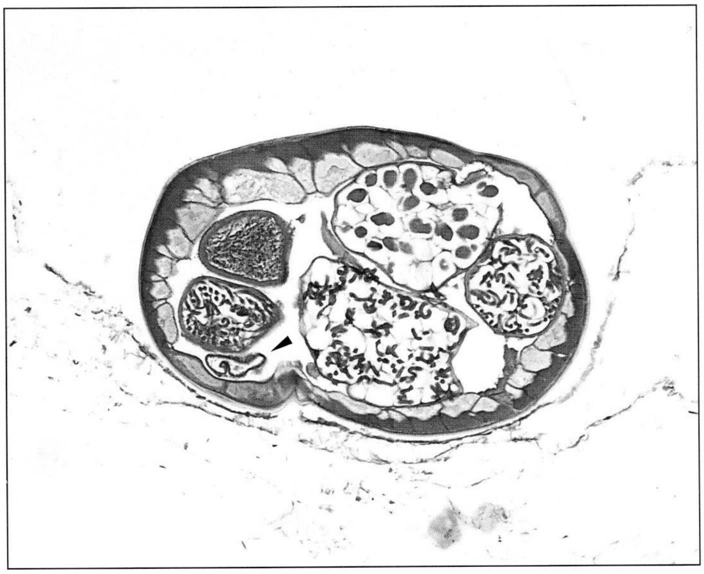

5

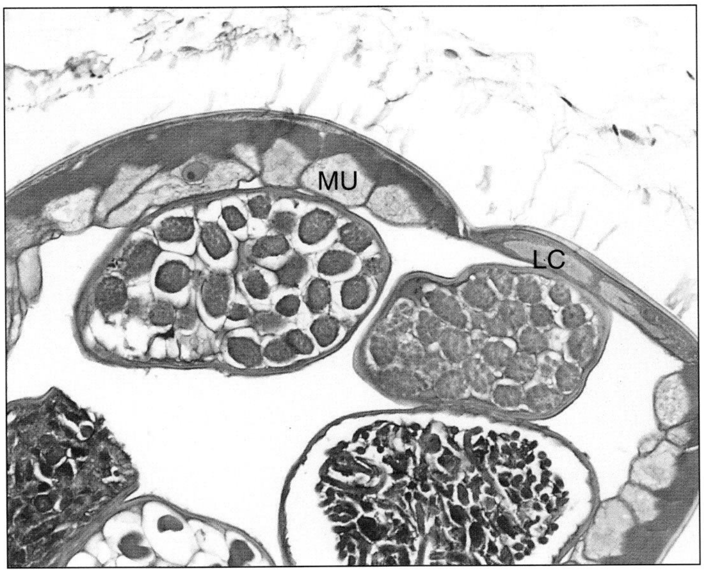

6

Dracunculus medinensis

Infection with *Dracunculus medinensis* was documented in ancient Egyptian medical literature dating back to the 15th century BC. Usually referred to as dracunculiasis, it is better known as the "Guinea worm," a name it received from a Swiss traveler who saw it in natives along the Guinea coast of West Africa (Nigeria) in the early 17th century. Today, the disease is distributed throughout India, Pakistan, and 17 African countries and afflicts about five million people. A consortium of US and international agencies has undertaken a major effort to eliminate the parasite from the human population by 1995.

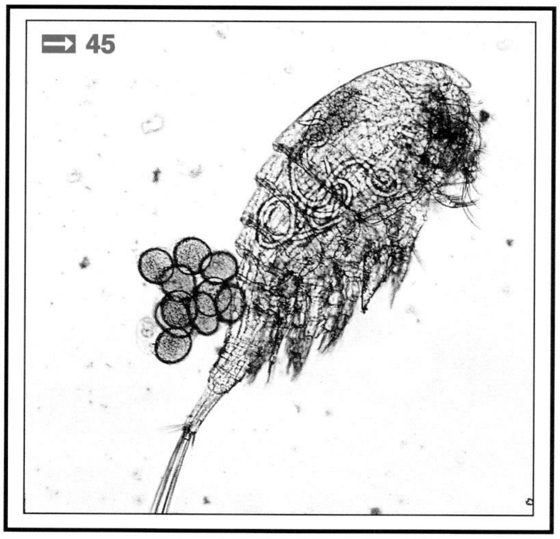

Biology and Life Cycle

Individuals acquire infection by drinking water containing copepods (*Cyclops*) infected with the parasite (45). The infective larvae are liberated from the copepod in the gut and make their way to deep body tissues of the host. Development to the adult stage requires about one year, at which time the female worm makes her way to the superficial tissues of the body, usually the extremities (46) but possibly the breast, scrotum, abdominal wall, etc. Development is essentially asymptomatic until the mature female worm reaches the surface of the skin. There, a blister forms, and the individual becomes aware of the presence of the parasite when, upon contact with water, the blister bursts and the anterior end of the worm emerges and spews thousands of larvae into the water. These larvae, which measure up to 750 µm in length, have a long, slender, whiplike tail. They are ingested by the copepods present in the water, and the cycle is repeated. As the female worm emerges it is typically wound on a small stick until it is totally extricated from the body. Dracunculiasis can be prevented and eradicated simply by providing safe sources of drinking water such as wells, which prevent human intrusion and seeding of the water with larvae.

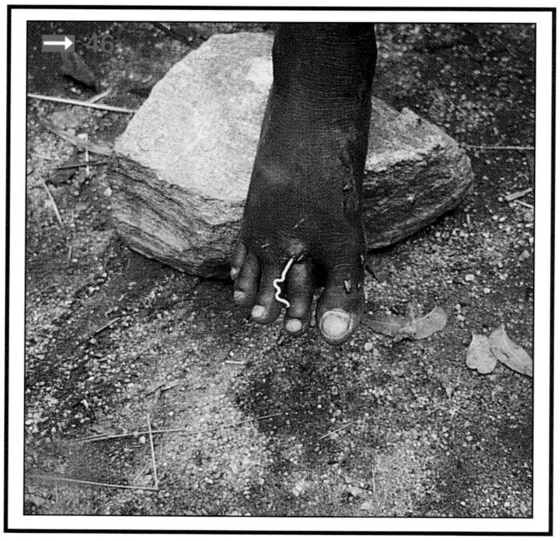

Pathology and Clinical Manifestations

The first indications of infection with *D. medinensis* are the systemic symptoms associated with the migration of the worm to the surface of the skin and the formation of the blister. Individuals may develop urticaria, dyspnea, fever, diarrhea, vomiting, and giddiness. The blister produces a painful, burning sensation. Individuals often seek relief by immersing the affected part in cool water, such as a pond or other standing water, where the blister ruptures and the worm discharges its larvae. Thereafter, the worm is carefully removed from the body. Breakage or rupture of the worm may cause a severe inflammatory response, and contaminated wounds can become septic. Infected individuals may be incapacitated for weeks until the worm(s) is removed from the body. No cure for the condition is available, other than removing the worms. Palliative drugs are used to reduce pain and minimize secondary infection. The secondary bacterial invaders may cause gangrene or focal suppuration. Some worms do not reach the surface of the skin and are not extracted; instead, they die in the tissues, where they cause abscesses and eventually are absorbed or calcified. Calcified worms may be found in almost any part of the body.

Parasite Morphology

Because animal reservoirs for *D. medinensis* are not known and because the species found in animals do not, as far as we know, infect humans, infected individuals will have a history of traveling to endemic areas and drinking water from potentially infective sources (eg, pools or ponds of standing water).

The adult female worm is large, reaching lengths of 60 to 120 cm with a diameter of 1.0 to 1.7 mm. Males are extremely small, measuring approximately 40 mm in length. Males also live in the subcutaneous tissues and are seldom seen. Some researchers believe that the male survives for only a short time in human tissues, just long enough to inseminate the female. However, experimental studies with animal species confirm that the male worm survives at least as long as the female. The typical living female worm possesses a relatively thick, smooth cuticle; usually conspicuous lateral chords; and strong bands of muscles that are polymyarian and coelomyarian (Plate 64:1 & 2). Overall, the body wall resembles that of typical filariae. However, the pseudocoelom is usually packed with larvae (Plate 64:1). The intestine may be present or atrophied; usually it is small in diameter and may contain pigmented granules. Fortuitous sections can be cut through the relatively short esophagus. The male worm has the same body-wall features that the female does, as well as a highly pigmented intestine (Plate 64:2). A single reproductive tube is filled with developing spermatozoa (Plate 64:2).

Dead worms are usually in a degenerate state, so that their body wall retains little of its normal architecture (Plate 64:4) or is no longer recognizable (Plate 64:4). However, the typical larvae may still be recognized by their slender whiplike tails in the lesion (Plate 64:6).

Although the body wall of *D. medinensis* is similar to that of the filariae, the uterine contents—rhabditoidlike larvae—clearly distinguish this species. In addition to the characteristics of the larval tail, the larvae have a well-differentiated esophagus and intestine lying within a pseudocoelom, unlike the more primitive microfilariae, which lack defined organ systems.

References

Allaire AD, Majmudar B. Dracunculosis of the broad ligament: a case of a "parasitic leiomyoma." *Am J Surg Pathol.* 1993;17:937-940.

Burnier M Jr, Hidayat AA, Neafie R. Dracunculiasis of the orbit and eyelid: light and electron microscopic observations of two cases. *Ophthalmology.* 1991;98:919-924.

Rohde J, Sharma BL, Patton H, et al. Surgical extraction of guinea worm: disability reduction and contribution to disease control. *Am J Trop Med Hyg.* 1993;48:71-76.

Smith GS, Blum D, Huttly SRA, et al. Disability from dracunculiasis: effect on morbidity. *Ann Trop Med Parasitol.* 1989;83:151-158.

Plate 64

Dracunculus species

Images 1 and 3

D. insignis, female. This dracunculid found in raccoons is morphologically indistinguishable from *D. medinensis* and demonstrates the typical morphology of *Dracunculus* species. Note the relatively thick cuticle, lateral chords (keyline), and well-developed muscles (MU). The intestine (dart) is a small tube. The pseudocoelom is filled by a branch of the uterus and is packed with rhabditoid larvae (H&E; 45x, 60x).

Image 2

D. insignis, male. This worm displays the strong musculature of the parasite, its highly pigmented intestine (IN), and a large reproductive tube (RT). Male worms are rarely found in the tissues (H&E, 30x).

Image 4

Dracunculus medinensis. This dead, degenerating female worm was found in a calcified mass in the scrotum of a patient from Nigeria. Although little of the body architecture is recognizable, remnants of muscles (MU) can be seen, and rhabditoid larvae are identifiable within the worm (darts) (H&E, 30x).

Image 5

D. medinensis. A fibrous, tumorlike mass was removed from the scrotum of a young Nigerian. Although no elements of the adult worm are recognizable, rhabditoid larvae are dispersed through the lesion (keyline) (H&E, 40x).

Image 6

D. medinensis. High magnification of keylined area in Image 5. The rhabditoid larvae are recognizable, with at least a portion of one displaying its long, whiplike tail (dart) (H&E, 200x).

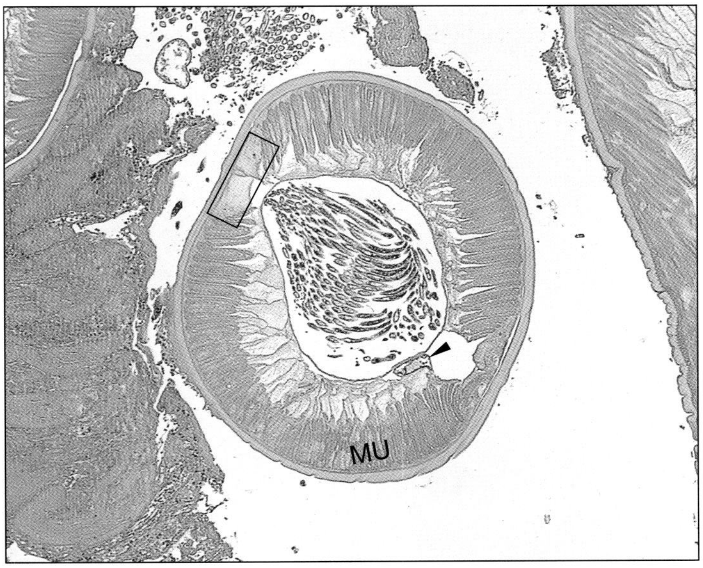

1

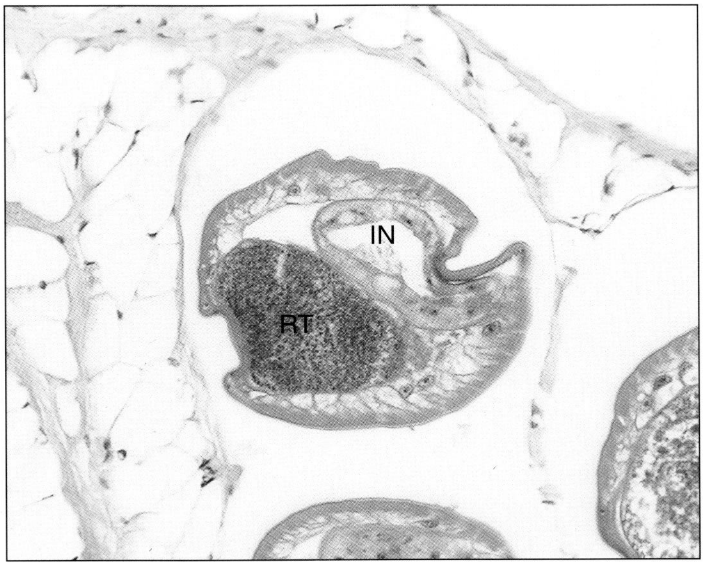

2

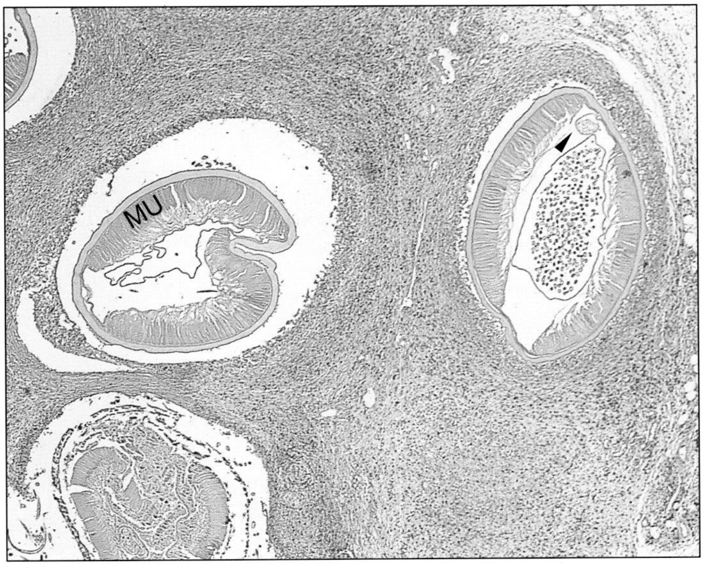

3

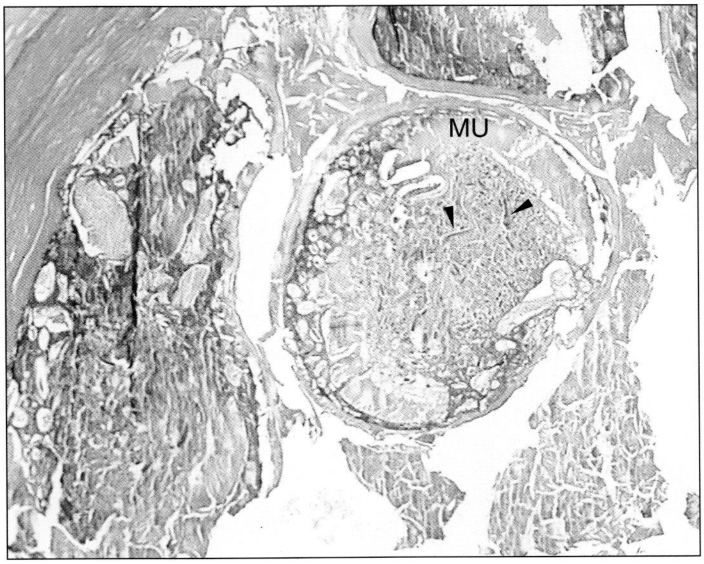

4

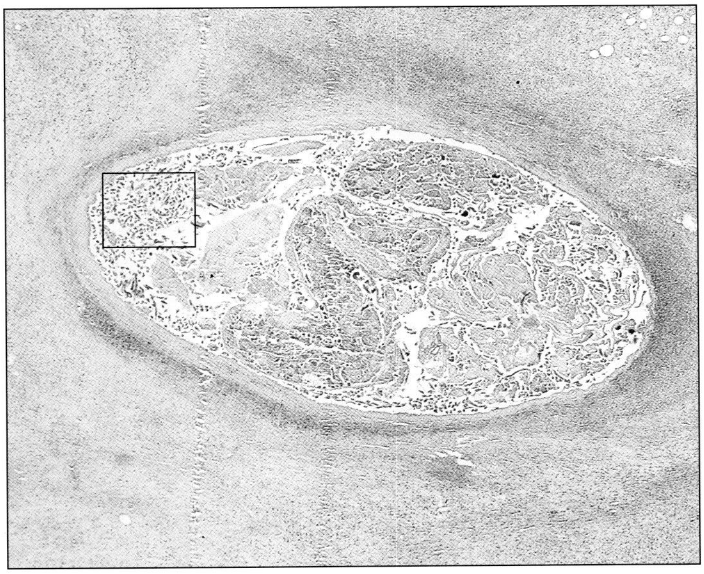

5

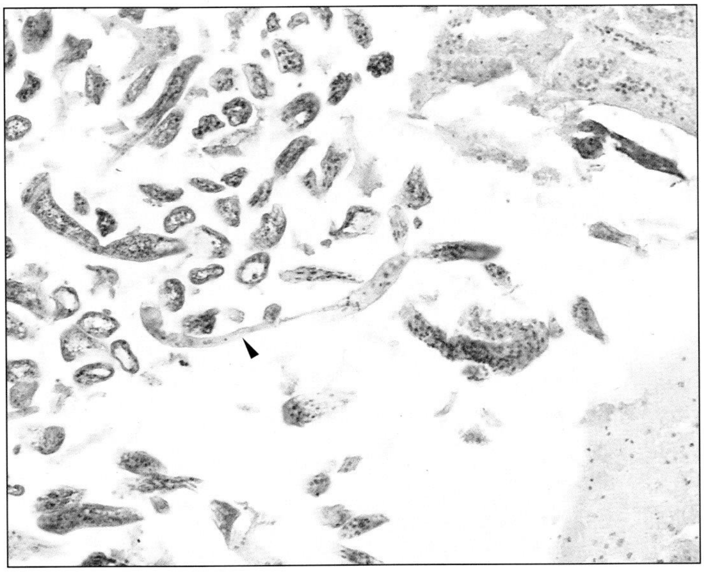

6

Strongyloides stercoralis

Strongyloides stercoralis is a common human parasite that has worldwide distribution throughout warm regions and is endemic in some temperate areas such as the southern United States. Approximately 75 million people are infected with the parasite. Strongyloidiasis has assumed new importance in recent years, primarily because of the widespread use of immunosuppressive drugs to prevent allograft rejection and treat malignancies and collagen vascular diseases. In these circumstances, individuals with latent or subclinical *Strongyloides* infections may develop disseminated infections that can be fatal if not diagnosed in time.

Another species, *S. fuelleborni*, is commonly found in apes and monkeys and has become established in human populations in parts of Asia and Africa. Still other species found in animals may cause a cutaneous larva migrans in humans. We limit our discussion to *S. stercoralis*.

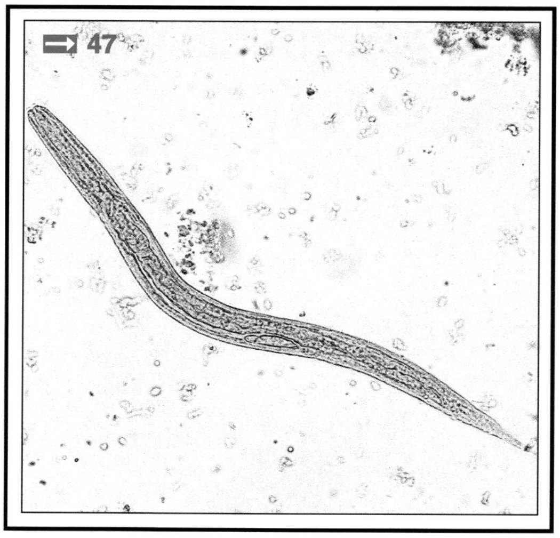

Biology and Life Cycle

Strongyloides is a unique parasite in terms of its behavior and biology. Parasitic adults are all females that reproduce parthogenetically. The female lives in the mucosal epithelium of the small intestine, especially the duodenum (Plate 65:1 & 2), and produces thin-shelled eggs that are deposited in the mucosa and develop into rhabditoid larvae. The larvae hatch, migrate into the intestinal lumen, and pass out of the body in feces. (➡ 47) Under proper conditions, rhabditoid larvae deposited on the soil develop rapidly to the infective (filariform) stage and are ready to infect a new host by penetrating exposed skin surfaces. Also, a free-living generation or two may be interposed—that is, some rhabditoid larvae may develop to free-living adults (males and females) in the soil. These females produce additional rhabditoid larvae, which in turn develop into infective (filariform) larvae. The infective larvae actively penetrate the skin, enter small blood vessels, and migrate rapidly to the pulmonary capillaries. Once they break out of these vessels, they enter the alveoli and migrate via the trachea to the mucosa of the small intestine. They develop through two molts to become mature females in about 14 days.

Variations in the cycle may produce significant complications in the host. For example, under some circumstances rhabditoid larvae in the intestine may develop to the infective stage and penetrate the perianal skin to start a cycle of internal or external autoinfection. A low-level autoinfection may occur in healthy individuals, and in this manner infections may be maintained for decades outside of endemic areas. In immunocompromised individuals or those taking long-term steroid therapy, autoinfection can progress at an accelerated rate, with extensive dissemination of the infection and frequently a fatal outcome.

Pathology and Clinical Manifestations

Patients with mild infections are generally asymptomatic. Some erythema, urticaria, and edema may be present at the site of entry into the skin, depending on the number of larvae that enter. Within a week, the individual may experience symptoms such as cough and bronchial irritation, which are related to the pneumonitis produced by larvae passing through the lungs and are followed a week later by mild gastrointestinal symptoms such as cramps and diarrhea. Chronic infection tends to produce some pain in the upper right quadrant, alternating diarrhea and constipation, along with moderate to high peripheral blood eosinophilia. A creeping eruption involving the skin in the region of the buttocks, thighs, and abdomen but originating near the anus has been termed *larva currens*. It has been reported with some frequency in individuals with chronic strongyloidiasis who also have gastrointestinal complaints. In individuals with hyperinfection, the migration of large numbers of larvae through tissues and organs of the body usually causes severe gastrointestinal and pulmonary symptoms. Sometimes, concurrent secondary bacterial infections and septicemia are noted. Infections with a few adult worms produce little or no irritation in these tissues.

Because migration through the lungs is rapid, pulmonary disorders are also minimal. However, in individuals with hyperinfection the bowel lining becomes congested and edematous, with possible ulceration. Chronic hyperinfection produces fibrosis of the bowel wall. Passage of large numbers of filariform larvae through the bowel wall and into various tissues and organs during migration to the lungs may damage the organs to the point that they may become nonfunctional. The presence of many larvae in the lungs causes pneumonitis, alveolar hemorrhage, and edema. Larvae and sometimes even adults may be found in the sputum (Plate 66:5 & 6). Penetration of the bowel wall may introduce bacteria into the tissues, causing septicemia.

Parasite Morphology

The parasitic female measures up to 2.7 mm in length by 30 to 40 µm in diameter. The anterior one-third of the body contains the esophagus, while the reproductive tube (which is reflected on itself) fills the posterior two-thirds. The paired, amphidelphic uteri contain several eggs (Plate 65:3). Most sections through the posterior two-thirds of the body contain the tubular intestine and, typically, two reproductive tubes (Plate 65:4). There are usually many eggs in the process of development adjacent to sections of adult worms (Plate 65:1–3). The eggs measure 50 to 58 mm by 30 to 40 µm and have a thin shell. Rhabditoid larvae measure 180 to 380 mm by 14 to 20 µm and may be found still within the egg membrane in the mucosa. In hyperinfections, both the eggs that contain a larva and free, rhabditoid larvae may be seen in samples of sputum (Plate 66:5). The filariform larva measures up to 500 to 600 mm in length by 15 to 16 mm in diameter. Key morphologic features include the long esophagus (about half of the total body length) and a notched tail. These features are usually easy to see and facilitate identification of the larvae found in samples from sputum (Plate 66:6). The larva also has double lateral alae, which are not always easy to see in transverse sections (Plate 66:2). In hyperinfections, larvae are visible in many tissues and organs (Plate 65:5 & 6; Plate 66:1 & 4).

The morphologic features of the adult female *Strongyloides stercoralis* are difficult to discern in the tissues, but the minute size of the worm and the presence of developing eggs and larvae in the immediate vicinity suggest the diagnosis. Based on purely morphologic criteria, adult *S. stercoralis* are not easily confused with *Trichinella spiralis* or *Capillaria philippinensis* in the same tissues. *Trichinella* larvae are more minute and primitive in structure than *S. stercoralis* and are generally not seen in the intestinal mucosa. A stichosome is present in *C. philippinensis*; also, eggs in the female uterus and in adjacent tissue have distinctive morphologic features, such as plugs, that immediately distinguish them from the thin-shelled eggs of *S. stercoralis*.

References

Davidson RA. Infection due to *Strongyloides stercoralis* in patients with pulmonary disease. *South Med J*. 1992;85:28-31.

DeVault GA, King JW, Rohr MS, et al. Opportunistic infections with *Strongyloides stercoralis* in renal transplantation. *Rev Infect Dis*. 1990;12:653-671.

Genta R. Global prevalence of strongyloidiasis: critical review with epidemiologic insights into the prevention of disseminated disease. *Rev Infect Dis*. 1989;11:755-767.

Morgello S, Soifer FM, Lin CS, et al. Central nervous system *Strongyloides stercoralis* in acquired immunodeficiency syndrome: a report of two cases and review of the literature. *Acta Neuropathol*. 1993;86:285-288.

Purvis RS, Beightler EL, Diven DG, et al. *Strongyloides stercoralis* hyperinfections. *Intl J Dermatol*. 1992;31:160-164.

Plate 65

Strongyloides stercoralis

Image 1

Small intestine of hyperinfected monkey. Developing eggs (darts) and larvae (arrows) are seen in the mucosa (H&E, 80x).

Image 2

Adult female worm in intestinal crypt (dart) (H&E, 45x).

Image 3

Section through the female worm shows eggs in utero (darts). Developing rhabditoid larvae are seen in the mucosa (arrow) (H&E, 200x).

Image 4

Transverse section through female worm shows its minute size. The intestine (IN) and two sections of the reproductive tube are visible (H&E, 750x).

Image 5

At low power, filariform larvae are seen deep in the intestinal wall (keyline) of the same monkey (H&E, 200x).

Image 6

At high magnification, transverse sections of filariform larvae are shown in a small blood vessel (H&E, 250x).

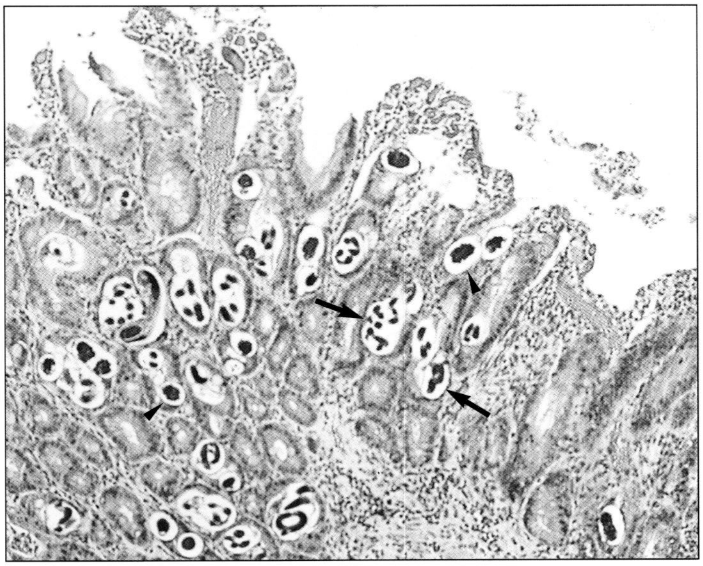

1

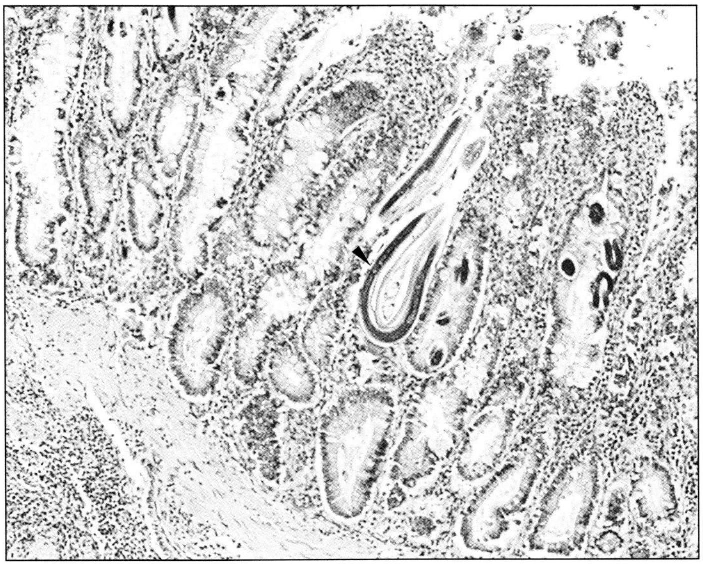

2

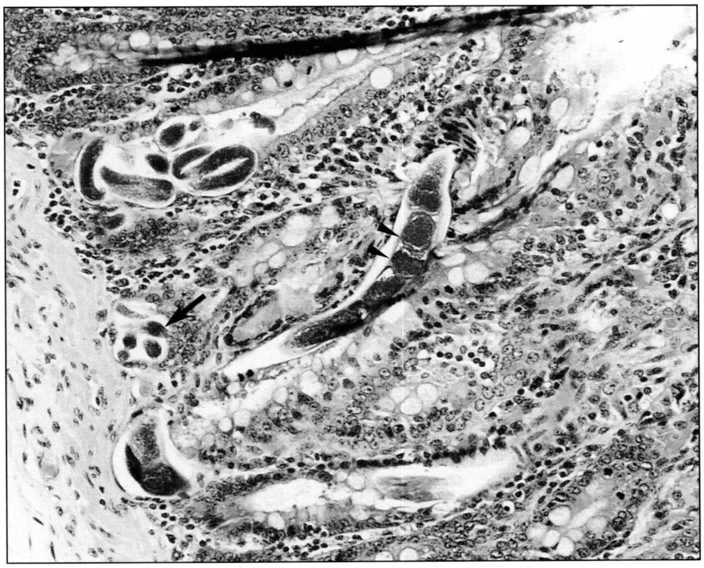

3

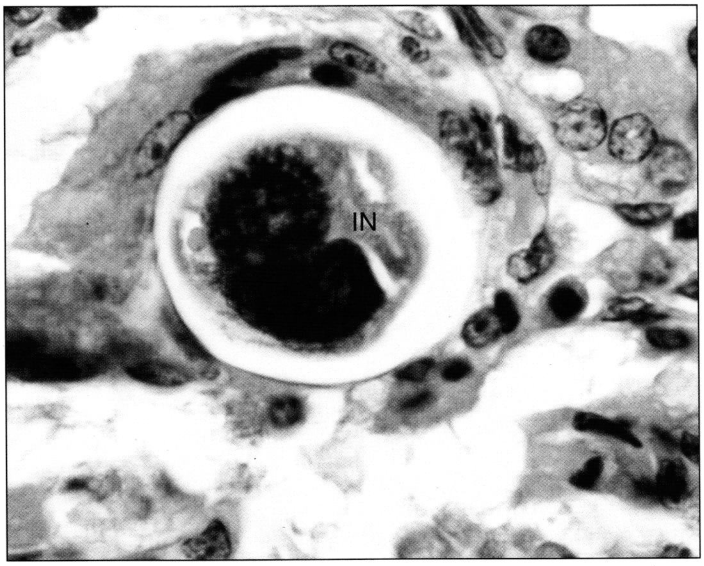

4

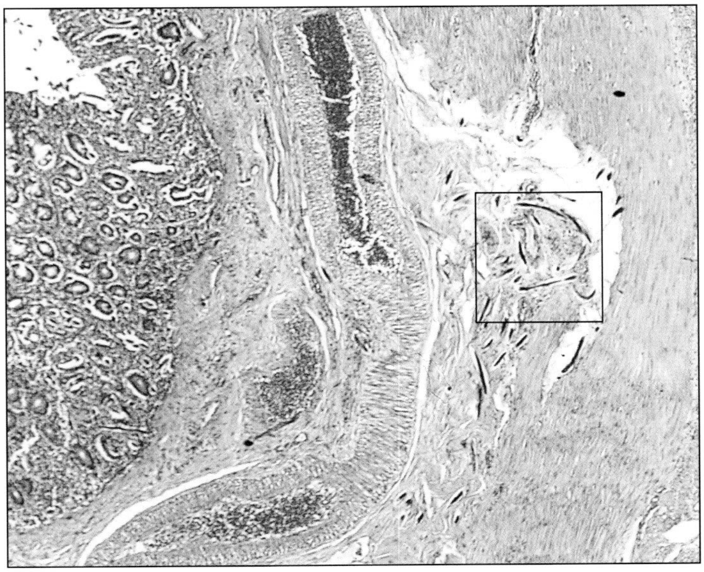

5

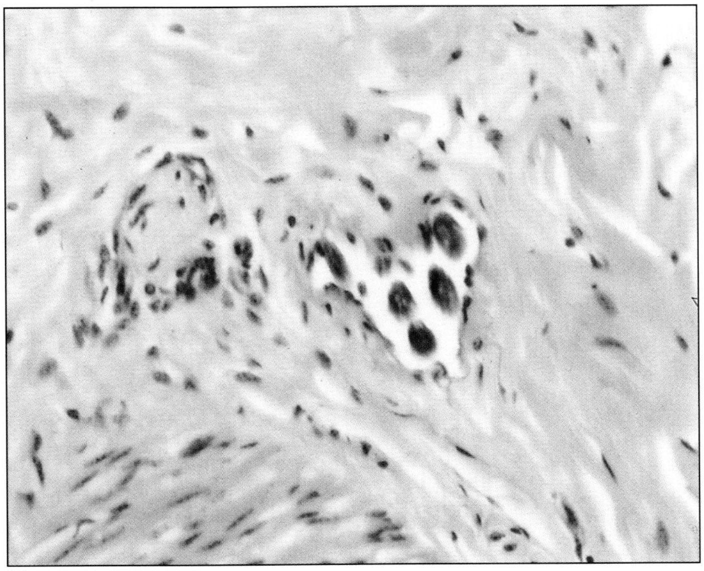

6

Plate 66

Strongyloides stercoralis

Image 1

Section of kidney from a monkey with disseminated infection shows larvae (darts) in the connective tissue capsule (H&E, 100x).

Image 2

At high magnification, transverse section through a filariform larva shows the double lateral alae (darts) (H&E, 800x).

Image 3

Several sections of filariform larvae in a blood vessel of the capsule of the kidney (H&E, 80x).

Image 4

A filariform larva in lung alveolus of a monkey with disseminated infection (H&E, 640x).

Image 5

Eggs containing rhabditoid larvae in a sputum sample from a 9-year-old child with disseminated strongyloidiasis (H&E, 200x). (Courtesy of M. D. Little.)

Image 6

Filariform larva in sputum from an infected individual (Giemsa, 530x).

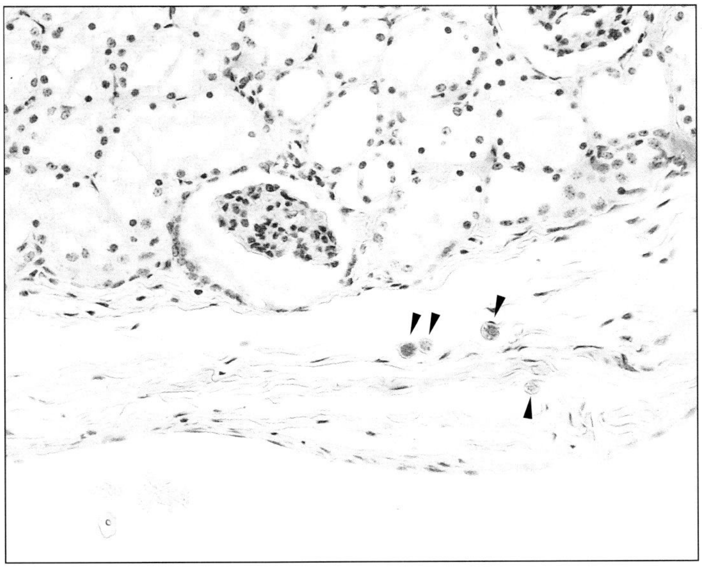

1

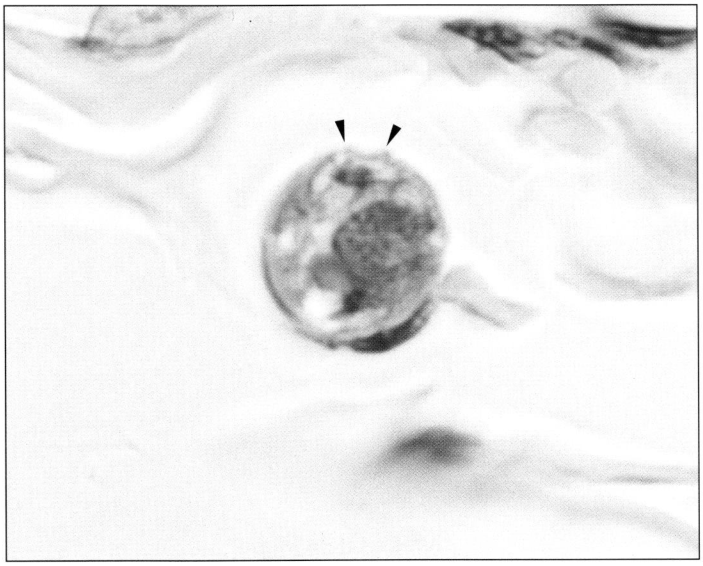

2

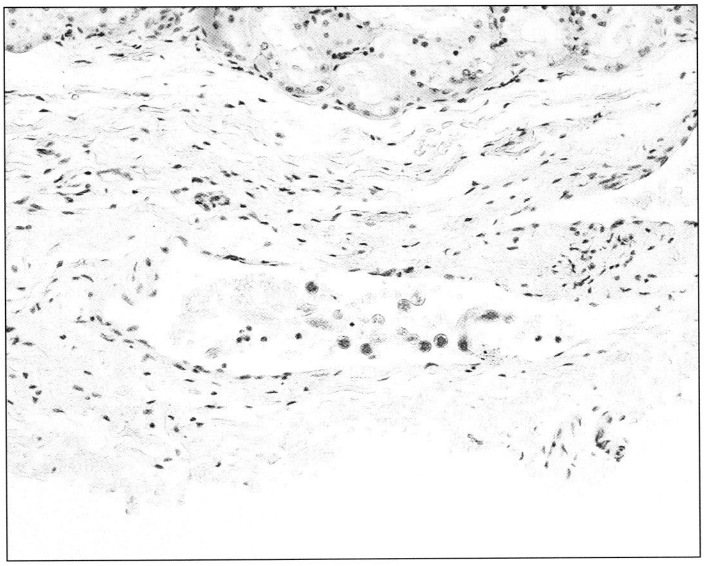

3

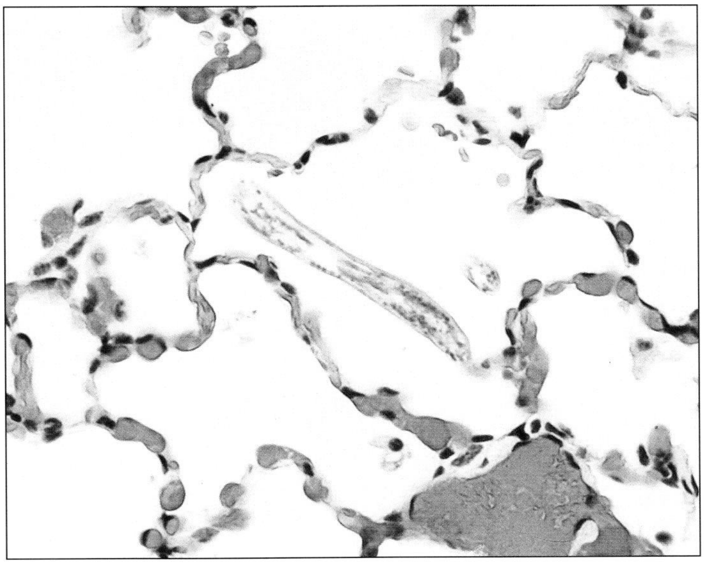

4

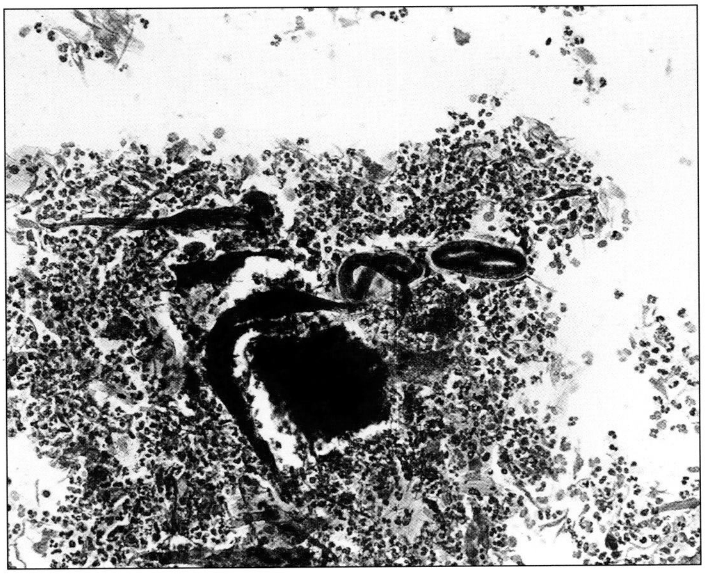

5

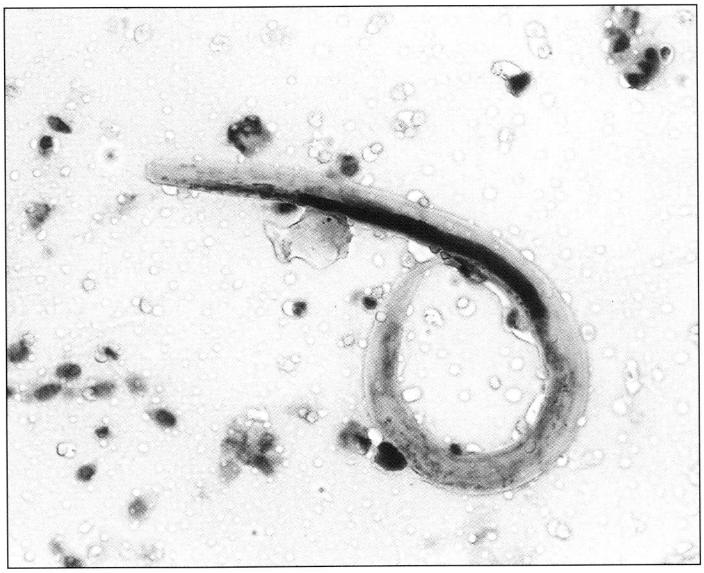

6

Halicephalobus and *Pelodera* species

Opportunistic Parasites

Some species of nematodes that are free living or saprophagous are able to infect animals and humans under certain conditions. *Halicephalobus* (= *Micronema*) *deletrix* is normally a saprophyte that lives in soil and decaying organic matter, but it is able to invade and multiply in mammalian tissues. The nematode appears to be able to enter the skin through existing lesions and disseminate to various organs and tissues, especially the central nervous system (Plate 67:1), where it multiplies rapidly. Such disseminated infections, usually with a fatal outcome, have been widely reported in horses in the United States, Europe, and the Middle East. At least three human cases, all fatal, have been described in the literature. In each case the organisms invaded the brain, causing meningoencephalitis. Diagnoses were made postmortem.

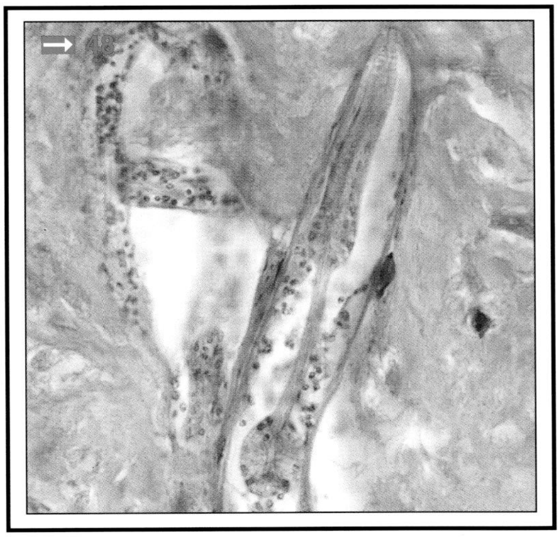

This rhabditoid nematode is minute in size. Only female worms have been found, and these measure from 250 to 465 μm in length with a maximum diameter of about 25 μm. Some investigators speculate that the female worm is parthenogenetic. A small buccal capsule is located at the anterior end, and the tail tapers to a point. The vulva is near the midbody. The body wall is thin, and it is not possible to separate the cuticle from hypodermis and muscle. The lateral chords can sometimes be seen (Plate 67:3A). The most characteristic feature of this worm is its rhabditoid esophagus, which is divided into a corpus, isthmus, and bulb (➡ 48). The intestine is tubular, typically with a compressed lumen (Plate 67:3). A single genital tube has a flexed ovary and usually no more than one fully developed egg in utero (Plate 67:5). Larvae in tissues are smaller than the female and have the same morphologic features except that they lack a reproductive system. The parasite is readily recognized in tissues by its preferred tissue habitat, the size of the adult worms, and especially their rhabditoid esophagus. No cuticular alae are present.

Pelodera strongyloides is another free-living nematode found in moist soil and decaying organic material. Under certain circumstances, it too may invade the skin of a variety of animals, including dogs, cattle, sheep, and rodents, producing possibly severe dermatitis. Both larvae and adults have been found in animal skin scrapings. The worms are small. Females reach a length of 1.5 mm and males reach a length of 1.2 mm. Larvae are about 600 μm in length and 36 μm in diameter. Both adults and larvae have a rhabditiform esophagus.

Two documented cases of dermatitis have been attributed to the larvae of *Pelodera strongyloides*. One involved a child in Poland, the other a 6-month-old infant in Alabama. In the infant's case, the skin bore hyperpigmented papulonodules scattered over the lower abdomen. Skin biopsy specimens showed focal hyperplasia of the epidermis and infiltration with polymorphonuclear leukocytes. The dermis showed extensive inflammation and granulomas with foreign body giant cells, epithelioid cells, and mononuclear cells (Plate 67:2 & 4). Lymphoid cells, plasma cells, and eosinophils were predominately dispersed through the dermis. Larvae seen in transverse sections measured about 25 μm in diameter (Plate 67:6). The body wall measured approximately 3 μm in thickness, and prominent, double lateral alae were present on each side of the body (Plate 67:6). In longitudinal sections, the rhabditiform esophagus and a long, tubular buccal capsule are visible. The long buccal capsule and the low double alae with widely separated crests are key morphologic features in differentiating between *P. strongyloides* and larvae of hookworms and *S. stercoralis*.

Reference

Dunn DG, Gardiner CH, Dralle KR, et al. Nodular granulomatous posthitis caused by *Halicephalobus* (syn. *Micronema*) sp. in a horse. *Vet Pathol.* 1993;30:207-208.

Gardiner CH, Koh DS, Cardella TA. *Micronema* in man: third fatal infection. *Am J Trop Med Hyg.* 1981;30:586-589.

Plate 67

Halicephalobus and *Pelodera* species

Image 1

Halicephalobus (= *Micronema*) *deletrix*. In this section of brain from a fatal human infection, longitudinal (arrow) and transverse (dart) sections of a female worm are visible (H&E, 75x).

Image 2

Pelodera strongyloides. Low-power view of a section of human skin shows epidermal hyperplasia and extensive granulomatous changes in the dermis. Some lesions contain larvae, which may not be evident at this magnification (keylines) (H&E, 80x).

Image 3

Halicephalobus deletrix. Transverse sections through a female worm.

A. Note the intestine (IN) and well-developed musculature of the body wall. Darts indicate lateral chords.

B. The intestine (IN) and the reproductive tube (RT) are evident (H&E, 500x).

Image 4

Pelodera strongyloides. Transverse section through larva (arrow) in granuloma (H&E, 400x).

Image 5

Halicephalobus deletrix. Longitudinal section through a female worm shows large developing egg. Typically only one mature egg is present in the uterus at any point in time (H&E, 400x).

Image 6

Pelodera strongyloides. Transverse section of larva at high magnification shows the double alae (darts) (H&E, 1500x).

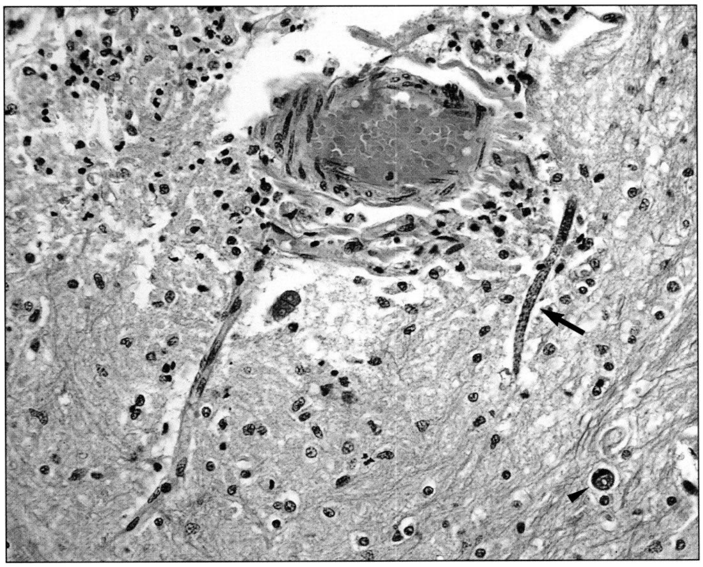

1

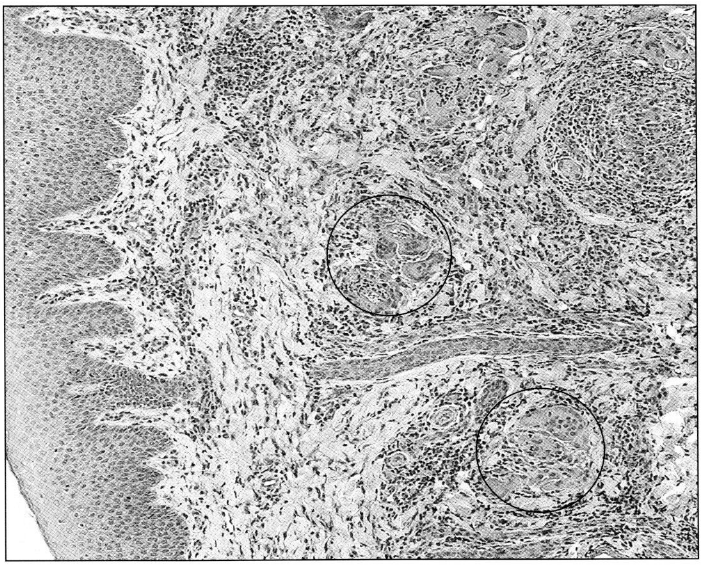

2

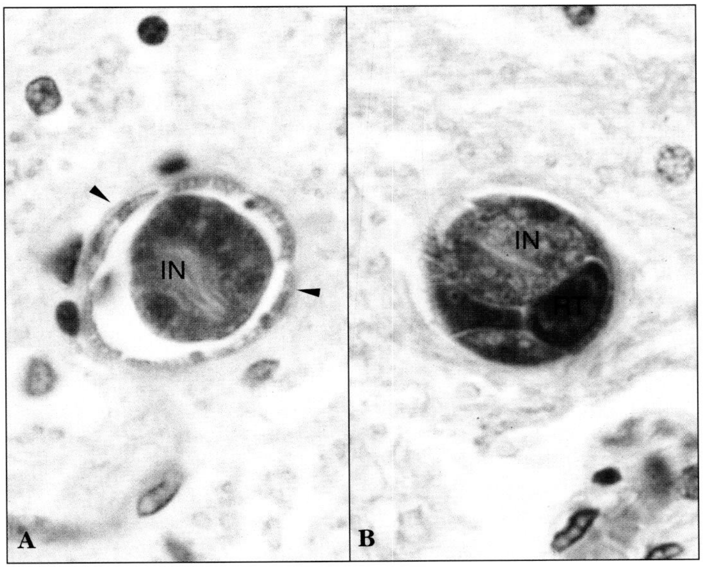

3

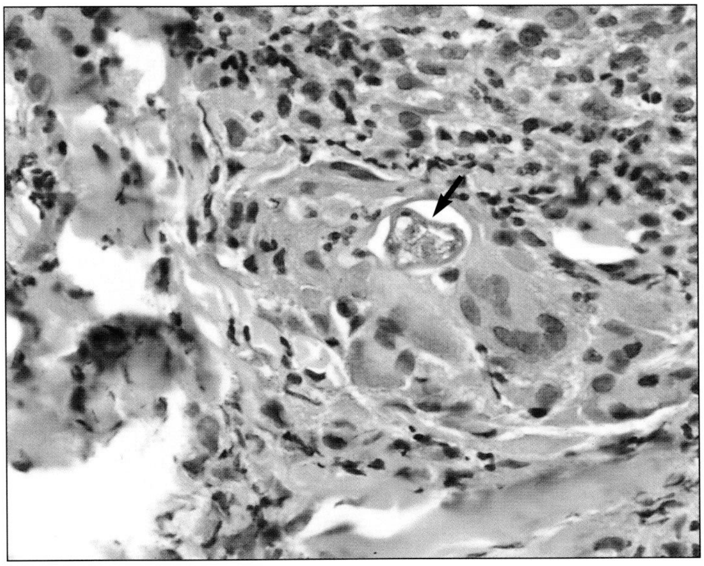

4

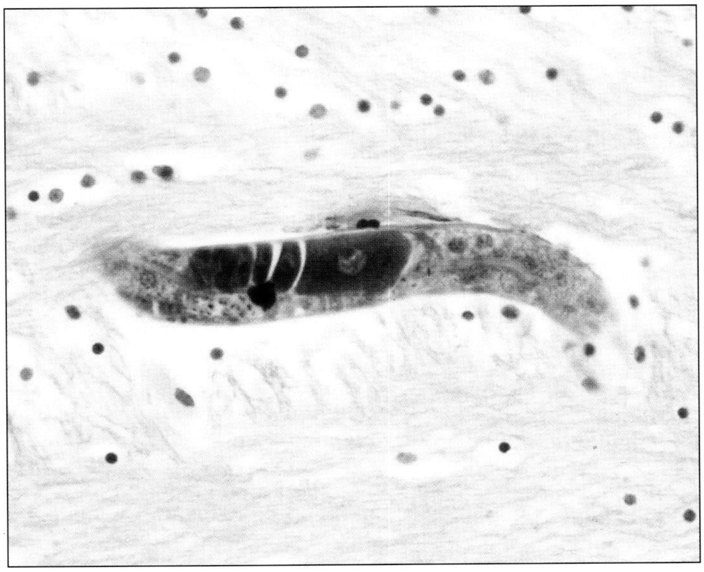

5

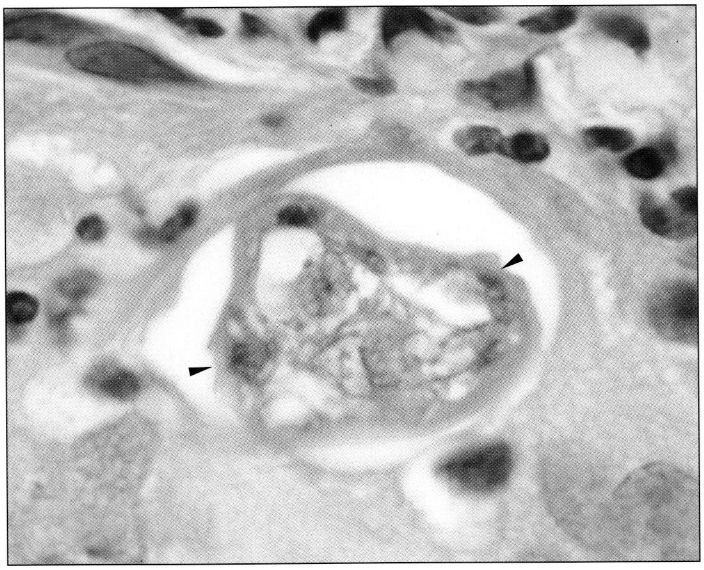

6

Trichuris trichiura

Trichuris trichiura, frequently referred to as whipworm, is a common helminth parasite of humans with worldwide geographic distribution. It is most prevalent in tropical and subtropical climates where sanitation is generally poor. Approximately one billion people worldwide are infected with this parasite. The infection is still seen in the United States, usually in rural areas of the Southeast. The adult parasites are found primarily in the colon, with the anterior end embedded in the mucosal epithelium and the remainder of the body lying free in the lumen. This parasite is not likely to be found in locations outside the intestine, but it may be encountered fortuitously when examining histopathologic sections of the colon.

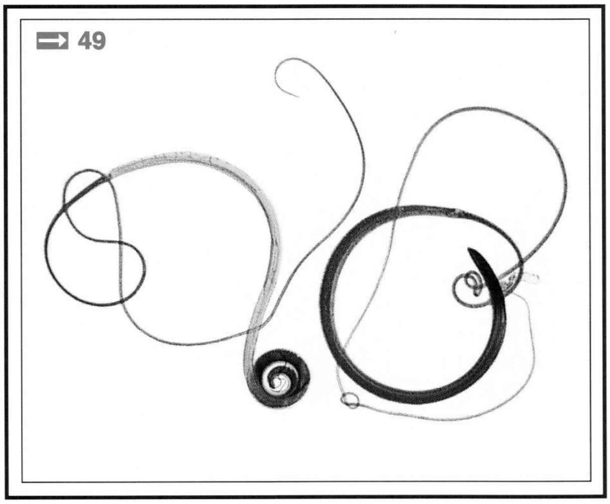

Biology and Life Cycle

Female worms produce and discharge as many as 10,000 eggs per day into the fecal stream. These eggs pass out of the body in an unembryonated condition and require at least three weeks of incubation in warm, moist soil to reach the infective stage. Transmission occurs when infective eggs from the soil are ingested by the human host, most commonly by eating fresh vegetables contaminated with infective eggs, or, in children, through pica. The eggs hatch in the small intestine, and the larvae invade the cells of the intestinal villi and undergo further development. Ultimately, they make their way to the colon and burrow into the mucosa, with much of the anterior end securely attached to the tissues. Infections become patent in about 90 days and may persist for several years.

Pathology and Clinical Manifestations

Infections with small numbers of worms are asymptomatic. However, severe infections may cause abdominal pain, diarrhea, and sometimes dysentery, weight loss, and tenesmus as well. Rectal prolapse may accompany chronic, severe infections in children. Often a moderate, peripheral eosinophilia occurs, and in dysenteric stools both eosinophils and Charcot-Leyden crystals may be present in large quantity.

Infections are diagnosed by finding typical eggs in the feces during the course of stool examination. Diagnosis does not depend on the demonstration of adult worms in the tissues.

Parasite Morphology

Trichuris has a unique body structure. Adult worms are large, with females reaching 50 mm in length and males about 45 mm. The worms are whiplike in appearance (49). The anterior three-fifths of the body is slender and firmly threaded into the mucosa. The remaining, thick portion of the body lies free in the lumen (Plate 68:1). The anterior portion of the body contains the unusual esophagus, which is a slender tube embedded in the stichosome (Plate 68:2 & 3). At this level, the worm has a diameter of 100 to 150 µm, and the body wall has a characteristic appearance. The cuticle and hypodermis are modified to form a single bacillary band (Plate 68:3). In both sexes the cuticle is thick and the hypodermis is thin, but hypodermal nuclei can be seen in the submuscular areas. The muscle layer is strong. Individual muscle cells are coelomyarian, and the cytoplasmic portion of the cell is as tall or taller than the contractile portion (Plate 68:3, 4, & 6). The remainder of the body, the thick portion lying in the lumen, measures up to 700 µm in diameter and contains the reproductive organs and the intestine.

In both sexes the reproductive system is a single tube that is flexed or looped. In the female, the vulva is positioned near the junction of the thick and thin portions of the body. In a transverse section of female worm through the posterior two-fifths of the body, the large saccular uterus is filled with eggs, and an ovary or oviduct can be seen (Plate 68:4). In the male worm, the thick posterior end of the body usually contains sections through the testis and vas deferens, or, more posteriorly, through testis and ejaculatory duct or cloaca (Plate 68:5). Because the male has a single, long, sheathed spicule, sections through the extreme posterior end usually display the cloaca and spicule (Plate 68:6). Finally, the intestine in both sexes is a single tubular structure with a lining of columnar cells of different heights, which gives the lumen an irregular shape. The intestinal cells have a microvillus, luminal border (Plate 68:4 & 5).

Trichuris is easily recognized in sections of intestine by its tissue habitat (cecum), its stichosome and bacillary bands in the anterior levels, and the structure of the body wall and the reproductive organs in the posterior levels.

Reference

Bundy DAP, Cooper ES. *Trichuris* and trichuriasis in humans. *Adv Parasitol.* 1989;28:107-173.

Plate 68

Trichuris trichiura

Image 1

Anterior end of adult worm embedded in the mucosa of the colon. Each transverse section of worm in the mucosa contains a stichocyte. A transverse section through the posterior end of the body of this female worm, which is lying in the lumen (arrow), illustrates the varying diameters of the worm at the different levels (H&E, 100x).

Image 2

Longitudinal section through the anterior end of the worm illustrates its relationship to the mucosa as well as the structural organization of the stichosome, ie, the individual stichocytes (H&E, 180x).

Image 3

At higher magnification, the anterior end of the worm shows the stichocyte, the esophageal tube (dart), the broad bacillary band (BB), and the remaining elements of the body wall (H&E, 360).

Image 4

Transverse section through the thick, posterior portion of a female worm. Especially evident are the thick cuticle (C), coelomyarian muscles (MU), the ovary (OV), the uterus, which contains developing eggs (UT), oviduct (dart), and the intestine (IN) (H&E, 200x).

Image 5

Transverse section through a male worm illustrates the male reproductive structures, the testis (TE) and the ejaculatory duct (EJ) (H&E, 200x).

Image 6

Transverse section through the posterior extremity of a male worm shows the thick-walled cloaca (CL), the spicule (dart), and a portion of the spicule that extends outside the body (arrow) (H&E, 165x).

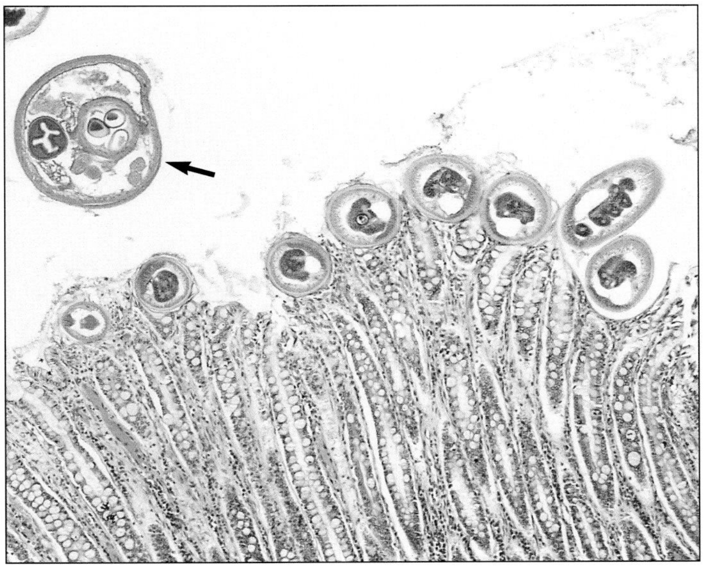

1

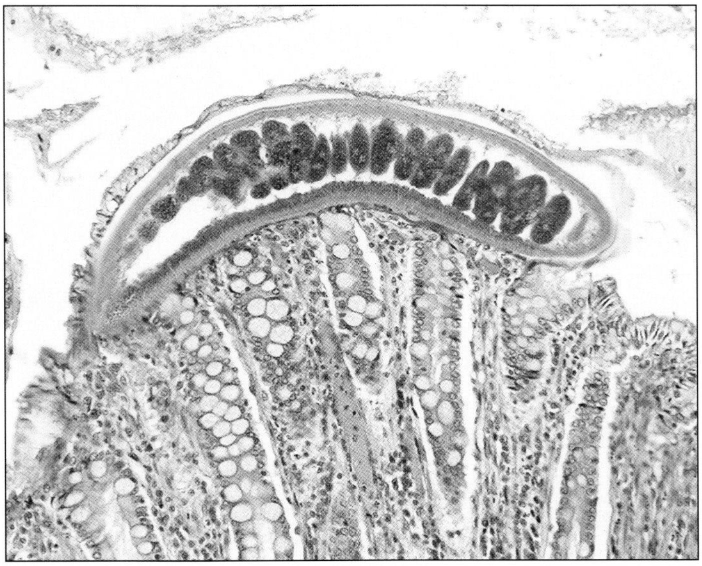

2

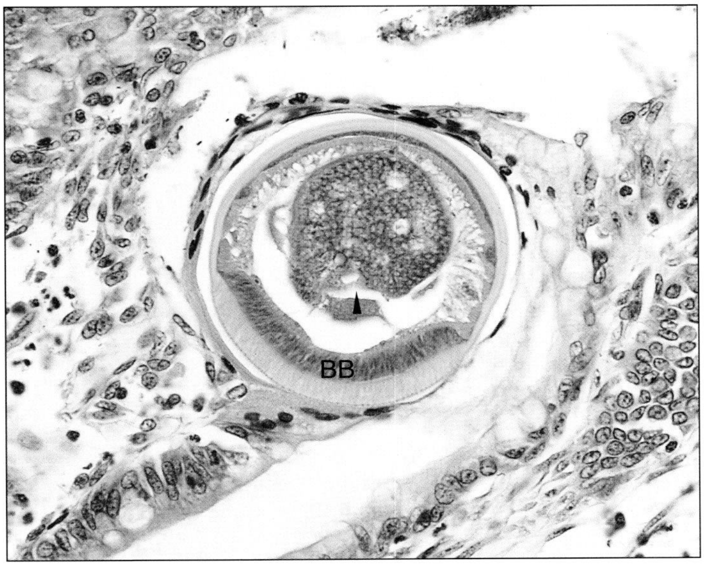

3

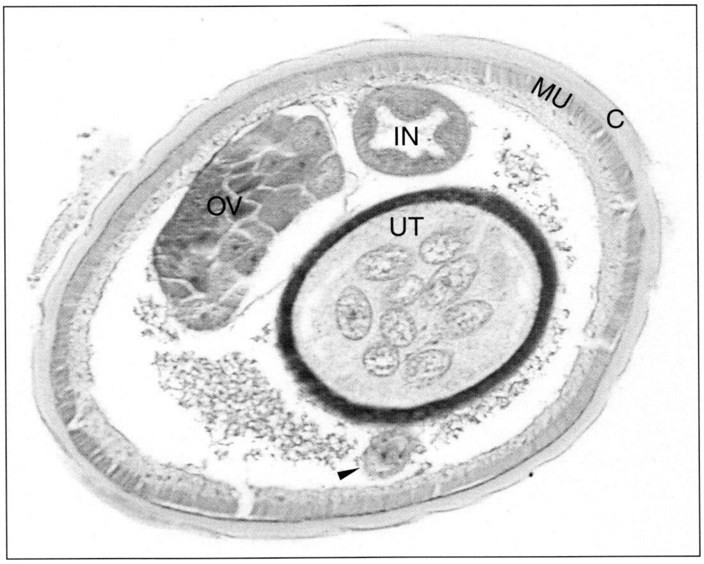

4

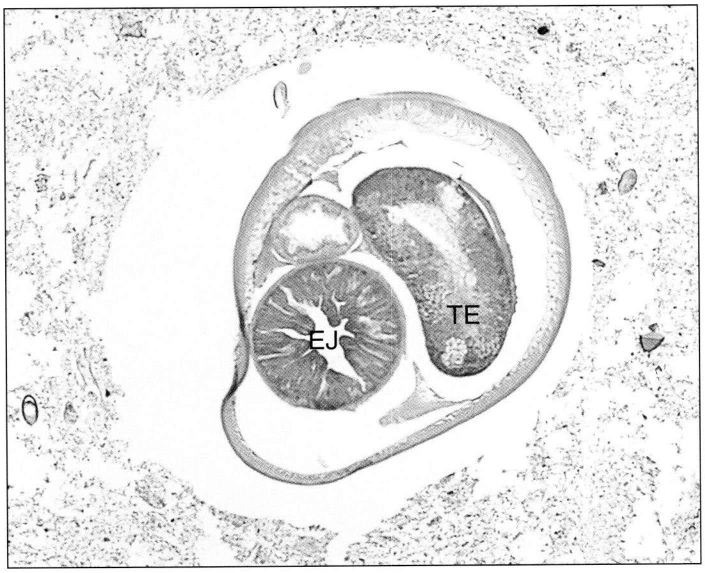

5

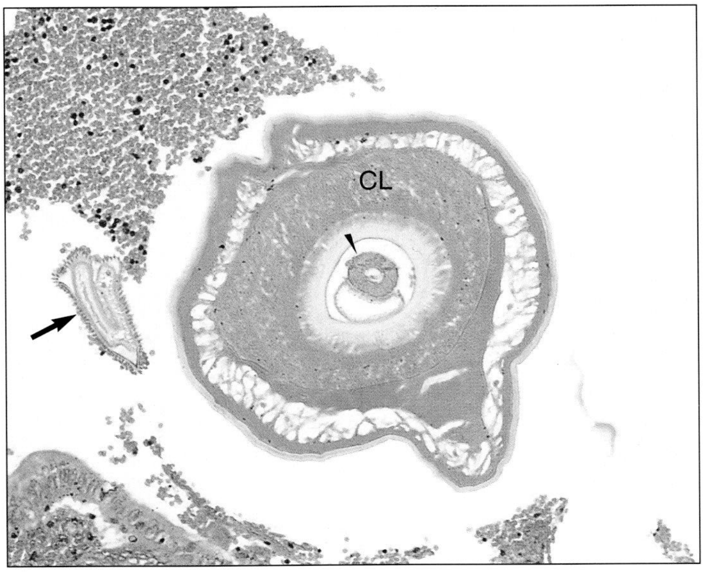

6

Trichinella spiralis

Trichinella spiralis, a close relative of *Trichuris* and *Capillaria* species, is a natural parasite of swine, rats, and a variety of wild animals. Humans are accidental hosts for the parasite. *Trichinella spiralis* has worldwide distribution but is most prevalent in humans in parts of Europe and North America (including Canada, Greenland, and the Arctic region), as well as East Africa, Asia, and parts of South America. Trichinosis is acquired by eating raw or insufficiently cooked meat products containing the encysted infective larva. Pork is the major source of infection in the United States, but game animals are also an acknowledged source. In Europe, horse meat has been identified as a source of outbreaks of human infections. Trichinosis was an important public health problem at the turn of the century. However, governmental regulations governing the feeding of garbage to pigs, the proper processing and treatment of commercial pork products, and the education of the public about the proper cooking of pork have drastically reduced its prevalence, especially in the United States. In recent years, an average of fewer than 60 cases of trichinosis have been reported per year in the United States; however, two large outbreaks in 1990, when 106 cases were reported, highlight the need for continued surveillance and control measures.

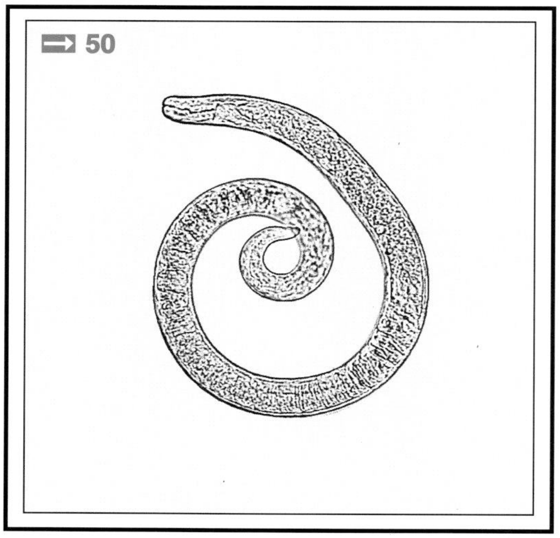

Biology and Life Cycle

The adult worms and the infective stages occur in the same host, but a two-host cycle is essential for transmission of the parasite. The tiny adult worms live in the intestinal mucosa (Plate 69:1). Females discharge minute larvae (100 by 6 µm) into the mucosal epithelium. From there, the larvae enter the bloodstream and are carried to the skeletal muscles and other internal organs, including the heart, lungs, and brain (Plate 69:2). The larvae mature only in striated muscles and reach infectivity in three to four weeks. They become encapsulated by host tissues and remain in this state alive and infective for many months and even years (Plate 69:3 & 4). Unless they are ingested by another carnivorous animal, the larvae eventually die and calcify in the tissues. Upon entering the new host, the infective larvae (➡ 50) escape from the capsule and immediately burrow into the intestinal epithelium, where they rapidly mature to the adult stage. Females begin to discharge larvae by the sixth day, with peak production occurring during the second week of infection and continuing for as long as 16 weeks. The adult worms live for a relatively short time and are expelled from the body after a few to several weeks or months.

Trichinella spiralis is not a uniform species. Strains of the parasite from Western Europe and the United States have biologic and behavioral characteristics different from those isolated in east and southern Africa and the Arctic regions. Genetic, biochemical, and epidemiologic studies have led many scientists to conclude that different species of *Trichinella* exist. These have been named *T. spiralis*, *T. nelsoni*, and *T. nativa*; they are from the temperate, tropical, and Arctic regions respectively. Recently, another species, *T. pseudospiralis*, was confirmed and reported for the first time in a woman living in New Zealand who may have acquired the infection in Tasmania.

Pathology and Clinical Manifestations

Mild infections may be asymptomatic. On the other hand, ingesting large numbers of larvae may produce abdominal pain and diarrhea. These first signs of infection begin within 48 hours and may continue for several days. The symptoms mimic food poisoning or influenza, and they mark the period during which the larvae invade the intestinal epithelium and subsequently mature to adults. Beginning in the second week, fever, myalgia, periorbital edema, and peripheral eosinophilia develop in response to larval invasion of the muscles and encystment. These symptoms usually persist for as long as larvae are being produced and invading the muscles—typically one month or longer. After the trauma and toxicity of the invasive phase, in about the fifth week of infection, the individual begins a period of convalescence during which myalgia, weakness, and residual periorbital edema may continue. Prognosis is usually good in mild infections but may be poor to grave in severe ones. The mortality rate is typically low, approximately 1% in the United States.

Adult worms in the crypts of the mucosal epithelium of the duodenum and jejunum cause chronic, interstitial inflammation with infiltrates of lymphocytes, polymorphonuclear cells, and eosinophilia. Larvae begin to invade skeletal muscles of the body by about the eighth day. Muscles most frequently involved include the diaphragm, tongue, larynx, masseters, intercostals, biceps, pectorals, deltoid, and gastrocnemius, among others. Larvae penetrate the individual cell, which undergoes degeneration and redifferentiation during the encystment process. A hyaline membrane forms around the larva, along with an infiltration of inflammatory cells, which are mostly eosinophils. The larva is fully developed and encapsulated by the fifth week. Myositis subsides and inflammatory cells disappear. The cyst is typically elongated or spindle shaped (Plate 69:3). Larvae that lodge in organs or tissues other than skeletal muscles provoke an acute inflammatory response. Larvae migrate through cardiac muscles, causing an acute inflammatory response and myocarditis, but they do not encyst. Typically, only a single larva occupies a cyst but more have been reported.

Parasite Morphology

Trichinella is closely related to *Trichuris* and *Capillaria* species. This is most apparent morphologically in the structure of the esophagus. As in *Trichuris* and *Capillaria*, *Trichinella* has a stichosome that can be seen in both the adult and the infective larva (Plate 69:1 & 5; ➡ 50). This structure makes identification of the parasite easy. Adults are small. Females measure up to 4.0 mm in length with a diameter of 150 µm, whereas males measure only 1.4 to 1.6 mm by 40 to 60 µm. Adult worms are rarely found in feces and are seen almost exclusively but fortuitously in situ in the small intestine. Females are readily identified by the stichosome and the presence of larvae in utero (Plate 69:1), whereas males are identified primarily by their size, the stichosome, and associated females.

The early larvae discharged by the female are minute, rarely more than 100 µm in length by 6 µm in diameter. They are undifferentiated in structure and somewhat resemble microfilariae (Plate 69:2). The infective larva measures up to 1 mm in length (➡ 50). Its tissue habitat, the capsule that surrounds it, and the stichosome facilitate identification (Plate 69:5 & 6). Clinical symptoms also aid in diagnosis. *Trichinella* is unlikely to be confused with any other trichuroid or capillarid, because its tissue habitat, stage of development, and related clinical presentation are distinctive. A species designation other than *T. spiralis* is unnecessary and impossible except on biologic and clinical grounds.

References

Abernethy D. *Trichinella pseudospiralis* in man. *Lancet*. 1993;342:298-299. Letter to the editor.

Bailey TM, Schantz PM. Trends in the incidence and transmission patterns of trichinosis in humans in the United States: comparisons of the periods 1975–1981 and 1982–1986. *Rev Infect Dis*. 1990;12:5-11.

Plate 69

Trichinella spiralis

Image 1

Sections through an adult female *T. spiralis* in the intestinal mucosa of a rat. Note especially the stichosome (arrow) and the larvae within the uterus (keyline) (H&E, 200x).

Image 2

A young larva (dart) found in the brain of an individual with severe infection, who died 20 days after the onset of symptoms of trichinosis (H&E, 400x).

Image 3

A press preparation of a small piece of fresh muscle from a rat shows the typical encapsulated larvae of *T. spiralis* (H&E, 60x).

Image 4

Sections of encapsulated larvae from the tongue of a rat (H&E, 125x).

Image 5

Section of encapsulated larva from the tongue of a rat illustrates the stichosome (H&E, 400x).

Image 6

At high magnification, the anatomic features of the larva in transverse sections are illustrated. Note the structure of the body wall and the presence of stichocytes (dart). In one section, both the intestine and reproductive tube can be seen (H&E, 400x).

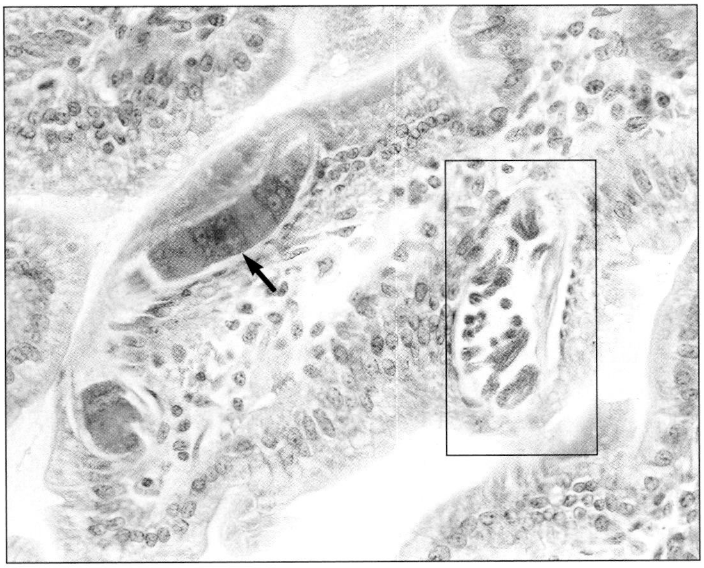

1

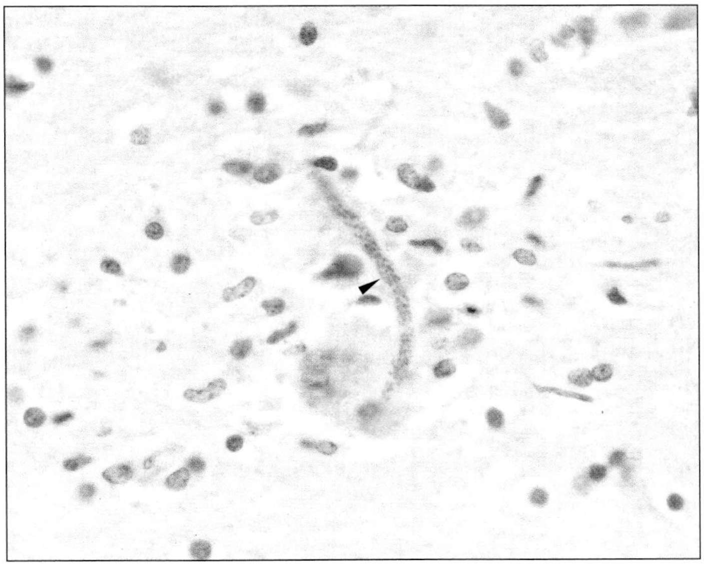

2

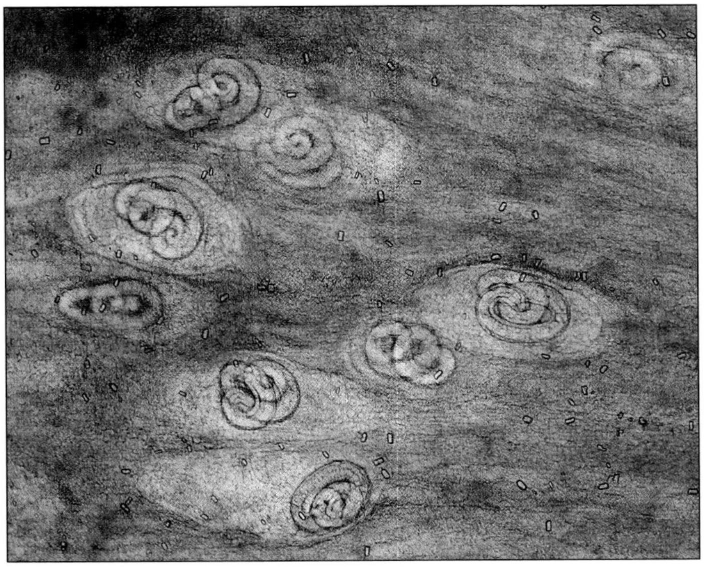

3

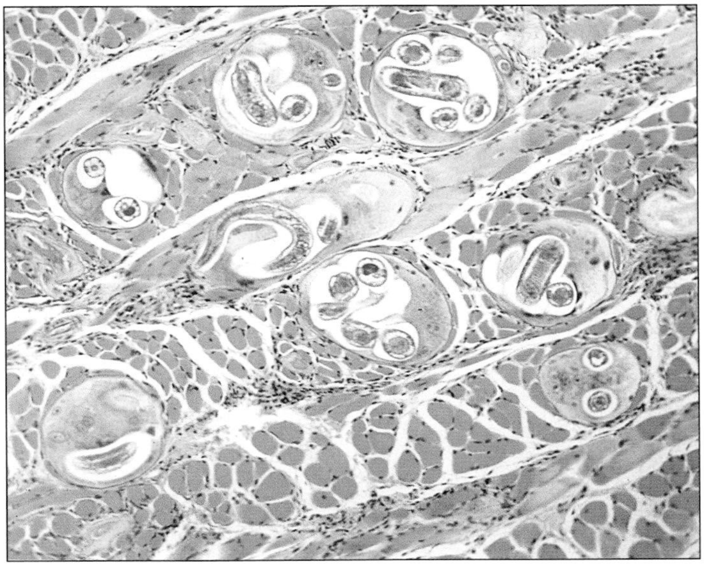

4

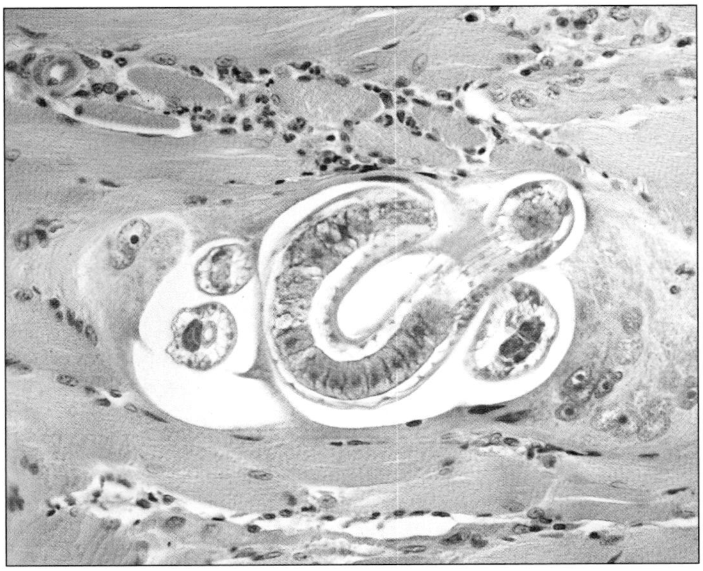

5

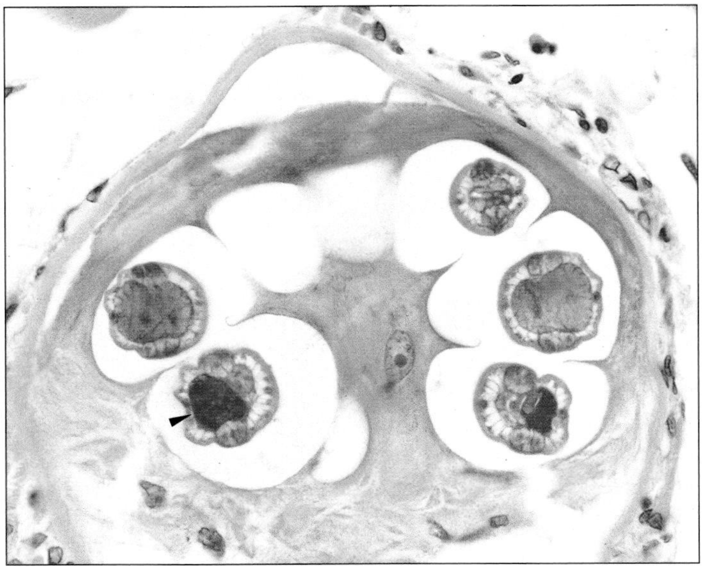

6

Capillaria (= Aonchotheca) philippinensis

Capillaria species

The capillarids, which are close relatives of *Trichuris*, parasitize a wide range of animals, including fish, amphibians, reptiles, and mammals. Only three of the nearly 300 species have a significant impact on human health. The taxonomy of this large group has often been revised, with many changes in generic groups and the assignment of species. We use the old taxons by which the parasites are known best but indicate the most recent changes where applicable.

Capillaria (= *Aonchotheca*) *philippinensis* is an intestinal parasite that was first seen in humans in the early 1960s in the Philippines. It has now extended its known geographic range considerably. *Capillaria* (= *Calodium*) *hepatica* is a liver parasite of rats and other wild animals. Human infections with this parasite occur infrequently, usually in children of dirt-eating age, and manifest clinically as a visceral larva migrans syndrome. Another zoonotic species, *C.* (= *Eucoleus*) *aerophila*, is a natural parasite of dogs, cats, foxes, and other carnivorous animals. It occasionally infects humans and produces pulmonary disease.

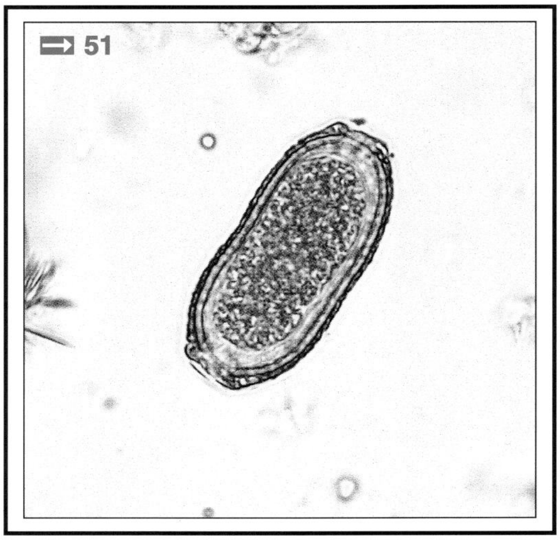

Capillaria philippinensis

Intestinal capillariasis was first reported in humans in the Philippines in 1962 and soon reached epidemic proportions. Between 1967 and 1990, almost 2000 people became infected and at least 110 died. Since its initial discovery, the disease has become widespread in Thailand and cases have been reported in Japan, Taiwan, Iran, and Egypt.

Biology and Life Cycle

The life cycle of the parasite in the natural environment has been difficult to document. Fish-eating birds are apparently the natural definitive hosts of the parasite, with small fishes serving as intermediate hosts and harboring the infective stage. Under experimental conditions, infective larvae rapidly develop into mature adults. Egg production typically begins in six to seven weeks but may start as early as three weeks. Experimental studies also reveal that internal autoinfection occurs, resulting in high worm burdens. Humans become infected when they eat raw fish harboring the infective stages. The adult worms are found in the small intestine, primarily the jejunum. The eggs produced by the female are passed in feces and bear a superficial resemblance to the *Trichuris* egg. They are peanut shaped, have flattened bipolar plugs and a striated shell, measure 36 to 45 µm by 20 µm, and may be embryonated or unembryonated, depending on the status of the infection (➡ 51).

Pathology and Clinical Manifestations

Capillaria philippinensis reportedly always causes illness and leads to death if left untreated. Symptoms include borborygmus, abdominal pain, and intermittent diarrhea that may persist for several weeks and is usually accompanied by weight loss. During this period, patients usually pass eggs, larvae, and even adult worms in feces. Early treatment is essential because of the potential for autoinfection and the buildup of massive numbers of adult worms. At autopsy, the intestine is congested and distended with fluid. Most disease typically occurs in the jejunum. Worms in all stages of development may be seen in the crypts of the mucosa (Plate 70:1). Villi are flattened and atrophic. On at least one occasion, an estimated 200,000 worms were recovered from 1 L of bowel fluid.

Parasite Morphology

The adult worms may be seen in large numbers in the jejunum and less frequently in the ileum and duodenum. They are small, delicate worms. Females measure up to 5.3 mm and have a maximum diameter of about 47 µm. Male worms are smaller, with lengths of up to 4.0 mm and diameters of up to 28 µm. The worm's small size, its tissue habitat, and the presence of a conspicuous stichosome are key diagnostic features (Plate 70:1 & 2). In transverse sections, the body wall is thin. A thin, smooth cuticle, discernible bacillary bands, and coelomyarian muscles are visible (Plate 70:3). In the female, the single uterine tube contains unembryonated eggs, embryonated eggs, or larvae. In the male worm, the single genital tube contains developing spermatozoa. The male also has a single spicule that occasionally will be evident in transverse sections through the extreme posterior end of the body. The typical *C. philippinensis* egg, with its peanut shape and flattened polar plugs, may be seen in utero as well as in host tissues (Plate 70:4).

Reference

Cross JH. Intestinal capillariasis. *Clin Microbiol Rev*. 1992;5:120-129.

Lee SH, Hong ST, Chai JY, et al. A case of intestinal capillariasis in the Republic of Korea. *Am J Trop Med Hyg*. 1993;48:542-546.

Capillaria (= Eucoleus) aerophila

This small, delicate nematode lives in the mucosal epithelium of the trachea, bronchi, and bronchioles of cats, dogs, foxes, and other carnivorous animals. Its geographic distribution is wide, including North and South America, Europe, Asia, Australia, and possibly other areas. We know of only 10 infections reported in humans, with the majority from the former Soviet Union, one from Morocco, and one from Iran.

Biology and Life Cycle

Female worms in the mucosal epithelium discharge eggs into burrows created by the worms. These are sloughed into the respiratory passages, coughed up, swallowed, and ultimately discharged in feces. Under favorable environmental conditions, the eggs become infective in the soil in about six weeks. Infective eggs are believed to be ingested by young children in the contaminated soil. Paratenic or transport hosts may be involved in transmission as well. Larvae hatched from the egg in the intestine make their way via the bloodstream to the lungs and develop to mature adults in five to six weeks. The egg is similar in appearance to eggs of *Trichuris* and *Capillaria* species. It measures 58 to 79 µm by 29 to 40 µm and has bipolar plugs. The shell is green-brown and its surface is pitted.

Pathology and Clinical Manifestations

Infection usually produces severe lower respiratory tract infection with acute bronchitis, asthmalike symptoms, and a productive cough. However, patients do not respond to anti-asthma medication. X-rays may show expanding hilar shadows with a reticulogranular pattern in the lung fields. Typical eggs may be found in the sputum or feces.

Parasite Morphology

Little histopathologic material from human cases is available for study. Our information has been supplemented with material from a natural host. Adult worms are small and have a uniform diameter through most of the length of the body. Female worms measure up to 4.0 cm in length and up to 180 µm in diameter. The anus is subterminal, and the tail has a truncate shape. The vulva is positioned near the esophago-intestinal junction in the ventral midline. The male is smaller than the female, measuring 1.5 to 2.5 cm in length with a maximum diameter of 60 to 100 µm. The cloaca is subterminal, and a single spicule is present. In both sexes the esophagus is long, with a well-developed stichosome. It may equal as much as one-third of the body length. The body wall has typical capillarid features. The cuticle is thin. Muscles are coelomyarian and are divided by three bacillary bands (Plate 70:6). The small size of the worm, its tissue habitat, and the key morphologic features of the stichosome and bacillary bands aid in identification. Fortuitous sections may also reveal the presence of the typical capillarid egg.

Reference

Aftandelians R, Raafat F, Taffozoli M, Beaver PC. Pulmonary capillariasis in a child in Iran. *Am J Trop Med Hyg*. 1977;26:64-71.

Plate 70

Capillaria philippinensis and *Capillaria aerophila*

Image 1

An adult *C. philippinensis* (dart) lying in a mucosal crypt in the jejunum of a patient from the Philippines (H&E, 30x).

Image 2

Longitudinal section through the anterior end of the same parasite shows the long stichosome (H&E, 230x).

Image 3

Transverse section of female *C. philippinensis* at high magnification shows a stichocyte (dart) in one section and the uterus, which contains developing eggs and larvae, in the others (H&E, 600x).

Image 4

A thin-shelled egg (dart) demonstrates the typical morphologic features of the *C. philippinensis* egg, including a plug (arrow) (H&E, 800x).

Image 5

A biopsy specimen of bronchiolar epithelium shows two portions of a minute worm identified as *C. aerophila* in an Iranian (H&E, 400x).

Image 6

High-magnification view of a transverse section of the worm in Image 5 shows a stichocyte (ST). Although not very clear, three bacillary bands (darts) are present. These characteristics, along with the location of the worm in the bronchiolar epithelium, lead to the identification of *C. aerophila* (H&E, 400x).

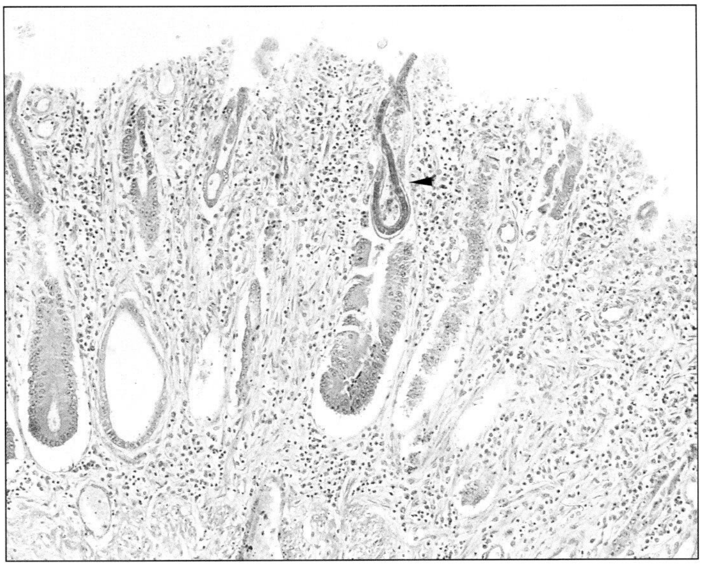

1

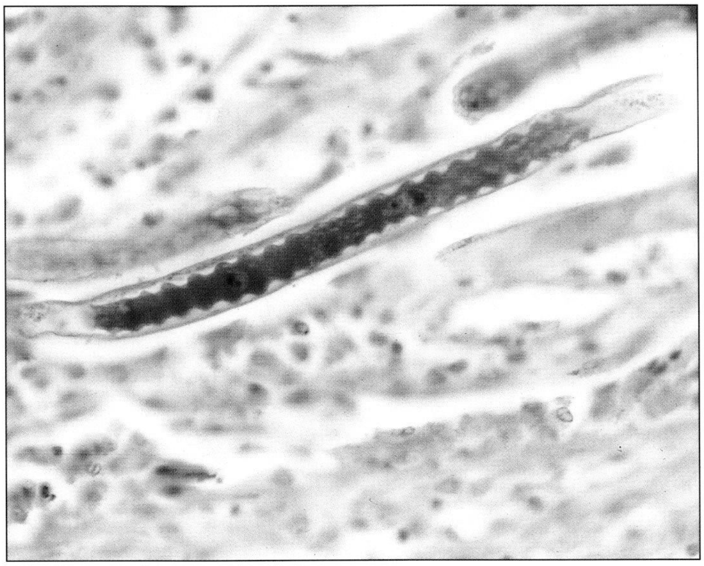

2

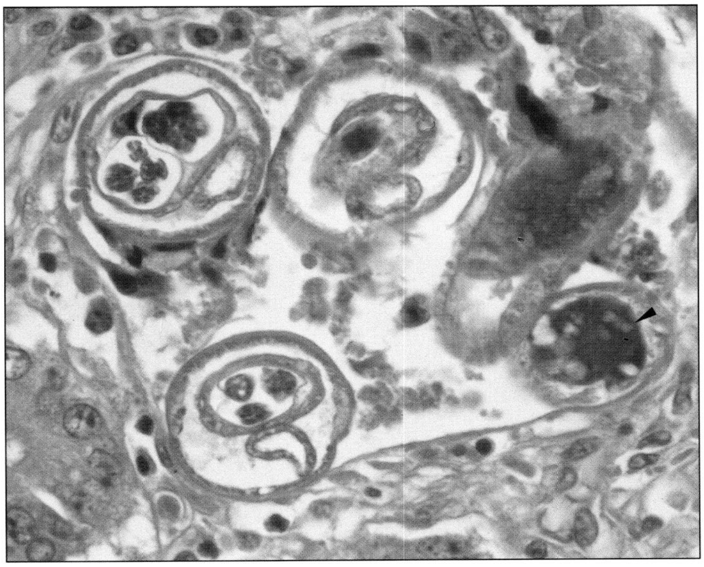

3

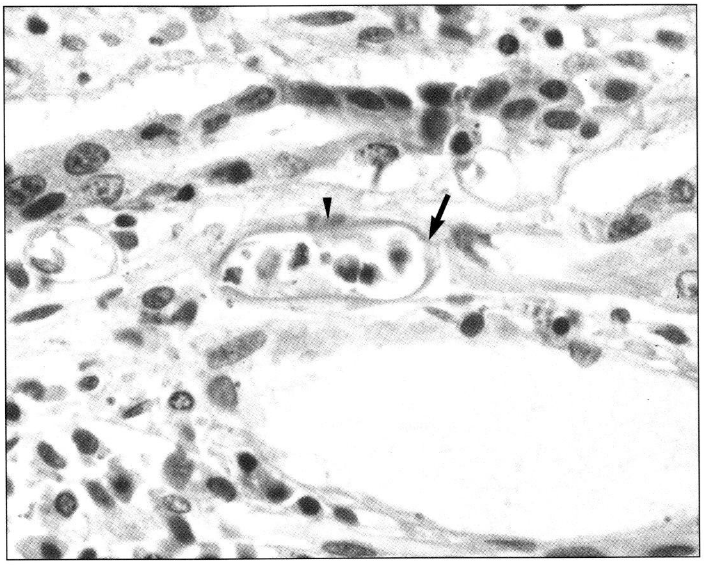

4

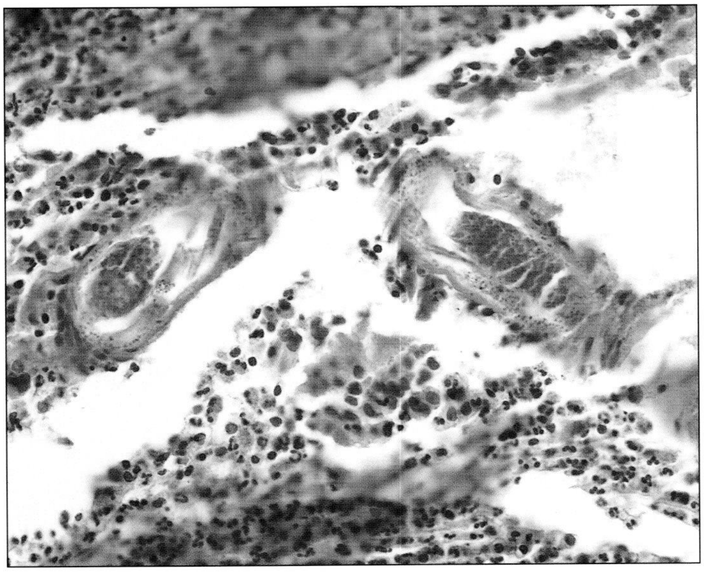

5

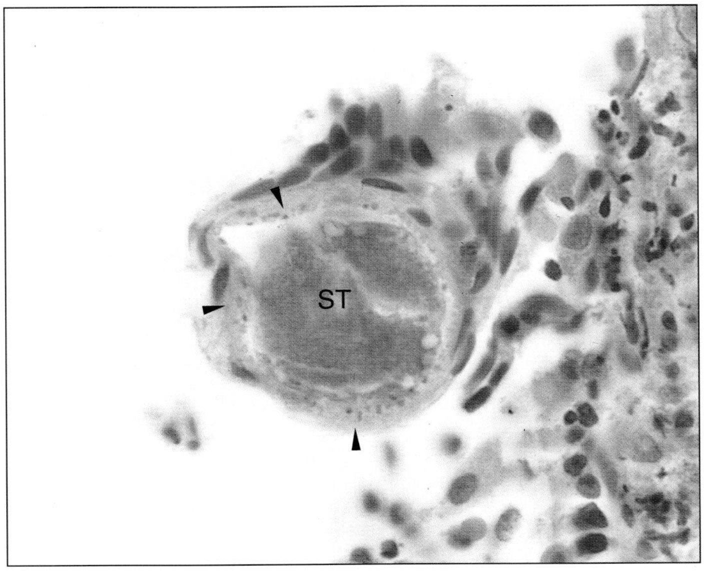

6

Capillaria (= Calodium) hepatica

This minute and fragile capillarid parasitizes the livers of a wide range of domestic and wild animals, especially rats. Infections in humans, which are acquired by accident, are rare. About 25 well-documented cases have been reported from all over the world. Most infections are found in children of dirt-eating age who present with a clinical picture of visceral larva migrans.

Biology and Life Cycle

The adult worms reside in the parenchyma of the liver, burrowing through the tissues, with the female depositing eggs in her wake (➡ 52). When an infected animal is eaten by a predator, unembryonated eggs are liberated from the liver and pass out of the predator in feces. An infected animal may simply die and decompose in the environment, which also liberates eggs. The eggs develop in the soil to the infective (larval) stage over a period of a few weeks. When infective eggs are ingested by another host, including a human host, they hatch in the intestine and larvae migrate via the bloodstream to the periportal tissues of the liver. Here they mature in about 3 to 4 weeks, completing the life cycle. The infection remains in an occult state. The adults die, and the only vestiges of infection are the eggs encased in fibrous tissues in the parenchyma of the liver. The eggs have a characteristic appearance, resembling *Trichuris* eggs with their bipolar plugs. The egg measures about 50 to 70 µm by 30 to 35 µm. Unlike *Trichuris* eggs, however, *Capillaria* eggs have a thick shell with a striated or pitted surface.

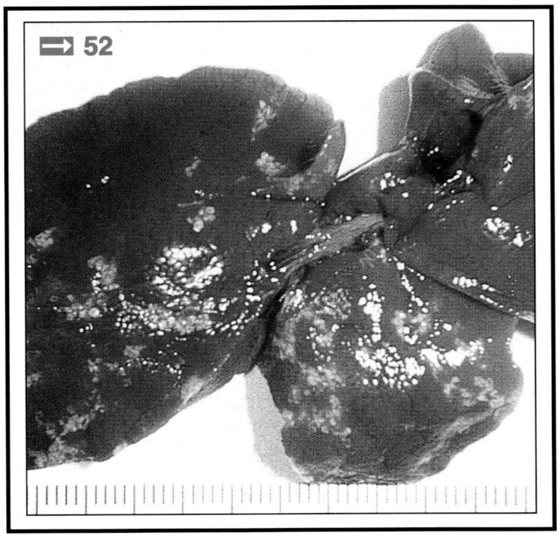

Pathology and Clinical Manifestations

Mild infections involving only a few worms probably go undetected. In severe infections, patients present with fever, hepatomegaly, and hypereosinophilia. The clinical picture is similar to that of visceral larva migrans. Diagnosis is confirmed by liver biopsy. Adult worms die within a few weeks of invading the liver. An infiltration and proliferation of fibrous connective tissue bind the worms and the eggs in diffuse nodules. The lesions are eventually and gradually replaced by scar tissue. Typically, only the eggs remain identifiable. However, the presence of eggs in human feces results from the ingestion of parasitized livers by the host, who probably ate squirrel or other animal livers. These are spurious infections, and eggs usually disappear from the feces in a few days.

Parasite Morphology

The adult worms are long, slender, and delicate. Females measure between 50 and 104 mm in length with a maximum diameter of 78 to 184 µm. Males are smaller, reaching a length of 22 mm and a maximum diameter of about 80 µm. Both sexes have a long esophagus with a prominent stichosome in the anterior portion of the body and reproductive structures in the posterior. In the female, the vulva is a short distance posterior to the end of the esophagus. The male has a single spicule. The body wall of the adult worms is thin and not strongly developed. The cuticle is thin. Two large bacillary bands are usually evident; a third, smaller one is much less conspicuous and difficult to identify (Plate 71:5). Muscle cells are of the coelomyarian type but are weakly developed. Muscle groups are separated by the bacillary bands (Plate 71:5).

The reproductive system in both sexes is a single tube, so that only one such tube is usually seen in a given section. However, both ovary and testis may be flexed (Plate 71:6). The reproductive systems in both sexes are confined to the posterior end of the body behind the esophagus. The intestine is a simple tube lined with a low epithelium throughout its length. Diagnosis of hepatic capillariasis does not usually depend on identification of the adult worms, which may be present in the liver. The fibrous tracts filled with eggs are the key features (Plate 71:1 & 2). All of the characteristics of the egg are evident in tissue sections: the general shape, the bipolar plugs, and the striated appearance of the thick shell (Plate 71:2). It would be difficult to misidentify hepatic capillariasis.

References

Attah EB, Magarajan S, Obineche EN, Gera SC. Hepatic capillariasis. *Am J Clin Pathol*. 1983;79:127-130.

Choe G, Lee HS, Seo JK, et al. Hepatic capillariasis: first case report in the Republic of Korea. *Am J Trop Med Hyg*. 1993;48:610-625.

Moravec F. Proposal of a new systematic arrangement of nematodes of the family Capillariidae. *Folia Parasitol (Praha)*. 1982;29:119-132.

Moravec F, Prokopic J, Shlikas AV. The biology of nematodes of the family Capillariidae, Neveu-Lemaine, 1936. *Folia Parasitol (Praha)*. 1987;34:39-56.

Plate 71

Capillaria hepatica

Image 1

Section of liver from a rat infected with *C. hepatica* shows fibrous tract containing typical eggs (H&E, 100x).

Image 2

At high magnification, the distinctive features of *C. hepatica* eggs are evident. The major morphologic characteristics of the egg are illustrated in the longitudinal section. Also shown are the pitted surface of the shell (darts) and the bipolar plugs (arrows) (H&E, 500x).

Image 3

Transverse section through a female worm. The uterus contains immature eggs (darts) (H&E, 270x).

Image 4

Transverse section of a gravid female worm. The thick-walled uterine tube contains maturing eggs. Eggs are also scattered about (arrows) in the burrow made by the female. The body wall of the worm is thin and weakly developed. The intestine (dart) is a simple tube (H&E, 400x).

Image 5

Transverse section through a female worm at the level of the ovary. In this section, bacillary bands (BB) are evident. Muscle can also be discerned between the bacillary bands. The intestine (IN) is the simple tube above the ovary (OV) (H&E, 500x).

Image 6

Transverse section through a male worm shows the reflexed testis (TE) and the intestine (IN) (H&E, 800x).

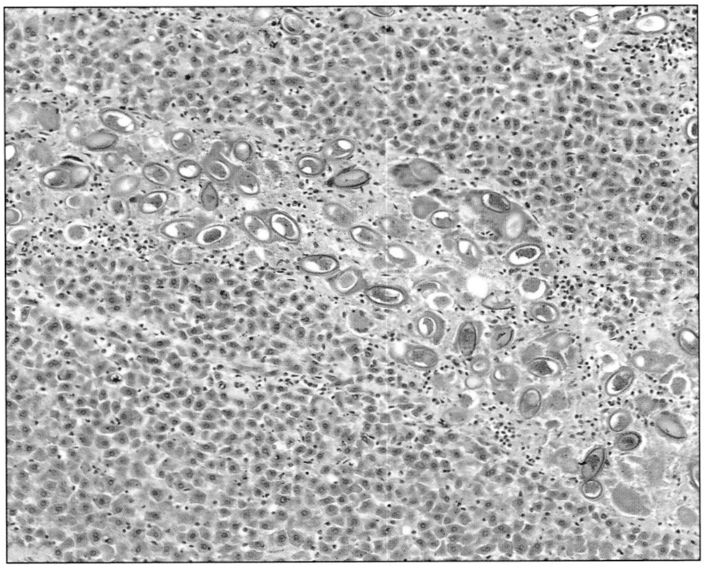

1

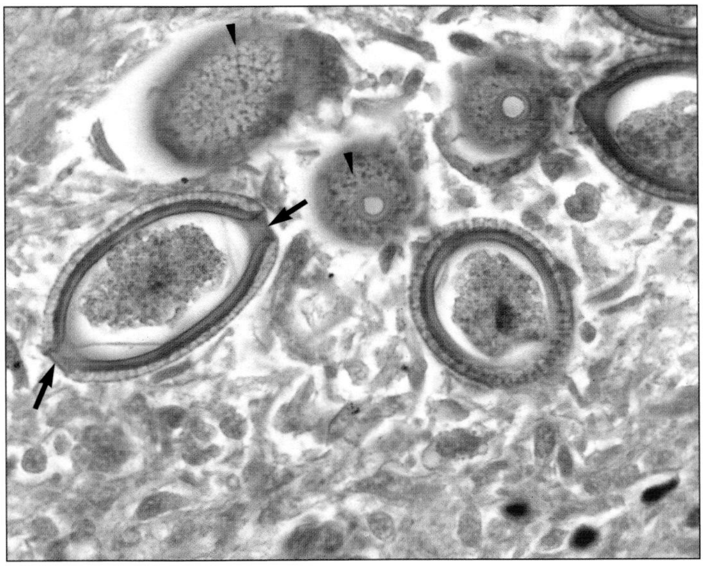

2

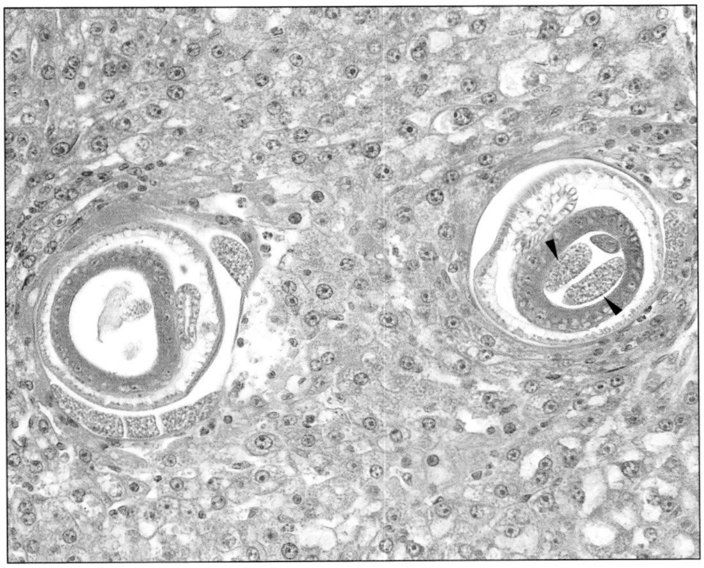

3

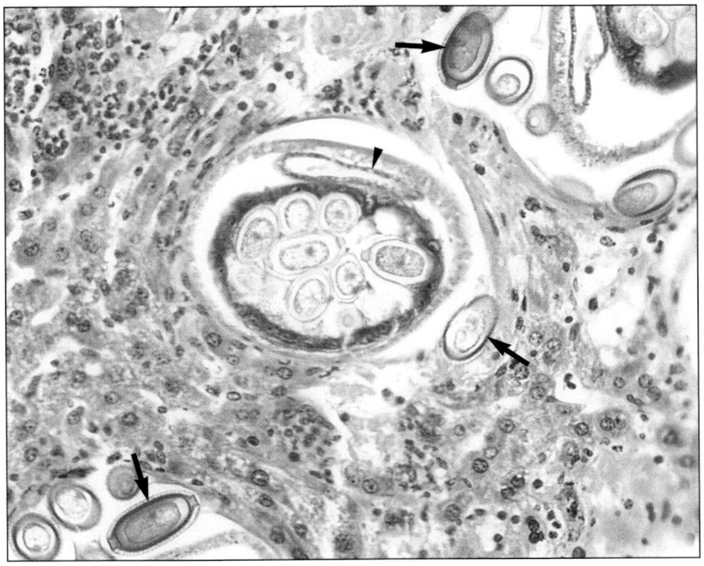

4

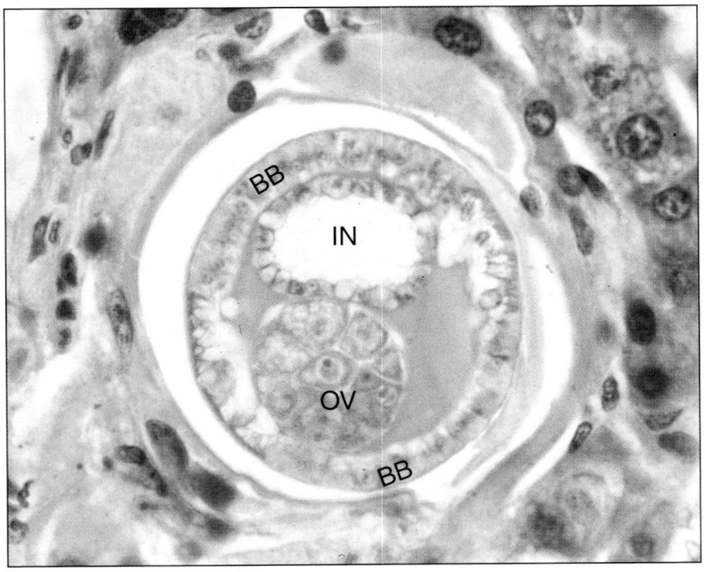

5

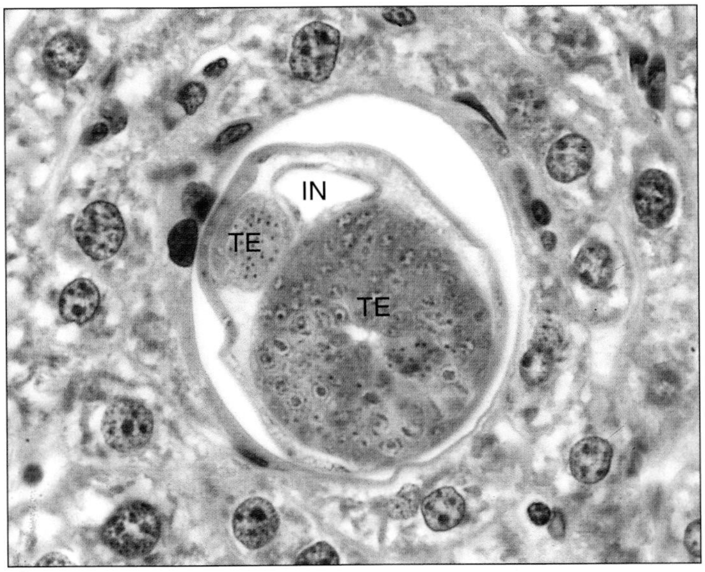

6

Anatrichosoma species

The anatrichosomes are an unusual and poorly known group of trichuroids found in prosimians, primates, marsupials, and, rarely, in dogs and cats. They appear to have worldwide distribution. These small, delicate worms burrow in the cutaneous and subcutaneous tissues of their hosts and on rare occasions infect humans.

Biology and Life Cycle

The worms, at least the females, actively migrate through the stratified layers of the squamous epithelium, forming burrows or tunnels in the tissues (Plate 72:1). The gravid female deposits eggs in these tunnels as she moves about. The tunnels, which are made up of epithelial cells, typically maintain their structural integrity and are sloughed with the superficial layers of the epithelium (⇒ 53). In monkeys, the parasite is typically found in the nasal vestibule and adjacent tissues. In the opossum, the parasite burrows in the tissues of the buccal cavity (palate and mandible), and in the prosimian, a tree shrew, it is found in the corneal and conjunctival epithelium. Eggs deposited in the nasal vestibule are most frequently liberated into the environment when the infected animal sneezes. Only small numbers are deposited in feces. Eggs in buccal tissues are typically recovered in feces, while those in ocular tissues apparently collect in ocular secretions and tears. Eggs liberated from skin lesions are sloughed in dander.

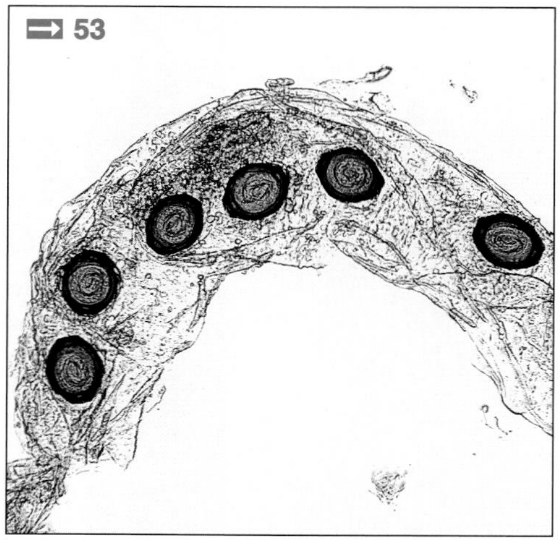

Although male worms are seen in the tunnels with the females, they are also found in deeper subcutaneous tissues (Plate 72:5). The reproductive behavior of at least some anatrichosome species is unusual in that the slender male worms enter the female reproductive tract, apparently to inseminate the female (Plate 72:4). This is similar to the behavior of *Trichosomoides* species, in which a much smaller male inhabits the female reproductive tract. The eggs produced by the anatrichosomes resemble those of the trichuroids. They measure approximately 76 by 58 µm but may be larger or smaller depending on the species. The egg is barrel shaped with bipolar operculae, and it contains a larva. The remainder of the life cycle and the mode of transmission of infection remain a mystery. Occasionally, outbreaks of anatrichosomiasis occur in primate colonies, but these have not aided in further elucidation of the transmission cycle.

Pathology and Clinical Manifestations

Extensive clinical observations do not exist; only three cases of human infection have been reported in the literature. In the published reports from Southeast Asia (Japan, Vietnam), the patients presented with symptoms similar to cutaneous larva migrans. Each had reddened, zig-zag lesions on the hand and foot, and, in one patient, additional lesions on the scrotum. These were associated with an intense pruritus, which ceased when the worms were removed from the terminal portions of the tracts. In both cases, the typical anatrichosome eggs were found, which were significant in the identification of the parasite. The third case, in a Malaysian aborigine, was an incidental finding during a survey for *Demodex*. In natural hosts such as the monkey or the opossum, no significant gross or microscopic indication of inflammation is generally associated with female worms in the epithelial layers (Plate 72:1, 3, & 4). Host response to the worms generally is limited to acanthotic thickening of the epithelium. Inflammatory infiltrates consist of few lymphocytes, macrophages, and eosinophils in the adjacent dermis, and they are more evident around male worms coiled in deeper subcutaneous tissues.

Parasite Morphology

These small, fragile worms typically measure less than 3.0 cm in length. Males tend to be of the same length or slightly larger than females, but females have a greater average diameter. The anatrichosomes have many typical trichuroid features that aid in identification. In tissue sections, female worms may measure up to 300 µm in diameter, depending on the species. Males are typically less than 100 µm in diameter. The body of the female is more slender anteriorly and of greatest diameter posteriorly (Plate 72:1). Males tend to be of uniform diameter through most of the length of the body and are about one-third the diameter of females. The cuticle is thick, and cephalic inflations may be present. Paired bacillary bands are noted through most of the length of the body (Plate 72:3, 4, & 6). Muscles are polymyarian and coelomyarian. As in other trichuroids, the esophageal tube is embedded along most of its length in the stichosome (Plate 72:2). The intestine is a simple tube, and the anus is terminal in position. In the female, the vulva is slightly postesophageal. The reproductive system is a single tube differentiated along its length into vagina, uterus, seminal receptacle, oviduct, and ovary.

In almost all sections of the worm the male reproductive tube is posterior to the esophagus (Plate 72:6). In *A. buccalis*, and possibly in other species, sections of male worms may be seen in the uterine canal (Plate 72:4). They are only slightly larger than the mature eggs, which already contain a larva. The male may have a spicule. The identification of anatrichosomes in histologic sections is aided by their small size, their cutaneous and subcutaneous habitat, the formation of burrows in which the parasite resides, the prominent stichosome, the paired bacillary bands, and the occasional presence of the male within the uterine canal. The anatrichosome egg, which may be fully developed in utero or scattered about the tunnels in the skin, quickly confirms the generic diagnosis. Given our current state of knowledge, specific identification is problematic.

References

Le-Van-Hoa, Duong-Hong-Ma, Nguyen-Luu-Vien. Premier cas de capillariose cutanee humaine. *Bull Soc Pathol Exot*. 1963;56:121-126.

Marivi MA, Omar B, Mohammod CG, Jeffery J. *Anatrichosoma* species egg and *Demodex folliculorum* in facial skin scrapings of Orang Aslis. *Trop Biomed*. 1990; 7:193-194.

Morishita K, Tani T. A case of *Capillaria* infection causing cutaneous creeping eruption in man. *J Parasitol*. 1960;46:79-83.

Plate 72

Anatrichosoma species

Image 1

Section through the nasal epithelium of a monkey shows transverse sections of *A. cynomolgi* at the level of the stichosome (keyline) and more posterior levels of the body of a female worm (H&E, 100x).

Image 2

Longitudinal section of the anterior end of *A. cynomolgi* shows the stichosome and the linear arrangement of the individual stichocytes (H&E, 200x).

Image 3

Transverse section through a mature female worm. Note the large uterine tube (UT), which contains an egg, and the smaller intestinal tube (H&E, 400x).

Image 4

Transverse section through a tunnel created by a female *A. buccalis* in the buccal cavity of an opossum (*Didelphis*). Note the well-developed body wall, with its thick cuticle, polymyarian musculature, and conspicuous bacillar bands (BB).The uterine tube (UT) of the female worm contains a transverse section of a male worm (dart) and three eggs. Operculae are evident in two of the eggs; a larva is present in the other egg. The tunnel itself contains two portions of a male worm (arrows) and five eggs (H&E, 230x).

Image 5

A male *Anatrichosoma* (keyline) coiled in the deep subcutaneous tissues of a piece of skin excised from the face of a patas monkey (*Erythrocebus*) (H&E, 60x).

Image 6

At high magnification, the structure of the male worm demonstrates the prominent bacillary bands (darts), the reproductive tube (RT), and the small, tubular intestine (H&E, 300x).

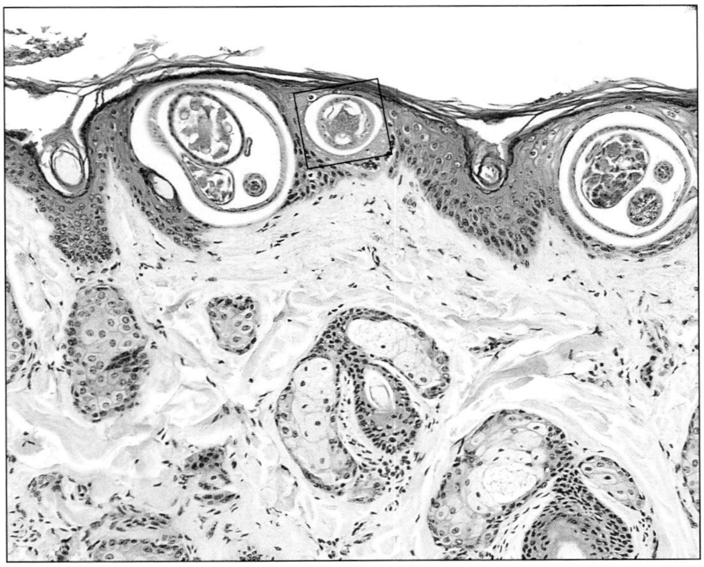
1

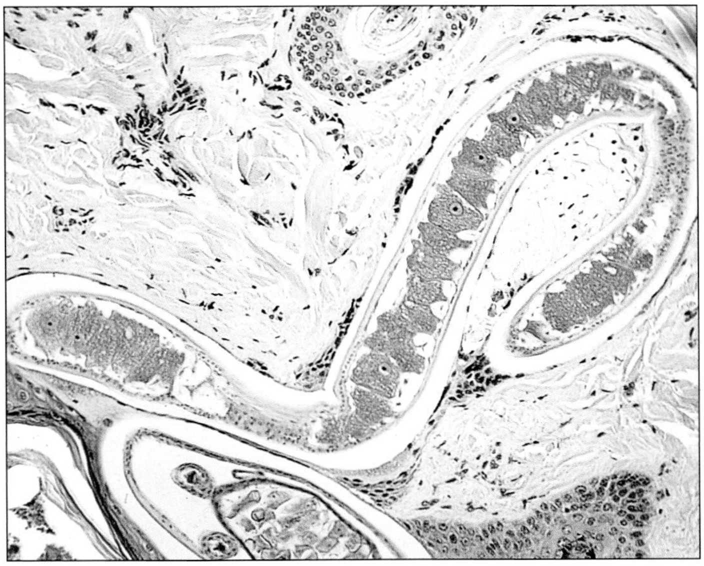
2

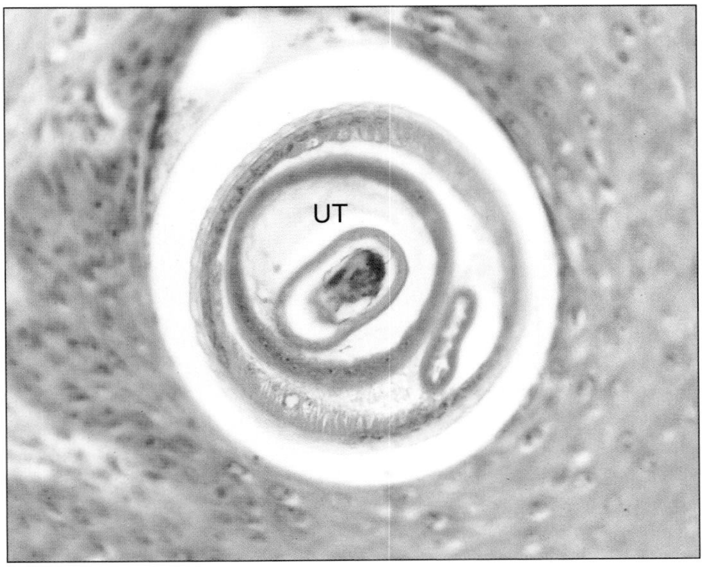

3

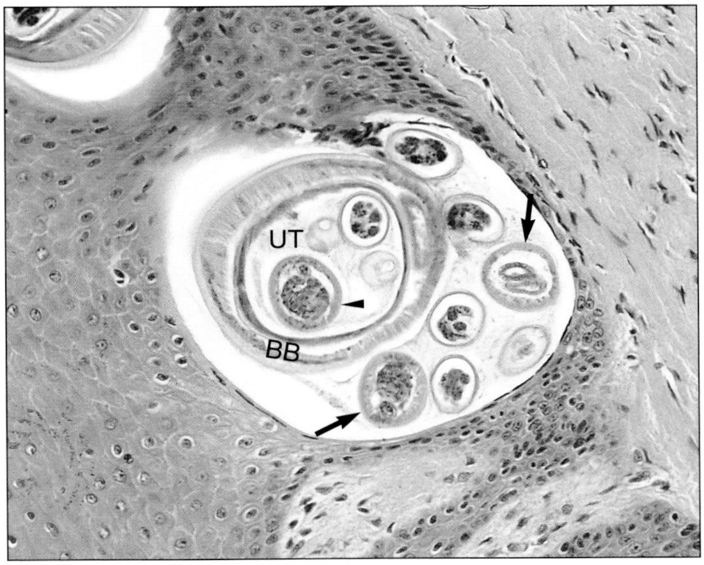

4

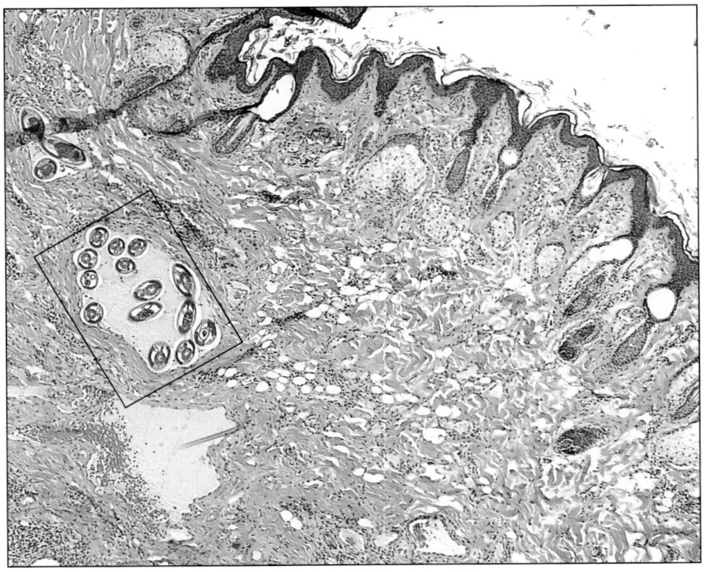
5

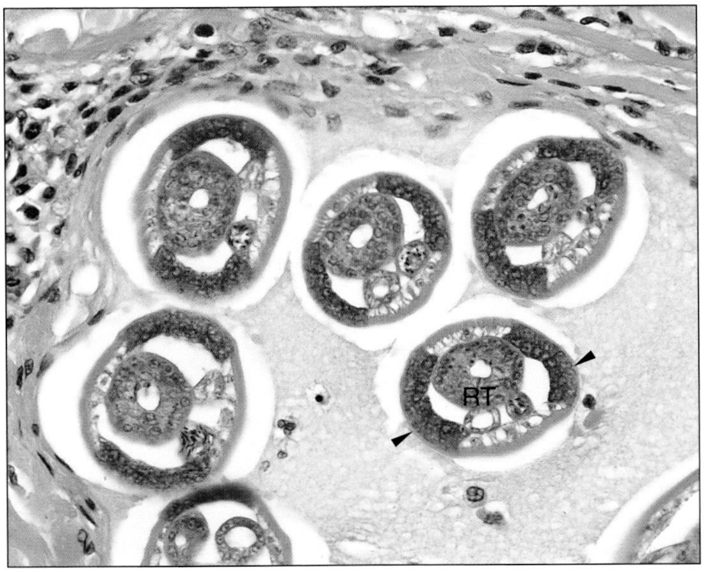

6

Dioctophyme renale

Dioctophyme renale, usually referred to as the giant kidney worm, parasitizes a wide range of predominately fish-eating, carnivorous mammals throughout the world such as mink, raccoon, and the domestic dog. As its common name implies, this bright-red worm may reach a length of 100 cm, but only in the female; the male reaches a maximum of 45 cm in length. The adults typically reside in the kidney, which they ultimately destroy, or they are found in the body cavity or other organs of the host. At least 12 cases of human infections have been reported, based primarily on the finding of eggs in urine or the recovery of adult worms. In recent years, larval stages have been identified in human tissues in residents of the United States and Thailand.

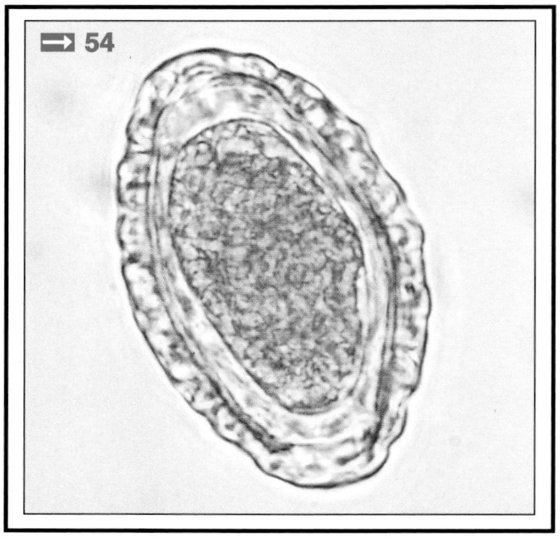

Biology and Life Cycle

This parasite has a long and unusual life cycle. Eggs produced by the female worm pass out of the body of the host in urine (⇨ **54**). They must be discharged into water, where it may take up to one month or more for them to embryonate and develop into first-stage larvae. Apparently, the larvae may survive within the egg for as long as two years until they are ingested by the first intermediate host, usually a branchiobdellid oligochaete that lives attached to the surface of crayfish. The eggs hatch, and the larvae make their way into the body cavity of the annelid host, encysting in the body cavity or associated organs. Fish such as the bullhead (*Ameirus*) serve as a second intermediate host, in which the larvae encyst in abdominal mesenteries or in the liver, where they develop to the infective stage. Paratenic hosts such as tadpoles, frogs, and other fish may be involved in the life cycle as well. Whether the final host is animal or human, it becomes infected when it ingests the infected fish or paratenic host. Apparently, the infective (third-stage) larva migrates directly from the intestine to the kidney of the host by actively penetrating the organs. The parasite typically invades the right kidney, ultimately destroying it. Usually only the capsule of the kidney remains intact and harbors the adult worms. The entire life cycle requires about two years to complete. Humans most likely become infected by eating inadequately cooked infected fish or possibly frogs.

Pathology and Clinical Manifestations

Of the dozen or so cases of *Dioctophyme* infections reported until 1979, six were diagnosed from worms passed in urine; five from worms recovered from kidneys at autopsy; one from a worm discharged through the body wall (fistula) from an abscessed kidney; and one from typical eggs found in urine. In the most recent reports, a third-stage larva of *Dioctophyme* was found in a nodule removed from the subcutaneous tissues of a resident of California; another in a migratory nodule in the abdominal subcutaneous tissues of a resident of Ohio (Plate 73:1); and a third in a subcutaneous nodule in the chest wall of a patient from Thailand. In two of the three cases, the nodules were migratory or disappeared and then reappeared. Microscopically, the worms could be identified at the generic level on the basis of their morphologic features. They were coiled in the lesions, surrounded by heavy infiltrates of inflammatory cells, and appear to have been alive when the tissues were fixed.

Parasite Morphology

The adult female worm may reach 100 cm in length and have a diameter of more than 1 cm. The male, by contrast, measures up to 45 cm in length with a diameter of 4 to 6 mm. Intact worms are not difficult to identify, because their size, color, and location are unique. Larvae in sections of human tissues are less well characterized. They measure up to 385 µm in diameter. The body wall has a somewhat unusual structure. The cuticle is multilayered but thin. The hypodermis is also thin, with a large ventral chord containing several nuclei arranged in a U or V pattern (Plate 73:2 & 6). Dorsal and lateral chords are inconspicuous. Hypodermal nuclei are evident in the interchordal (submuscular) regions as well (Plate 73:6). The muscles are polymyarian and coelomyarian. They are divided into four longitudinal bands by the dorsal, lateral, and ventral chords and further subdivided by four somato-intestinal muscles that extend from the intestinal wall to the body wall. Individual muscle cells vary in their appearance at different levels of the body. The cytoplasmic portions of the cell may appear reduced or expanded (Plate 73:2 & 5).

The esophagus, which has a distinct triradiate lumen (Plate 73:2), is not divided into muscular and glandular portions; glandular elements are interspersed among the muscle fibers. The intestine is tubular and often rectangular rather than round, in part because of the tension produced by the attachment of the mesenteries (Plate 73:3). The cells lining the intestine are uninucleate and cuboidal, with exceptionally long, uneven microvilli. Sphaerocrystals are found in the cytoplasm (Plate 73:3 & 4).

The reproductive system is a single tube in both sexes, although the male is diorchic (two testes). Histologic structure of the developing reproductive systems in larval *Dioctophyme* has not been described in any detail to date.

The division of the muscles into eight bands, the four rows of somato-intestinal muscles, the pseudocoelomic membranes, the dispersal of glandular elements among the muscle cells in the esophagus, and the features of the intestine (sphaerogranules and uneven microvilli) facilitate reliable diagnosis of the larval dioctophymid in tissues. However, on at least two occasions Liesegang rings found in human kidneys have mistakenly been identified as eggs of *D. renale,* even though Liesegang rings have no similarity to this species (Plate 105:3).

References

Beaver PC, Khamboonruang C. *Dioctophyma*-like larval nematode in a subcutaneous nodule from man in northern Thailand. *Am J Trop Med Hyg*. 1984;33:1032-1034.

Beaver PC, Theis JC. Dioctophymatid larval nematode in a subcutaneous nodule from man in California. *Am J Trop Med Hyg*. 1979;28:206-212.

Gutierrez Y, Cohen M, Machicao CN. *Dioctophyme* larva in the subcutaneous tissues of a woman in Ohio. *Am J Surg Path*. 1989;13:800-802.

Sun T, Turnbull A, Lieberman PH, et al. Giant kidney worm *(Dioctophyma renale)* mimicking retroperitoneal neoplasm. *Am J Surg Path*. 1986;10:508-512.

Plate 73

Dioctophyme renale

Image 1

A coiled larva of *Dioctophyme* in a subcutaneous nodule in the abdominal wall of an Ohioan. The worm is cut through several levels of the body (H&E, 40x). (Case courtesy of Y. Gutierrez.)

Image 2

Transverse section through the level of the esophagus shows its triradiate lumen and the interspersion of glandular elements among the muscle fibers. Note the conspicuous ventral hypodermal chord (dart) and the subventral position of the pseudocoelomic membranes (arrows). The coelomyarian muscles display few of the cytoplasmic elements of the muscle cells (H&E, 260x).

Image 3

In transverse section the intestine appears almost rectangular in shape. Note the dorsally placed pseudocoelomic membranes (darts) (H&E, 220x).

Image 4

High-power view of the intestine shows its low cuboidal cell lining, the uneven microvilli, and spherogranular inclusions. The cell nuclei are conspicuous (H&E, 1100x).

Image 5

Transverse section of a larva in a subcutaneous nodule from the chest wall of a Thai. The section is cut at the level of the esophagus. Visible are the muscle cells with distinct cytoplasmic elements, the prominent ventral chord (dart), and submuscular hypodermal nuclei in the interchordal areas. Note also the subventral position of the pseudocoelomic membranes (arrows) (H&E, 300x).

Image 6

At higher magnification, the "U" pattern of distribution of nuclei is apparent in the ventral chord. Hypodermal nuclei in the submuscular interchordal regions are also evident (darts) (H&E, 600x).

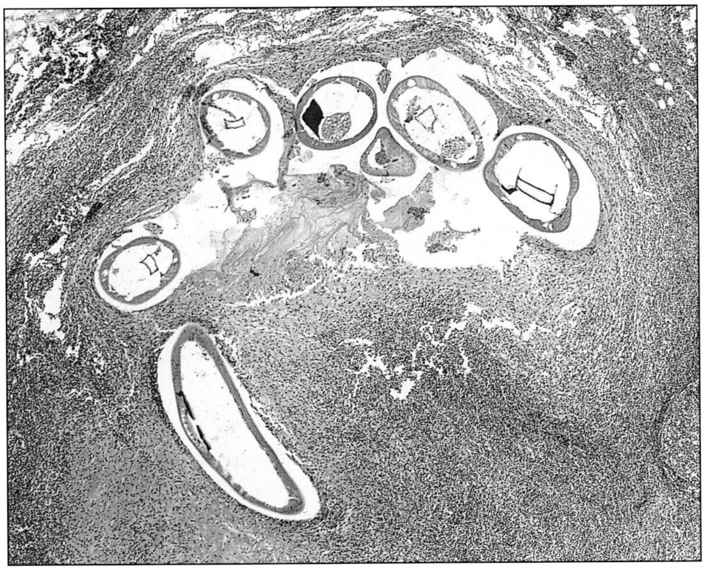

1

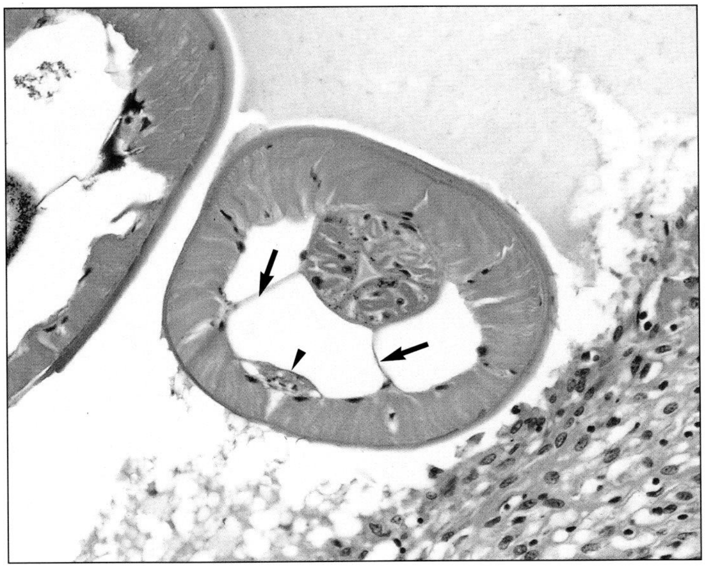

2

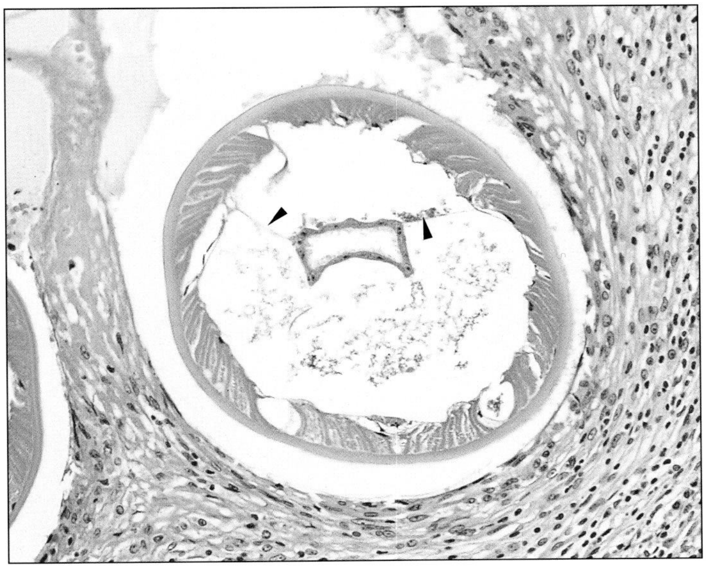

3

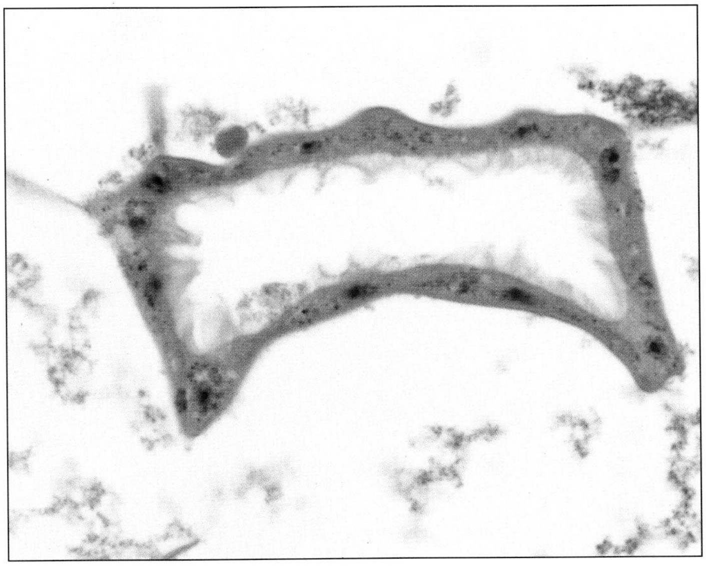

4

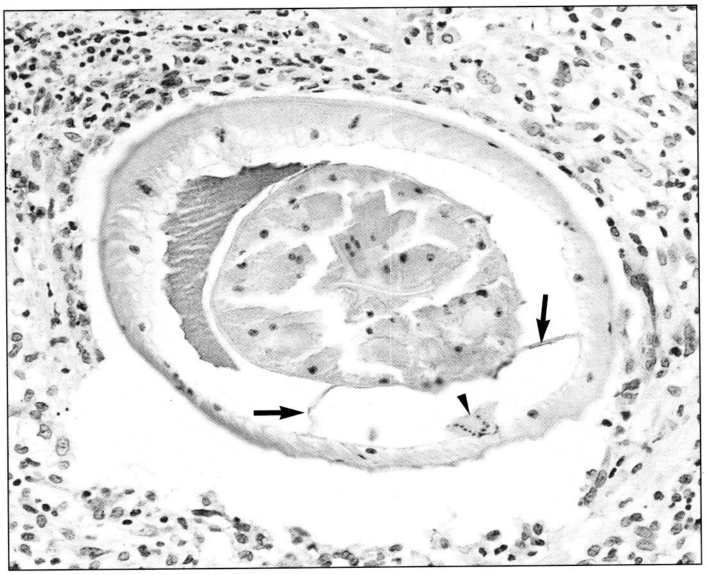

5

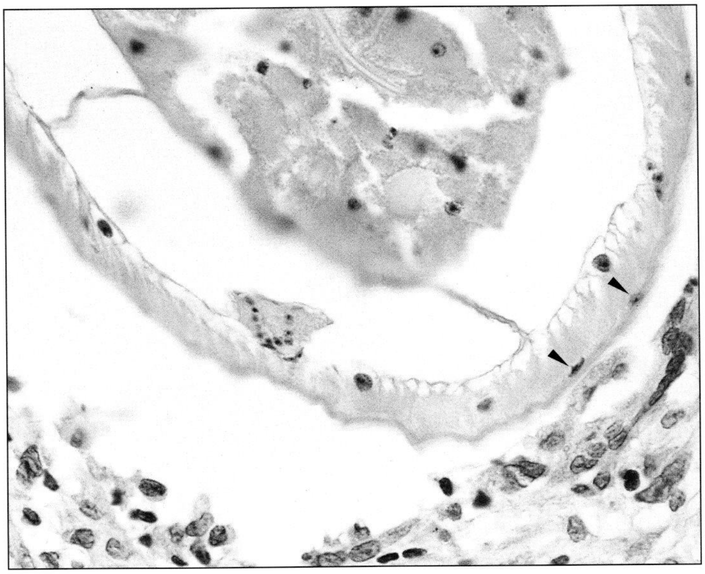

6

Eustrongylides species

Eustrongylides species are dioctophymatoid nematodes that are closely related to *Dioctophyme renale.* They are a small and poorly known group of nematode parasites. The adults are found in the mucosa of the esophagus, proventriculus, and intestine of a variety of piscivorous water birds. Only a few cases of human infection have been documented, all from the United States.

Biology and Life Cycle

More than 12 species of *Eustrongylides* have been described, but recent studies have reduced the number of valid species to only three, two of which have been recorded from the United States. They parasitize a wide range of bird species. Their life cycles are not completely documented but appear to be similar to that of *Dioctophyme.* An aquatic oligochaete serves as the first intermediate host, and various fish are second intermediate hosts. Other fish, amphibians, and reptiles serve as transport or paratenic hosts. The infective stage is presumed to be the fourth-stage larva.

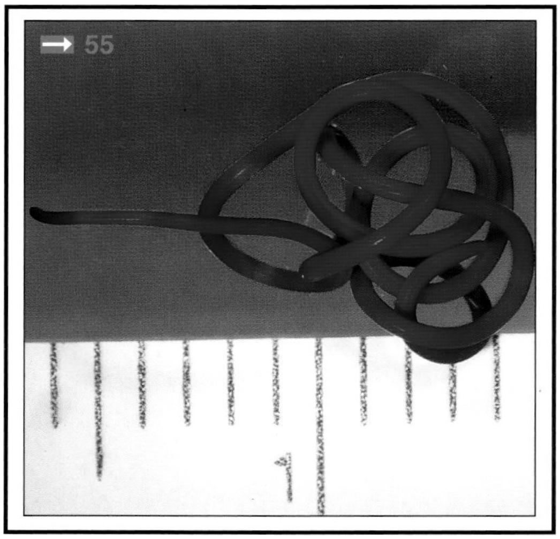

Humans become infected by ingesting larvae encysted or encapsulated in an intermediate host. In four of the five human infections documented, the individual acquired infection by ingesting bait minnows; the fifth person ate raw fish used to prepare sushi and sashimi. In cases where the worms were subjected to critical examination, they were determined to be larvae rather than adults.

Pathology and Clinical Manifestations

Patients with infections developed severe abdominal pains within 24 hours of eating fresh fish or minnows. Four of five patients required exploratory surgery; at least one had a preoperative diagnosis of appendicitis. In three patients, two or more worms were crawling about in the peritoneal cavity. In the other, a worm crawled onto the surgical drapes during the surgical procedure. Removal of the worms resulted in cessation of any further pain or discomfort.

Parasite Morphology

As adults in their normal hosts, these bright-red worms reach lengths of 15 cm with diameters of 0.4 mm, depending on the species (➞ 55). Larvae recovered from patients have measured between 4.2 and 15 cm in length, with most between 4 and 6 cm.

The worms have a moderately thick cuticle that is transversely striated. The anterior end has two circles of six papillae each. The mouth is variable in shape, usually in the form of a dorsoventral slit. The posterior end is blunt in both sexes. In the female, the anus and vulva are terminal; in the male, the tail is expanded into a muscular sucker. A single, needlelike spicule is present. Both sexes have a single reproductive tube.

Most often, these worms are removed from the patient intact. However, it is possible that some will be sectioned as a routine procedure. The microscopic features of the parasite are unique and facilitate accurate diagnosis.

In transverse sections, the cuticle is multilayered and moderately thick, although its appearance may vary at different levels of the body (Plate 74:1–3). The hypodermis is thin but is expanded slightly to form dorsal, lateral, and ventral chords. The ventral chord, which is fan shaped, is the most conspicuous (Plate 74:2 & 3). Subdorsal and subventral chords divide the muscles into eight bands (Plate 74:2). Unlike the subdorsal and subventral chords in other nematodes, these are slender and relatively inconspicuous. Hypodermal nuclei are present in the interchordal (submuscular) areas as well (Plate 74:2). The musculature is strong and well developed. Muscle cells are coelomyarian, with a well-developed contractile portion and a reduced cytoplasmic portion (Plate 74:1–3). Four somatic intestinal muscles link the body wall to the alimentary tract, particularly in the posterior end of the worm. These muscles are often difficult to identify in a given transverse section of the parasite (Plate 74:6). A pair of pseudocoelomic mesenteries extend from the body wall to the alimentary tract at most levels of the body (Plate 74:1–3).

The esophagus is club shaped and round in transverse sections, multinucleate and glandular throughout. It has a triradiate lumen and prominent dorsal and subventral glands (Plate 74:1). The intestine is tubular and sometimes irregular in shape with a large lumen. The intestinal wall is made up of a large number of tall, slender, columnar cells with individual nuclei positioned near the base of the cell. Their luminal borders have microvilli (Plate 74:4).

The reproductive system in both sexes is a single tube that typically is flexed and may be coiled. Other than the ovary or testis, the anatomic components of *Eustrongylides* species are difficult to recognize in the larval stages. They do not facilitate identification, except perhaps in the male, where the single spicule may be seen in the extreme posterior end.

References

Eberhard ML, Hurwitz H, Sun AM, Coletta D. Intestinal perforation caused by larval *Eustrongylides* (Nematoda: Dioctophymatoidea) in New Jersey. *Am J Trop Med Hyg*. 1989;40:648-650.

Measures LN. Revision of the genus *Eustrongylides* Jargerjkiöld, 1909 (Nematoda: Dioctophymatoidea) of piscivorous birds. *Can J Zool*. 1988;66:885-895.

Spalding MG, Forrester DJ. Pathogenesis of *Eustrongylides ignotus* (Nematoda: Dioctophymatoidea) in Ciconiiformes. *J Wldlf Dis*. 1993;29:250-260.

Wittner M, Turner JW, Jacquette G, et al. Eustrongylidiasis: a parasitic infection acquired by eating sushi. *N Engl J Med*. 1989;320:1124-1126.

Plate 74

Eustrongylides species

Image 1

Section through the anterior end of a female worm shows the esophagus with its triradiate lumen. Note also the pseudocoelomic mesenteries (arrows) and the ventral hypodermal chord (dart) (H&E, 100x).

Image 2

Section through the posterior end of a male worm near the intestinal-rectal junction. Two sections through the reproductive system are shown: one through the spicule within its sheath (dart), although detail is lacking at this magnification, and the other through the ejaculatory duct. The ventral hypodermal chord is conspicuous (arrow) (H&E, 130x).

Image 3

Section through a female worm illustrates the moderately thick cuticle, coelomyarian muscles, ventral hypodermal chord (arrow), and, in the pseudocoelomic cavity, the ovary (OV) and vagina (dart). Some hypodermal nuclei are evident in interchordal areas (H&E, 130x).

Image 4

At high magnification, the structure of the intestine is especially clear, particularly the narrow columnar epithelium, with nuclei near the base of the cells, and the microvillus border of the intestinal cells (H&E, 260x).

Image 5

Section through a female *E. ignotus* shows typical morphologic characteristics of *Eustrongylides*. The cuticle has detached from the hypodermis (H&E, 100x).

Image 6

Section through a worm recovered from the abdominal cavity of a patient in New Jersey. Note the typical *Eustrongylides* morphologic features (H&E, 150x). (Case courtesy of M.L. Eberhard.)

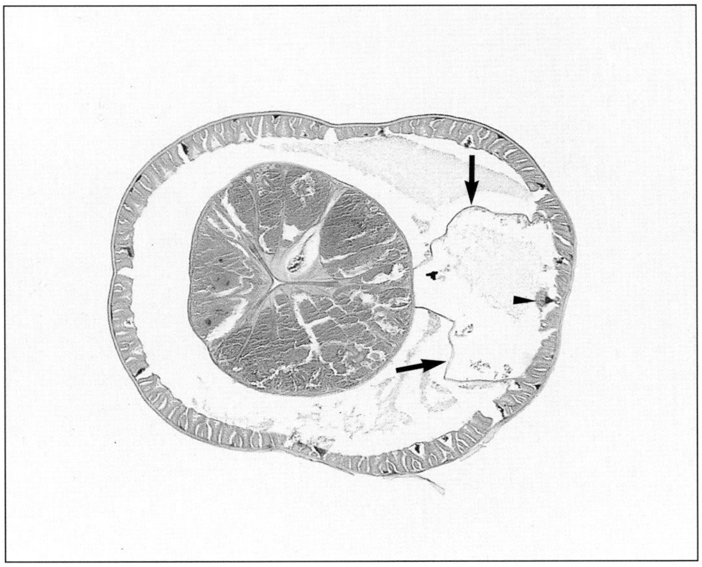

1

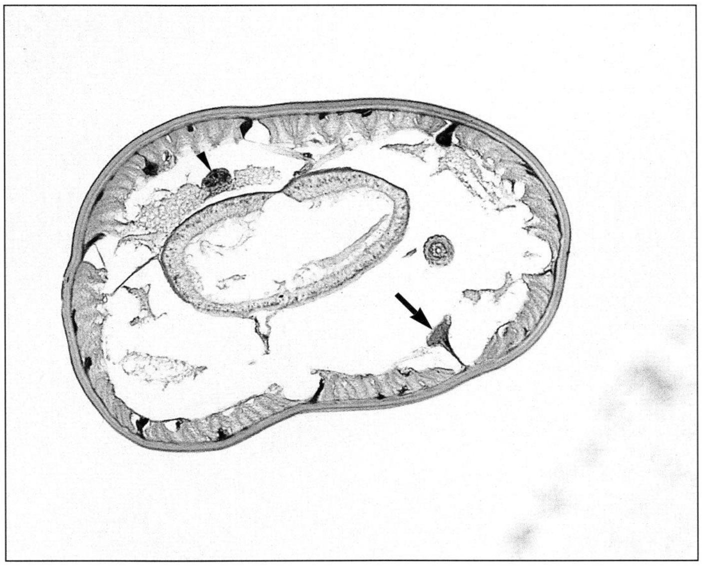

2

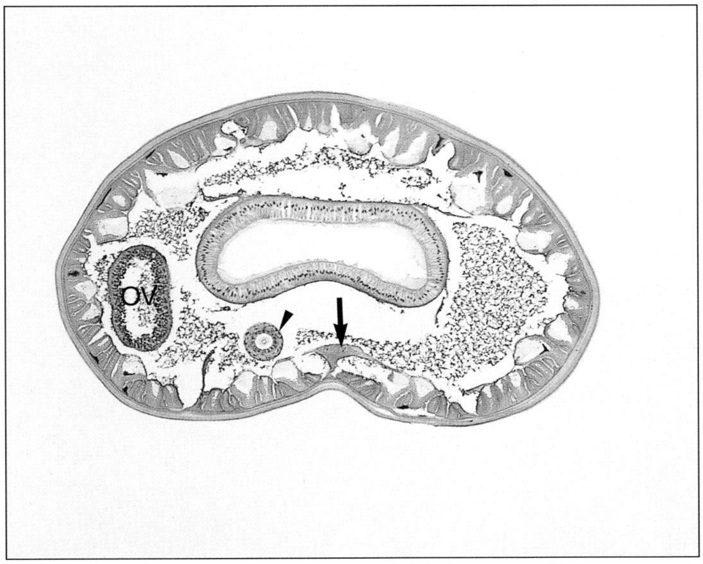

3

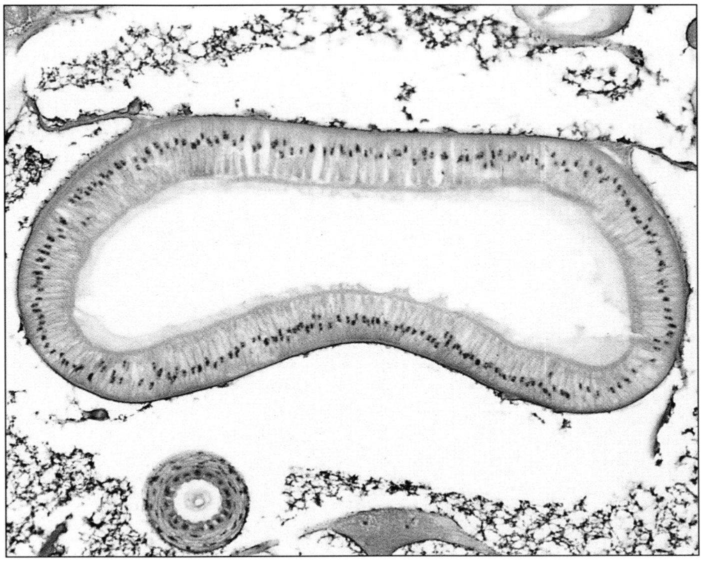

4

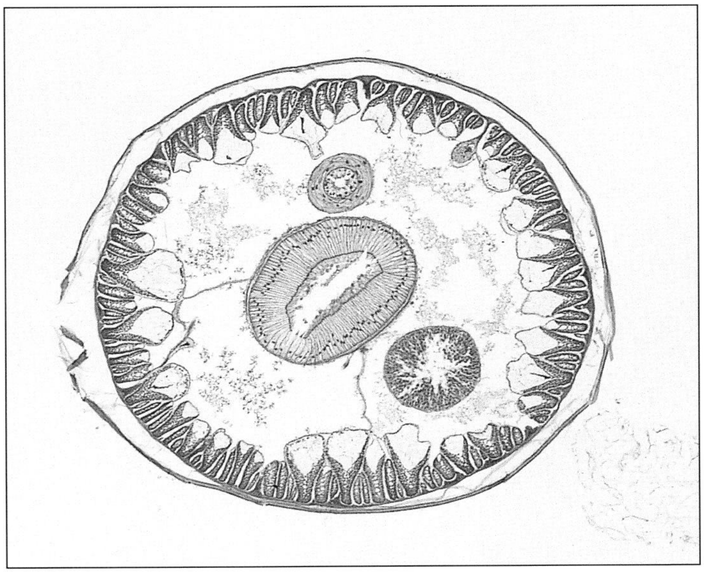

5

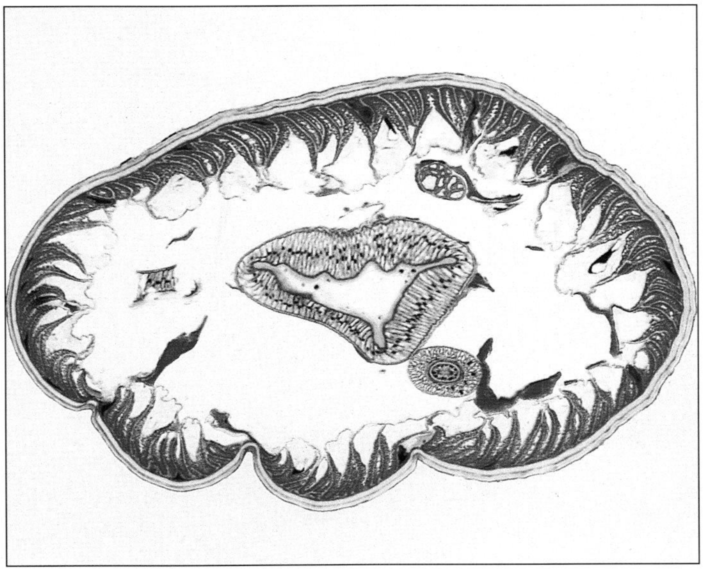

6

Trematoda

Trematodes, which are commonly referred to as flukes, belong to the Phylum Platyhelminthes. They have complex life cycles involving one, two, or occasionally more intermediate hosts. All of the flukes that parasitize humans require a freshwater snail as a first intermediate host and thus are referred to as snail-transmitted diseases. The flukes of human importance belong to the Order Digenea, a group of more than 40,000 species with extremely diverse morphology and life cycles. Coombs and Crompton (1991) list 113 species of flukes belonging to more than 50 genera as agents of human infection.

Trematode Life Cycles

The eggs produced by the adult fluke contain a ciliated larva called a miracidium at the time they are discharged or shortly thereafter. This larva penetrates a snail host and undergoes considerable morphologic change and extensive multiplication. The result is the production of large numbers of the infective stage, the cercaria, which the snail sheds into the water. These free-swimming larvae may infect an additional intermediate host or, as in the case of the schistosomes (*Schistosoma* species), may infect humans directly by skin penetration. In other species (*Fasciola* and *Fasciolopsis*), cercariae attach to and encyst as metacercariae on aquatic vegetation. In still others, cercariae attach to and encyst as metacercariae in fish (eg, *Clonorchis, Heterophyes*), in crabs and other crustaceans (*Paragonimus* species), or in other mollusks (*Echinostoma* species). Definitive hosts for flukes include not only humans but all vertebrate species. Trematodes are generally not host specific, and many will infect a broad range of mammalian hosts that serve as reservoir hosts for human infections.

Although the intestinal tract is the most common site of adult trematode infections, in some human and animal infections the adult worms live in the liver *(Fasciola, Clonorchis*), lung (*Paragonimus*), and mesenteric blood vessels (schistosomes). To reach such extraintestinal locations, larval trematodes must make a tissue migration in the definitive host to arrive at the site where they will complete maturation. Eggs and worms may be found in unusual tissue locations, because flukes such as *Fasciola, Paragonimus,* and others will occasionally end up in aberrant locations and die. In addition, eggs produced by adult worms may enter the bloodstream and be carried to the brain, spinal cord, lungs, and other tissues. Identification of these eggs in tissues is facilitated by a knowledge of their characteristic morphology (ie, size, spines, operculum, or other features).

Trematode Relationships

As might be expected with such a large group of diverse organisms, the classification and taxonomy of the trematodes vary considerably. Although most of this variation is not particularly relevant here, it is useful to have some knowledge of relationships among trematode species because the life cycles, biology, morphology, and pathology of related organisms are often similar. In general, the flukes of human importance all belong in the Class Trematoda, Order Digenea. Descriptions of family groupings place the species that infect humans in their proper perspective and provide a synopsis of their most relevant morphologic and biologic characteristics. Many families of trematodes, including some human parasites (eg, *Dicrocoelium, Echinostoma),* are not included here either because they are rarely reported or because they do not invade human tissues.

Family Heterophyidae

Small, ovoid, or pyriform flukes of the Family Heterophyidae live in the intestinal tract of a wide range of mammalian and avian definitive hosts. The tegument of these flukes usually has small spines. Eggs are typically small and operculate and contain a miracidium when excreted in feces. Freshwater snails are the first intermediate host, and fish, which harbor metacercariae, serve as the second intermediate host. Adult worms usually live in the crypts of the small intestine or within the mucosal epithelium, and they typically have short lifespans. A wide variety of genera and species cause human infections, and animals or birds serve as reservoirs of infection. Species that infect humans and are included here are *Heterophyes heterophyes* (➡ 56) and *Metagonimus yokogawai.*

Family Fasciolidae

These large, flat, leaflike flukes parasitize humans and herbivorous animals. Some members have a cone-shaped anterior end; others do not. The tegument may be spiny or aspinous.

In *Fasciola* and *Fascioloides,* the intestinal cecae are long and dendritic, and reproductive structures are branched. Eggs are large, operculate, and unembryonated when passed in feces. Freshwater snails are the intermediate host. Metacercariae, the infective stage for the definitive host, encyst on vegetation. Adult worms live in the liver, although *Fasciolopsis buski* resides in the intestinal tract. Both *Fasciola hepatica* (➡ 58) and *Fascioloides magna* infect humans.

Family Opisthorchiidae

These small to medium-sized, usually elongated flukes are found primarily in the bile ducts of the liver. Testes are branched or ovoid at the posterior end of the body. Eggs are small and operculated and contain a miracidium when excreted in feces. Freshwater snails are the first intermediate host, and fish, which harbor metacercariae, are the second intermediate host. Canine and feline hosts are frequent reservoirs for human infection. *Clonorchis sinensis* (➡ 60) and *Opisthorchis viverrini* are two common Asiatic species covered in this atlas.

Family Paragonimidae

Medium-sized, thick, ovoid trematodes of the Family Paragonimidae have a spiny tegument. These lung flukes parasitize humans and many species of carnivorous animals. Adult worms usually occur in pairs within a well-developed tissue capsule in the lung parenchyma. Testes and ovary are lobed or branched. Eggs are medium to large, operculated, and unembryonated when passed into the external environment via sputum or feces. Freshwater snails are the first intermediate host, and crabs and crayfish are the typical second intermediate hosts. Numerous species of *Paragonimus* infect humans in many parts of the world, but we focus on *P. westermani* (➡ 62).

Family Schistosomatidae

Schistosomes are the only human trematodes in which the sexes are separate. Males are more robust than females, and they form a gynecophoral canal within which the slender female worms lie in permanent or semipermanent copula. Eggs are typically large, are not operculated, and contain a miracidium when excreted to the external environment. Freshwater snails are the intermediate host. Infections are acquired by direct penetration of the skin by fork-tailed cercariae. Adults live in blood vessels. Because schistosomes are important causes of human disease, we discuss three major species: *Schistosoma mansoni* (➡ 65), *S. japonicum,* and *S. haematobium.*

Family Diplostomatidae

These trematodes usually parasitize the intestinal tracts of birds and mammals. Advanced larval stages known as mesocercariae are rarely found migrating in human tissues. Some species may also attain maturity in the human intestine. Freshwater snails are the first intermediate host, and fish, amphibians, and snails serve as second intermediate hosts. We discuss *Alaria* species (Plate 83:2).

Family Philophthalmidae

These elongated, medium-sized trematodes are usually found in the cloaca, intestine, or conjunctival sac of birds. Human infections are rare but thus far have always been characterized by the presence of adult worms in the eye. We discuss *Philophthalmus* species (Plate 83:6).

Trematode Morphology

Gross Morphology

Adult flukes (with the exception of the schistosomes, which are discussed separately) are flattened dorsoventrally and vary greatly in size, from a few millimeters to 75 mm or more.

The most characteristic feature of trematodes is their two suckers. The oral sucker surrounds the mouth opening at the anterior end, and the ventral sucker (acetabulum) is typically found at or anterior to the midbody. The simple alimentary tract consists of an oral opening leading to a pharynx (sometimes absent), followed by the esophagus, which bifurcates into a pair of blindly ending intestinal ceca. The parasite has no anus.

Most flukes are hermaphroditic (ie, both male and female reproductive systems occur in the same individual), and the reproductive organs usually begin at or posterior to the ventral sucker. The male system is generally composed of two testes. Arising from the testes are two vasa efferentia, which unite to form a single vas deferens. This structure enlarges as it enters a cirrus sac to form a seminal vesicle, which ends in a muscular cirrus organ that is protrusible through a genital pore, the terminus of the male system. The female system usually is single, with one ovary and an oviduct that receives both a duct from a seminal receptacle and a duct from the vitelline glands located on both sides of the worms. The oviduct then enters into the ootype where eggshell formation begins. From the ootype, eggs pass into the long, coiled uterus, which leads through the genital atrium to open externally via the common genital pore. The vitelline glands located along the lateral fields of the adult worms secrete yolk material for the developing eggs.

Details of the excretory and nervous systems of the trematodes are not relevant for diagnosis in histologic sections. Eggs of the trematodes vary substantially in size and, with the exception of the schistosomes, have an operculum. They may be unembryonated or contain a miracidium when discharged from the body.

Schistosomes differ from the other flukes that infect humans in that they have separate sexes. Male worms have a short anterior portion and a much longer and wider part posterior to the ventral sucker. The posterior part of the body is folded ventrally to form the gynecophoral canal. Males have multiple testes, with the number varying among species. The tegument of male worms may be finely (*S. haematobium*) or grossly (*S. mansoni*) tuberculate, or it may lack tuberculations (*S. japonicum*). Female worms are filiform and round in transverse section. The tegument of female worms lacks tuberculations. Eggs of the schistosomes are large, lack an operculum, have large or small spines, and contain a miracidium when excreted (➡ 66, 67, & 69).

Microscopic Morphology

The external body surface of a trematode is referred to as a tegument—it is a living and metabolically active layer. The tegument is a continuous syncytial epithelium bounded externally by a plasma membrane that is approximately 10 μm thick and internally by another trilaminated plasma membrane. Spines of the tegument, when present, are found on this outer layer (Plate 75:2 & 3). Beneath the internal laminated membrane is an outer layer of circular muscle and an inner layer of longitudinal muscle (Plate 75:1–4). Tegumental cell bodies (also called epidermal cells) are found beneath the muscle layers, but they have cytoplasmic connections that extend to the tegument. The rest of the body of the fluke between the tegument and organ systems is filled with cells of the parenchyma and interstitial fibers that serve as a kind of connective tissue

(Plate 75:1). Dorsoventral muscle fibers also course through the parenchyma and surround the internal organs.

The histologic appearance of the alimentary canal and various parts of the reproductive system vary somewhat from species to species. Sections through the anterior portion of most trematodes may contain a transverse section of the pharynx or esophagus. Sections through the oral and ventral sucker are frequent (Plate 75:1 & 5). In sections posterior to the ventral sucker, the paired intestinal ceca are usually visible as narrow ducts lined with epithelial cells (Plate 75:1). In flukes such as *Fasciola,* the intestinal ceca are branched. Prominent structures of the reproductive system that are usually encountered posterior to the ventral sucker include sections through ovary (Plate 75:1), testis, uterus containing eggs (Plate 75:1), and the vitellaria in the lateral fields (Plate 75:2).

In schistosomes, it is typical to find transverse sections of the female worm partially surrounded by the folding of the male gynecophoral canal (Plate 75:4). In *S. mansoni* (Plate 75:4) and *S. haematobium,* it may be possible to see tuberculations on the surface of the tegument.

In immature flukes migrating in tissues, the appearance of anatomic structures seen in section may differ significantly, since reproductive organs have not yet developed and the excretory system may be especially prominent (Plate 75:5).

Reference

Fried B, Haseeb MA. Platyhelminthes: Aspidogastrea, Monogenea, and Digenea. In: Harrison FW, Bogitish BJ, eds. *Microscopic Anatomy of Invertebrates, Vol III: Platyhelminthes and Nemertinea.* New York, NY: Wiley-Liss Inc; 1991.

Plate 75

Trematode Anatomy

Image 1

Transverse section through an adult *Clonorchis sinensis* shows features that are representative of trematode species: the coiled uterus (UT) containing eggs, lobed ovary (OV), intestinal ceca (IC), and excretory canals (EC). Note the large ventral sucker (VS).

Image 2

Tegument of *Paragonimus westermani* demonstrates characteristic spines. Vitelline glands appear as dark red structures within the underlying parenchyma. Muscle is visible between the external surface and vitelline glands (Trichrome).

Image 3

Section through tegument of *Fasciola hepatica*. This fluke also has spines (darts) on the tegument, but the spines are broader and flatter than those seen in *P. westermani*.

Image 4

Transverse section through a male and female *S. mansoni* shows the smaller, round female almost completely surrounded by the folds of the male gynecophoral canal. Tuberculations (darts) on the dorsal surface of the male tegument are readily visible.

Image 5

Longitudinal section of a migrating immature *Paragonimus* seen in boar muscle. The oral and ventral suckers (dart) are seen, as are two portions through one of the intestinal ceca (IC) that has folded on itself. The large structure at the posterior end is part of the excretory bladder, which is strikingly prominent in larval stages. Reproductive structures are not visible. (Case courtesy of I. Miyazaki.)

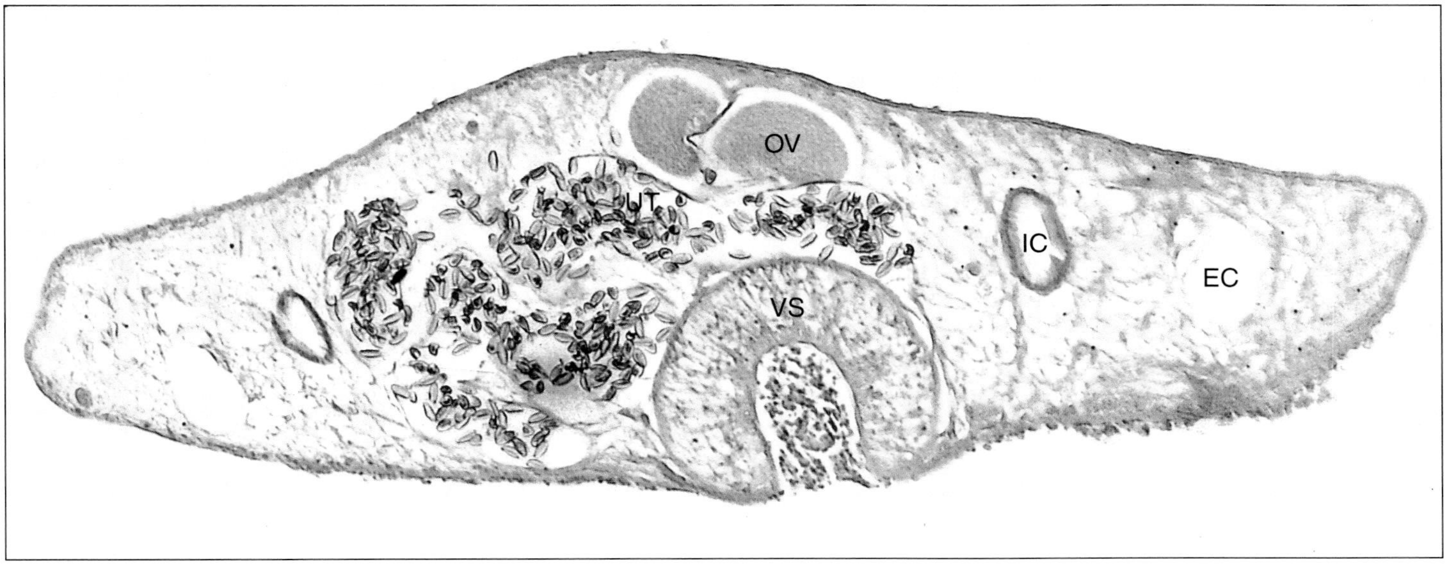

1

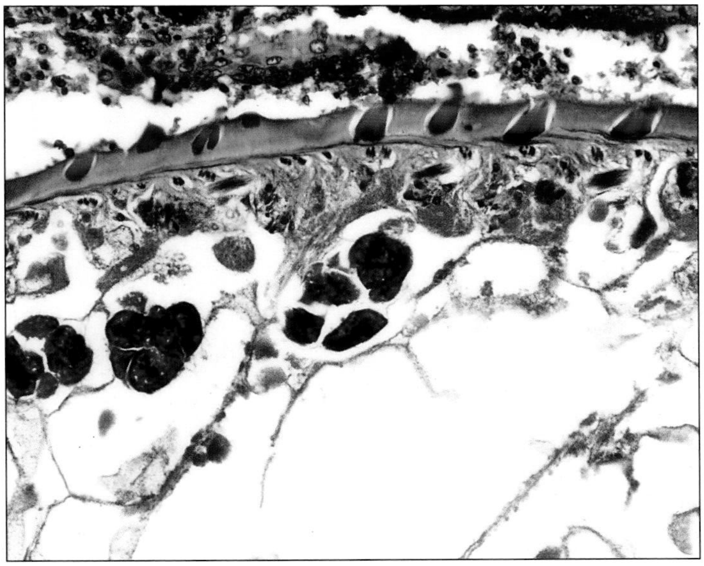

2

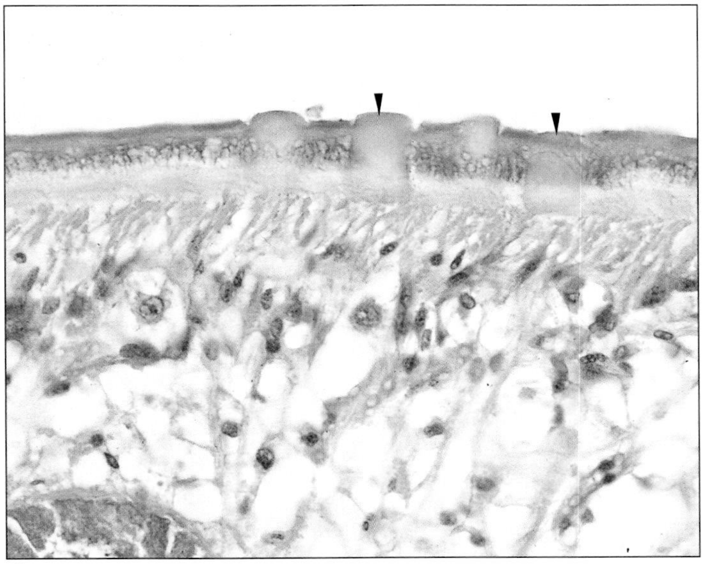

3

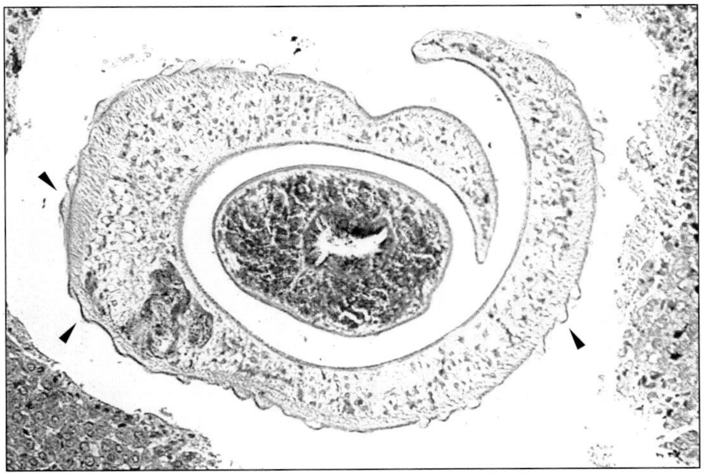

4

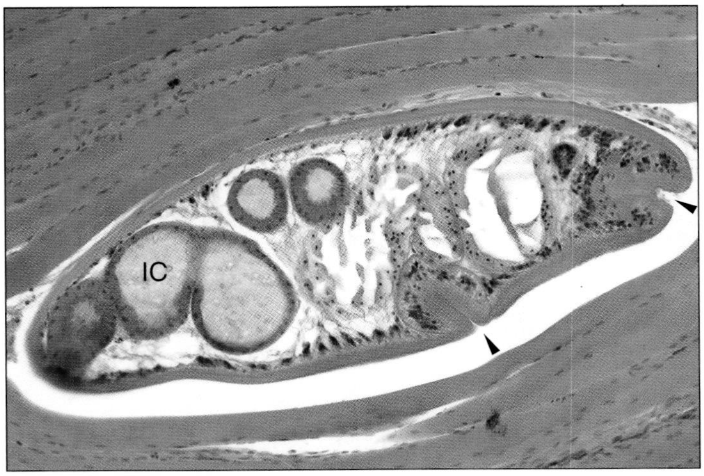

5

Heterophyes heterophyes

Heterophyiasis

Heterophyes heterophyes and *Metagonimus yokogawai* are two of the common species of heterophyid and similar intestinal flukes that parasitize humans. Many genera and species of these small trematodes mature not only in the human small intestine but also in a wide range of animal reservoir hosts, including birds, rodents, canids, felids, and many wild mammals. Many of these parasites are classified as heterophyids, but a large number belong to other, obscure families of trematodes that are normally parasites of mammals and birds and are minimally involved in human infections. Most lack host specificity, so that any one of these species may develop in a number of different hosts, including humans. Although many heterophyids have a wide geographic distribution, others may be localized. Human infections usually reflect the species that are prevalent in animal reservoirs in the geographic area.

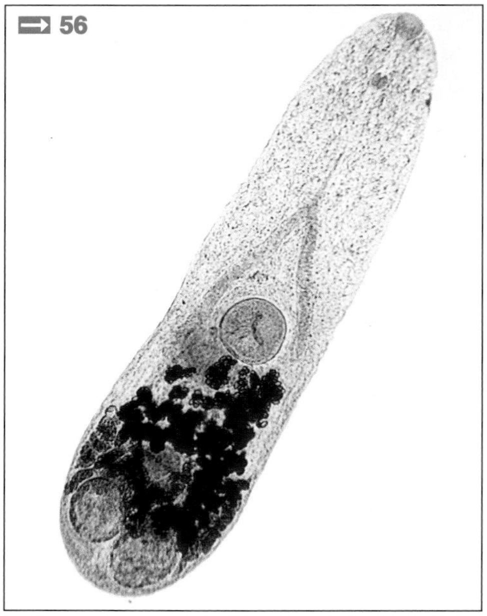

56

Biology and Life Cycle

Most of these small intestinal flukes live in the lumen or the crypts of the duodenum and jejunum of the small intestine (Plate 76:1–5). Some of the minute adult worms may burrow into the superficial mucosal epithelium. These organisms, which may be discovered inadvertently in intestinal biopsy specimens or at autopsy, have similar life cycles. For example, adult worms of *Heterophyes* and *Metagonimus* living in the crypts of the intestine produce small operculated eggs that contain a developed miracidium when excreted in feces. Freshwater snails and fish serve as first and second intermediate hosts, respectively. In fish, the infective metacercarial stage encysts under the scales, and the definitive host is infected by eating raw fish. Adult worms mature rapidly, typically within one or two weeks; their lifespan is usually only a few months.

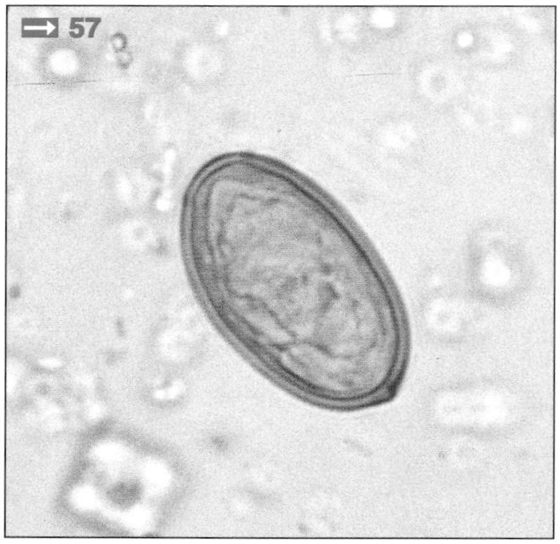

57

Pathology and Clinical Manifestations

Mild to moderate infections with small flukes are usually asymptomatic. Severe infections may produce abdominal tenderness, colicky pain, and mucous diarrhea. In general, these clinical manifestations pertain to most small fluke infections. Abnormalities associated with small fluke infections, primarily *Heterophyes* and *Metagonimus* infections, appear to be limited to mild inflammation and some necrosis in cases where the adult flukes are attached to or have burrowed into the mucosal epithelium. When adults lie within the epithelium near the vascular supply, the small eggs they produce may enter the bloodstream and become embolized in various organs and tissues, including the myocardium and central nervous system. Instances of such embolization in humans have been reported rarely in recent literature.

Parasite Morphology

Adult flukes such as *Heterophyes* and *Metagonimus* typically are minute, 1.0 to 2.5 mm in length by 0.3 to 0.7 mm in width (56). Eggs of the heterophyids and closely related species usually measure between 18 to 30 µm in length by 14 to 18 µm in width (57). Species of *Echinostoma* and related genera may attain lengths of up to 8 mm. Specific anatomic details for each species have been well described.

Many of these flukes have a spiny tegument (Plate 71:2 & 3). This feature, in conjunction with the small size of the parasite and the presence of embryonated eggs in sections through the uterus, facilitates a correct diagnosis.

The only other common human intestinal fluke is *Fasciolopsis buski*. It is much larger than any of the heterophyids, with a length of up to 75 mm, a width of 8 to 20 mm, and a thickness of 0.3 to 3.0 mm. Although infections with *Fasciolopsis* may result in inflammation and intestinal ulceration as well as abscesses in the intestinal wall, no pathologic descriptions or reports in the literature have depicted sections through parasites in tissue. Although it may not be possible to specifically identify small flukes encountered in tissue sections of the intestinal tract, a general diagnosis of trematode infection should be sufficient.

References

Africa CM, de Leon W, Garcia EY. Visceral complications in intestinal heterophyidiasis of man. *Acta Med Philipp.* 1940;1:1-122.

Collomb H, Deschiens REA, Demarchi J. Sur deux cas de distomatose cerebrale a *Heterophyes heterophyes. Bull Soc Pathol Exot.* 1960;53:144-147.

Kean BH, Breslau RC. Cardiac heterophyidiasis. In: *Parasites of the Human Heart.* New York, NY: Grune & Stratton; 1964.

Plate 76

Heterophyes heterophyes and Other Heterophyids

Image 1

Parasites in the mucosal epithelium of the small intestine of a patient from the Philippines. The largest section demonstrates the typical tegument and, internally, coils of the uterus, which contains eggs (H&E, 100x).

Image 2

An adult worm within a crypt of the small intestine. Among the anatomic features are the spiny tegument, the oral sucker (dart), typical parenchyma, and the muscular genital sucker (GS) which is just anterior to the coiled uterus containing eggs (H&E, 125x).

Image 3

At higher magnification, the oral sucker and spiny tegument are prominent (H&E, 500x).

Image 4

An adult heterophyidlike fluke in a crypt of the small intestine of a raccoon. The most prominent feature of this small fluke (0.5 mm long) is the coiled uterus (UT) containing many small eggs (H&E, 125x).

Image 5

At high magnification, the spiny tegument and the typical heterophyid eggs (20 µm x 10 µm) are seen (H&E, 500x).

Image 6

A small intestinal fluke lies within a crypt of the small intestine. This is a different fluke from that seen in Image 4 and Image 5. At the anterior end, several prominent spines (darts) at the level of the oral sucker are suggestive of, but different from, the collar spines associated with small intestinal flukes of the genus *Echinostoma*. Several species of *Echinostoma* are human parasites that might be encountered in the small intestine. In histologic section, a generic or specific designation is often impossible (H&E, 500x).

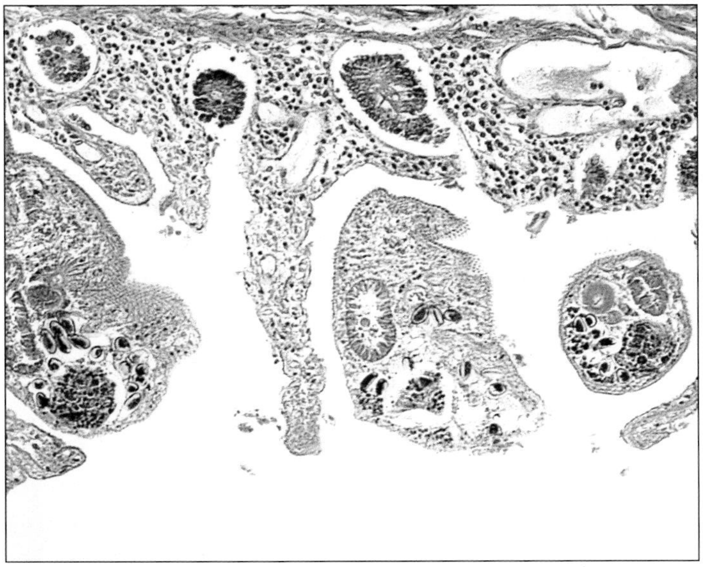

1

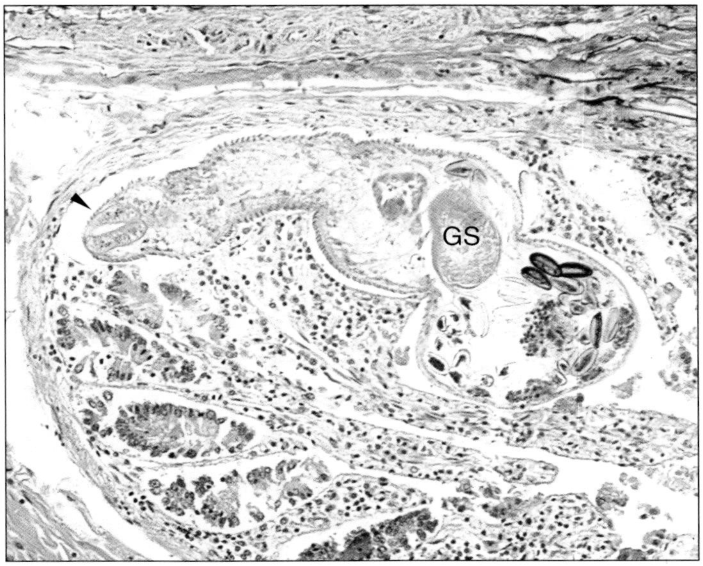

2

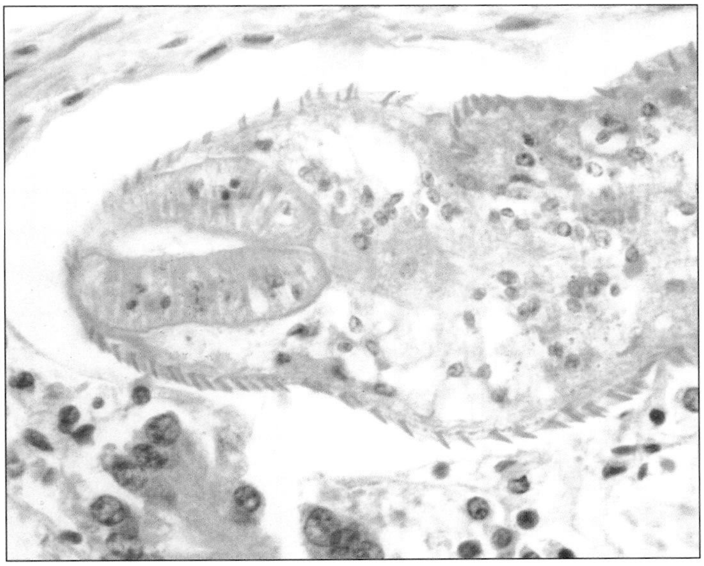

3

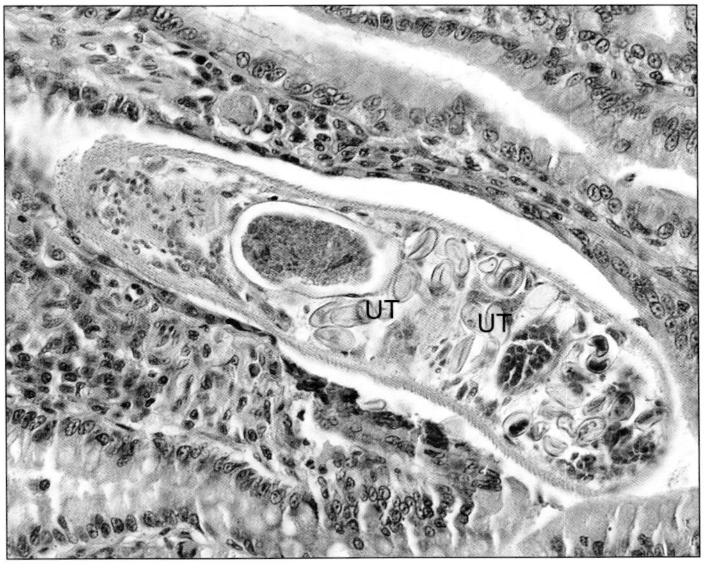

4

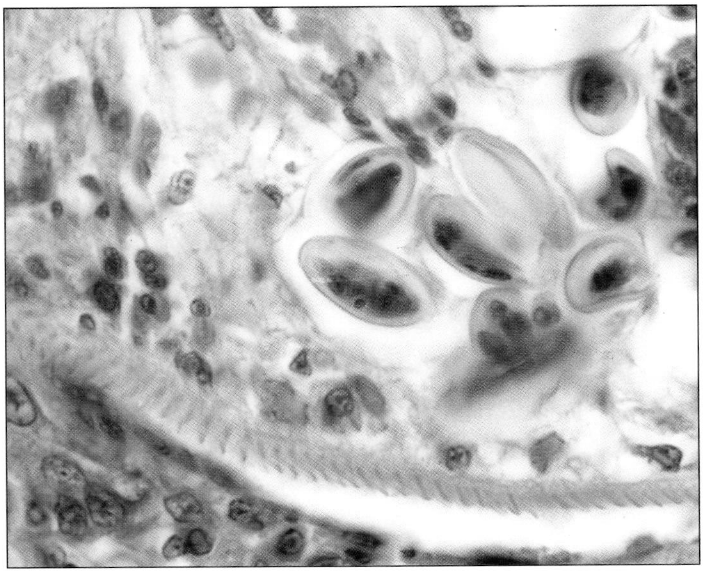

5

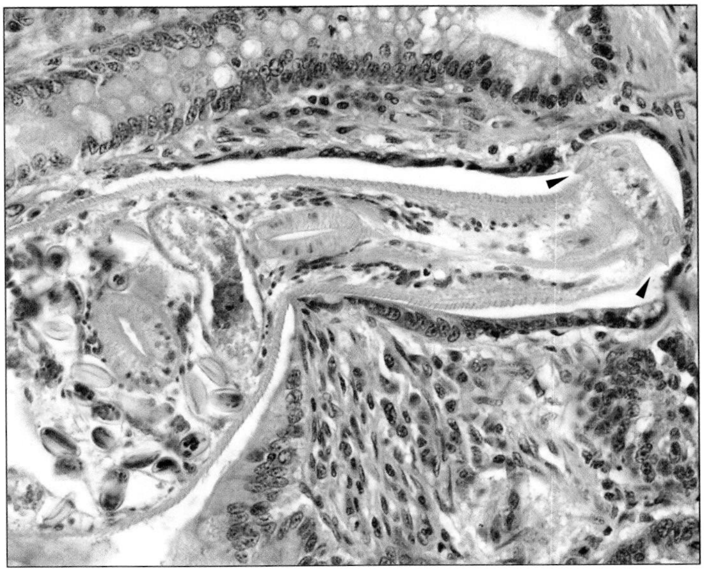

6

Fasciola hepatica

Fascioliasis

Fascioliasis is an important liver disease of sheep, cattle, and other herbivorous animals. It has worldwide distribution. The extensive liver disease produced in these animals by *Fasciola hepatica* is often referred to as liver rot and may have considerable economic impact in livestock-raising areas. Human infections are common, may occur in epidemic fashion, and have been reported from areas where there are infections in animals. Human cases in the Western Hemisphere are seen frequently in Puerto Rico, Mexico, and Latin America. In the United States, cases have been reported primarily from Hawaii. A closely related parasite, *Fasciola gigantica*, also parasitizes ruminants in the Americas, Africa, Asia, and the former Soviet Union, and causes human infections in Hawaii as well as other parts of the world. Another related parasite, *Fascioloides magna,* also causes severe infections in herbivorous animals in many areas of the world, but no cases of human infection have been described.

⇨ 58

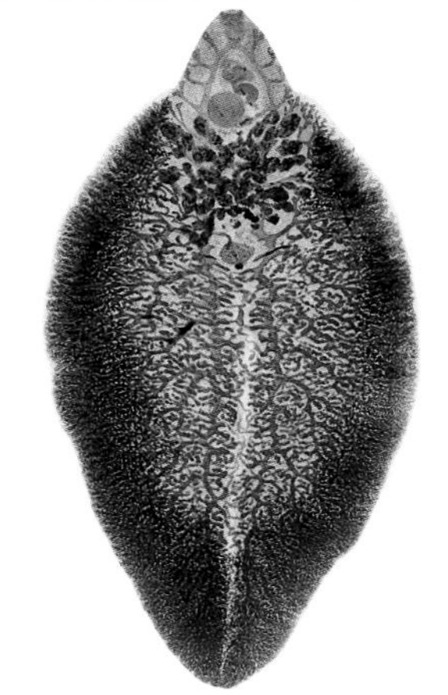

Biology and Life Cycle

The large, leaflike adult flukes (⇨ 58) normally live in the bile ducts of their definitive hosts, where they produce large, unembryonated eggs (⇨ 59) that are excreted in feces. Eggs develop in fresh water and miracidia invade appropriate snail intermediate hosts. Cercariae liberated from snails attach to various types of aquatic vegetation (eg, watercress, grass) and encyst to become metacercariae, which are infective for the definitive host. After ingestion, the metacercariae burrow through the wall of the intestine into the abdominal cavity, come in contact with the liver, and penetrate through Glisson's capsule to enter the parenchyma and then the bile ducts, where they reach maturity in approximately two to four months. A similar course of migration occurs in humans who accidentally ingest metacercariae on vegetation.

⇨ 59

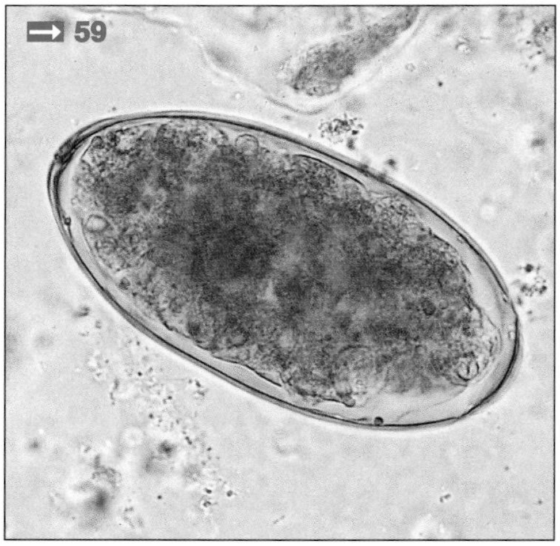

Pathology and Clinical Manifestations

Early infection in humans is characterized by abdominal tenderness, epigastric pain, fever, nausea, and vomiting. Migration of the parasite through the liver parenchyma to the bile ducts results in leukocytosis, severe eosinophilia, and hepatomegaly. Once the parasites are established in the biliary tree, chronic infection manifests as diarrhea, anemia, and cholelithiasis. Pathologically, the presence of parasites within the bile ducts results in fibrosis and extensive proliferation of bile duct epithelium. Erosion of bile duct epithelium by the flukes often results in invasion of the parenchyma, where abscesses are produced and the adult worms die and disintegrate. As a result, frequently only eggs are found in histologic sections. In addition to the liver manifestations, the migration of metacercarial stages through the intestinal wall in the initial stages of human infection may result in worms ending up in ectopic locations, including the abdominal wall, subcutaneous tissues, lungs, and brain. The dead or dying worms produce abscesses in these locations.

Parasite Morphology

Adult *F. hepatica* worms are large and fleshy, measuring up to 50 mm long by 13 mm wide. The fluke tapers to form a cephalic cone anteriorly and has a broadly rounded posterior end (⇨ 58). The tegument is spinose with fewer spines on the posterior portion of the body (Plate 77:1, 2, & 4). The oral and ventral suckers are near each other in the anterior end; the ventral sucker is somewhat larger. The ovary is anterior to the paired testes, which lie one behind the other in the posterior half of the body. These organs are highly branched. The uterus is short and coiled and opens at the genital pore slightly anterior to the ventral sucker. The extensive vitelline follicles are highly branched and extend along the lateral margins from the ventral sucker to the posterior end. Eggs are large (130 to 150 µm long by 70 to 90 µm wide), are unembryonated when laid, and have a moderately thick shell and an indistinct operculum (⇨ 59). *Fasciola gigantica* is a larger organism, up to 75 mm long, and the eggs range from 150 to 200 µm long by 90 to 100 µm wide. Adults of *Fascioloides magna* may reach 100 mm long, and their eggs range from 100 to 170 µm long by 75 to 100 µm wide.

In microscopic sections, fasciolids have a thick tegument with spines, sometimes scalelike, which are spaced irregularly and are fewer posteriorly (Plate 77:1, 2, & 4). Due to the extensive branching of the various organs, multiple sections of intestinal ceca, testes, and ovary are characteristic findings within the parenchyma (Plate 77:1–3). Eggs appear moderately thick shelled. Because of their large size, it is not common to see whole eggs in histologic section. Instead, eggs are often collapsed or otherwise distorted or seen in oblique or cross-sections (Plate 77:5 & 6). These eggs, which demonstrate typical fasciolid egg morphology, are those of *Fasciolides magna*, a parasite of herbivores and not reported from humans. Because migration into the liver parenchyma or ectopic locations casues the worms to die and disintegrate, only eggs are seen in the abscesses that the parasites produce.

Other liver flukes such as *Clonorchis*, *Opisthorchis*, and *Dicrocoelium* are smaller and more delicate than *Fasciola*. The presence in bile ducts of large flukes that have spines on their tegument, multiple sections through various organs, and large eggs suggests a diagnosis of fasciolid infection. When flukes occur in ectopic locations, one must consider whether the diagnosis is fascioliasis, paragonimiasis, or some other, rarer type of zoonotic trematode infection.

References

Acosta-Ferreira W, Vercelli-Retta J, Falconi LM. *Fasciola hepatica* human infection: histopathological study of sixteen cases. *Virchows Arch A Pathol Anat*. 1979;383:319-327.

Dawes B, Hughes DL. Fascioliasis: the invasive stage of *Fasciola hepatica* in mammalian hosts. *Adv Parasitol*. 1964;2:97-165.

Park CI, Ro JY, Kim H, et al. Human ectopic fascioliasis in the cecum. *Am J Surg Pathol*. 1984;8:73-77.

Stemmermann GN. Human infestation with *Fasciola gigantica*. *Am J Pathol*. 1953;29:731-753.

Swales WE. Further studies on *Fascioloides magna* (Bassi, 1875) Ward, 1917, as a parasite of ruminants. *Can J Res*. 1936;14:83-95.

Plate 77

Fasciola hepatica

Image 1

Adult *Fasciola hepatica* in the pancreatic duct of a goat. At this magnification, the thick tegument bearing spines and multiple sections through the highly branched intestinal ceca (keyline) and testes (TE) within parenchyma can be seen (H&E, 35x).

Image 2

At higher magnification, irregularly spaced spines (darts), with underlying muscle and tegumental cells, are seen. A single section through an intestinal cecum and multiple sections through branched testes (TE) are found (H&E, 100x).

Image 3

Ectopic location of an adult *Fasciola* in the wall of the colon of a Korean. At scanning magnification, the spines in the tegument are not readily visible, but intestinal ceca and portions of the testes are clear (H&E, 20x).

Image 4

Fascioloides magna, adult worm. This section shows the typical tegument, the underlying muscle layers, tegumental cells, and the parenchyma. The spines (darts) are dark pink and scalelike (H&E, 125x).

Image 5

Eggs of *F. magna* in the liver of a sheep (H&E, 250x).

Image 6

At higher magnification, note the thickness of the shell. This partial section of an egg measures approximately 80 µm x 50 µm. Eggs of this size suggest a fasciolid (H&E, 400x).

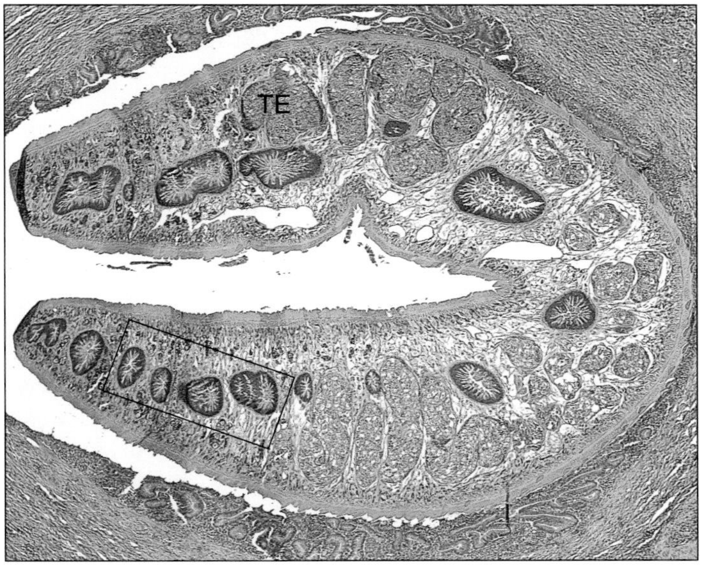

1

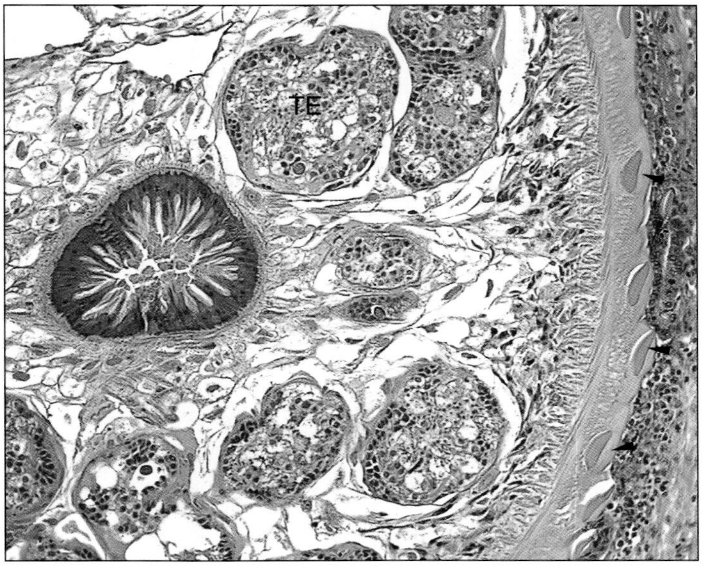

2

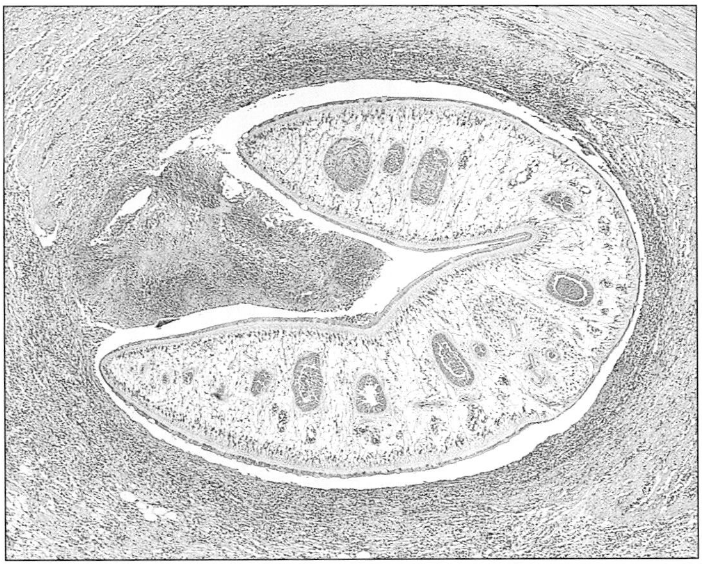

3

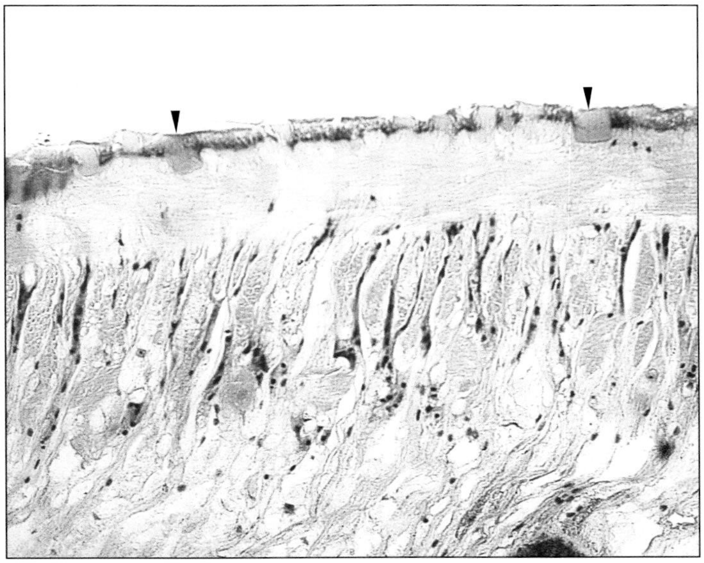

4

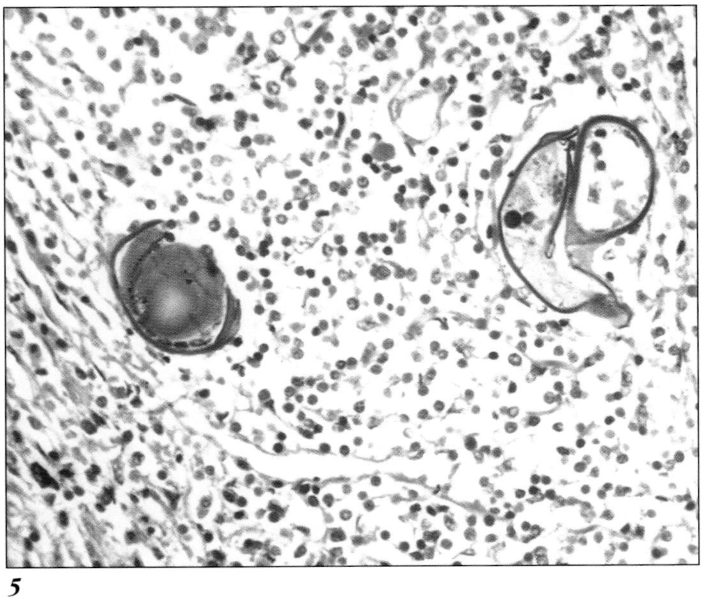

5

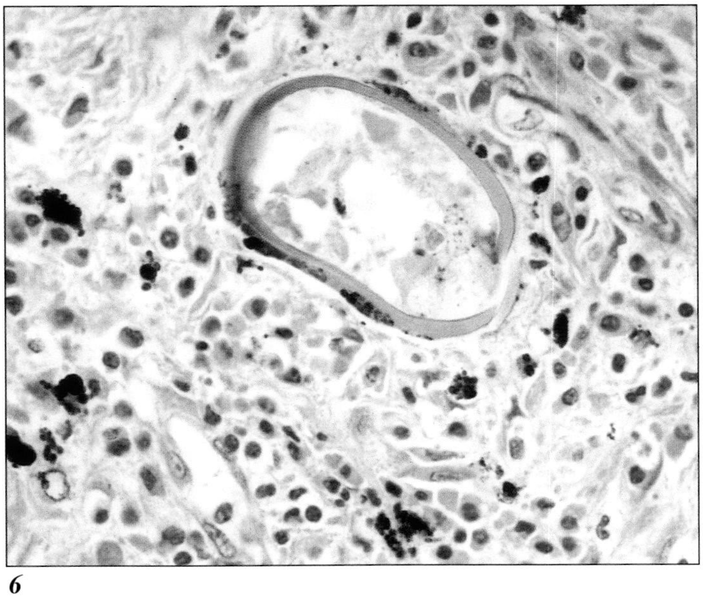

6

Clonorchis sinensis

Clonorchiasis

Both *Clonorchis sinensis*, the Chinese liver fluke, which is endemic to Asia, and species of the related genus *Opisthorchis* (*O. viverrini* and *O. felineus*), which occur in Asia and Europe, live in the bile ducts of humans and animals. Prevalence rates in humans may be high in geographic areas where raw or inadequately cooked fish are commonly consumed.

Biology and Life Cycle

These hermaphroditic adult trematodes live within the bile ducts of the liver of their definitive hosts (most frequently humans, cats, and dogs) (Plate 78). Embryonated, operculated eggs are shed into the bile ducts and are excreted in feces. Freshwater snails and fish serve as first and second intermediate hosts, respectively. Metacercariae, the infective stage, become encysted under the scales and in the skin and flesh of fish. Infection is acquired by ingesting inadequately cooked, infected fish. In the final host, the larval flukes migrate from the intestine to the liver via the common bile duct and develop into egg-laying adult worms in approximately three months. The life span of adult worms may exceed one to two decades.

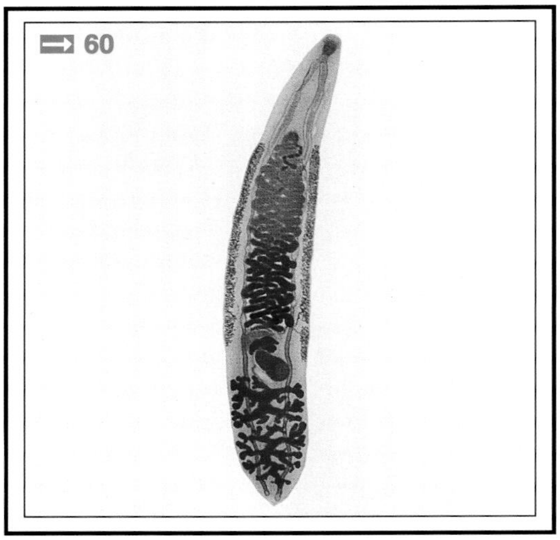

⇒ 60

Pathology and Clinical Manifestations

Clinical manifestations of clonorchiasis or opisthorchiasis depend on the number of parasites present and the duration of the infection. Individuals infected with few parasites are often asymptomatic, whereas those with heavy worm burdens of long duration may have anorexia, diarrhea, fever, jaundice, and moderate eosinophilia. Pathologic changes in heavy infections of *Clonorchis* include liver enlargement, fibrotic thickening of the bile ducts, proliferation of biliary epithelium, and cholelithiasis. Invasion of the gall bladder and pancreatic duct by adult worms is frequent in severe infections. Infections produced by *Opisthorchis viverrini* differ from those produced by *Clonorchis* in that invasion of the gall bladder is a common feature of severe infections. In several epidemiologic studies, long-term liver fluke infections resulting in hyperplasia of bile duct epithelium have been associated with the development of cholangiocarcinoma.

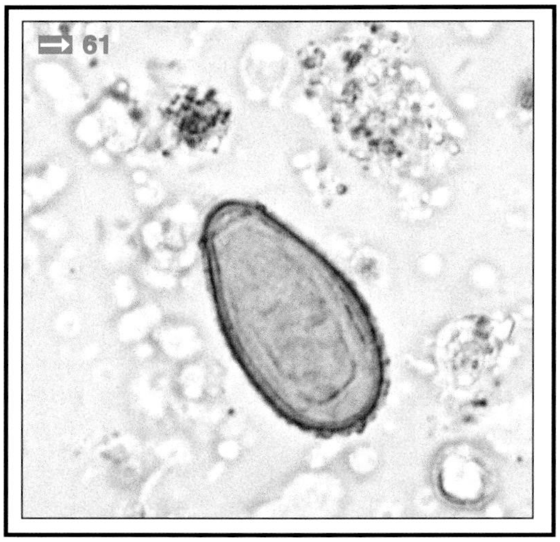

⇒ 61

Parasite Morphology

Adult *C. sinensis* parasites are transparent, flattened, and attenuated anteriorly, measuring 10 to 25 mm long by 3 to 5 mm wide (⇒ 60). The tegument lacks spines. The oral and ventral suckers are small, with the ventral sucker and the opening of the genital pore in close apposition in the lower portion of the anterior third of the body. Coils of the uterus are located between the ventral sucker and the ovary. The paired, greatly branched testes are positioned one behind the other in the posterior third of the body. Vitellaria occupy the lateral fields in the middle third of the body. Eggs of *Clonorchis* are small (27 to 35 µm long by 12 to 19 µm wide) and yellow-brown. They have a seated operculum, a moderately thick shell, and a small knob or protuberance at the abopercular end (⇒ 61). Eggs are embryonated and contain a miracidium when passed in feces. Adults of *O. viverrini* and *O. felineus* are approximately half the size (5.5 to 10.0 mm by 0.8 to 1.5 mm) of *Clonorchis*, and their testes are not as deeply branched.

In microscopic sections, adult worms have typical trematode features. The tegument is a cytoplasmic syncytium that lacks spines and overlies a spongy parenchyma consisting of parenchymal cells and fibrous interstitial tissue that fills the body. Sections through the uterus of the worm show characteristic eggs, with at least some demonstrating typical size and a seated operculum (Plate 78:2–4). In some instances, eggs alone may be found within the bile ducts. Dead parasites may exhibit marked degenerative changes in their histologic morphology.

Histologic sections showing adult trematodes in bile ducts of the liver may suggest several possible parasites, including *C. sinensis*, *Opisthorchis* species, *Dicrocoelium dendriticum*, and *Fasciola* species. *Fasciola* are large flukes that produce large, thin-shelled, unembryonated eggs and can be readily distinguished from other, smaller species. Although adults of *Dicrocoelium* are similar to the opisthorchid flukes in size, their eggs are larger, thicker shelled, and have no seated operculum. The identification of the parasite as *Clonorchis* or *Opisthorchis* depends to a great extent on the geographic location in which the infection was acquired. *Clonorchis, Opisthorchis*, and *Fasciola* adults may be found in the gall bladder and pancreatic ducts in severe infections.

References

Chan PH, Teoh TB. The pathology of *Clonorchis sinensis* infestation of the pancreas. *J Pathol Bacteriol.* 1967;93:185-189.

Hou PC. The pathology of *Clonorchis sinensis* infestation of the liver. *J Pathol Bacteriol.* 1955;70:53-64.

Koompirochana C, Sonakul D, Chinda C, et al. Opisthorchiasis: a clinicopathologic study of 154 autopsy cases. *Southeast Asian J Trop Med Public Health.* 1978;9:60-64.

Mohamed ARE, Mummery V. Human dicrocoeliasis: report on 208 cases from Saudi Arabia. *Trop Geogr Med.* 1990;42:1-7.

Plate 78

Clonorchis sinensis

Image 1

In this parasagittal section of an adult *Clonorchis*, the parasite is seen within a dilated human bile duct that has undergone considerable proliferation of the biliary epithelium. Five sections through the branched, blue-staining testes are seen, the largest of which lies next to a portion of the excretory canal (EC). Two small tubules with an epithelial lining and prominent lumina represent the intestinal ceca (darts) (H&E, 50x).

Image 2

In this transverse view of a *Clonorchis* adult situated within a human bile duct, the muscular ventral sucker (VS) is visible. Coils of the uterus containing eggs can be seen between the sucker and the two lobes of the ovary. Intestinal ceca (darts) with their epithelial lining and excretory tubules near to each side are also visible (H&E, 50x).

Image 3

Clonorchis adult in a human bile duct demonstrates the typical appearance of trematode parenchyma. Coils of the uterus containing eggs are seen. The two large tubules with an epithelial lining (darts) are the intestinal ceca (H&E, 50x).

Image 4

At higher magnification, typical eggs in the uterus are seen. One egg (dart) is in almost perfect sagittal section. The size and morphology of these eggs facilitate identification of the parasite (H&E, 500x).

Image 5

Clonorchis adult in a bile duct. At this magnification, details of typical trematode morphology are visible: the smooth tegument, muscle layers, and the spongiform parenchyma. In this plane of section, no reproductive structures are seen. The two tubular structures represent sections through the two intestinal ceca (H&E, 125x).

Image 6

Adult *Opisthorchis viverrini* in the bile duct of a cat. Although smaller than *Clonorchis*, the adults of this and other *Opisthorchis* species have a similar histologic appearance. In this section, coils of the uterus, a few vitellaria (keyline), and the paired intestinal ceca (darts) can be seen within the parenchyma (H&E, 50x).

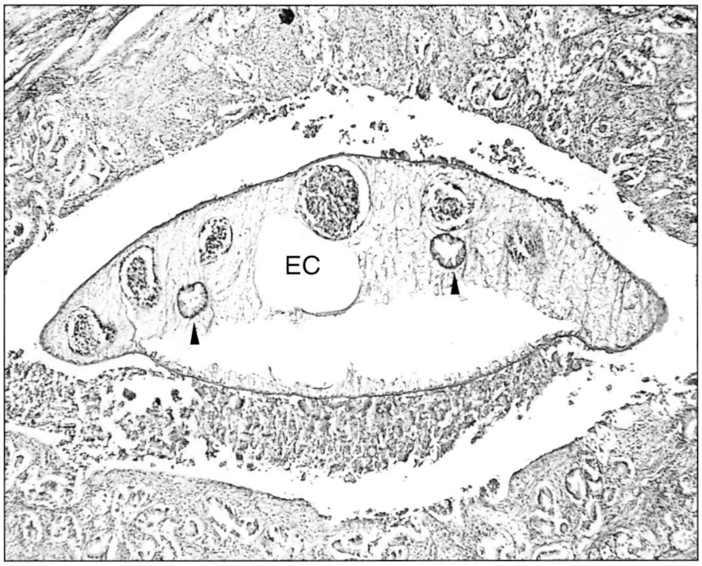

1

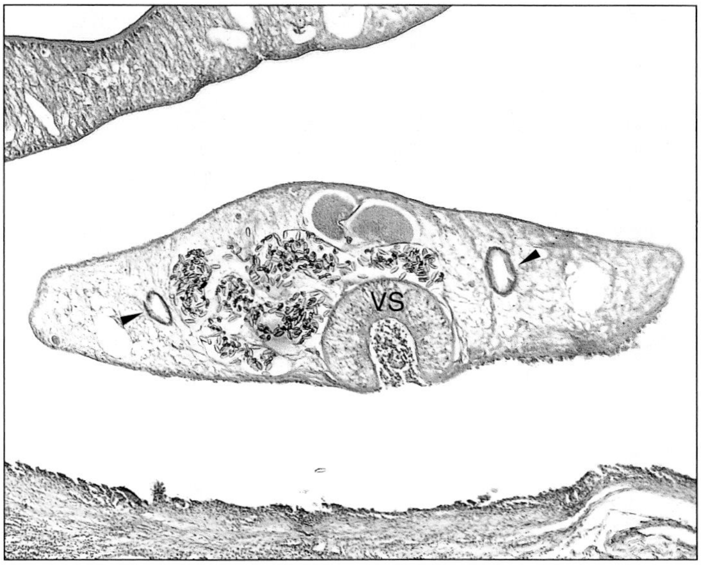

2

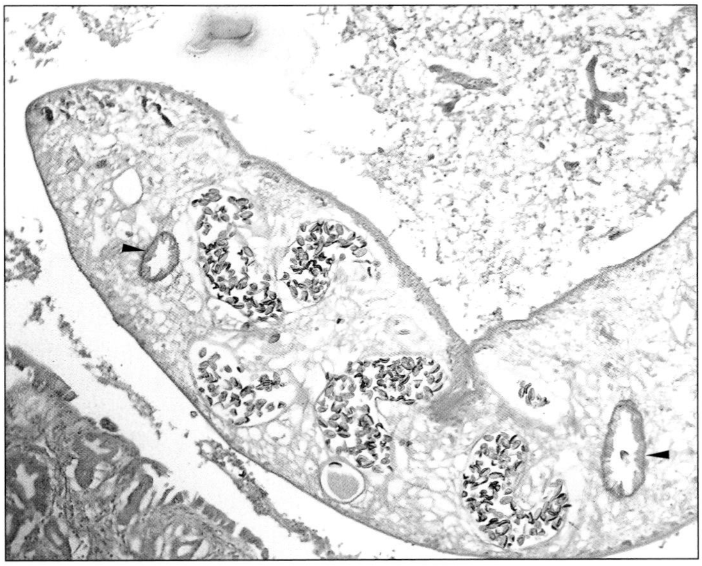

3

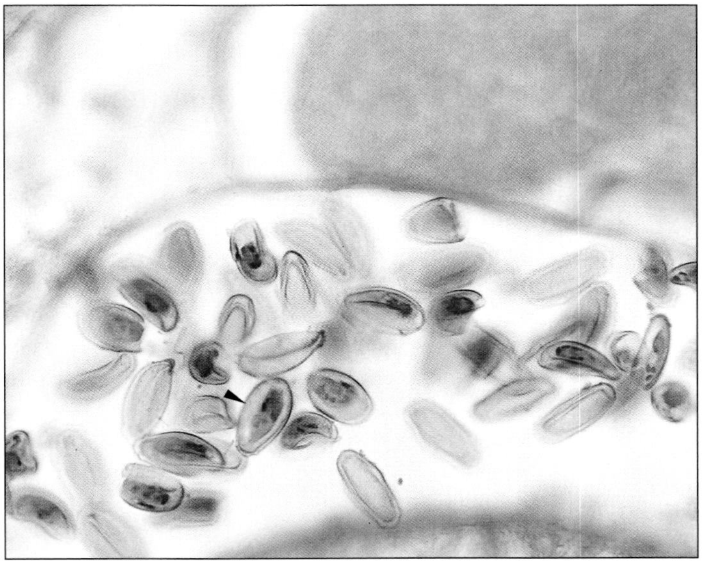

4

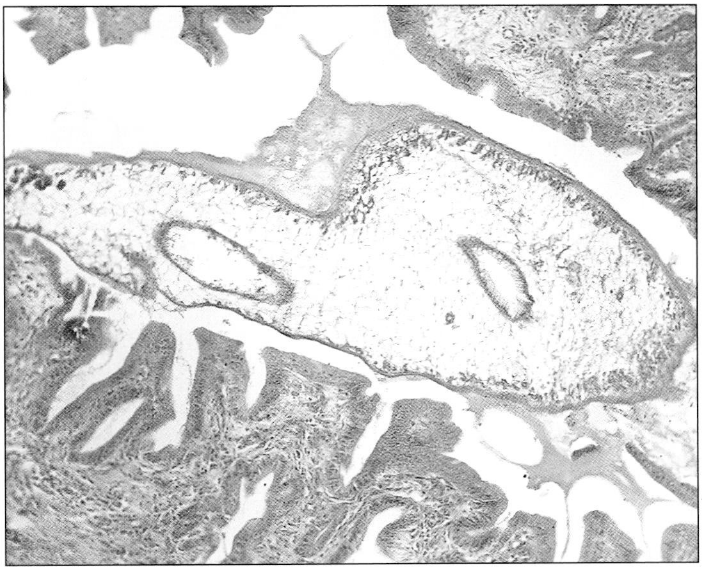

5

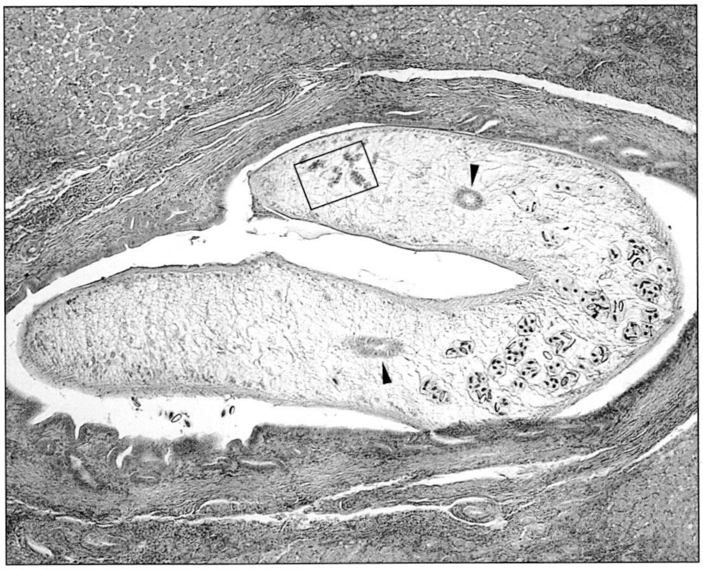

6

Paragonimus westermani

Paragonimiasis

Human paragonimiasis is caused by many species of lung flukes of the genus *Paragonimus*, the most important of which is *P. westermani*. The disease is distributed in Asia, India, Latin America, and Africa, where various types of canids and felids serve as significant animal reservoirs for human infection. Among the species causing human disease are *P. westermani, P. miyazakii*, and *P. heterotremus* in Asia; *P. africanus* and *P. uterobilateralis* in Africa; and *P. mexicanus* and *P. ecuadoriensis* in Latin America.

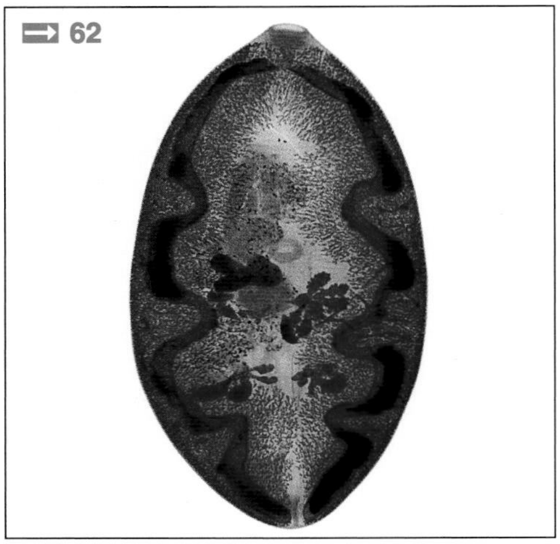

⇒ 62

Biology and Life Cycle

These adult lung flukes typically live encapsulated in the parenchyma of the lung, usually in pairs. Unembryonated eggs are discharged by the adult and move up the bronchial tree; they are subsequently found in sputum or are swallowed and excreted in feces. Eggs must embryonate in water for several weeks or longer before miracidia are produced. Crabs and crayfish serve as the usual second intermediate hosts; human or animal infections are acquired by ingesting the infective metacercarial stage in raw or inadequately cooked crustaceans. The consumption of infected crustaceans by wild boars and perhaps other food animals results in metacercarial invasion of tissues by *P. westermani*. Some human infections may be acquired by eating inadequately cooked meat of infected animals. In definitive hosts, the larval fluke migrates through the intestinal wall, enters the abdominal cavity, migrates through the diaphragm to the thoracic cavity, and invades the lung parenchyma. Worms reach maturity and become encapsulated in the lung in approximately three months. Infections may persist for 10 years or longer.

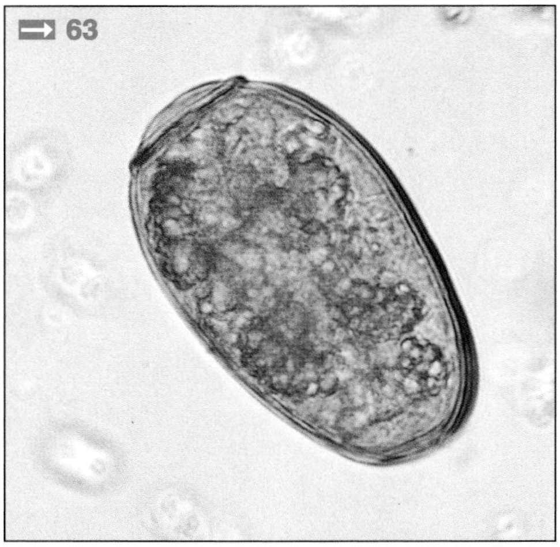

⇒ 63

Pathology and Clinical Manifestations

Pulmonary manifestations may be nonspecific, but pleural pain, persistent cough (especially in the morning), and hemoptysis are common. Sputum is characteristically viscous and tinged with blood and flecks of rusty brown material, which when examined microscopically is found to contain eggs of the parasite. Eosinophilia often accompanies the infection.

Pathologic findings vary considerably. Thick, fibrous cysts containing adult worms are characteristically present. When worms die and undergo degeneration, large abscess cavities may form in which only eggs, sometimes calcified, may be found. Sections of typical eggs also may be found in granulomas in the vicinity of cysts. Aberrant migration of larval *Paragonimus* is a common feature of infection in humans (Plate 79:5). Worms develop in the intestinal wall or migrate from the abdominal cavity to the wall of the abdomen or to other tissues, including the brain, where they reach maturity, produce eggs, and subsequently die. Resulting abscesses, when examined histologically, show dead worms or necrotic tissue in which only eggs remain identifiable. Abscesses in the central nervous system are often fatal.

Parasite Morphology

Living *P. westermani* are red-brown, thick, robust, and ovoid. They measure 7.5 to 12.0 mm in length, 4 to 6 mm in width, and are 3 to 5 mm thick (⇒ 62). The tegument has spines on its surface (Plate 79:3 & 4). The lobed ovary is slightly anterior to the paired, branched testes, which are nearly side by side in the upper portion of the posterior third of the body. Vitellaria occur as extensively branched follicles from the lateral margins toward the midline of the flukes. The operculated, unembryo-nated eggs are moderately large, thick shelled, and broadly ovoid, measuring 80 to 120 μm by 45 to 70 μm (⇒ 63). At the abopercular end of the egg, the shell is thickened. Adult worms of the various species of *Paragonimus* are similar in basic morphology, but their size and shape may vary considerably. Eggs of the different species are also similar, but they show variations in size, shape, and the appearance of the operculum.

In microscopic sections, *Paragonimus* adults typically present as paired or sometimes single large trematodes surrounded by a fibrous tissue capsule (Plate 79:1). When only eggs are found in sections, their size, shell thickness, and the presence of the operculum usually allow for at least an identification of the genus (Plate 79:6).

The presence of large flukes in a fibrous capsule of the lung is a strong indication of *Paragonimus* infection. Spines in the thick tegument, typical eggs in the surrounding tissue, and the other features described above make diagnosing lung fluke infection relatively easy. When flukes are present in aberrant tissue locations, the correct diagnosis of paragonimiasis may be less clear cut. Eggs cut in transverse sections make it difficult to estimate size and overall appearance. Other rare trematode infections (eg, *Achillurbainia* and *Poikilorchis*) can be found in human tissues, and their eggs may be difficult to distinguish from those of *Paragonimus*.

References

Diaconita G, Goldis G. Investigations on pathomorphology and pathogenesis of pulmonary paragonimiasis. *Acta Tubercul Scand.* 1964;44:51-75.

Oh SJ. Cerebral and spinal paragonimiasis: a histopathological study. *J Neurol Sci.* 1969;9:205-206.

Oh SJ. Paragonimiasis in the central nervous system. In: Vinken PJ, Bruyn GW, eds. *Handbook of Clinical Neurology, Part III: Infections of the Nervous System.* 1978;35:243-266.

Yokogawa M. *Paragonimus* and paragonimiasis. *Adv Parasitol.* 1965;3:99-158.

Paragonimus westermani

Image 1

A pair of *P. westermani* adult worms in a fibrous capsule in the lung of an experimentally infected dog. At this magnification, one can see the dark-staining clumps of vitelline glands (H&E, 20x).

Image 2

Another section of *P. westermani* from the same experimentally infected dog. Five sections through the branched testes (TE) and a few coils of uterus (arrow) containing eggs are seen. The intestinal ceca (darts) are evident, each one near the small, brown-staining vitelline follicles (H&E, 25x).

Image 3

In this section of *P. westermani*, the thick tegument containing spines (keyline) overlies the muscle layers and the parenchyma. The prominent, dark-staining structure in the center is a section through one of the intestinal ceca (H&E, 100x).

Image 4

At high magnification, the prominent, red-staining spines on the tegument are readily visible. Muscle can be noted beneath the tegument. Within the parenchyma, prominent, dark-staining vitelline follicles are evident (Trichrome, 125x).

Image 5

A developing *Paragonimus*, species unknown, is seen in human subcutaneous fatty tissue of a Honduran. The prominent muscular sucker is the ventral sucker, and intestinal ceca (darts) are present within the parenchyma (H&E, 20x).

Image 6

A *P. westermani* egg in an abscess. In longitudinal section, this egg demonstrates the typical size, shell thickness, and operculum (dart) (H&E, 450x).

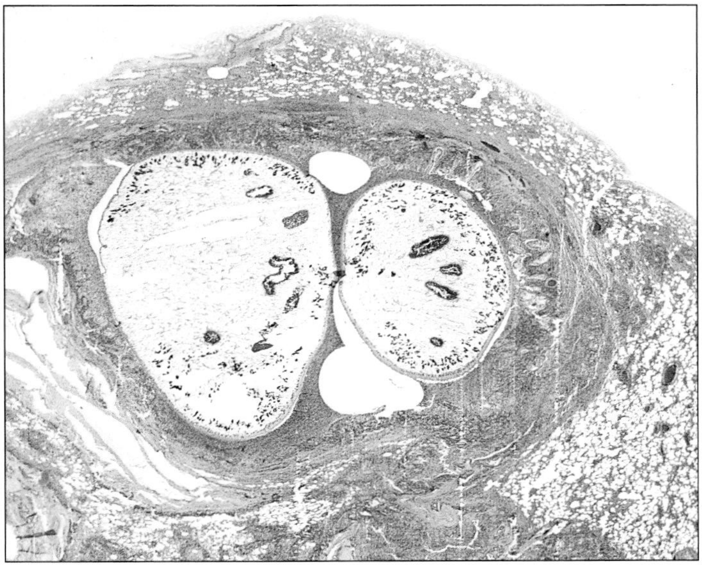

1

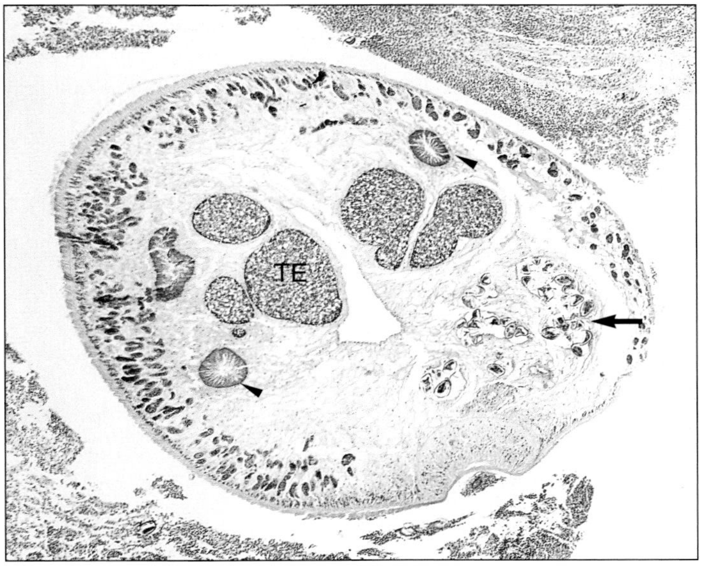

2

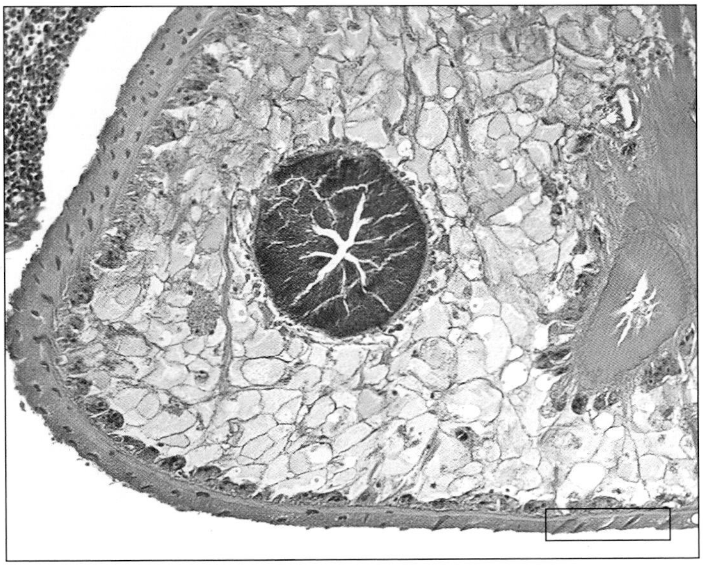

3

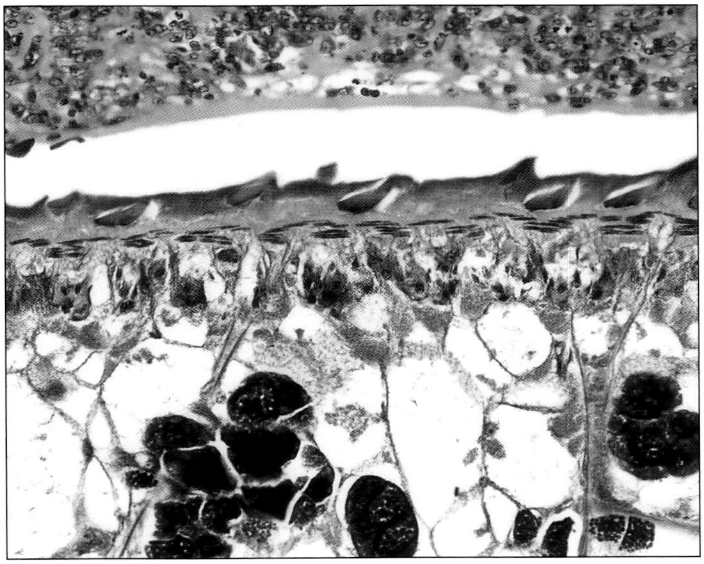

4

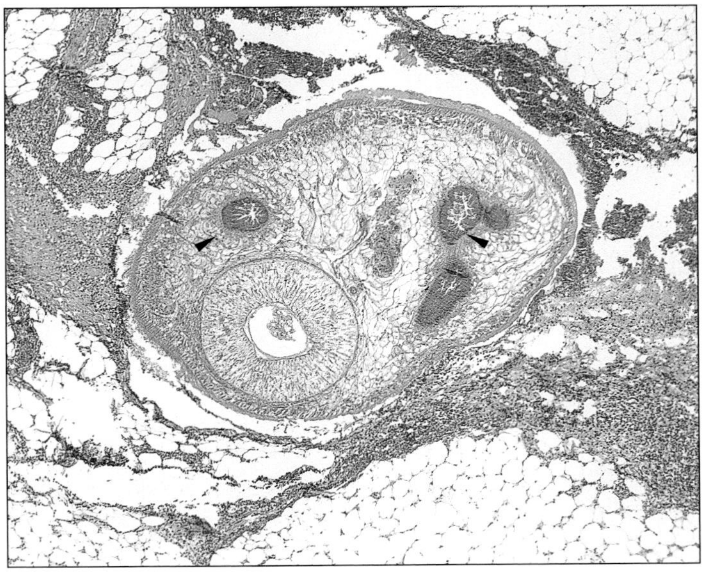

5

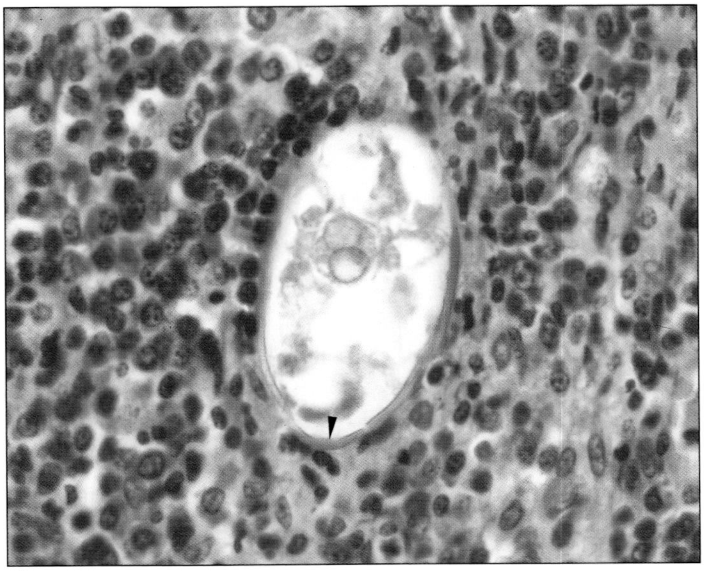

6

Schistosoma mansoni

Schistosomiasis mansoni

Schistosoma mansoni is one of the three major human schistosome parasites and the only one that occurs in the Western Hemisphere as well as Africa and the Arabian peninsula. In the Americas, it is prevalent in Brazil, many islands of the West Indies, and a few foci in Puerto Rico. The parasite is distributed widely in Africa, including the Nile River valley, much of West and East Africa, and South Africa. Human disease is often referred to as intestinal schistosomiasis or bilharziasis. As with the other schistosomes, the worms have separate sexes and live within blood vessels.

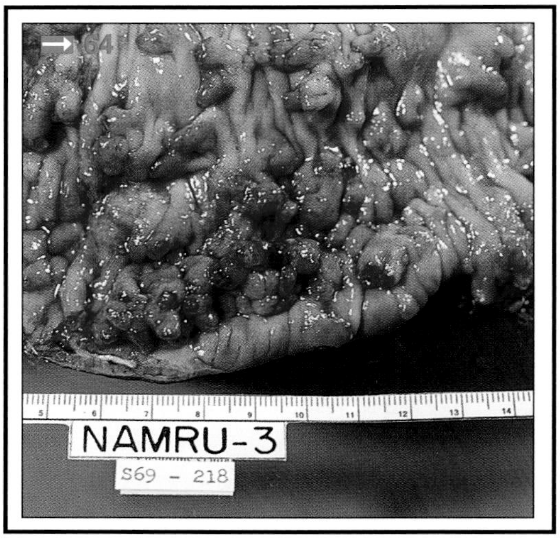

Biology and Life Cycle

Adult male and female *S. mansoni* parasites live primarily in the hemorrhoidal venous plexus draining the lower ileum and colon, but they also are found in the portal system of the liver. Eggs are laid in small venules near the mucosa of the rectum and sigmoidal region of the colon. They make their way through the wall of the intestine to reach the lumen and pass out of the body in feces. In fresh water, miracidia hatch and undergo further development in snails of the genus *Biomphalaria*. Liberated cercariae produced after several weeks of intramolluscan development are fork tailed and active in water. They initiate human infection by direct invasion through the skin. In the human host, the larval stage (now called a schistosomulum) migrates via the bloodstream to the lungs, liver, and mesenteric venules to complete maturation. Worms require six to eight weeks before they mature and begin laying eggs. Adult worms live for two decades or more.

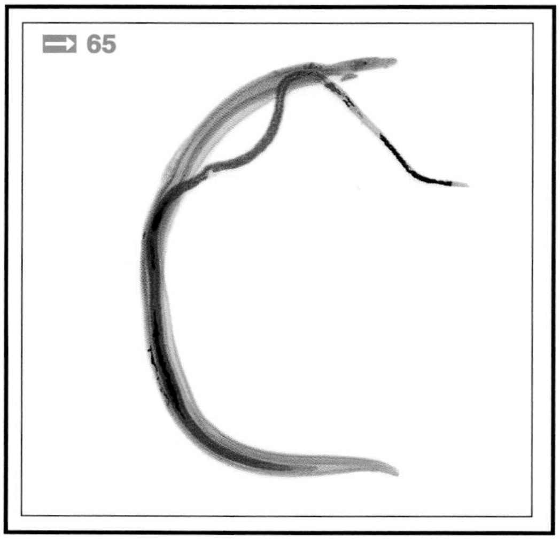

Pathology and Clinical Manifestations

As with all of the human schistosomes, both clinical expression of disease and pathologic events can be divided into acute and chronic phases. Symptomatically, early and mild infections may go unrecognized unless eggs are found in fecal examinations. More severe infections can cause skin rash and pruritus, diarrhea, fever, cough, eosinophilia, diffuse lymphadenopathy, general malaise, and hepatomegaly and splenomegaly over the course of several months. With the beginning of egg deposition, symptoms include abdominal pain and diarrhea followed by dysentery. Host response to eggs deposited in tissues is the most important event in the complex series of pathophysiologic reactions associated with chronic schistosomiasis. In tissues, circumoval granulomas form around eggs. Granulomata that first develop consist of a cellular infiltration of neutrophils and eosinophils. These cells are followed by a proliferation of lymphocytes and macrophages and giant cell formation. The lesions heal by fibrosis.

Lesions occur initially in the wall of the intestinal tract, resulting in inflammation, thickening, fibrosis, and polyp formation (➡ 64). The concentration of eggs within the polyps is much higher than elsewhere in the intestine. Eggs in the liver infiltrate the intrahepatic portal system, resulting in granuloma formation that can cause classic Symmers' pipestem fibrosis and hepatomegaly. Hepatosplenic involvement is the most important cause of morbidity in this infection. Calcification of *S. mansoni* eggs in human tissues is not seen as commonly as calcification of *S. japonicum* and *S. haematobium* eggs. Eggs provoking typical granulomatous lesions disseminate to many tissues and organs, including the lungs, spleen, kidneys, myocardium, spinal cord, and other sites. Within the fibrous lesions, eggs often appear collapsed or distorted in various stages of degeneration .

Parasite Morphology

Adult worms are usually found in copula (➡ 65). Male worms are robust, measuring 6.4 to 12.0 mm long. The posterior portions of their bodies are folded ventrally to form a gynecophoral canal. The slender female worms, measuring 7.2 to 17.0 mm long, lie within the gynecophoral canal. Males have a grossly tuberculate tegument, two small suckers in the anterior part of the body, and six to nine testes that lie slightly posterior to the ventral sucker. Female worms lack tuberculation on their tegument, have a single ovary near the ventral sucker, and have a short uterus that contains only one or a few large, lateral-spined eggs. Vitelline glands occur in the lateral fields in the posterior part of the female body. The intestinal tract in both sexes bifurcates at the level of the ventral sucker. Mature eggs are 114 to 175 µm long and 45 to 70 µm wide. They have a transparent shell with a large lateral spine and contain a miracidium when passed in feces (⇨ 66).

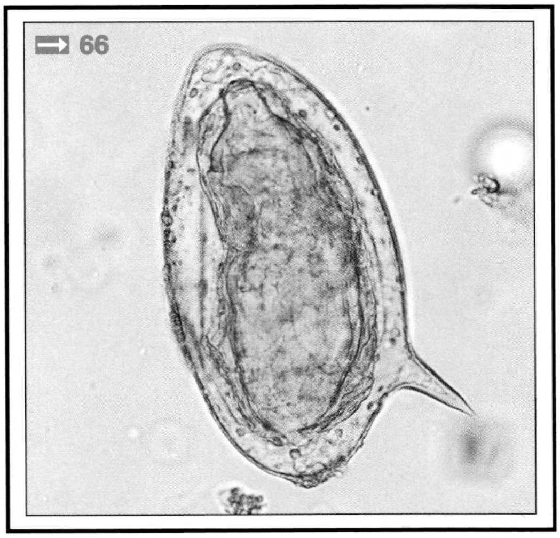

In microscopic sections the elongated adult worms, either singly or in copula, are seen most frequently as transverse sections within blood vessels in the wall of the intestine or in the liver (Plate 80:1 & 2). When in copula, the larger sections of the male worms surround the more slender females lying within the gynecophoral canal. In histologic sections male worms not only are larger but the intestinal ceca and, less frequently, the testes and the suckers are most often seen within the parenchyma. Prominent tuberculations on the tegument are characteristic of *S. mansoni*. Females in section usually demonstrate intestinal ceca and, more rarely, portions of the reproductive system. It is more common to find eggs than adult worms in tissue (Plate 80:3–6). Eggs within the characteristic-appearing pseudotubercle (egg granulomas) (Plate 80:6) indicate a possible diagnosis of schistosomiasis, but specific identification depends on morphologic features and epidemiologic considerations. The large lateral spine may be seen in whole or in part in some of the eggs (Plate 80:4 & 5). In many instances, only collapsed and distorted eggshells are found, which often do not give a true impression of size. The miracidium is clearly visible in some eggs, whereas in others it cannot be seen.

Schistosome eggs within granulomas in the intestinal wall are usually *S. mansoni* or *S. japonicum,* although rarer and more geographically localized infections with *S. mekongi* or *S. intercalatum* are a possibility. In tissue section, *S. mansoni* eggs can usually be distinguished from those of *S. japonicum* on the basis of size and the lateral spine. In the liver, eggs of *S. japonicum* are often more numerous because the species has a greater egg-laying capacity. The eggs are smaller, and their shell wall is usually more distorted. Calcified eggs in the liver are seen less frequently with *S. mansoni* than with *S. japonicum*.

References

Mousa AH, Ata AA, El Rooby A, et al. Clinicopathological aspects of hepatosplenic bilharziasis. In: Mostofi FK, ed. *Bilharziasis*. New York, NY: International Academy of Pathology; 1967:15-29.

Warren KS, Domingo EO, Cowan RBT. Granuloma formation around schistosome eggs as a manifestation of delayed hypersensitivity. *Am J Pathol*. 1967;51:735-756.

Winslow DJ. Histopathology of schistosomiasis. In: Mostofi FK, ed. *Bilharziasis*. New York, NY: International Academy of Pathology; 1967:230-241.

Plate 80

Schistosoma mansoni

Image 1

S. mansoni adult male and female worms in copula in the mesenteric blood vessels of a hamster. Two sections of a smaller female worm (intense dark staining) lie within the gynecophoral canal of a male worm. The tegument of the male shows irregularly spaced tuberculations (arrows) (H&E, 100x).

Image 2

S. mansoni adult worms in copula in the blood vessel of a hamster intestine. Two sections of a darker-staining female worm (darts) lie within the male gynecophoral canal (H&E, 50x).

Image 3

S. mansoni eggs in hamster liver. The large size of the eggs and their elongate shape are evident (H&E, 125x).

Image 4

S. mansoni eggs in the wall of a hamster intestine. These eggs demonstrate different aspects of the large lateral spine (darts) in histologic section. The dark- and differential-staining characteristics of the miracidia within these eggs indicate that they were viable when the tissue was removed for fixation (H&E, 100x).

Image 5

Cluster of *S. mansoni* eggs in a human liver. These eggs are distorted and collapsed, a result of tissue fixation and processing. In one of the eggs, a typical lateral spine (dart) is seen (H&E, 500x).

Image 6

S. mansoni egg granuloma in the liver of an infected mouse demonstrates a characteristic pseudotubercle, or granuloma with fibrous tissue, surrounding three eggs. In the larger egg, the lateral spine (dart) is faintly visible (H&E, 100x).

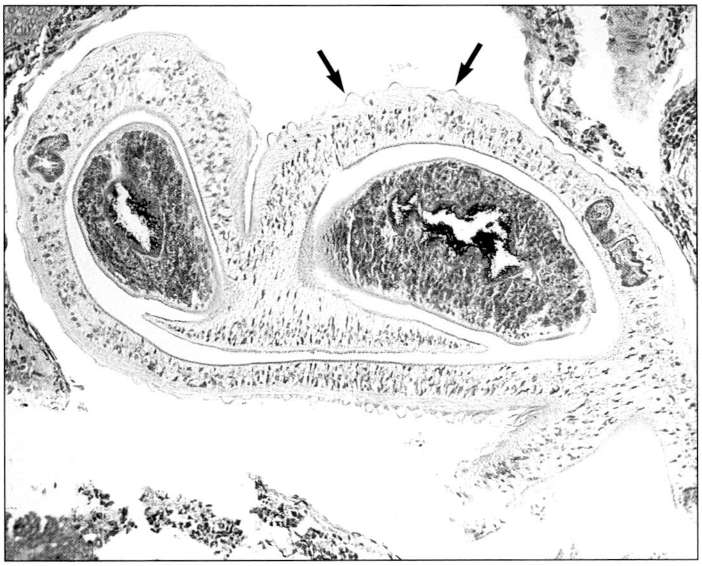

1

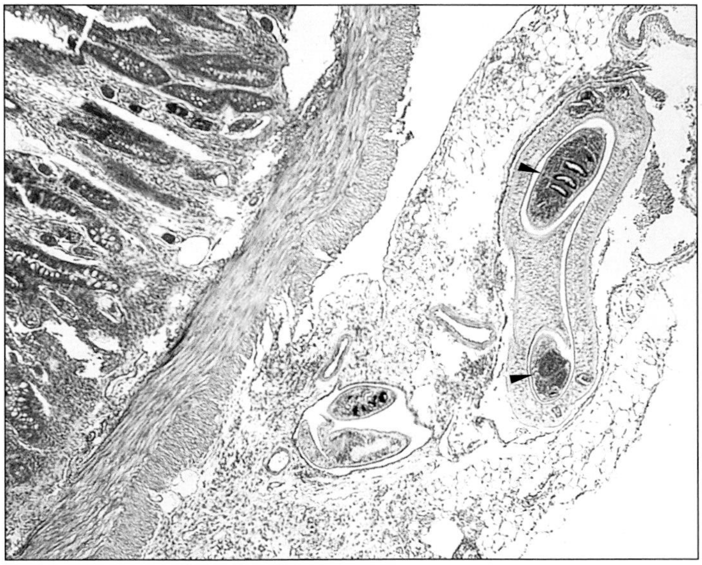

2

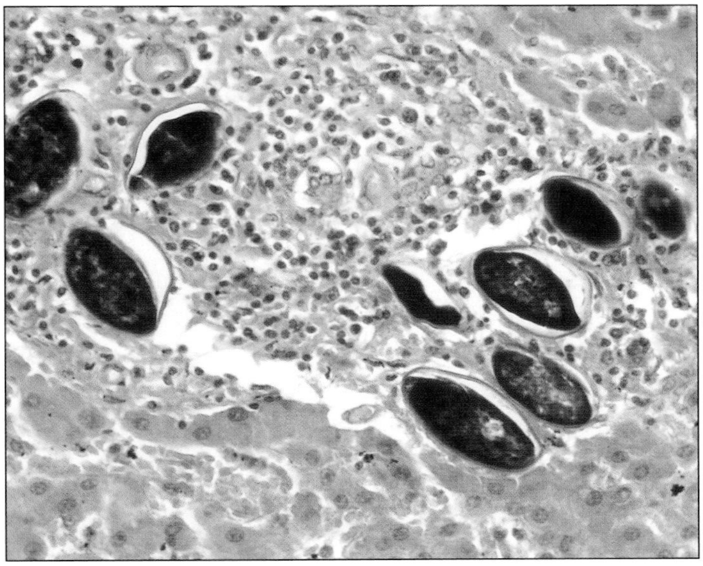

3

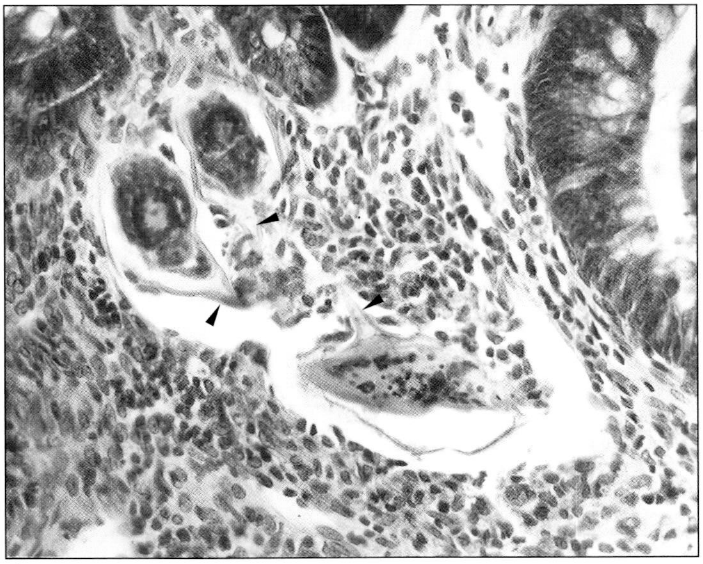

4

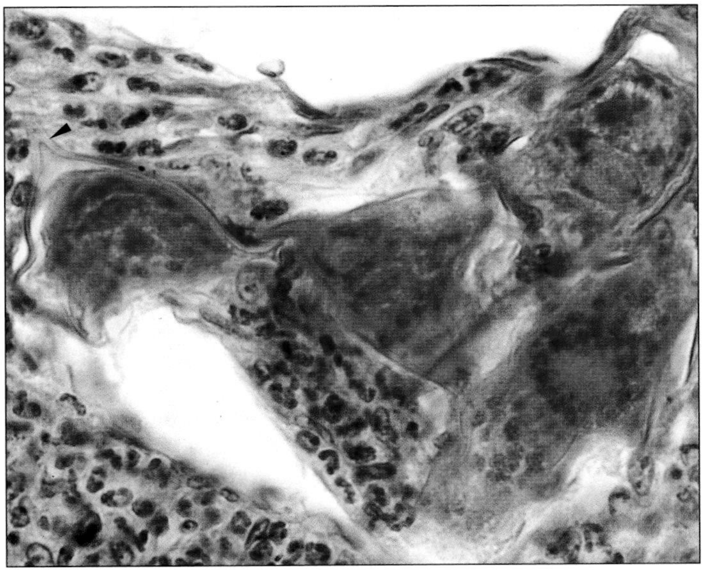

5

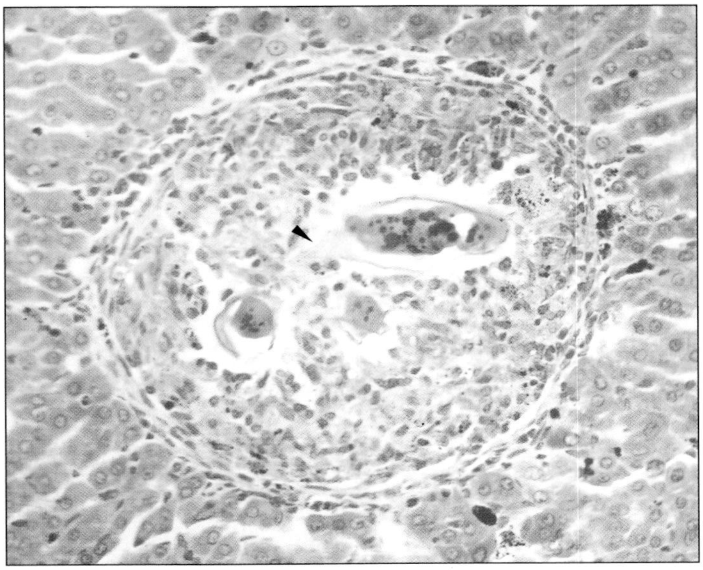

6

Schistosoma japonicum

Schistosomiasis japonica

Schistosoma japonicum, often referred to as the Oriental blood fluke, is another of the three major human schistosome parasites. Human and animal infections occur principally in Asia, including Japan, China, and the Philippines. Infection in Japan has been largely eradicated, and infection in Taiwan is limited to animals. *Schistosoma mekongi*, also a human and animal schistosome parasite, is found in countries along the Mekong River (Laos, Cambodia, and northern Thailand). This species produces eggs that are morphologically similar to those of *S. japonicum* except that they are smaller. Both species produce intestinal schistosomiasis. As with the other schistosomes, the sexes are separate.

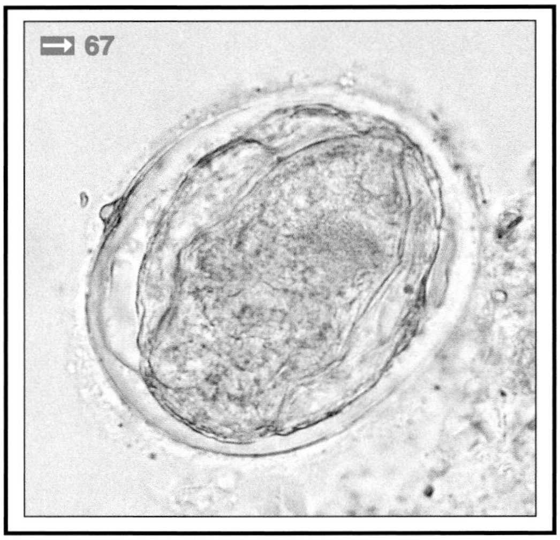

Biology and Life Cycle

Adult *S. japonicum* parasites primarily inhabit the radicles of the superior mesenteric vein, which drains the small intestine, but worms also occur in intrahepatic portal vessels. Their life cycle is essentially similar to that of *S. mansoni* and the other schistosomes. Embryonated eggs excreted in feces into water infect small, amphibious snail species of the genus *Oncomelania*. Cercariae liberated into water penetrate human skin to establish infection, and worms mature and begin egg production in five to six weeks. The tiny snail that acts as intermediate host for *S. mekongi* belongs to the genus *Neotricula*. Of all the major human schistosome parasites, *S. japonicum* is the most prolific in egg production, with female worms producing up to a few hundred eggs daily. *Schistosoma mekongi* is similar to *S. japonicum* in its location in the host, maturation time, and egg production. Animals play a significant role as reservoirs of human infection for *S. japonicum* and *S. mekongi*. Dogs, cats, water buffalo, cattle, other domesticated animals, and rodents can all be infected with *S. japonicum*. Infections with *S. japonicum* can last for decades.

Pathology and Clinical Manifestations

Clinical manifestations are similar to those seen in *S. mansoni* infections, except that the incubation period is characterized by more intense urticaria, fever, and cough. This condition has been referred to as the Katayama syndrome (named after the prefecture in Japan in which the condition was first described). The major differences between pathologic manifestations of *S. japonicum* infection and *S. mansoni* infection relate to the greater egg production by the former. The small intestine is the organ primarily affected, but eggs may be found throughout the intestinal tract and in large numbers in the liver as well. The eggs' smaller size and increased number allows for wide dissemination throughout the body via the vascular system. Eggs of *S. japonicum* enter the brain and spinal cord in particular. In the Philippines, epileptic-type seizures caused by the presence of these eggs in the brain are common.

Parasite Morphology

Male worms are 10 to 20 mm long. Lying within their gynecophoral canal are the longer and more slender female worms, which range from 16 to 26 mm in length. Male worms lack tuberculations on the tegument, but they do have many minute spines along the edge of the gynecophoral canal and around the inner surfaces of the oral and ventral suckers. The esophagus in both sexes bifurcates into paired intestinal ceca at the level of the ventral sucker. Near the posterior end, the ceca reunite to form a cecum that ends blindly. Males have seven testes aligned one behind the other slightly posterior to the ventral sucker. The ovary is situated slightly posterior to midbody, and the straight uterus extends anteriorly to the genital pore, which opens near the ventral sucker. The uterus contains 50 or more eggs, which far exceeds the number in utero for both *S. mansoni* and *S. haematobium*. Vitellaria occupy the lateral fields in the posterior fourth of the body. Eggs in utero are not yet mature and are somewhat smaller (approximately 67 by 50 µm) than mature eggs, which are excreted in feces and measure 70 to 100 µm by 50 to 70 µm (➡ 67). The eggs have a transparent shell, contain a miracidium, and have a small, inconspicuous spine that is often difficult to see. Some strains of the species appear to have a more prominent spine than others. Eggs of *S. mekongi* are morphologically similar to those of *S. japonicum*, but they are usually smaller (51 to 78 µm by 39 to 66 µm).

As with all schistosomes, in sections of tissue the elongate adult worms are usually seen within blood vessels (Plate 81:6). The tegument of the males is smooth, but minute spines along the gynecophoral canal are often visible. The uterus of females often contains several eggs in section. Eggs of *S. japonicum* are frequently collapsed or considerably distorted in tissue section due to the thin shell wall (Plate 81:1–5). Viable eggs as well as some undergoing degeneration or calcification are often numerous in sections of the intestine and liver. Eggs are often seen in many other organs and tissues, including the lungs and the central nervous system. It is rare to see the small spine on the eggshell in histologic section.

The schistosome eggs most likely to be encountered in granulomas in the intestinal wall or the liver are those of *S. mansoni* or *S. japonicum*. The geographic origin of the infection may be such that *S. mekongi* or *S. intercalatum* should also be considered. The deposition of larger numbers of *S. japonicum* eggs often results in clusters of eggs in tissue, many of which have thin shells that are considerably distorted or collapsed. In addition, many of the eggs may be undergoing calcification.

References

Hsu HF, Davis JR, Hsu SYL. Histopathological lesions of rhesus monkeys and chimpanzees infected with *Schistosoma japonicum*. *Ztschr Tropenmed Parasitol*. 1969;20:184-205.

Warren KS, Boros DL, Hang LM, et al. The *Schistosoma japonicum* egg granuloma. *Am J Pathol*. 1975;80:279-294.

Plate 81

Schistosoma japonicum

Image 1

Eggs of *S. japonicum* in the intestinal wall of an experimentally infected mouse. Many thin-shelled eggs (darts), some collapsed and distorted, are visible (H&E, 100x).

Image 2

At higher magnification, these two viable eggs have thin shells that have collapsed around miracidia (H&E, 300x).

Image 3

S. japonicum eggs in a human liver. Many elongate eggs are clustered in portal triads. The darkly stained ones have calcified (H&E, 100x).

Image 4

S. japonicum eggs in the wall of a human rectum. The egg near the center (dart) has retained its oval shape, and the differential staining of the miracidium indicates that it is a viable egg. Collapsed shells of degenerated eggs are scattered in the field (H&E, 300x).

Image 5

Appendix of a patient from the Philippines shows numerous eggs of *S. japonicum*. Features that suggest a diagnosis include the large size of the eggs and the relatively thin collapsed shells (Trichrome, 250x).

Image 6

A pair of dead adult worms of *S. japonicum* in the lung of an experimentally infected rabbit. The small female worm is within the gynecophoral canal of the male worm. Although degenerated, the tissue is typical of a trematode, and the presence of both a male and female worm suggests a diagnosis of schistosomiasis (H&E, 50x).

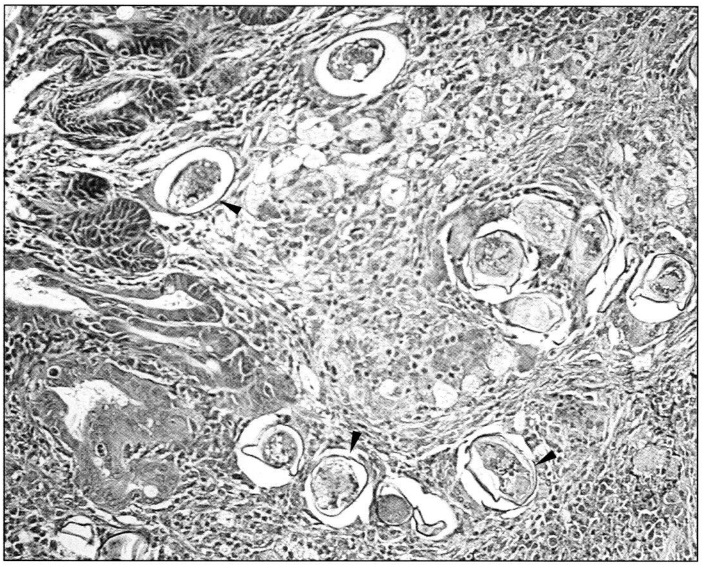

1

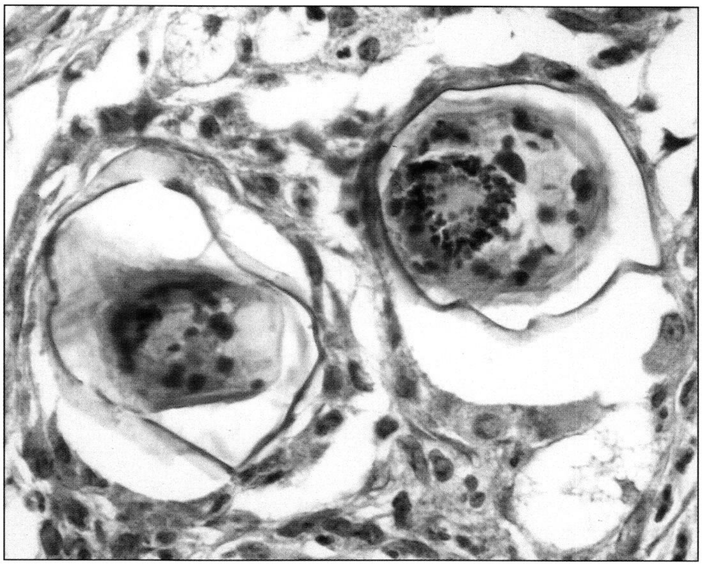

2

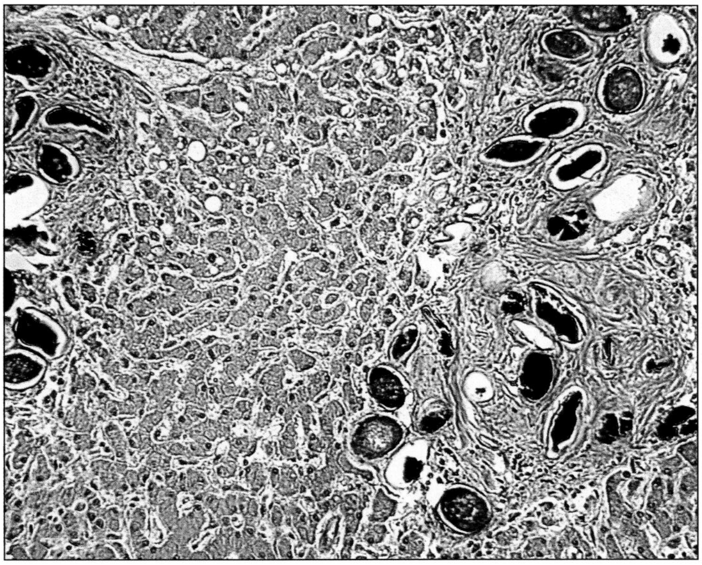

3

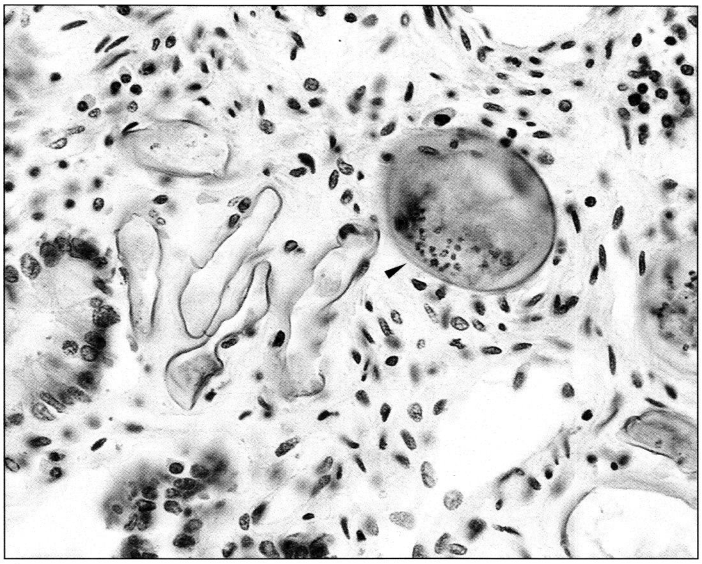

4

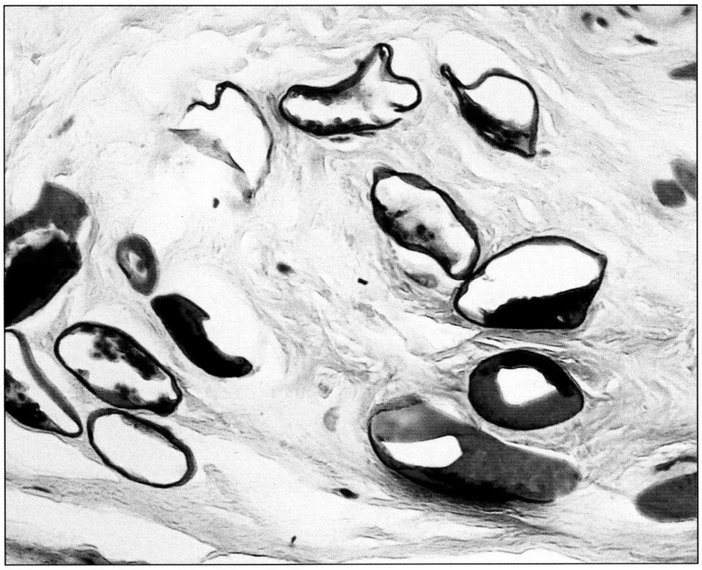

5

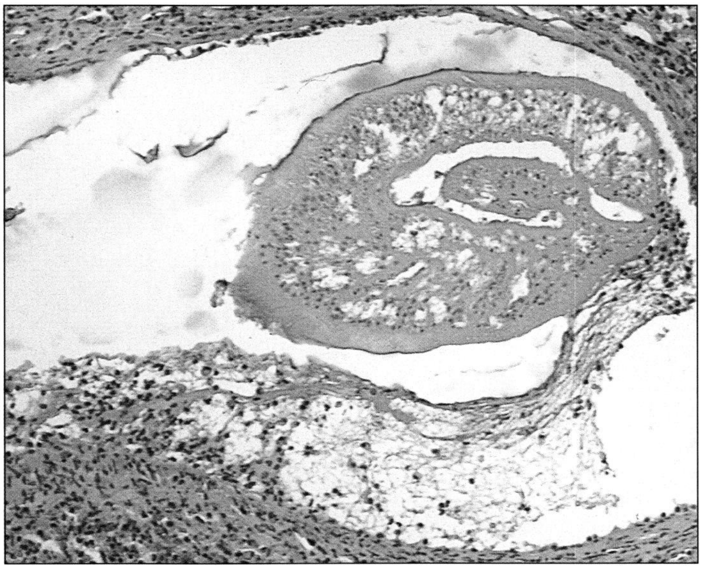

6

Schistosoma haematobium

Urinary schistosomiasis

Urinary tract schistosomiasis, or vesical bilharziasis, is caused by *Schistosoma haematobium*, the third of the major schistosome parasites of humans. It has wide geographic distribution throughout most of Africa and extends into southern Europe (southern Portugal) and into western Asia (Iraq, Iran, Lebanon, Syria, the Arabian peninsula, and southern Turkey). A small focus appears to occur in Maharashtra State of India, south of Bombay, and is thought to have been introduced from Portugal.

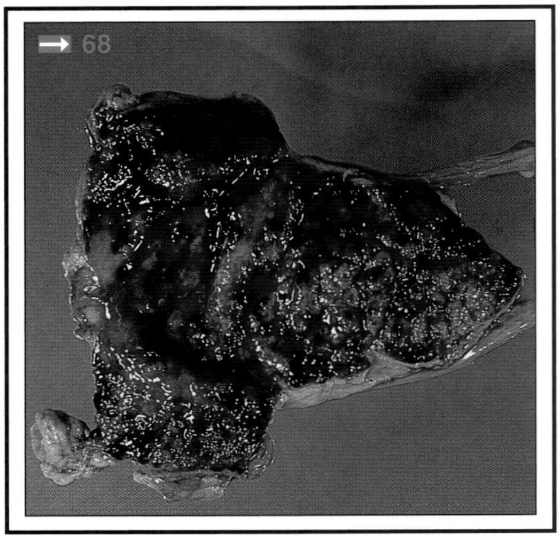

Biology and Life Cycle

Adult *S. haematobium* parasites normally live in the vesical and pelvic plexuses of the venous system and rarely in the portal system or other venous vessels. Immature eggs are discharged primarily in venules in the submucosa of the urinary bladder. These eggs mature as they make their way into the lumen of the bladder, and the terminal-spined eggs are voided in urine. Eggs of this species can also be found in the wall of the rectum and in feces. Freshwater snails of the genus *Bulinus* serve as intermediate hosts. Human infections are established by direct penetration of the skin by free-swimming cercariae, and the prepatent period is 10 to 14 weeks. Adult worms live for up to 15 to 20 years, though longer life spans have been reported.

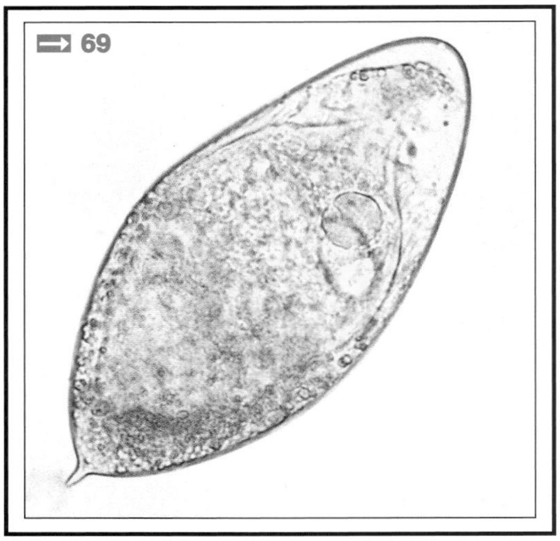

Pathology and Clinical Manifestations

Skin rash associated with initial infection is not a prominent feature of cercarial invasion. Usually, clinical symptoms will not appear until the end of the prepatent period, when general malaise, headache, fever, night sweats, and back and leg pains occur. When egg deposition begins, eosinophilia, liver and spleen hypertrophy, a burning sensation with micturition, and hematuria may occur. Long-term symptomatology includes hematuria, difficulty with micturition, and development of hydroureter and hydronephrosis, leading to renal complications and renal failure.

Pathologically, the urinary bladder is the organ most consistently and severely damaged. Granulomatous response to the eggs deposited in the wall of the bladder results in cystitis, ulcer and polyp formation, and fibrosis and contraction of the bladder (➡ 68). Other tissues and organs demonstrating pathologic lesions include the ureters, kidney, prostate gland, urethra in both sexes, and the wall of the rectum. In endemic areas, *S. haematobium* infection is believed to be one of the major predisposing factors to squamous cell carcinoma of the bladder.

Parasite Morphology

Adult males are 10 to 15 mm long and have a finely tuberculate integument dorsally behind the ventral sucker (Plate 82:2). Minute spines occur on the inner surfaces of the suckers as well as in the gynecophoral canal. Testes number four or five, one behind the other and posterior to the ventral sucker. Female worms are elongate and slender, 16 to 20 mm long, and lack tuberculations on the tegument. They have minute spines in the cavities of the suckers and at the posterior end. The ovary is situated slightly posterior to midbody, and the uterus courses anteriorly from it to the genital pore, which is slightly posterior to the ventral sucker. The uterus usually contains 20 to 30 eggs. Vitellaria occupy the lateral fields in the posterior fourth of the body. Eggs are 112 to 170 µm long by 40 to 70 µm wide, have a transparent shell with a terminal spine, and contain a miracidium when voided in urine (➡ 69).

As with the other human schistosomes, in microscopic sections the adults of *S. haematobium* are seen within blood vessels, often those in or near the urinary bladder. Adult worms possess typical trematode anatomy. Like the other schistosomes, the female worms are frequently seen lying in the gynecophoral canal of male worms (Plate 82:1, 2, & 6). The small tuberculations on the dorsal surface of the tegument may be seen, but these tuberculations are not as prominent as those in *S. mansoni*. Eggs of this species are found in the wall of the bladder and in a variety of organs and tissues, including the rectum (Plate 82:5 & 6), appendix, cervix, ureters, mesenteries, prostate, seminal vesicles, and urethra. Eggs are often collapsed and distorted, but it is frequently possible to see the typical terminal spine (Plate 82:4). Calcified eggs are frequently found in tissues. Such eggs stain dark blue or black with hematoxylin and eosin stain (Plate 82:3).

The tissues and organs in which adults and eggs of *S. haematobium* predominantly occur vary from those in which *S. mansoni* and *S. japonicum* occur. In geographic areas where *S. mansoni* and *S. haematobium* overlap in distribution, finding schistosome egg granulomas without the characteristic spines can make diagnosis difficult. When a modified Ziehl-Nielsen staining technique is used, the eggs of *S. haematobium* are not acid fast, whereas those of both *S. mansoni* and *S. japonicum* are. *Schistosoma intercalatum*, a terminal-spined, intestinal schistosome species in Africa, produces eggs found in feces. In tissue, the eggs of this species are acid fast when stained after use of Bouin's fixative. The small tuberculations on the tegument of *S. haematobium* are useful in distinguishing the adult worms from those of *S. mansoni*, which have much larger tuberculations. Eggs of both *S. haematobium* and *S. japonicum* are found calcified in tissues more frequently than those of *S. mansoni.*

References

Lichtenberg F, Lindenberg M. An alcohol-acid-fast substance in eggs of *Schistosoma mansoni. Am J Trop Med Hyg.* 1954;3:1066-1076.

von Lichtenberg F, Edington GM, Nwabuebo I, et al. Pathologic effects of schistosomiasis in Ibadan, western state of Nigeria, II: pathogenesis of lesions of the bladder and ureters. *Am J Trop Med Hyg.* 1971;20:244-254.

Smith JH, Christie JD. The pathobiology of *Schistosoma haematobium* infection in humans. *Hum Pathol.* 1986;17:333-345.

Plate 82

Schistosoma haematobium

Image 1

S. haematobium adult worms in venules associated with the wall of a human urinary bladder. In the larger of the two worm pairs, the dark-staining intestine is visible. Small tuberculations are present, but difficult to see, on the dorsal tegument of the larger male worm. In the smaller of the worm pairs, only a small portion of a female worm (dart) is seen within the gynecophoral canal of the male (H&E, 25x).

Image 2

At higher magnification, the small portion of a female worm (dart) is visible within the gynecophoral canal of the male worm. Small tuberculations (arrows) are visible on the dorsal tegument of the male worm (H&E, 100x).

Image 3

A large number of eggs are seen in this heavily infected human bladder (H&E, 40x).

Image 4

Eggs of *S. haematobium* in a granuloma in the wall of a urinary bladder. At this magnification, the terminal spine characteristic of the species is clearly visible (dart) in one of the eggs and slightly less so in another. The appearance and staining characteristics of the miracidia within the eggs indicate that they are viable (H&E, 250x).

Image 5

A cluster of eggs and egg fragments of *S. haematobium* in a snip from the rectal mucosa. An intact egg (dart) is in the center of the field (H&E, 100x).

Image 6

Adults of *S. haematobium* in venules within a papilloma of the rectum. Eggs are also seen in the mucosal tissue. The presence of eggs in the wall of the rectum is not uncommon in this infection, although eggs of this species are usually thought of as occurring in urine rather than in feces (H&E, 40x).

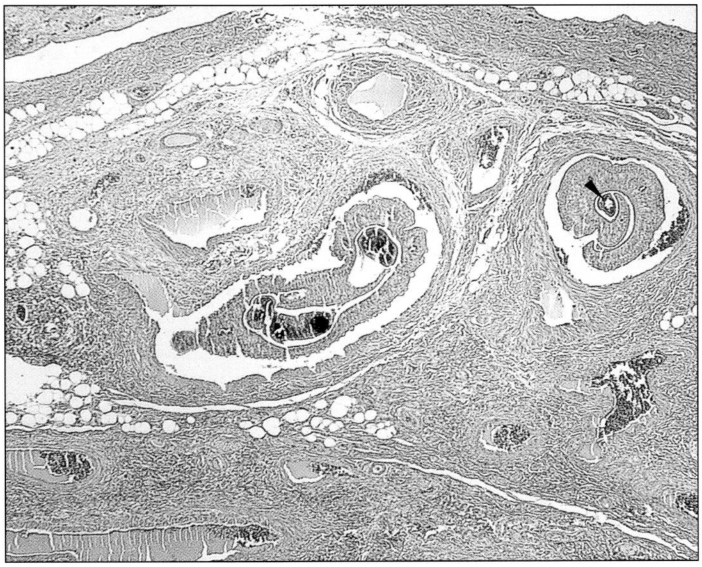
1

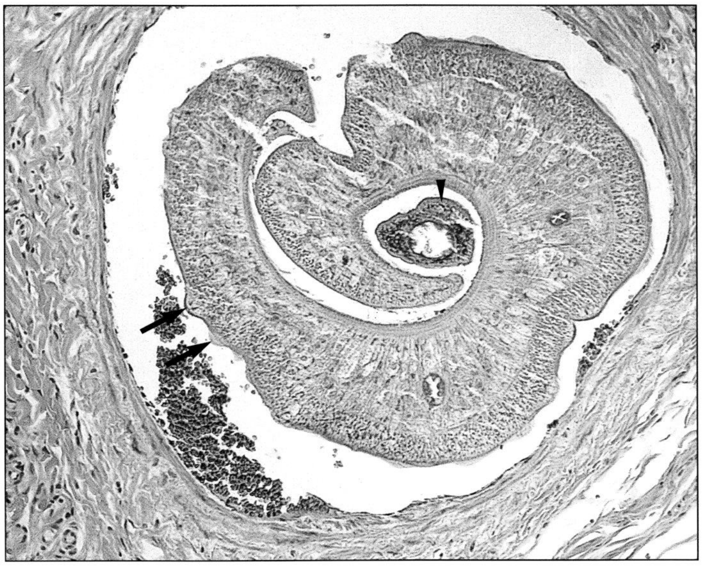
2

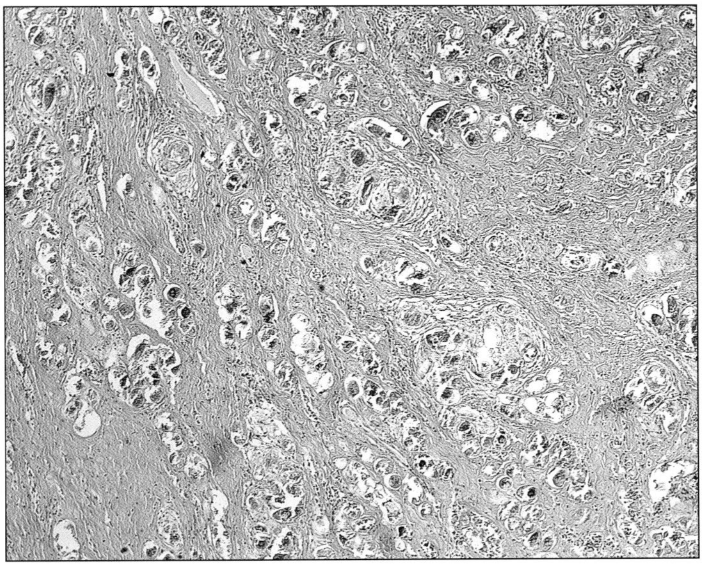
3

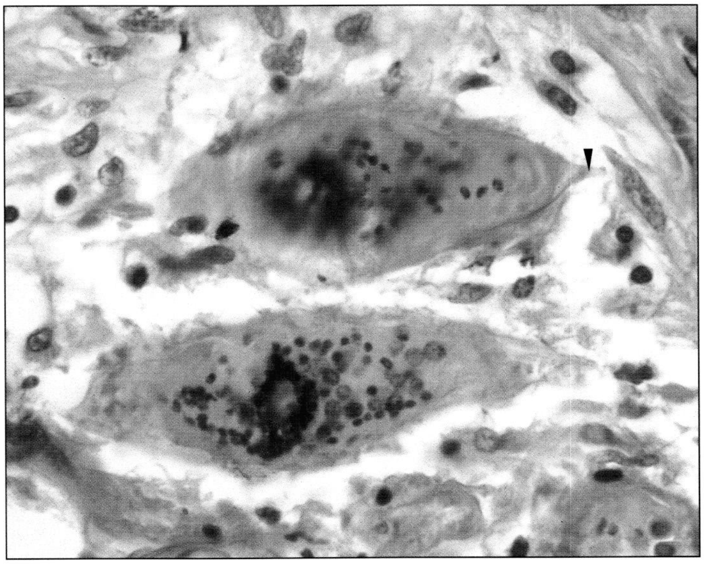
4

5

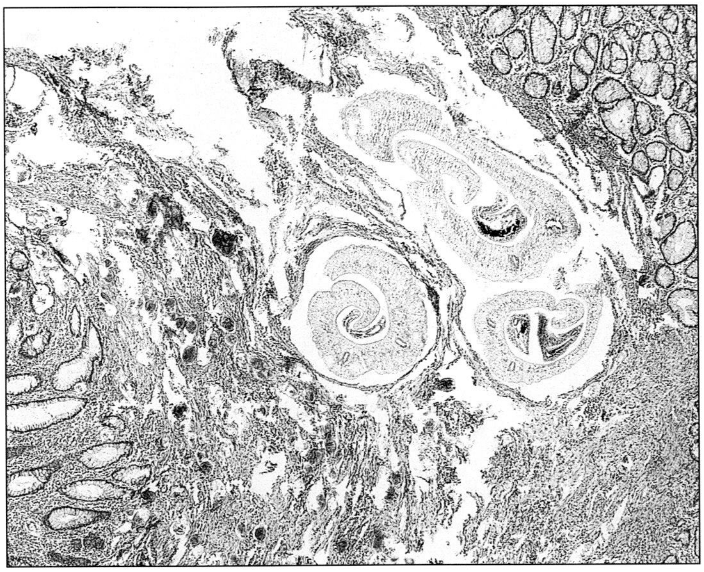
6

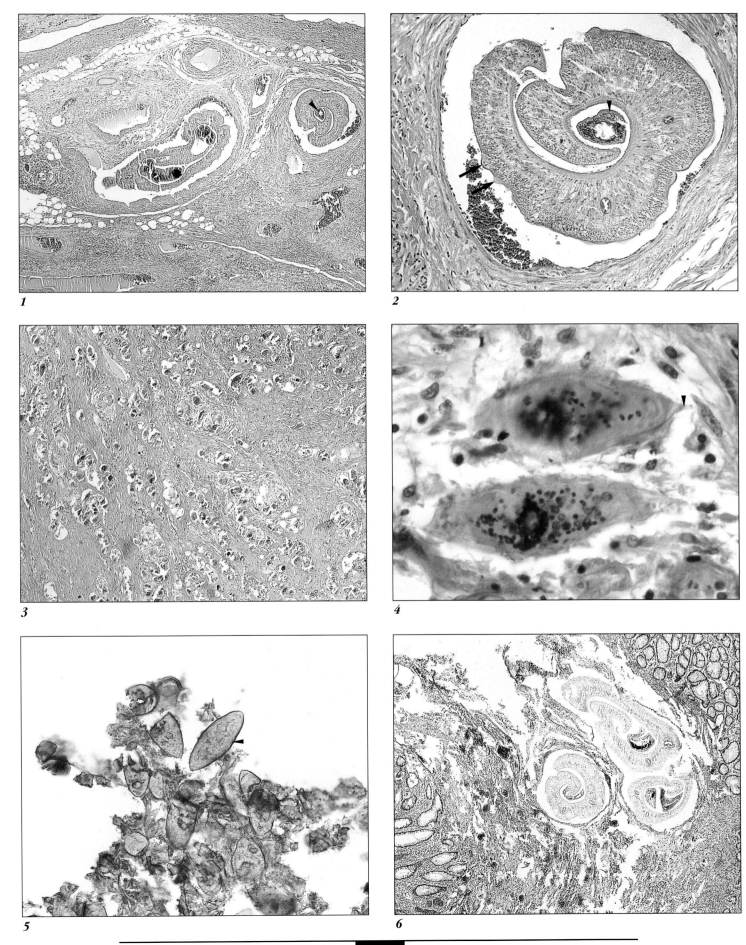

Other Trematodes in Human Tissues

Diplostomatid trematodes are commonly found in the intestines of raccoons, dogs, cats, and other animals. Their life cycles are different from many trematodes in that they have a morphologic stage, the mesocercaria, between the cercaria and metacercaria. This mesocercarial stage develops when a tadpole becomes infected via skin penetration by the free-swimming cercaria of parasites of the genera *Alaria, Procyotrema,* and *Pharyngostomoides.* This nonencysted larval stage migrates in the tissues, and when ingested by frogs, small mammals, or humans, the mesocercarial stage leaves the intestine and migrates in the tissues of these hosts. The mesocercaria retains in its body large penetration glands from the cercarial stage, which facilitate identification of these parasites (Plate 83:1–4).

References

Beaver PC, Little MD, Tucker CF, et al. Mesocercaria in the skin of man in Louisiana. *Am J Trop Med Hyg.* 1977;26:422-426.

Gold D, Lang Y, Lengy J. *Philophthalmus* species, probably *P. palpebrarum,* in Israel: description of the eye fluke from experimental infection. *Parasitol Res.* 1993;79:372-377.

Gutierrez Y, Grossniklaus HE, Annable WC. Human conjunctivitis caused by the bird parasite *Philophthalmus. Am J Ophthalmol.* 1987;104:417-419.

McDonald HR, Kazacos KR, Schatz H, et al. Two cases of intraocular infection with *Alaria* mesocercaria (Trematoda). *Am J Ophthalmol.* 1994;117:447-455.

Plate 83

Other Trematodes

Image 1

In this section of a skin biopsy specimen taken from the upper thigh of a Louisianan, a mesocercaria (dart) of *Alaria* can be seen in an area of inflammation (H&E, 50x).

Image 2

At higher magnification, the large gland cells on either side of a section through the ventral sucker (VS) of this larval trematode can be identified. A portion of an intestinal cecum is just above the sucker (H&E, 250x).

Image 3

A skin biopsy specimen in another case from Louisiana again demonstrates at low magnification the presence of a small, migrating mesocercaria (dart) surrounded by an inflammatory reaction (H&E, 50x).

Image 4

At higher magnification, more morphologic details of the parasite are seen. Although not as clearly seen as in Images 1 and 2, this organism can still be recognized as a small trematode, possibly suggestive of a mesocercaria on clinical and epidemiologic grounds (H&E, 400x).

Image 5

In this section of sputum that was being examined for the presence of cancer cells, a small subadult trematode was found. It has characteristics of a heterophyidlike fluke that is contained within a capsule. A section through the ventral sucker (dart) and possibly part of the oral sucker (arrow) can be recognized (H&E, 400x).

Image 6

A trematode removed from the eye of a patient with conjunctivitis was sectioned longitudinally. The worm is approximately 2.4 mm long by 0.73 mm in breadth at the region of the ventral sucker (VS), which is located just posterior to the oral sucker in this section. Other visible morphologic features of this fluke are the pharynx between the oral and ventral suckers, eggs in utero, and a lobed testis (TE) at the posterior end. This fluke is identifiable on morphologic grounds as *Philophthalmus*, a parasite that normally lives in the conjunctival sac or cloaca of birds. Its presence in humans is rare (H&E, 40x).

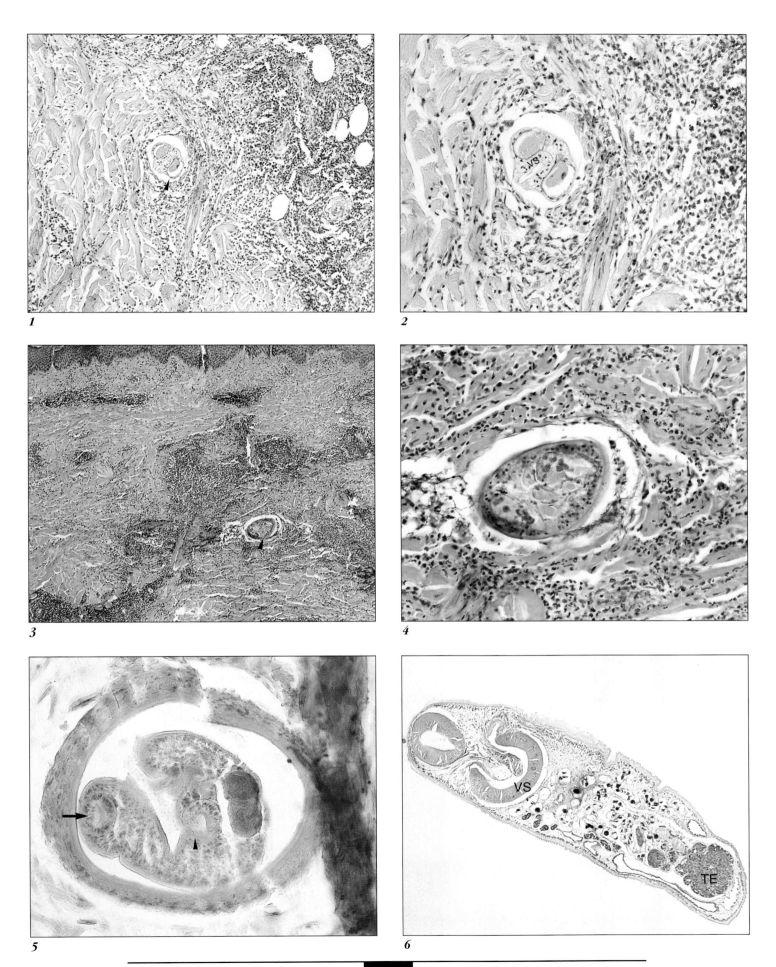

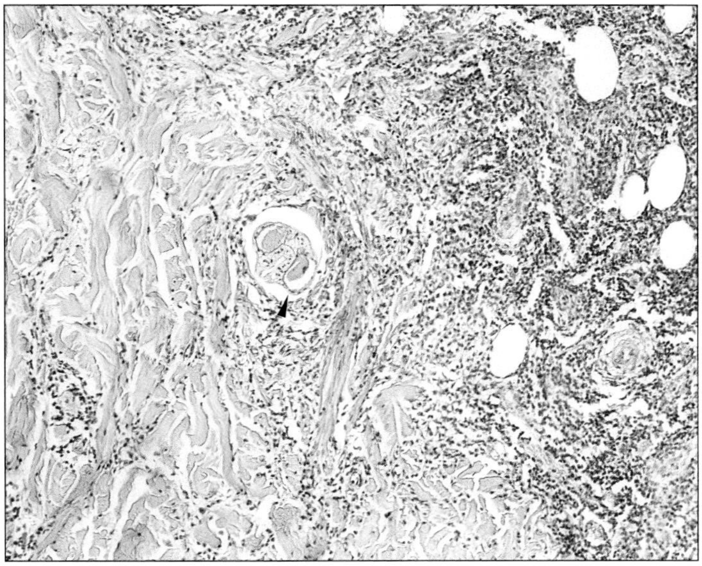

1

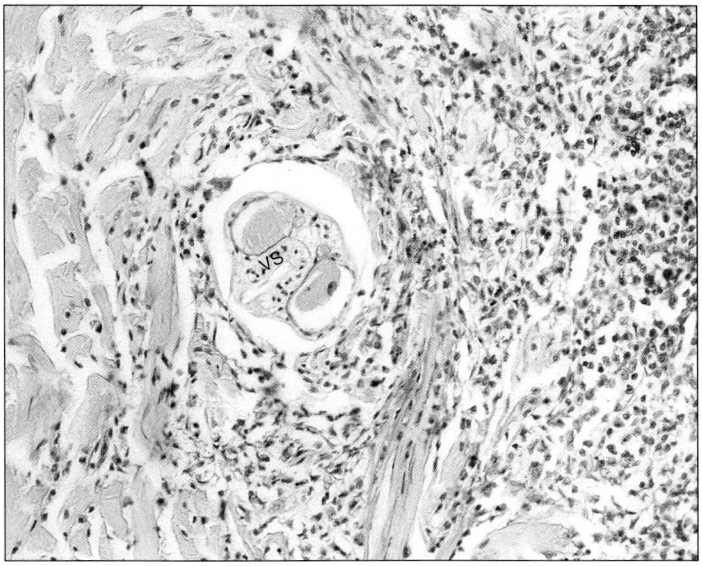

2

3

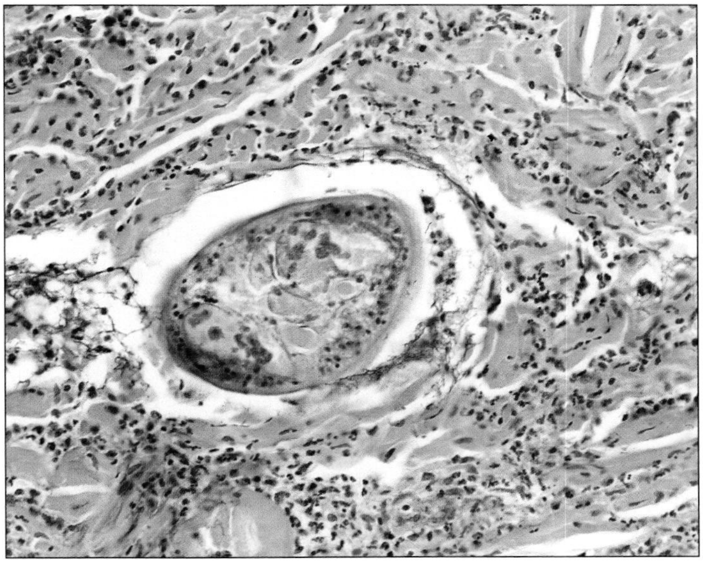

4

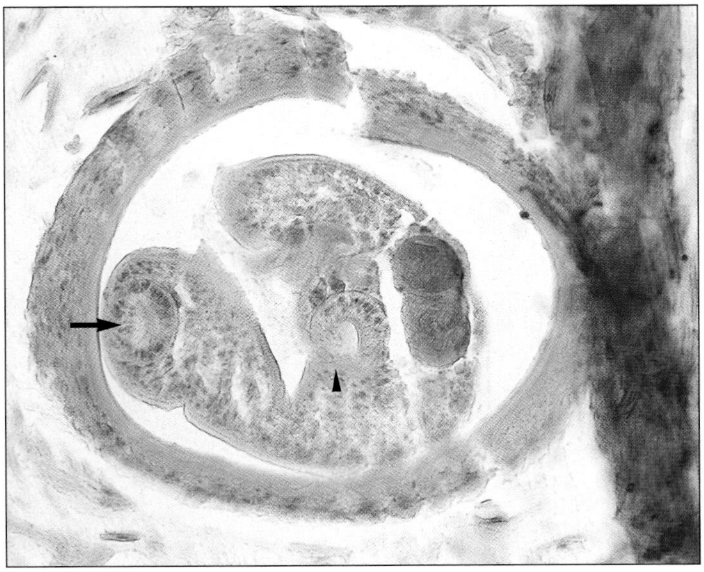

5

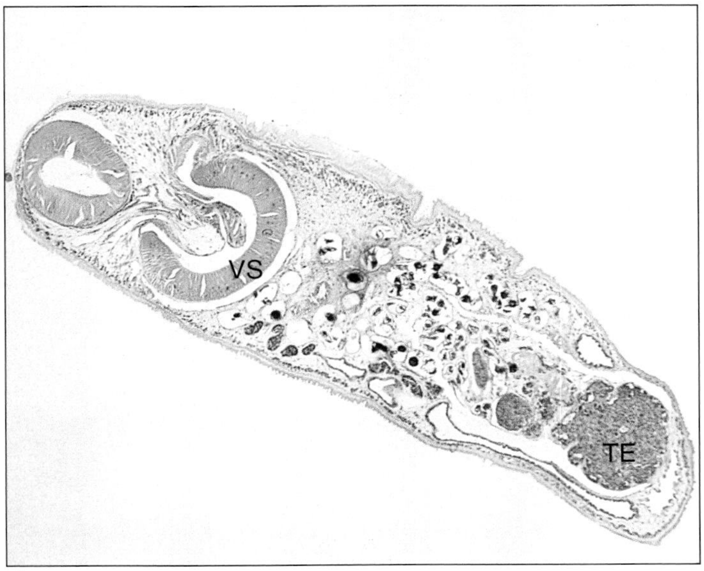

6

Cestoda

The cestodes, usually referred to as tapeworms, are segmented, ribbonlike flatworms of varying sizes that normally reside in the small intestine of vertebrate hosts, including humans. Like the trematodes, they are acoelomate organisms and belong to the Phylum Platyhelminthes. Those of medical importance are placed in two orders: the Pseudophyllidea and the Cyclophyllidea. The intestinal, adult stages of these parasites are of comparatively minor interest and importance. The larval stages, on the other hand, are intimately associated with the tissues and can cause serious disease in humans.

Relatively few species produce disease in humans. However, knowledge of the life histories of the two major groups (which are markedly different) is crucial to understanding how people acquire these infections. Also, the structure of the larval stages is significantly different, so that a review of their morphologic features will aid in their recognition.

Cestode Life Cycles

The two major groups of cestodes have significantly different larval stages and intermediate host requirements.

Pseudophyllidea

The species that infect humans belong either to the genus *Diphyllobothrium,* which as adults live in the small intestine, or to the genus *Spirometra*, which occur in human tissues only as larvae. In both genera, the life cycle begins with the passage of unembryonated, operculated eggs into water, where they develop into a ciliated, six-hooked larval stage—a coracidium. After hatching, the coracidium is actively motile in water and must be ingested by the first intermediate host, a copepod, where it develops into a larva known as a procercoid. When infected copepods are ingested by fish, the procercoids, liberated in the intestine, migrate to the musculature where they grow into a plerocercoid larva, also known as a sparganum. When spargana in the flesh of small fish are ingested by other fish, they have the ability to re-enter the muscles of these fish. Moving up the food chain gives the spargana an enhanced opportunity to be ingested by a definitive host such as a human or a fish-eating mammal.

More than 20 species of *Diphyllobothrium* have been described as agents of human intestinal infection, but invasion of human tissues by spargana of this genus is unknown. Adult tapeworms of the genus *Spirometra* parasitize canid and felid intestines but not human intestines. Human sparganosis is caused by several species of *Spirometra*, including *S. mansoni, S. mansonoides, S. ranarum, S. erinacei,* and others. Infection is acquired by accidentally ingesting copepods that contain procercoids or by eating raw or undercooked fish flesh that contain spargana.

Cyclophyllidea

Although several cyclophyllidean tapeworms parasitize the human small intestine, we discuss only those whose larval stages invade human tissues. The most important of these species belong to the genera *Taenia* and *Echinococcus.* As adults these tapeworms produce eggs that contain six-hooked embryos called oncospheres or hexacanth embryos. Depending on the species of tapeworm, the hexacanth embryo develops into a cysticercus, a coenurus, or a hydatid. All of these larval types are situated in host tissues and usually cause extensive disease in the human host. In vertebrate hosts, including humans, they are found in many organs (liver, lungs, brain) and tissues (subcutaneous tissues, mesenteries), where they encyst, grow, and sometimes multiply extensively (hydatids, coenurus). After the infected intermediate host is ingested, the adult tapeworm develops in the intestine of the definitive host. Humans who become infected with larval stages, such as a cysticercus, coenurus, or hydatid, are considered "dead-end" hosts.

Cestode Relationships

The tapeworms are grouped together in the Class Cestoda within the Phylum Platyhelminthes. The most important genera from the human perspective are *Diphyllobothrium, Taenia,* and *Echinococcus*, which account for more than half of the species recorded from humans. The Cestoda are divided into two orders, the Pseudophyllidea and Cyclophyllidea. Within each order is one family that plays a significant role in human infection, the Diphyllobothriidae in the former and Taeniidae in the latter.

Family Diphyllobothriidae

Pseudophyllidean tapeworms have a scolex with two bothria (sucking organs), one on the dorsal surface and one on the ventral surface. Male and female genital pores are midventral in the anterior half of the proglottids. Eggs have an operculum and are unembryonated when passed in feces. Although *Diphyllobothrium latum* matures in the human intestine, we focus on sparganosis caused by *Spirometra* species.

Family Taeniidae

Cyclophyllidean tapeworms have a scolex bearing four suckers and usually a rostellum at its apex that may bear hooks. A genital pore is usually situated at the lateral margin of the proglottid. Eggs lack an operculum and contain a hexacanth embryo when passed in feces. We focus on the larval stages of species of *Taenia* and *Echinococcus.*

Cestode Morphology

Adult Tapeworms

Gross Morphology

The typical adult tapeworm has a scolex at the anterior end bearing bothria (in pseudophyllideans) or suckers (in cyclophyllideans), followed by a short "neck" region of undifferentiated tissue that gives rise to a chain of proglottids (sometimes called segments). Each proglottid contains both male and female reproductive organs. Proglottids nearest to the anterior end are immature, but by progressing distally in the chain of segments (known as the strobila), they become mature and are finally known as gravid proglottids, which contain many eggs in utero. Tapeworms lack a digestive tract. The male reproductive system may have few to hundreds of testes, vasa efferentia, a sperm duct, and a cirrus. The female reproductive system has a single, sometimes lobed ovary, an oviduct, and a vagina. Pseudophyllidean eggs resemble trematode eggs in that they have a shell with an operculum. Cyclophyllidean eggs lack an operculum.

Microscopic Morphology

Microscopic sections of tapeworm proglottids in the intestinal tract are rarely encountered. For example, proglottids of *T. solium* or *T. saginata* are sometimes found in routine sections of the appendix. In proglottids of cyclophyllidea, the outer layer of tegument appears to be noncellular and homogeneous by light microscopy, although electron microscopy reveals the surface to be covered with hairy projections known as microtriches. Beneath the basement membrane of this layer is a subtegumental layer of nuclei and cytoplasm interspersed with thin layers of outer circular and inner longitudinal muscles (Plate 85:1). The rest of the proglottid is filled with a loose accumulation of cells and fluid-filled spaces that comprise a parenchymal meshwork.

The parenchyma is divided into distinct cortical and medullary portions by a prominent system of longitudinal and transverse muscle fibers (Plate 85:1 & 4). Reproductive structures are found within the medullary portion (Plate 85:2). Scattered throughout the parenchyma are round or oval bodies called calcareous corpuscles (Plate 85:6). These bodies frequently have a whorled appearance and a complex chemical composition that includes calcium carbonate (Plate 85:7). Calcareous corpuscles are unique to the parenchyma of cestodes and are especially prominent in larval stages. Their presence in tissue sections is diagnostic for tapeworms.

Larval Tapeworms

Of the many types of larval tapeworms, we describe only those that are often found in human tissues.

Sparganum

Spargana are typically white, ribbonlike, solid-bodied larvae (Plate 84:1). They are unsegmented and measure up to 20 mm or more in length by 1.0 to 1.5 mm in width. The scolex is not yet developed. A rare, proliferating type of larva, *Sparganum proliferum,* lacks a definitive scolex and develops branching processes that may detach and become separate larval stages.

In microscopic sections, the typical cestode tegument has dark nuclei beneath the basement membrane. The parenchyma is fibrous and contains numerous, irregularly scattered bundles of longitudinal muscle fibers. Numerous small ducts of the excretory channels are seen in the parenchyma. Calcareous corpuscles are numerous and usually are easily seen (Plate 85:6 & 7).

Cysticercus

This larval stage consists of a fluid-filled bladder into which a single protoscolex is inverted (Plate 84:2). The cysticerci with which we are most concerned are those of *Taenia solium* (*Cysticercus cellulosae*) and *T. saginata* (*Cysticercus bovis*). These cysticerci are filled with a clear fluid, have a thick bladder wall, and measure up to 10 mm in diameter. The protoscolex of *C. cellulosae* has a rostellum bearing two rows of hooklets (13 large and 13 smaller ones), but *C. bovis* lacks an armed rostellum. The cysticercus of *C. cellulosae* develops in the tissues of humans as well as in the tissues of its normal intermediate host, the pig. *Cysticercus bovis* only develops in cattle. A "racemose" type of cysticercus is occasionally reported in humans. This rare, proliferating, invasive larva lacks a scolex and may be an aberrant form of *T. solium* or some other cestode species. Other rare types of cysticercuslike larvae are occasionally found in human tissues, but their specific identification is often impossible.

Microscopically, the moderately folded spiral canal is often seen leading to a well-developed protoscolex, which has suckers, rostellum, and hooklets. The surface of the spiral canal is folded, with the underlying parenchyma containing fibrous and muscle tissue and numerous calcareous corpuscles. The neck region of the spiral canal is more markedly folded, and the parenchyma has fewer calcareous corpuscles. The bladder wall is moderately thick and has warty protrusions on its surface. The underlying fibrous parenchyma lacks calcareous corpuscles. Depending on the plane of section, only the bladder, the region of the spiral canal, or the large or small portions of the scolex with or without suckers or hooks may be visible.

Coenurus

Certain species of *Taenia* tapeworms, formerly classified in the genus *Multiceps,* have a larva called a coenurus. Like a cysticercus, this bladder worm has a fluid-filled, thick-walled bladder; however, unlike a cysticercus it has hundreds of protoscoleces inverted into its bladder (Plate 84:3). The protoscoleces are often randomly scattered on the surface of the bladder (*T. multiceps*) or arranged linearly (*T. serialis*).

Microscopically, sections of a coenurus usually demonstrate many views of protoscoleces or spiral canals surrounded by the bladder wall. These protoscoleces have an armed rostellum, and sections of hooklets are commonly seen in one or more of the scoleces.

Hydatid

Several types of hydatids occur in humans. The unilocular type is produced by *Echinococcus granulosus,* the alveolar type by *E. multilocularis,* and the polycystic type by *E. vogeli.* Unilocular cysts vary in size, depending on their age in the intermediate or dead-end host. They tend to be round or oval, but when they occur in confined spaces, such as bone, they ramify and conform to the shape of the structure they occupy. Masses of cells are budded internally into the cystic cavity. These masses become stalked and vacuolate to become brood capsules. Some brood capsules break free and undergo degeneration, whereas others grow and create daughter cysts. Large cysts may attain sizes up to 20 cm or more in diameter and harbor many daughter cysts that contain large numbers of viable protoscoleces (Plate 84:4).

Microscopically, the wall of a hydatid cyst typically consists of a surrounding host tissue capsule, a laminated, acellular layer, and an inner, nucleated, germinal layer that gives rise to brood capsules (Plate 90:1–3).

In rodents, their normal intermediate hosts, alveolar cysts of *E. multilocularis* occur principally in the liver, contain many protoscoleces, and are multicompartmented (Plate 93:2 & 3). In humans, exogenous budding of the germinal membrane results in highly folded and convoluted hyaline membranes infiltrating throughout the liver tissue (Plate 92:6; Plate 93:1). Metastasis to lung and brain occurs when larval tissue invades blood vessels.

Microscopically, in rodents, the compartments harbor many brood capsules and calcareous corpuscles are abundant (Plate 93:3). In humans, brood capsules are not commonly seen, calcareous corpuscles are difficult to find, and areas of calcification may occur.

Polycystic hydatid cysts typically occur in the liver of large rodents (paca, nutria), which are the natural intermediate hosts. The cyst wall is surrounded by host fibrous tissue and is composed of a thick, laminated layer and a germinal layer. Endogenous proliferation of the germinal layer creates folds and pockets within the primary cyst. A similar presentation is seen in cases of human infection with this parasite.

In microscopic sections, multiple cavities are composed of collapsed and folded laminated membranes and germinal epithelium (Plate 93:4 & 5). Scoleces and brood capsules are frequently present in small numbers. Calcareous corpuscles are not abundant, and calcification occurs in some of the degenerated vesicles.

Reference

Coil WH. Platyhelminthes: Cestoidea. In: Harrison FW, Bogitsh BJ, eds. *Microscopic Anatomy of Invertebrates, Vol III: Plathyhelminthes and Nemertinea*. New York, NY: Wiley-Liss Inc; 1991.

Plate 84

Larval Cestodes

Image 1

Numerous spargana of *Diphyllobothrium* species digested from the musculature of fish. Note the variation in size and thickness.

Image 2

Typical cysticercus removed from pork. The dense, central area represents the invaginated scolex and spiral canal within the fluid-filled bladder of *Cysticercus cellulosae*, which is the larval stage of *Taenia solium*.

Image 3

A coenurus (*Taenia* species) of 1 cm in diameter removed from the eye of a Ugandan child. Note the protoscoleces that project from the outer surface of the fluid-filled bladder. The dense white areas on the surface represent other protoscoleces that are invaginated into the bladder.

Image 4

A unilocular hydatid cyst of *Echinococcus granulosus* contains multiple, round, daughter cysts within it.

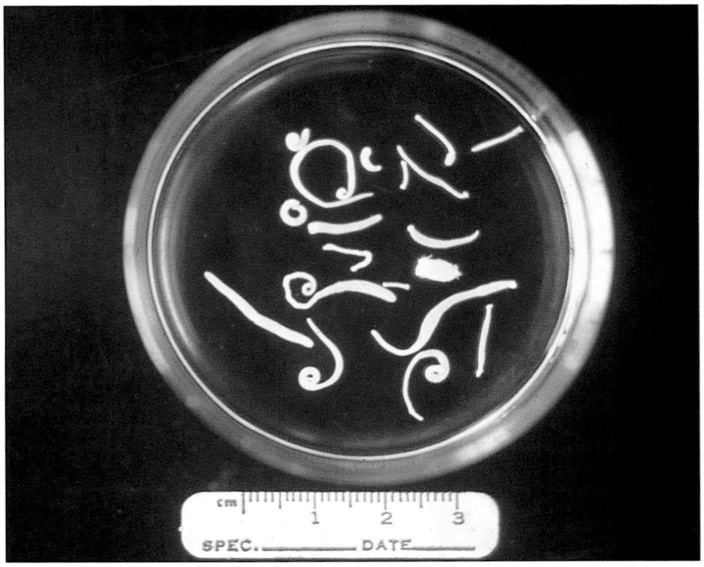

1

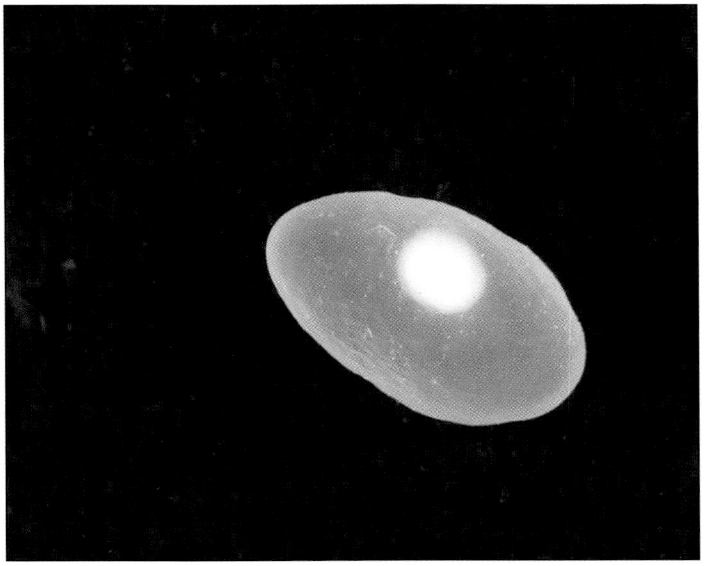

2

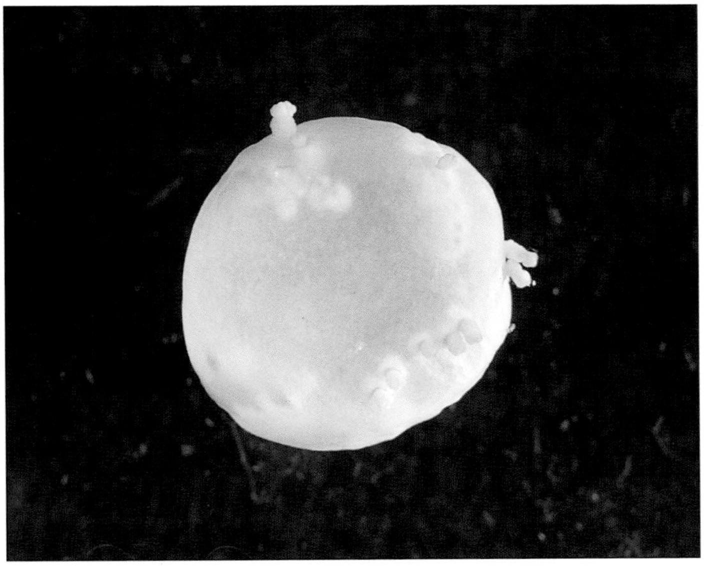

3

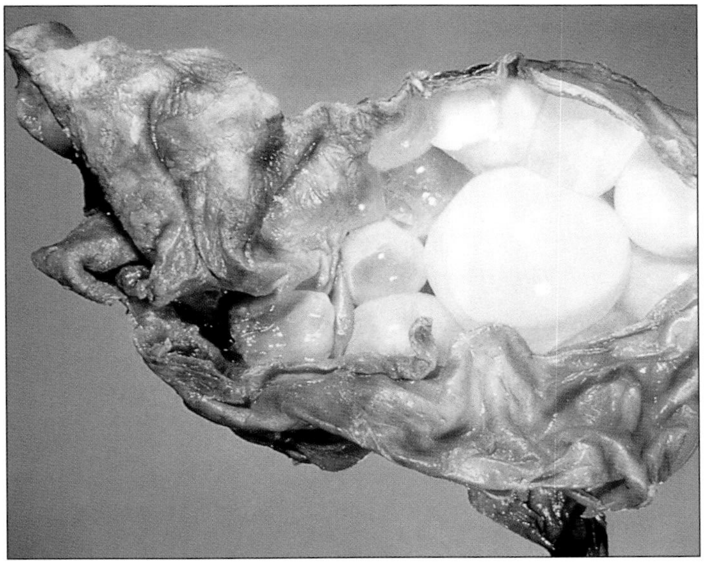

4

Plate 85

Cestode Anatomy

Image 1

Transverse section of a *Taenia saginata* proglottid. Beneath the thick tegument, the underlying parenchyma is divided into cortical (CO) and medullary (ME) layers by a thick band of longitudinal muscles. Prominent excretory trunks (EC) are readily visible on both sides of the proglottid. Smaller nerve trunks lie adjacent to the large excretory trunks. Branches of the uterus (UT) are evident in the medullary portion of the parenchyma (H&E).

Image 2

Longitudinal section through a proglottid of *Spirometra erinacei*. Nuclei in the subtegumentary layer stain darkly. Just beneath these nuclei are clusters of vitelline glands (keyline). Although the division into cortical and medullary layers of the parenchyma by longitudinal muscles (MU) can be seen, it is not as evident as in Image 1. The rounded structures in the medullary region represent the testes (TE) (H&E).

Image 3

At higher magnification, details of the tegument, vitelline glands, and parenchyma are more clearly seen. Note the longitudinal muscle fibers (MU) (H&E).

Image 4

In this section of the *Spirometra* proglottid, note the parenchyma with diagonal muscle fibers coursing through it (H&E).

Image 5

Eggs of *T. saginata* are seen in the uterus of this section through a gravid proglottid. Several of the eggs have the typical prismatic appearance of *Taenia* eggs (H&E).

Image 6

In this section of a sparganum, *Spirometra* species, the thick tegument and underlying parenchyma are seen. The numerous ovoid holes in the parenchyma represent spaces where calcareous corpuscles were present. With acid fixatives, the calcareous corpuscles are dissolved (H&E).

Image 7

In a different sparganum, fixed with buffered formalin, the calcareous corpuscles retain their morphologic integrity and appear as whorled structures composed of concentric layers of calcium carbonate and other elements (H&E).

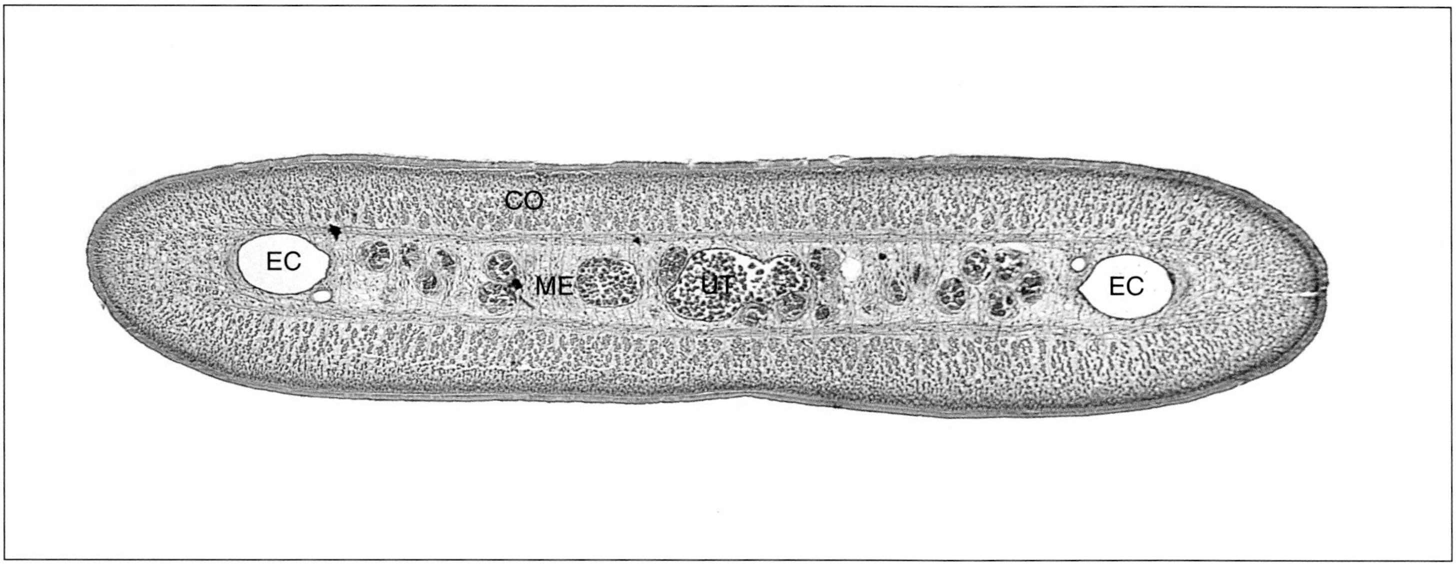

1

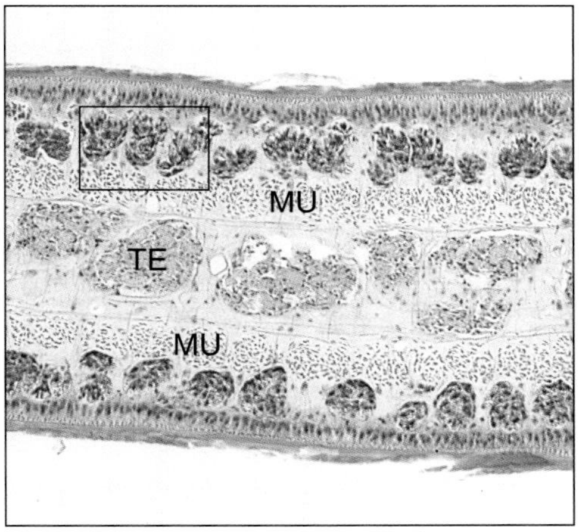

2

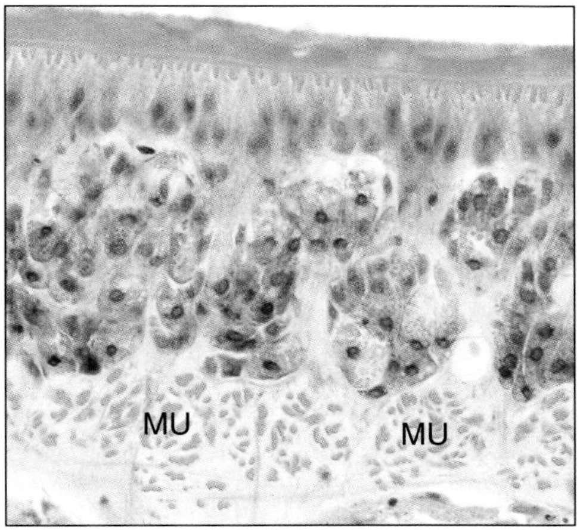

3

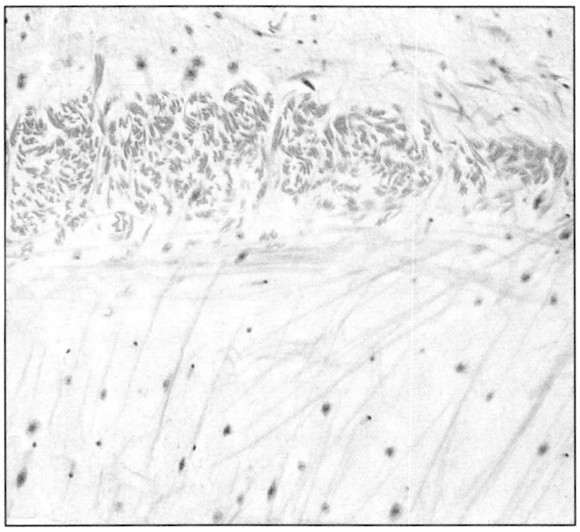

4

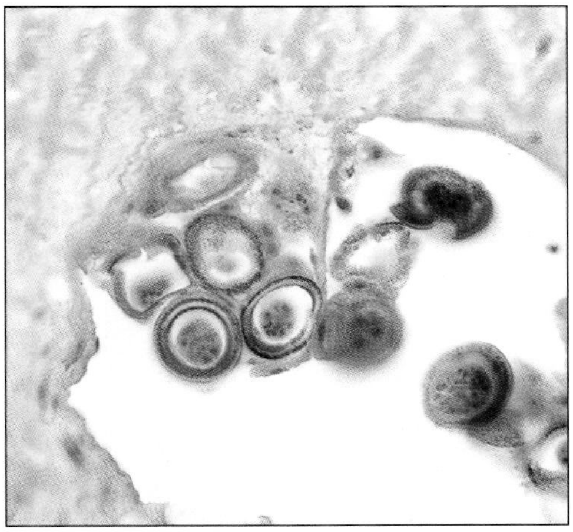

5

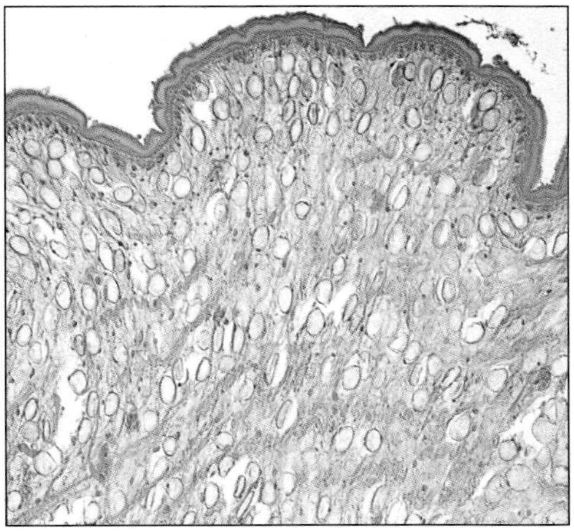

6

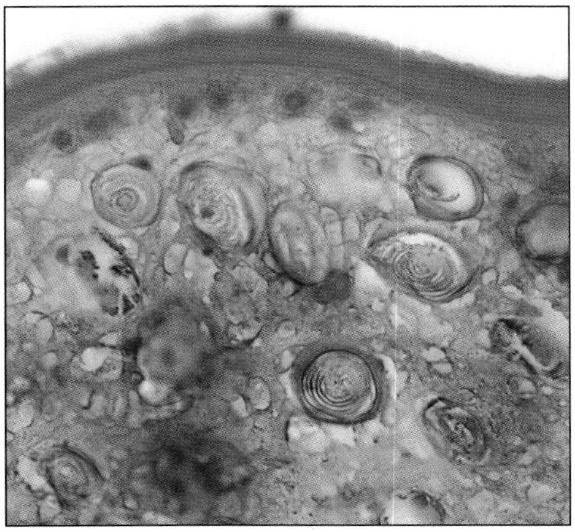

7

Spirometra species

Sparganosis

Human sparganosis is caused by the larval stages of various species of pseudophyllidean tapeworms of the genus *Spirometra*. Species reported as causing human infection include *S. mansonoides* in the United States and *S. mansoni*, *S. erinacei*, and *S. ranarum* in various parts of Asia. Other species may also be involved in human disease. *Spirometra* is related biologically and morphologically to the fish tapeworm of humans, *Diphyllobothrium latum*; however, *D. latum* develops to the adult stage in the human small intestine and does not cause human sparganosis.

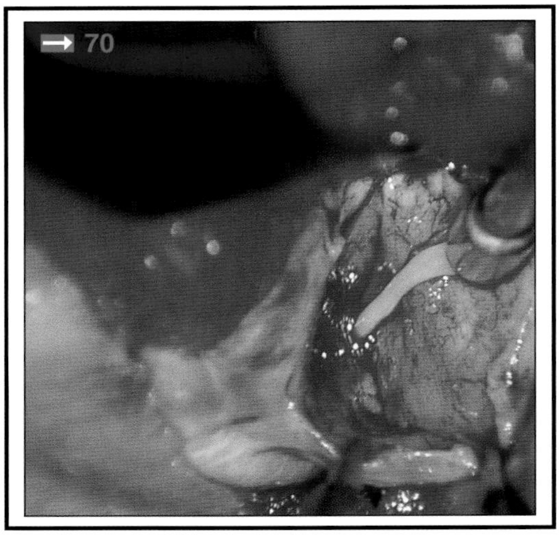

Biology and Life Cycle

Adult tapeworms of *Spirometra* reside in the small intestine of their canid and felid hosts and produce operculated eggs that are unembryonated when excreted in feces. Copepods are the first intermediate host, and fish and other cold-blooded vertebrates serve as second intermediate hosts. Humans acquire sparganosis by accidentally ingesting infected copepods in water or by eating the raw or poorly cooked flesh of infected fish, amphibians, or reptiles. In Asia, where frogs are used as poultices for ocular injuries, ocular sparganosis can result when spargana migrate from the abdominal cavity of the amphibians directly into the orbit of the eye. When spargana are ingested by pigs, boars, and other animals, they migrate into host tissues and cause sparganosis if the flesh of these animals is subsequently cooked inadequately and eaten by humans. Spargana appear to move frequently and with ease in the tissues and organs of their hosts.

Pathology and Clinical Manifestations

Spargana can migrate widely in the human body. The resulting symptoms of their presence depend on the particular tissues or organ systems involved. Migration to subcutaneous locations is painless and may go unnoticed. Frequently, spargana are discovered incidentally during unrelated surgical procedures. However, subcutaneous nodules may develop that are often transient or migratory and painful. Cerebral sparganosis has been reported with increasing frequency in humans, especially in Asia, and is often characterized by convulsions. Ocular sparganosis frequently results in inflammation, severe pain, and marked edematous swelling of the eyelids. Peripheral blood eosinophilia is often absent but occasionally may be marked. Pathologically, nodules containing living spargana usually show little histologic reaction, but spargana that die in tissue elicit the typical eosinophilic granulomas associated with dead or dying tissue helminths. In cerebral sparganosis, lesions may occur in deep regions of the brain, but in most instances they occur in the cortex or subcortex of the cerebral hemispheres. (➡ 70).

Parasite Morphology

Living spargana are white or ivory and have a ribbonlike shape. They range in size from a few millimeters to more than 30 cm long by approximately 3 mm wide (➡ 70). They are actively motile when removed from tissues and placed in saline. The flattened, anterior portion of the worm has a ventral pit or groove that constitutes the rudimentary scolex. Although the body appears to be transversely ridged or folded, it is not truly segmented. In living spargana, large numbers of calcareous corpuscles appear throughout the tegumental surface as refractile, sandlike particles (Plate 86:1).

In histologic section, the anterior end is a cleftlike invagination. The noncellular tegument varies in thickness from 5 to 15 µm. Deep folds of the tegument are usually visible (Plate 86:1, 2, & 5). Beneath this lies a cellular subtegument, which also varies in thickness but is thinner than the tegument. Beneath the subtegument is the parenchyma, a meshwork of fluid-filled spaces formed by parenchymal cells. Bundles of longitudinal muscle fibers and small to large excretory channels are scattered throughout the parenchyma (Plate 86:3 & 6). Although muscle bands in adult cestodes clearly divide the parenchyma of proglottids into cortical and medullary regions, this does not occur in spargana. Transverse sections of spargana do not show the bands of longitudinal muscle fibers in the parenchyma as clearly as longitudinal sections of the larvae do. Calcareous corpuscles, which are unique to cestode tissue and are not present in the parenchyma of flukes, have round or oval bodies with a whorled appearance. They usually measure between 10 and 25 µm. With hematoxylin and eosin, the calcareous corpuscles stain a dark blue (Plate 86:4). Because these corpuscles dissolve in acid fixatives, in acid-fixed tissues they appear as holes in the parenchyma.

In tissue sections, the organisms from which spargana must be distinguished are primarily trematodes and other tissue-invading cestode larvae, including cysticerci, coenuri, hydatid, and some zoonotic larval cestodes, which may infiltrate human tissues and are difficult to identify specifically. The solid-bodied sparganum lacks the suckers and the surrounding bladder wall that are typical of cyclophyllidean tapeworms. Irregularly scattered bundles of longitudinal muscle fibers, the presence of excretory channels, the typical folded tegument, and calcareous corpuscles in the parenchyma suggest a sparganum. Trematodes in section have a thinner, nonfolded tegument and circular, longitudinal, and diagonal muscle layers. Portions of the digestive tract and reproductive organs are also visible.

Although it is possible to see sections of cysticerci and coenuri without a visible bladder wall, one or more suckers or a portion of them are usually visible. If only the bladder wall of a cysticercus is visible, it is much thinner and lacks many of the typical features of the sparganum. *Sparganum proliferum* is a rare form of sparganosis in which many sections of numerous larvae exhibit characteristic sparganum morphology. Within the parenchyma, however, follicle and vesicle formation is common, and excretory channels may be large and form cavities. No sign exists of even a rudimentary pseudophyllidean scolex in these organisms. Proliferating cestode larvae, other than *S. proliferum*, that invade human tissues include racemose cysticercosis (caused by *Taenia solium* or other *Taenia* species), various zoonotic species, and the larval stage of *Mesocestoides,* which produces a tetrathyridium type of larva (Hubbard et al, 1993). Most of these proliferating larval stages lack a scolex (acephalic) and show exogenous budding of the tissue.

References

Beaver PC, Rolon FA. Proliferating larval cestode in a man in Paraguay: a case report and review. *Am J Trop Med Hyg.* 1981;30:625-637.

Chan ST, Tse CH, Chan YS, et al. Sparganosis of the brain: report of two cases. *J Neurosurg.* 1987;67:931-934.

Chang KH, Chi JG, Cho SY, et al. Cerebral sparganosis: analysis of 34 cases with emphasis on CT features. *Diagnost Neuroradiol.* 1992;34:1-8.

Hubbard GB, Gardiner CH, Bellini S, et al. *Mesocestoides* infection in captive Olive baboons (*Papio cynocephalus anubis*). *Lab Anim Sci.* 1993;43:625-627.

Huh S, Wang KC, Hong ST, et al. Histopathological changes of the cat brain in experimental sparganosis. *Path Res Pract.* 1993;189:1181-1186.

Mueller JF. Studies on *Sparganum mansonoides* and *Sparganum proliferum*. *Am J Trop Med.* 1938;18:303-328.

Noya O, Alarcon de Noya B, Arrechedera H, et al. *Sparganum proliferum*: an overview of its structure and ultrastructure. *Int J Parasitol.* 1992;22:631-640.

Yamashita K, Akimura T, Kawano K, et al. Cerebral *Sparganosis mansoni*: report of two cases. *Surg Neurol.* 1990;33:28-34.

Plate 86

Spirometra species

Image 1

A three-week-old sparganum of *Spirometra erinacei* recovered from the flesh of a tadpole. Although this is a young sparganum and is still small, it nicely illustrates the typical appearance of calcareous corpuscles in living larval cestodes. They appear as refractile, sandlike particles scattered throughout the parenchyma. The tegument and subtegument are slightly darker than the parenchymal region, and a slight depression (cleft) or pitlike structure is noted at the large end, indicating the region of the developing scolex. As a sparganum grows, it becomes ribbonlike. (Courtesy of J. Chai.)

Image 2

Sparganum in the parenchyma of the brain of a Chinese patient. Three sections of a single sparganum are present. Even at this low magnification, the infolding of the tegument in the larger section is visible. Longitudinal muscle fibers and holes representing excretory channels are apparent, although faint, within the parenchyma (H&E, 10x).

Image 3

At higher magnification, the folded tegument, longitudinal muscle fibers, and excretory channels within the parenchyma are readily seen (H&E, 50X).

Image 4

At still higher magnification, details of the thick tegument, underlying cellular subtegument, and the parenchyma are visible. Many calcareous corpuscles are present, appearing as round spheres with concentric whorls (darts). Some corpuscles stain more darkly than others (H&E, 250X).

Image 5

Sparganum from the brain of an Indian patient. Following a left parietal craniotomy, a worm measuring 2.5 cm in length was removed from the patient's brain. This case was initially reported in the literature as *Angiostrongylus cantonensis* infection. Subsequent examination of histologic sections revealed a sparganum with typical morphologic characteristics. In this section, the pseudoannulated tegument, cellular subtegument, and parenchyma are seen. The longitudinally oriented muscle fibers (darts) and excretory channels (EC) are quite visible. Calcareous corpuscles are not evident (H&E, 125x).

Image 6

Sparganum in tissue from a raccoon. Two portions of the same worm are present. In the larger portion, the tegument, cellular subtegument, and parenchyma containing calcareous corpuscles (arrows) are visible (H&E, 100x).

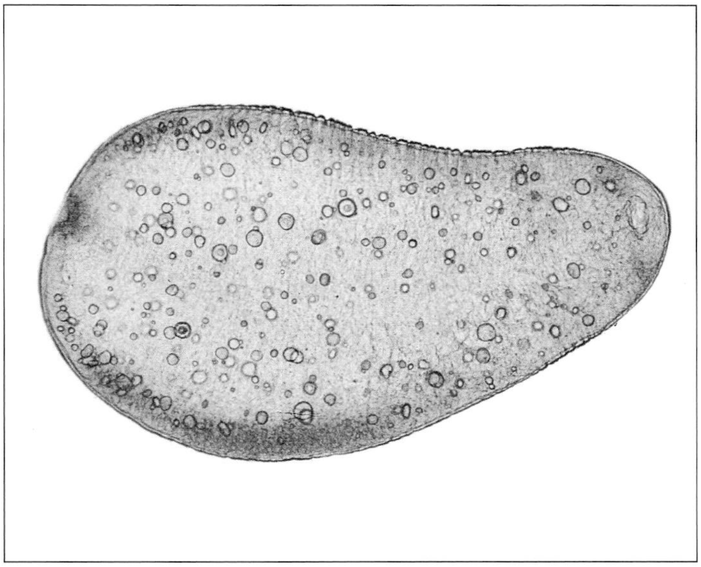

1

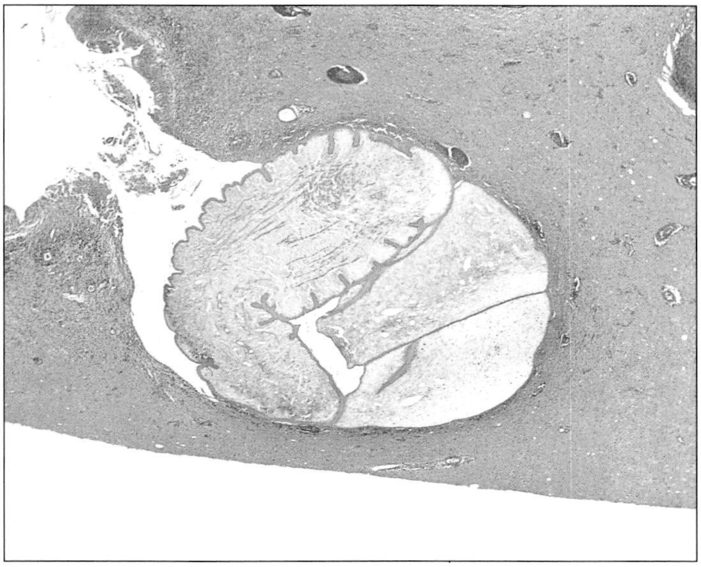

2

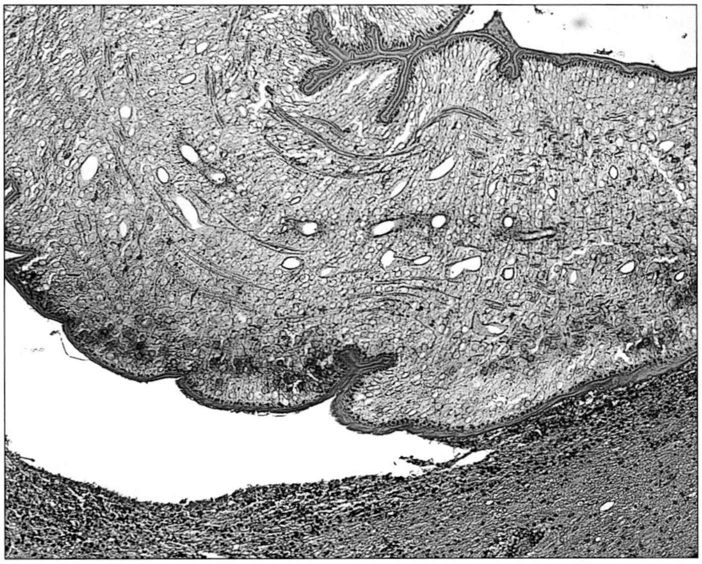

3

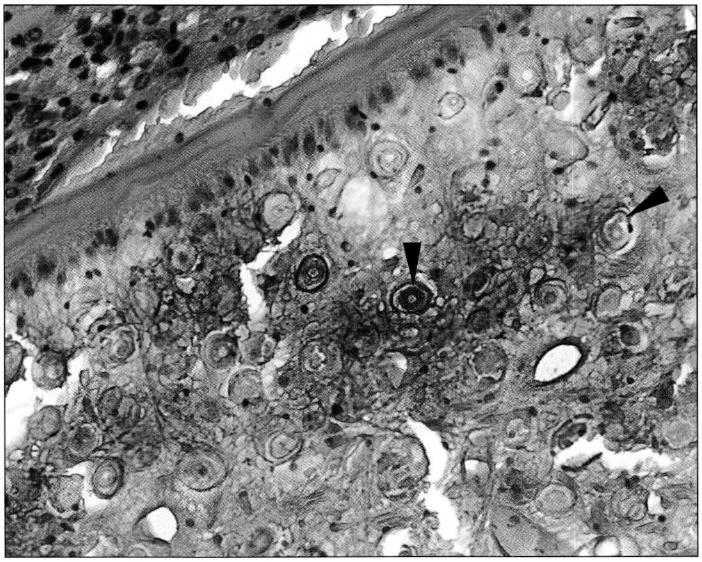

4

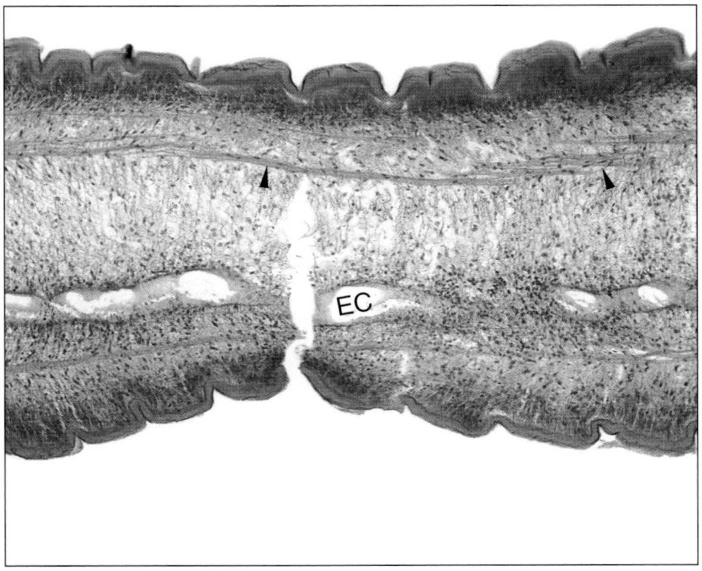

5

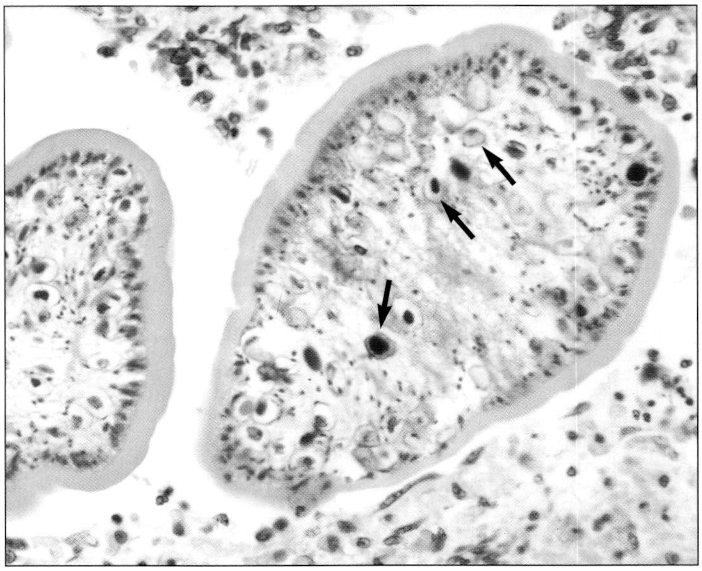

6

Taenia solium

Cysticercosis

Cysticercosis is caused by *Taenia solium*, the pork tapeworm, which is a common human parasitic infection in many parts of the world, particularly Latin America, Africa, and Asia. Invasion of the central nervous system by the larval parasite (neurocysticercosis) is an especially important cause of human morbidity and mortality. In the United States, reported cases of cysticercosis have increased markedly in the last decade, particularly in California and other western states. This increase corresponds directly to an increase in the number of immigrants from Mexico and other parts of Latin America where *T. solium* infection is widespread. Although the majority of these infections have been acquired outside of the United States, an increasing number of cases are acquired locally, often from infected immigrants who work in households or as food handlers.

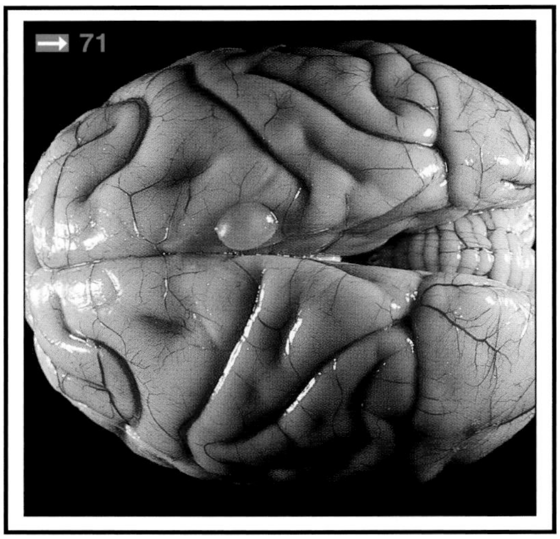

Biology and Life Cycle

Both the adult tapeworm and the cysticercus can be found in the human host. The adult tapeworm develops in the small intestine after the human host ingests cysticerci present in the flesh of infected pigs, which are the intermediate host. Maturation to the adult stage takes approximately 1 to 3 months. Adult worms may reach lengths of up to 7 m and have lifespans of one to two decades or more. The anterior end of the adult tapeworm attaches to the wall of the intestine by means of a scolex equipped with four suckers and a rostellum armed with a double row of small hooklets. Diagnosing this infection by finding eggs in feces is uncommon, because eggs are not routinely liberated from proglottids. Instead, one or more of the terminal, gravid proglottids may break off from the posterior end of the tapeworm and spontaneously make their way out of the anus or pass out of the body in feces. Diagnosis is based on recognition of the characteristic morphologic features of the gravid proglottids. Because the eggs of *T. solium* and *T. saginata* are indistinguishable from each other and from other taeniid tapeworms, a specific diagnosis cannot be made from eggs found in human feces. Ingestion of *T. solium* eggs by swine or humans results in the growth and development of cysticerci (referred to as *Cysticercus cellulosae*) in various tissues. Cysticerci reach the infective stage in swine after approximately two months.

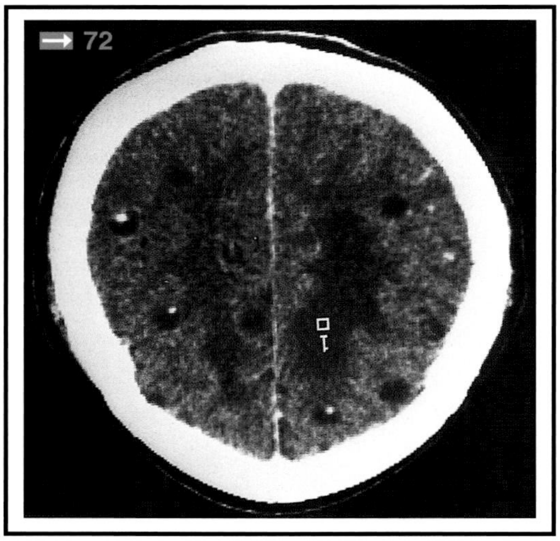

Pathology and Clinical Manifestations

The severity of pathologic manifestations associated with human cysticercosis often depends on the quantity and location of the larvae in the body. Cysticerci develop mostly in subcutaneous and muscle tissues, where they become encapsulated in fibrous tissue and ultimately die and undergo calcification. Although cysticerci have been reported from most tissues and organs, the eye and central nervous system are the next most common sites of infection (➡ 71). In these two sites, the larval tapeworm does not become encapsulated. In Mexico, an important focus of human cysticercosis, the parasite is the main cause of seizures and late-onset epilepsy. Inflammatory lesions in the brain are caused by both living and dead or dying worms.

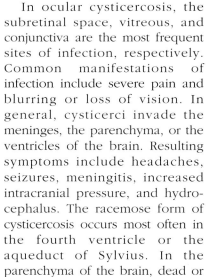

In ocular cysticercosis, the subretinal space, vitreous, and conjunctiva are the most frequent sites of infection, respectively. Common manifestations of infection include severe pain and blurring or loss of vision. In general, cysticerci invade the meninges, the parenchyma, or the ventricles of the brain. Resulting symptoms include headaches, seizures, meningitis, increased intracranial pressure, and hydrocephalus. The racemose form of cysticercosis occurs most often in the fourth ventricle or the aqueduct of Sylvius. In the parenchyma of the brain, dead or dying parasites elicit severe inflammatory reactions. The organisms usually calcify and when dead are often surrounded by a thin layer of fibrous tissue. Diagnosing cysticercosis is not easy: it frequently requires complex serodiagnostic procedures and imaging procedures such as computed axial tomography (➡ 72) and magnetic resonance imaging.

Parasite Morphology

Fully developed cysticerci are round or elongated, measure from 5 to 15 mm in length by 4 to 12 mm in diameter, and generally have a volume of a few milliliters (Plate 87:1). The size and shape of these bladder worms often depend on where they occur in the bodies of swine and humans. In some cerebral sites such as cavities or spaces, cysticerci attain diameters of 4 to 5 cm and their volume may exceed 60 mL. Inside the translucent bladder wall and near the surface is a large opaque mass that constitutes the invaginated scolex and the surrounding parenchyma. A moderately convoluted spiral canal leads to the invaginated scolex, which bears four suckers, and to the rostellum, which usually has 26 hooks (half of which are somewhat larger than the other half).

Morphologic variants of the usual *T. solium* cysticercus have been described in the human central nervous system. A racemose cysticercus can be large, round, or lobulated, or it may appear as a grapelike cluster with digitiform exogenous buds (Plate 88:6). It may reach up to 20 cm in length. The racemose cysticercus lacks a macroscopically visible scolex. A progressive morphologic evolution of the usual cysticercus to a racemose form may occur. In human neurocysticercosis, the usual as well as an intermediate form may be found in the same individual. In the intermediate form, the cysticercus is large and forms smaller bladders, but the scolex still remains visible and in some cases may be partially evaginated. Neither the racemose nor the intermediate forms have been found in animals other than humans.

In tissue sections the cysticercus typically has a dark-staining spiral canal and a scolex surrounded by a thin, lightly staining bladder wall (Plate 87:2 & 3). The tegument of the bladder wall may be smooth, or it may have wartlike protuberances (up to 40 µm in width and 20 µm in height) on its surface (Plate 88:3 & 5). Fine, hairlike processes (microtriches) are discernible on the surface of the tegument. Beneath the tegument of the bladder are bundles of muscle fibers. Below is a layer of subcuticular cells with small, evenly distributed pyknotic nuclei; this layer overlies the main fibrillar network, which contains scattered bands of muscle fibers, ducts, and canals (Plate 88:3 & 5). The thickness of the bladder wall ranges from 50 to 200 µm.

The parenchymatous portion of the cysticercus consists of the invaginated scolex with its spiral canal, four suckers, and a rostellum armed with hooks (Plate 87:2, 3, & 6; Plate 88:5). The surface of the spiral canal is deeply folded, and its tegumental surface is thicker than that of the bladder wall. Beneath the tegument are muscle fibers and subcuticular cells. The parenchyma is usually filled with calcareous corpuscles (Plate 87:4).

In tissue sections, small to extensive portions of the spiral canal, one or more of the four suckers, and the rostellum with hooks may be visible. In many instances, only small portions of the hooks are visible, and on some occasions neither the rostellum nor the hooks are seen within the plane of section. When only the bladder wall is observed, the identification of the parasite as a cysticercus is often difficult. Finding necrotic or calcifying cysticerci in human tissues also complicates the identification process. In such cases, the remnants of hooks or calcareous corpuscles aid in the correct diagnosis (Plate 88:1 & 2).

The racemose form of cysticercosis usually appears in histologic sections as multiple sections of characteristic bladder wall tegument with its underlying subcuticular cells, pyknotic nuclei, and bands of muscle fibers, ducts, and canals (Plate 88:4 & 5). The tegumental surface may be smooth or it may have prominent, wartlike protuberances. The scolex and spiral canal of a typical cysticercus are not seen in the racemose form.

Cysticerci in histologic section are unlikely to be confused with other cestode larvae such as spargana or unilocular or alveolar hydatids. The morphologic appearance of a bladder worm with a single invaginated scolex is different from that of a solid-bodied larva such as a sparganum. Hydatid cysts characteristically have a laminated layer and underlying germinal epithelium. Although the bladder wall of a coenurus is similar to that of a cysticercus, the coenurus has multiple scoleces. In the racemose form of cysticercosis, the proliferation of the bladder wall and the lack of a scolex make it difficult to distinguish from the proliferating bladder tissue of other, rarer acephalic tapeworm larvae that occur in human tissues.

References

Beaver PC, Rolon FA. Proliferating larval cestode in a man in Paraguay: a case report and review. *Am J Trop Med Hyg*. 1981;30:625-637.

Jung RC, Rodriguez MA, Beaver PC, et al. Racemose cysticercus in human brain: a case report. *Am J Trop Med Hyg*. 1981;30:620-624.

Rabiela MT, Rivas A, Flisser A. Morphological types of *Taenia solium* cysticerci. *Parasitol Today*. 1989;5:357-359.

Shandera WX, White AC Jr, Chen JC, et al. Neurocysticercosis in Houston, Texas: a report of 112 cases. *Medicine*. 1994;73:37-52.

Slais J. The morphology and pathogenicity of the bladder worms *Cysticercus cellulosae* and *Cysticercus bovis*. Prague, Czechoslovakia: Academia Publishing House of the Czechoslovak Academy of Sciences; 1970.

Slais J. The morphology of *Cysticercus racemosus* and the determination of the *Cysticercus* species. *Folia Parasitol*. 1967;14:27-34.

Voge M. Observations on the structure of cysticerci of *Taenia solium* and *Taenia saginata* (Cestoda: Taeniidae). *J Parasitol*. 1963;49:85-90.

Plate 87

Taenia solium

Image 1

Cysticerci isolated from pig muscle. The invaginated scolex and spiral canal appear as dense, opaque areas in several of these fluid-filled bladders.

Image 2

Typical section through a cysticercus in human brain. The bladder wall (dart) completely surrounds the parenchymatous portion, demonstrating the folded spiral canal (SC) and a portion of one of the suckers of the scolex (arrow). A narrow band of host tissue forms a fibrous capsule around the organism (H&E, 20x).

Image 3

At high magnification, the parenchymatous portion of a cysticercus is seen. The extensively folded spiral canal and a scolex with two suckers and the denser tissue of the rostellum (dart) are clear. Hooklets on the rostellum are not in the plane of section (H&E, 50x).

Image 4

At much higher magnification, the outer tegument and underlying calcareous corpuscles are found in the branches of the spiral canal. Numerous, rounded to elongate, blue calcareous corpuscles are present within the fibrillar tissue. If acid tissue fixatives were used, the calcareous corpuscles would be dissolved and only empty spaces would remain where the corpuscles had been (H&E, 250x).

Image 5

Section through the scolex region of a cysticercus demonstrates two of the four suckers and numerous portions of hooklets on the rostellum (H&E, 125x).

Image 6

Occasionally an entire hook may be seen. This section shows a typical taeniid hooklet in sagittal section as well as some of the parenchymatous portion of the cysticercus. Usually only portions of hooklets are seen in histologic sections (H&E, 400x).

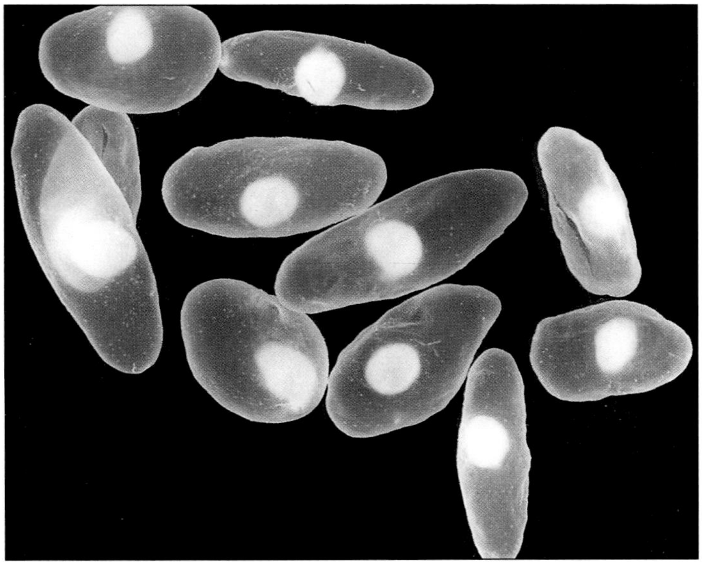

1

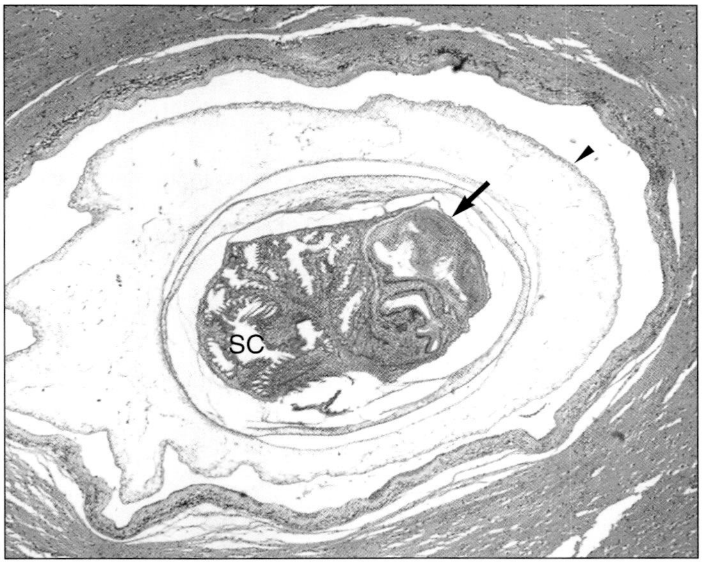

2

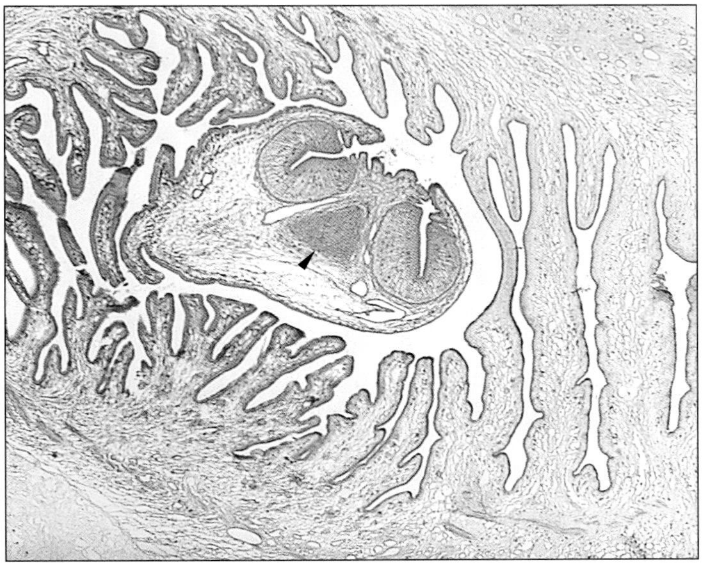

3

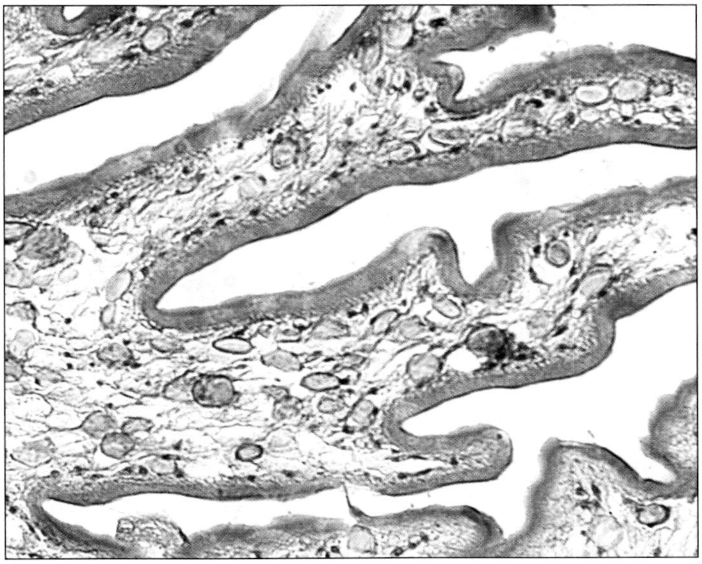

4

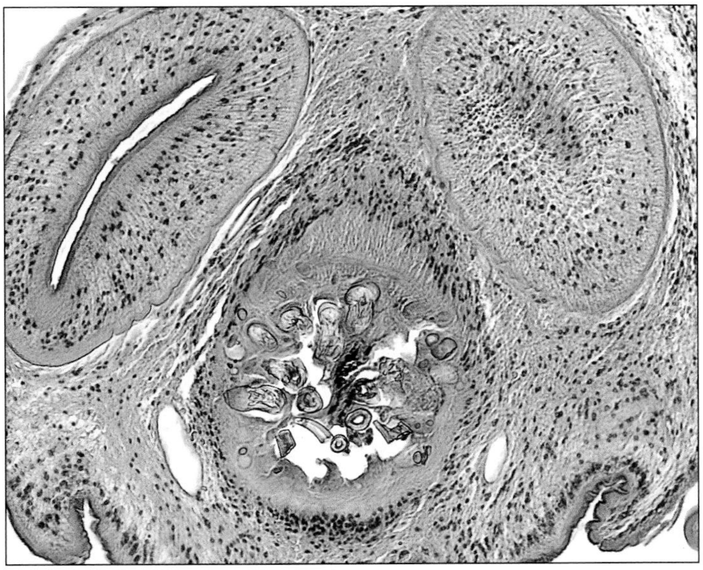

5

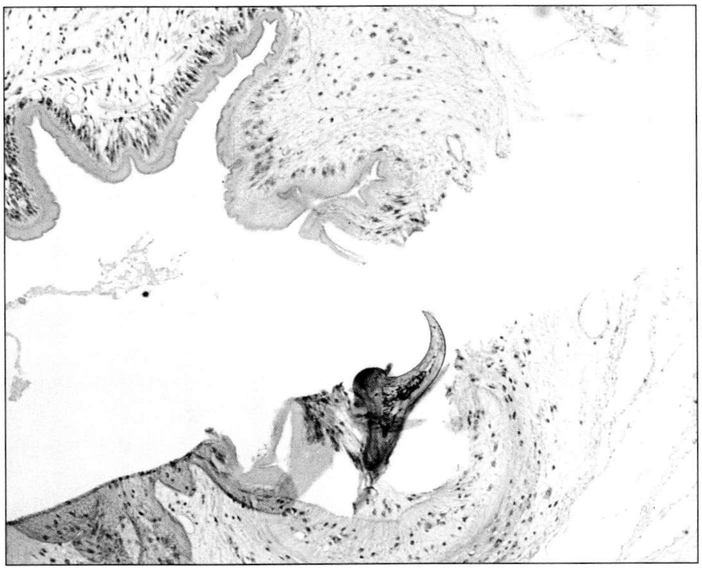

6

Plate 88

Taenia solium

Image 1

Section through a necrotic cysticercus in the brain of a Hispanic man who died after a seizure. This field contains an elongate section through a rostellar hook (dart) and small, oval, calcareous corpuscles (arrrows). No other characteristic remnants of a cysticercus are present (H&E, 250x).

Image 2

In another field from the same case, one can see the faint outlines of the branches of the spiral canal (SC). In addition, cross-sections of some of the rostellar hooklets (darts) and blue-staining calcareous corpuscles are evident (H&E, 500x).

Image 3

The bladder wall of a racemose type of cysticercus demonstrates three distinct layers. The tegumental surface has wartlike protuberances and is acidophilic. Directly beneath the tegument are small, rounded, pyknotic nuclei. The innermost layer is made up of loose connective tissue (H&E, 125x).

Image 4

Section of brain from a Thai patient shows a degenerating cysticercus. Only the thin bladder wall is present (H&E, 100x).

Image 5

A portion of the spiral canal demonstrates the characteristic folding of the tegument, the layer of dark-staining nuclei, and the loose connective tissue (H&E, 25x).

Image 6

In another section of a racemose cysticercus, different sections of buds from the bladder wall are evident. Even at this low magnification, the warty protuberances on the tegument, pyknotic nuclei, and loose connective tissue strongly suggest a larval tapeworm (H&E, 125x).

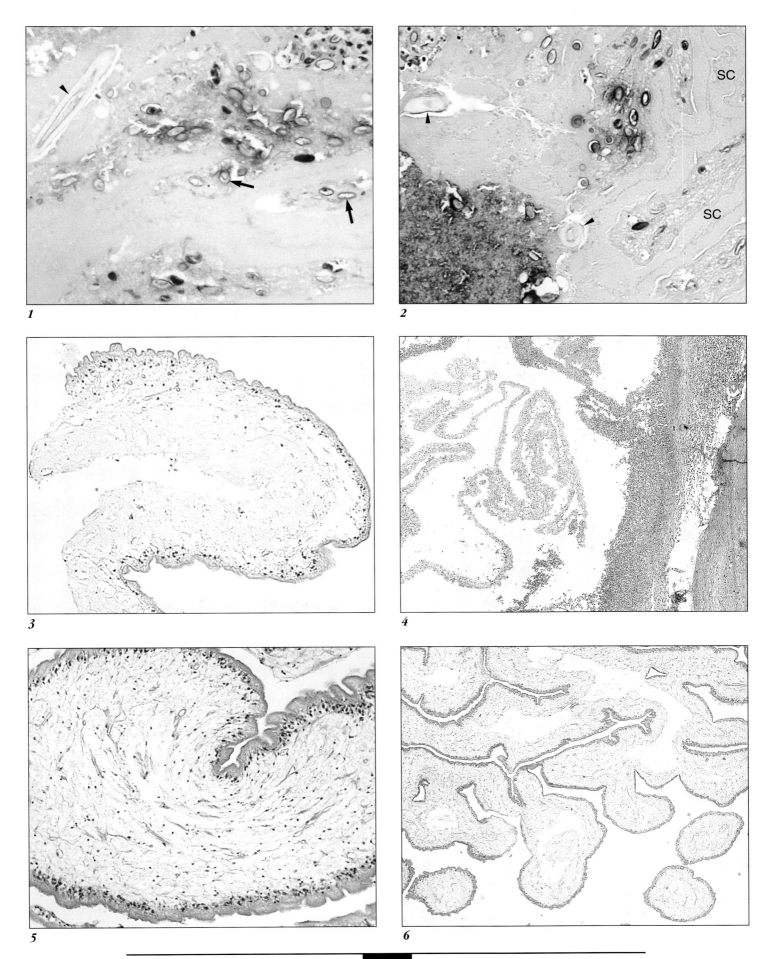

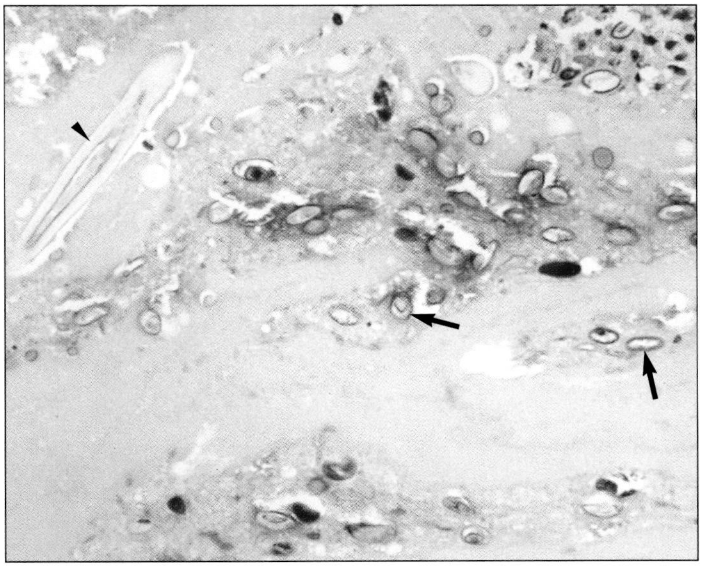

1

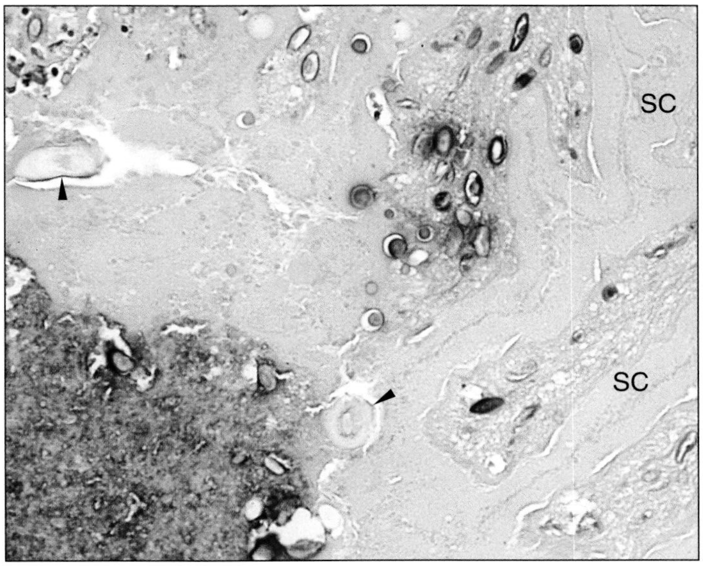

2

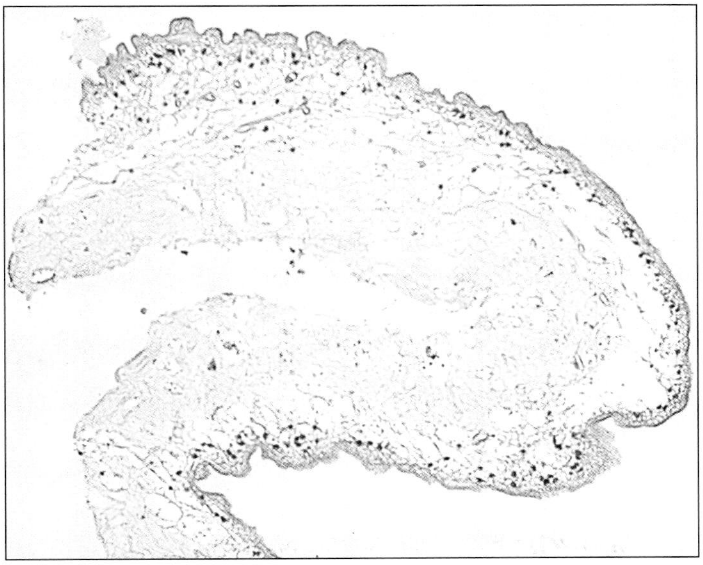

3

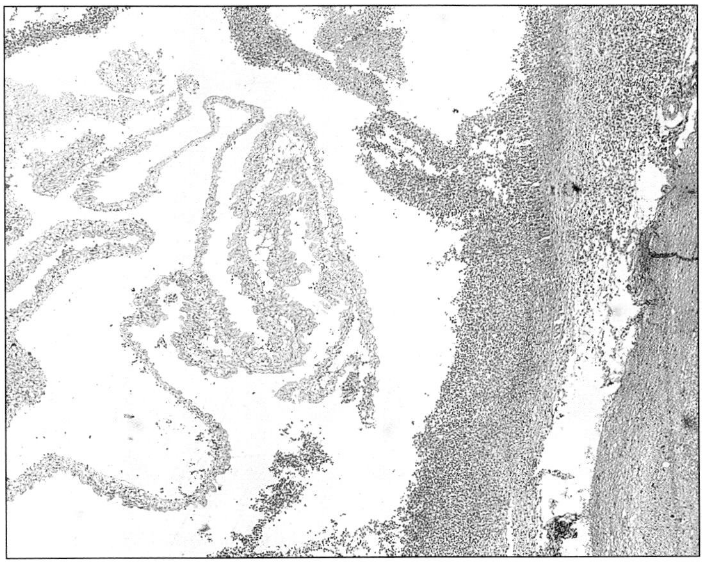

4

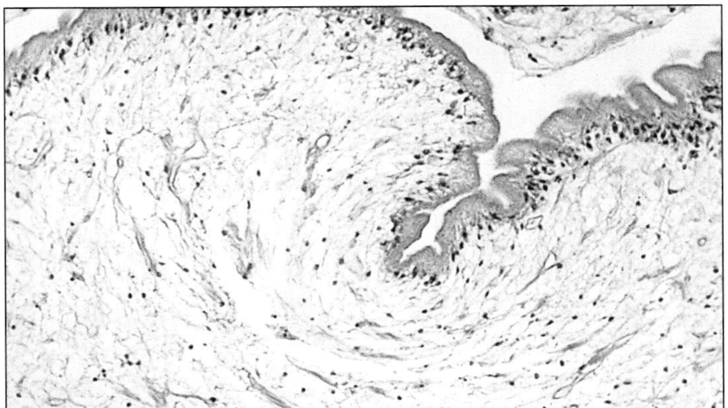

5

6

Taenia multiceps and *Taenia serialis*

Coenurosis

The larval stage of several species of *Taenia* is called a coenurus. A coenurus is a bladder worm that has multiple protoscoleces invaginated into a fluid-filled bladder. The two principal species that have a coenurus-type larva are *Taenia multiceps* and *T. serialis*, both of which use various canids as definitive hosts for the adult tapeworm. These two species were formerly classified within the genus *Multiceps* as *M. multiceps* and *M. serialis*. Numerous cases of human coenurus larvae have been reported. Larvae have been found in muscle tissue, the central nervous system, and the eye. Geographically, *T. multiceps* has been reported from the Americas, parts of Europe, and Africa; *T. serialis*, on the other hand, is found in the United States and Canada. A third species, *T. brauni*, has been reported from Africa. Coenurus infection in humans is rare compared to the incidence of cysticercus infection.

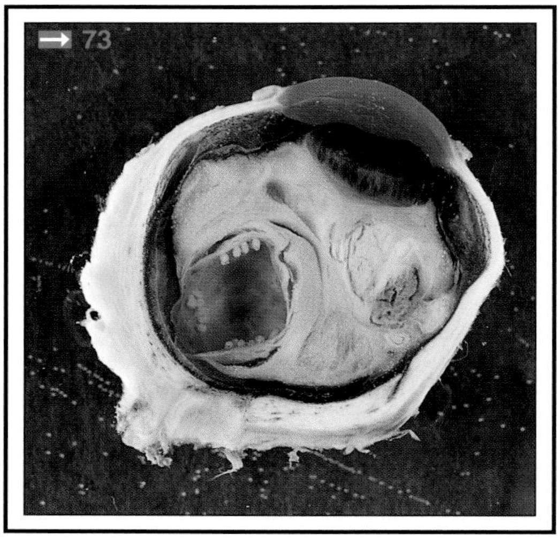

Biology and Life Cycle

All species of *Taenia* have similar life cycles. Adult tapeworms develop in dogs or other canids after ingesting a coenurus in the tissues of various intermediate hosts, including sheep, goats, and other herbivores (*T. multiceps*); hares, rabbits, and other rodents (*T. serialis*); and gerbils (*T. brauni*). Each protoscolex within a coenurus has the potential to mature into an adult tapeworm when the coenurus is eaten by a canid host. Eggs produced by the adult tapeworms are shed in feces and are morphologically typical taeniid eggs. Ingestion of eggs by appropriate intermediate hosts or by humans results in development of a coenurus.

Pathology and Clinical Manifestations

Clinical manifestations of human infection usually depend on the location of the coenurus. In the brain, coenuri are present more often in the subarachnoid space than in the ventricles. Invasion of the cerebral parenchyma also occurs. Typical meningeal symptoms include headache, transient hemiparesis, and epileptiform seizures. Imaging techniques often demonstrate space-occupying lesions, but a specific diagnosis cannot be made without removing the parasite. In the eye, the coenurus most frequently occurs in the posterior chamber, where it causes blurred vision (→ 73).

Clinical symptoms frequently suggest the presence of a neoplasm. When the coenurus develops in muscle tissue a painful nodule often results. Nodules that contain a coenurus and are located in the deep fascia or muscle may be confused with lipomas and neurofibromas. Pathologically, a living coenurus does not stimulate much cellular response, but dead organisms provoke an intense cellular infiltration of lymphocytes, plasma cells, and eosinophils.

Parasite Morphology

A coenurus measures from a few millimeters to several centimeters or more in diameter. It consists of a milky, viscous, fluid-filled bladder into which multiple protoscoleces are invaginated. Cysts are translucent, white to pearl-gray, and thin-walled. They have a globular or elongate shape, and their surface is studded with clumped or irregularly scattered grapelike masses, the scoleces (Plate 84:3). In coenuri of *T. multiceps*, the protoscoleces are scattered irregularly, often in clusters, and are attached to the inner surface of the cyst. The protoscoleces of *T. serialis* and *T. brauni* coenuri are usually arranged more linearly. Internally, cysts found in the subcutaneous tissues and the eye are usually unilocular, whereas those developing in the central nervous system are often multilocular. More rarely, the cysts take on a racemose form in which daughter bladders bud off externally and are attached by stalks to the cyst. Protoscoleces number up to one hundred or more, each having four suckers and a rostellum armed with a double row of hooklets. The spiral canal formed by the invaginated scolex is tortuous in appearance. In living cysts, the protoscoleces can apparently evert and then reinvert into the cyst cavity.

In histologic section, a coenurus typically has a thin bladder wall with multiple protoscoleces (Plate 89:2 & 3). The bladder wall itself is similar histologically to that of a cysticercus. The tegument is 0.5 to 1.0 mm thick and may have a smooth or wartlike surface with hairlike extensions (Plate 89:6). Beneath the surface of the tegument are irregularly scattered, circular muscle fibers and a layer of evenly distributed, dark-staining nuclei that covers the fibrillary network of the parenchyma. The parenchymatous layer, the thickest portion of the bladder wall, is approximately 25 to 30 µm thick. It contains longitudinal and transverse muscle fibers, ducts that have an excretory function, and large nuclei of cells without distinct cytoplasm. Multiple protoscoleces with typical hooks and suckers are present, each with its own spiral canal (Plate 89:2–5). The parenchyma of the spiral canal is similar histologically to that of the bladder wall, except that the parenchyma has a thicker tegumental surface and contains many calcareous corpuscles (Plate 89:6). In sections of a typical coenurus with multiple protoscoleces, short or long portions of the spiral canals are associated with each of the protoscoleces. Depending on the plane of section, the protoscoleces show none, one, or more suckers; the number of hooklets on the rostellum varies. The hooklets are acid-fast and birefringent when viewed with polarized light. Calcareous corpuscles are readily visible with standard hematoxylin and eosin stain and Von Kossa's stain for calcium.

Of the tapeworm larvae that are encountered in tissue sections, a coenurus is unlikely to be confused with a sparganum, which is a solid-bodied larva without a bladder. However, it may be confused with a cysticercus or a hydatid cyst. A section of a bladder worm containing multiple scoleces immediately identifies the worm as a coenurus, because a cysticercus has only a single invaginated scolex. Although a unilocular hydatid cyst in human tissues usually contains many protoscoleces and brood capsules, they proliferate from a germinal epithelium that underlies a laminated membrane, a structure that is found in a hydatid but not in a coenurus. Some other bladder-type cestode larvae reproduce asexually by both exogenous and endogenous budding at the end opposite the scolex. The larval stage of *Taenia crassiceps,* which has been occasionally reported from human tissues, proliferates in this fashion.

References

Freeman RS, Fallis AM, Shea M, et al. Intraocular *Taenia crassiceps* (Cestoda), part II: the parasite. *Am J Trop Med Hyg*. 1973;22:493-495.

Kurtcyz DFI, Alt B, Mack E. Incidental coenurosis: larval cestode presenting as an axillary mass. *Am J Clin Pathol*. 1983;80:735-738.

Orihel TC, Gonzalez F, Beaver PC. Coenurus from neck of Texas woman. *Am J Trop Med Hyg*. 1970;19:255-257.

Templeton AC. Human coenurus infection: a report of 14 cases from Uganda. *Trans R Soc Trop Med Hyg*. 1968;62:251-255.

Plate 89

Taenia multiceps and *T. serialis*

Image 1

A coenurus in a sagittal section of eye from a Ghanian. The organism lies between the choroid and the displaced retina and contains multiple, somewhat linearly arranged protoscoleces (darts). A specific identification of the organism is not possible.

Image 2

Section through a coenurus shows numerous protoscoleces (darts) within a bladder. At this low magnification, one can see the wartlike surface of the bladder wall (unknown stain, 20x).

Image 3

In this section of a coenurus from the neck of a Texan, several protoscoleces are present. There is an exogenous bud (dart) outside the bladder wall (H&E, 40x).

Image 4

In this section of the coenurus shown in Image 3, a protoscolex with two suckers and hooklets on the rostellum is visible (H&E, 125x).

Image 5

In this section through one protoscolex, portions of three suckers and the rostellum bearing refractile hooks are visible (H&E, 125x).

Image 6

At higher magnification, the warty surface of the bladder is clearly evident. In parenchymatous tissue surrounding a protoscolex, a prominent layer of blue-staining calcareous corpuscles is seen (H&E, 125x).

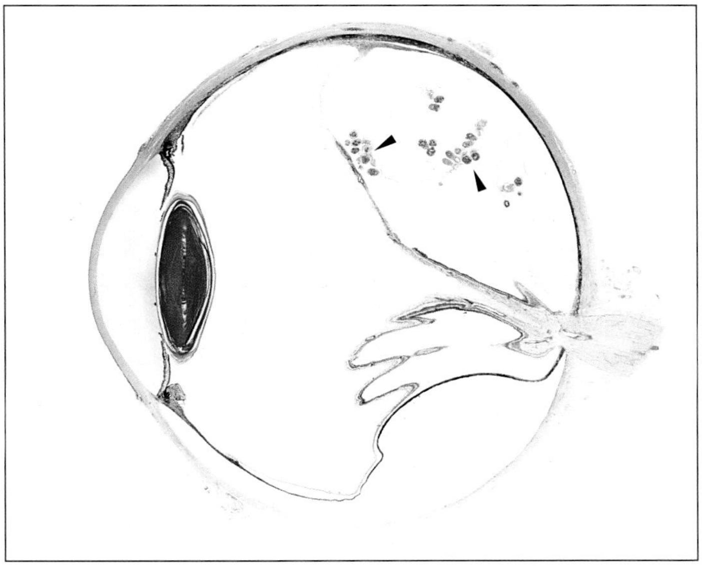
1

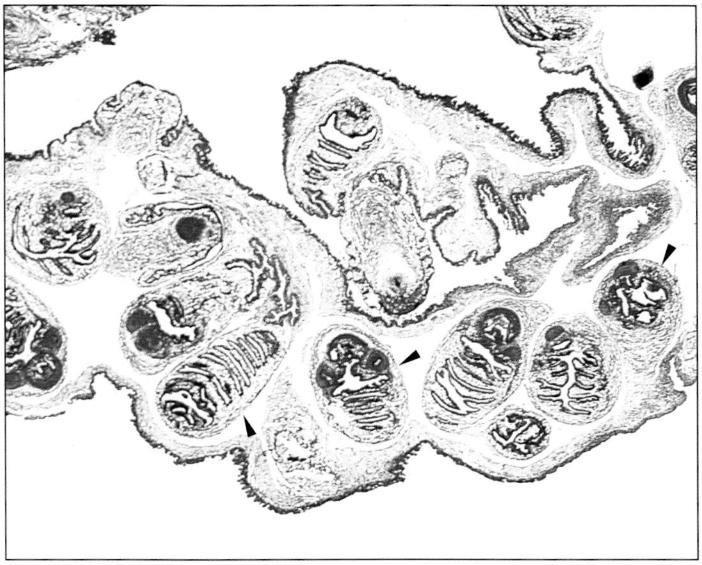
2

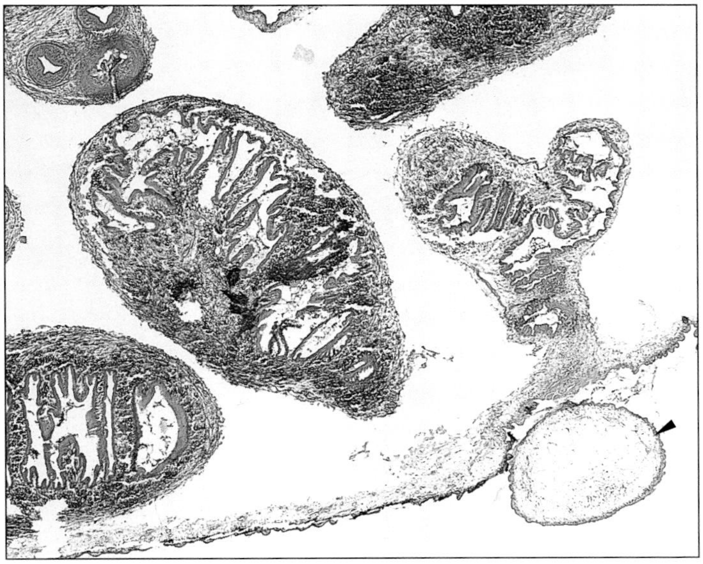
3

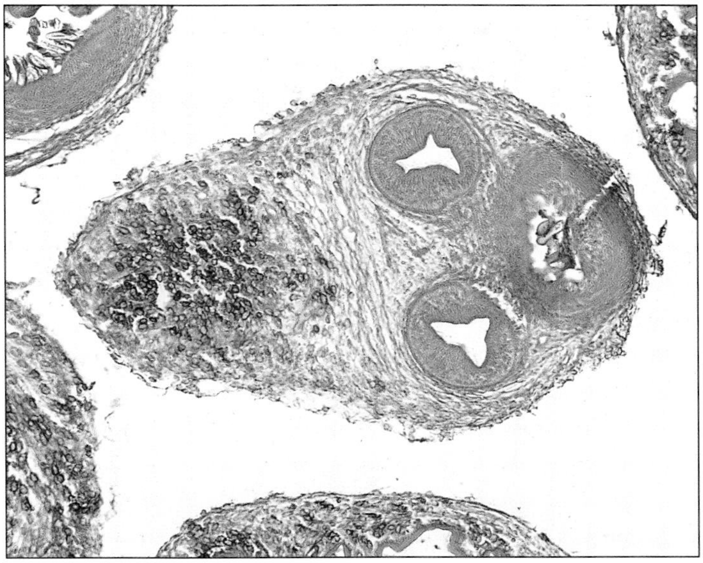
4

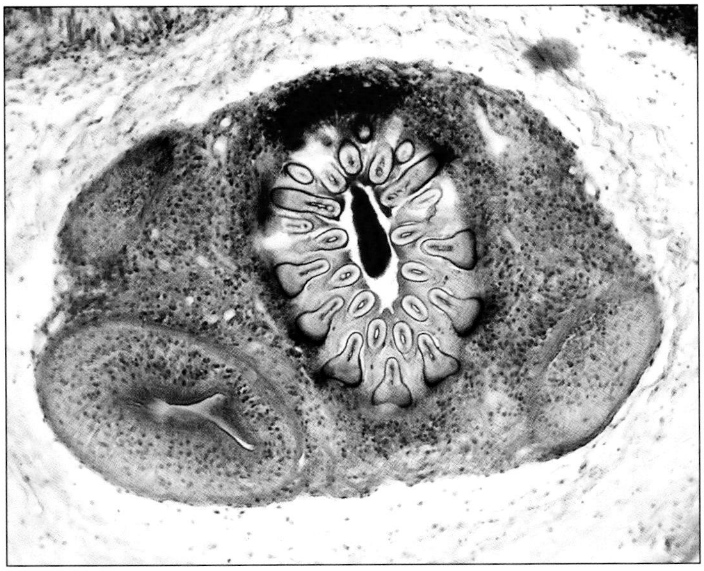
5

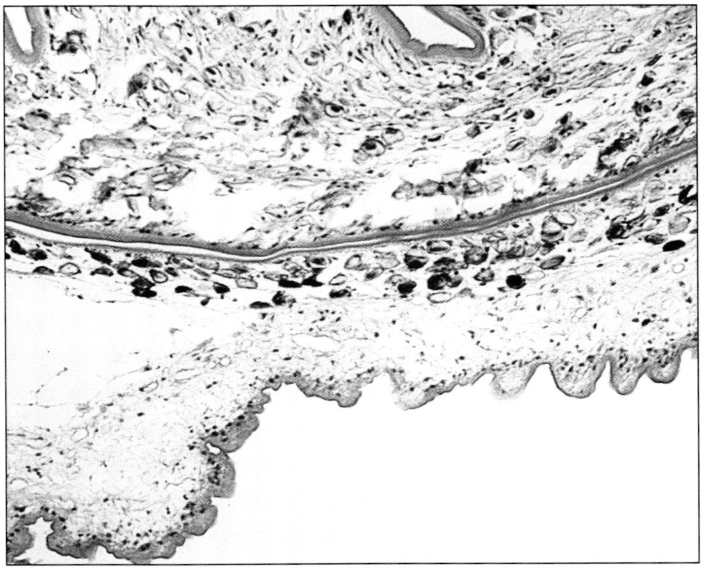
6

Echinococcus granulosus

Unilocular Hydatid Disease

Infection with the larval stage of *Echinococcus granulosus* is called unilocular hydatidosis. The normal definitive hosts for this parasite are canids, including dogs, wolves, hyenas, and others. The larval stage of the parasite, a hydatid cyst, develops in a wide range of intermediate and dead-end hosts, including humans, domesticated herbivorous animals, wild ungulates, and, in Australia, kangaroos, wallabies, and related species. *Echinococcus granulosus* has an extensive geographic distribution but infects humans mostly in sheep- and cattle-raising areas. Many biologic cycles in nature involve strains or subspecies of the parasite, which are associated both with specific types of canid definitive hosts and particular intermediate hosts. In each of these situations, human infections may be acquired accidentally through involvement or contact with the particular canid host or its environment.

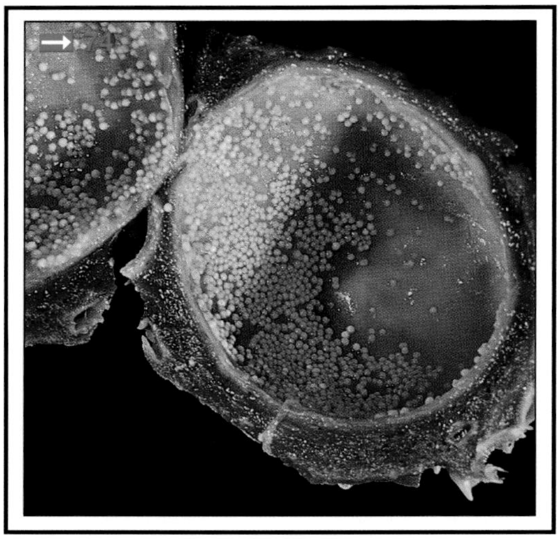

Biology and Life Cycle

The small adult tapeworms attain maturity in the small intestine of canid hosts. Humans are infected solely with the larval (metacestode) stage of the parasite, a unilocular hydatid cyst. Canids become infected by ingesting the protoscoleces present within hydatid cysts that develop in a wide range of intermediate hosts. The most familiar cycle involves domestic dogs as final hosts and sheep and cattle as intermediate hosts.

Adult tapeworms, often present in large numbers, reach maturity 5 to 8 weeks after the host ingests the tissue cysts. Typical taeniid-type eggs are produced and then shed in feces. When eggs are ingested by herbivorous or omnivorous intermediate hosts, the oncospheres hatch and penetrate the wall of the stomach or small intestine, enter the blood vessels or lymphatics, and are carried to extraintestinal sites. The hydatid cysts develop within various organs and tissues, particularly the liver and lungs. Cysts may require six or more months to develop to the infective stage in dogs. In humans, hydatid cyst growth and development is highly variable: cysts of some strains grow slowly, while cysts of other strains grow more rapidly. According to experiments, increases in cyst diameter range from 1 to 5 cm per year. However, many factors affect cyst growth rates, including the strain of parasite and the type of intermediate host. Although cysts are often less than a few centimeters in diameter, they can attain diameters of more than 20 cm and contain 1 L or more of fluid.

Pathology and Clinical Manifestations

Human hydatid cysts have been reported from most tissues and organs. The liver and lung are the two most important sites of infection, but cysts often occur in the kidneys, heart, central nervous system, bone, orbit and eye, muscles, and soft tissues. Clinical symptomatology and pathology are directly related to the cyst's size and location. In confined locations (ie, cranial case, bone), mechanical pressure may result in early clinical symptomatology, but cysts developing in the liver or the abdominal cavity can be present for years or even decades before symptoms develop. Often, infected individuals emigrate from an endemic area to a nonendemic area before symptoms occur, and proper diagnosis may be hampered by the lack of a complete history of residence and travel. Tissue reaction to the presence of cysts usually results in host fibrous tissue response in most organs and tissues, except in the brain and bone. Cysts rupturing spontaneously or because of mechanical trauma can cause fluid to spill and result in anaphylactic shock (Plate 41:3 & 4), the dissemination of free protoscoleces to other sites, or bacterial contamination.

Parasite Morphology

Adult tapeworms of *E. granulosus* are found only in the small intestine of canids; they are never found in humans. The hermaphroditic adult worms are small, 3 to 6 mm in length. They have a scolex that has a rostellum with approximately 30 to 36 taeniid-type hooklets, a short neck region, and typically only three proglottids—one immature, one mature, and one gravid. Eggs within the gravid proglottid are morphologically identical to the eggs of all species of *Taenia*, having a prismatic shell surrounding the 6-hooked embryo (oncosphere) and measuring 30 to 43 μm in diameter (➡ 75).

The size of the hydatid cyst varies depending on the age of the cyst, its location, and the type of intermediate host. Mature cysts containing brood capsules and protoscoleces typically range from a few centimeters to more than 20 cm in diameter (➡ 74). Brood capsules arising from the germinal layer each contain several protoscoleces, which are invaginated and protrude into the cavity of the brood capsule (Plate 90:1-3). In large cysts, daughter cysts with their own laminated and germinal layers develop within the unilocular mother cyst. Degeneration of brood capsules results in the presence of "hydatid sand," or degenerating protoscoleces and free hooklets in the cyst fluid (Plate 91:5; Plate 93:5 & 6). Some cysts are sterile and do not produce brood capsules.

At the microscopic level, the hydatid cyst wall is composed of a tough, elastic, acellular, laminated external layer and a thin, germinal or nucleated inner layer from which brood capsules develop and protrude into the cavity of the cyst (Plate 90:1–5). A host-produced fibrous layer surrounds the cyst. Brood capsules that arise from the germinal layer and protrude into the cystic cavity are stalked and contain several invaginated protoscoleces. In cysts that have ruptured and extruded their contents, histologic sections demonstrate only a much-folded laminated layer (Plate 91:1 & 2) and a thin, germinal, epithelial layer, which often lacks brood capsules. In osseous hydatidosis, the cyst wall may lack a laminated layer or it may be thin.

The morphology of the unilocular hydatid cyst is unique, so it is unlikely to be confused with other cestode larvae that produce bladders (cysticercus and coenurus). In some instances, the unilocular hydatid cyst might be confused with alveolar hydatid disease caused by *Echinococcus multilocularis* or other more rare species. In human alveolar hydatid infection, however, brood capsules are not produced, and the laminated membrane is invasive and more diffusely spread in the tissue (usually the liver). Staining qualities of the hydatid cyst, in particular the laminated membrane, are useful for differentiating it from other cestode larvae and even from other structures in human disease, such as the lipid pseudomembranes seen in membranous lipodystrophy (Plate 90:5 & 6). Of the routine histologic stains used in the laboratory, Gomori methenamine silver stain (GMS) is perhaps the best for distinguishing the laminated layer of the cyst from surrounding host tissue. With GMS, the concentric laminar layers stain black and the rest of the tissue stains a light green. With hematoxylin and eosin, the surrounding host tissue and the laminated layer stain a uniform pink. Movat and periodic acid–Schiff stains differentiate the laminated layer from surrounding host tissue somewhat better but not as dramatically as GMS stain. Although lipid pseudomembranes sometimes resemble the walls of hydatid cysts or cysticerci in histologic appearance, they lack the typical laminations of the hydatid cyst wall and the typical morphology of the bladder wall of cysticerci. The use of GMS and Oil Red O stains helps differentiate lipid pseudomembranes from these structures.

References

Cameron TWM, Webster GA. The histogenesis of the hydatid cyst (*Echinococcus* species), part 1: liver cysts in large mammals. *Can J Zool.* 1969;47:1405-1410.

Marty AM, Hess SJ. Tegumental laminations in echinococci using Gomori's methenamine silver stain. *Lab Med.* 1991;22:419-420.

Smyth JD, Heath DD. Pathogenesis of larval cestodes in mammals. *Helminth Abst A.* 1970;39:1-23.

Vercelli-Retta J, Manana G, Reissenweber NJ. The cytologic diagnosis of hydatid disease. *Acta Cytol.* 1982;26:159-164.

Plate 90

Echinococcus granulosus

Image 1

Typical appearance of a unilocular hydatid cyst of *E. granulosus* in the lung of a camel demonstrates the three layers of the cyst wall. The outer, bright-red–staining, thick fibrous wall (FW) produced by the host surrounds the thinner, pink-staining, laminated layer. Beneath the laminated layer (LL) is the thin, germinal epithelial layer (dart), from which arise the brood capsules. Portions of four brood capsules containing multiple protoscoleces are visible (H&E, 20x).

Image 2

At higher magnification, one can see that the middle laminated layer (LL) is acellular, and the thin germinal layer (dart) contains some calcareous corpuscles. Eight protoscoleces are visible in the brood capsule (H&E, 125x).

Image 3

A hydatid cyst of human origin shows a thick, acellular, light-pink–staining laminated layer and a cellular germinal layer that contains numerous calcareous corpuscles (darts). Several protoscoleces are visible (H&E, 125x).

Image 4

This section of a human hydatid cyst shows the thick laminated layer that stains uniformly and demonstrates the difficulty in distinguishing surrounding host tissue from the laminated layer (H&E, 90x).

Image 5

In this section of a human hydatid cyst, Gomori methenamine silver stain nicely demonstrates the laminar layers of the cyst, allowing for distinction of the parasite cyst wall from the host tissue. It appears that the wall of a hydatid cyst incorporates a chitinlike material that reacts with GMS to give this distinctive appearance (GMS, 100x). (Courtesy of AFIP.)

Image 6

The pathologic condition known as membranous lipodystrophy has occasionally been confused with cysticercosis or hydatid disease. In this GMS-stained section of a nodular mass removed from an arm, the lipid pseudomembrane does superficially resemble the wall of a hydatid cyst. However, the distinctive laminar layer of a hydatid cyst, as seen in Image 5, is lacking. The presence of what is obviously lipid material should suggest the correct diagnosis. In addition, lipid pseudomembranes stain positive with 72-hour oil red O, whereas hydatid cysts do not (GMS, 100x).

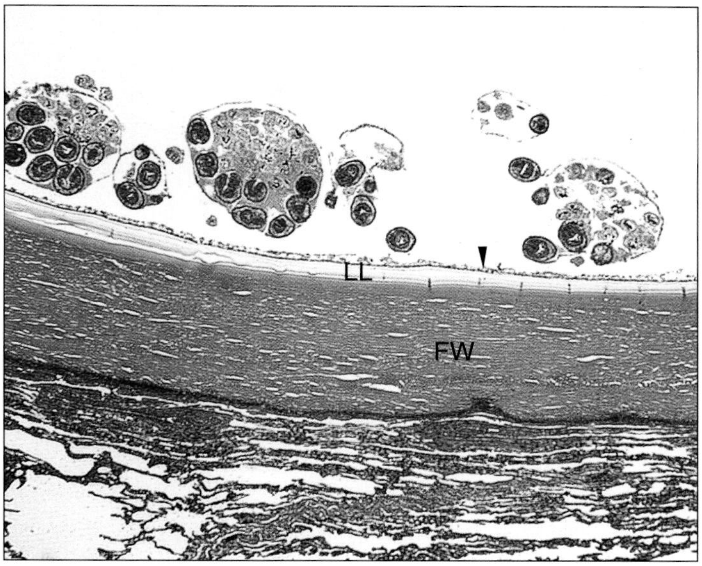

1

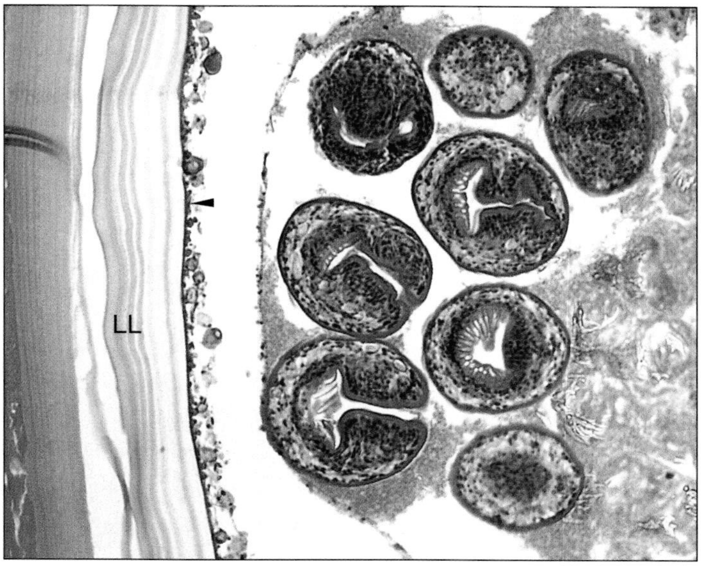

2

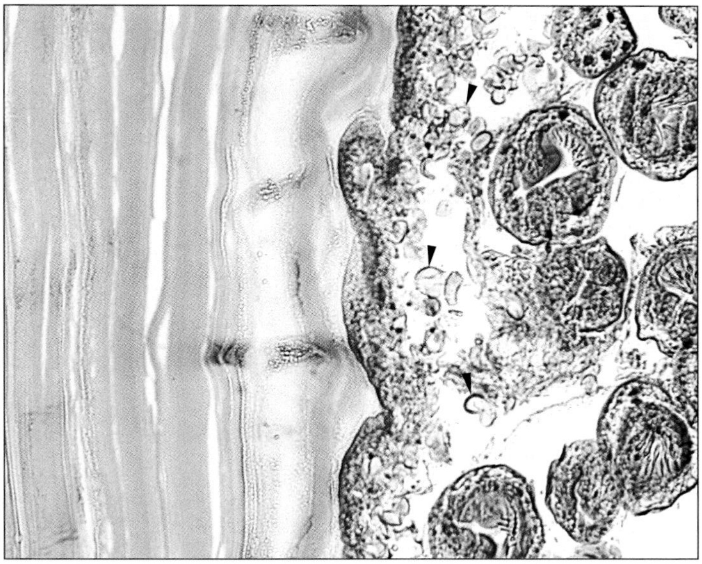

3

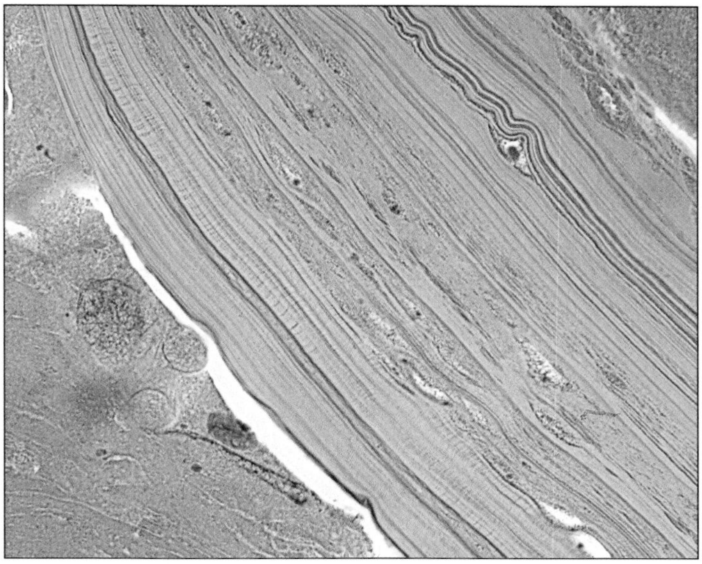

4

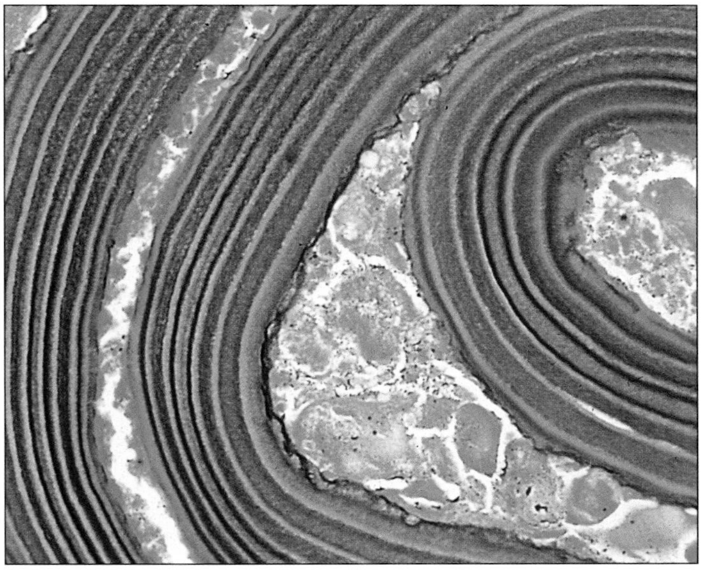

5

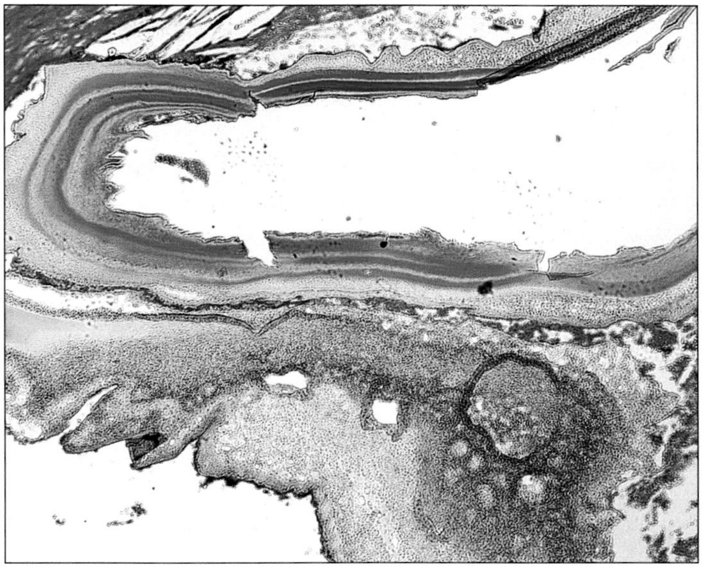

6

Plate 91

Echinococcus granulosus

Image 1

Following surgical resection of a unilocular hydatid cyst, preparations of histologic sections of the collapsed cyst are not uncommon. The most prominent structures are folds of the laminated layer. The germinal epithelial layer is difficult to discern, but a few protoscoleces (darts) are visible (H&E, 50x).

Image 2

In another hydatid cyst, Gomori methenamine silver clearly demonstrates the dark-red–staining lamellar layers, which aid in the diagnosis (GMS, 50x).

Image 3

A section of human lung shows multiple protoscoleces (keyline) liberated from a ruptured hydatid cyst (PAS, 50x).

Image 4

At higher magnification, two protoscoleces show portions of the hooklets present on the rostellum (PAS, 500x).

Image 5

In this section through a hydatid cyst, free hooklets from disintegrated protoscoleces are present. These structures have the typical appearance of taeniid-type hooklets. Fluid, disintegrating protoscolex material, and free hooklets are collectively known as hydatid sand. Such material can establish the diagnosis of hydatid infection when aspirated from hydatid cysts (H&E, 500x).

Image 6

In this section through a degenerate hydatid cyst, all that is visible in a pink-staining coagulum are numerous blue-staining calcareous corpuscles (H&E, 190x).

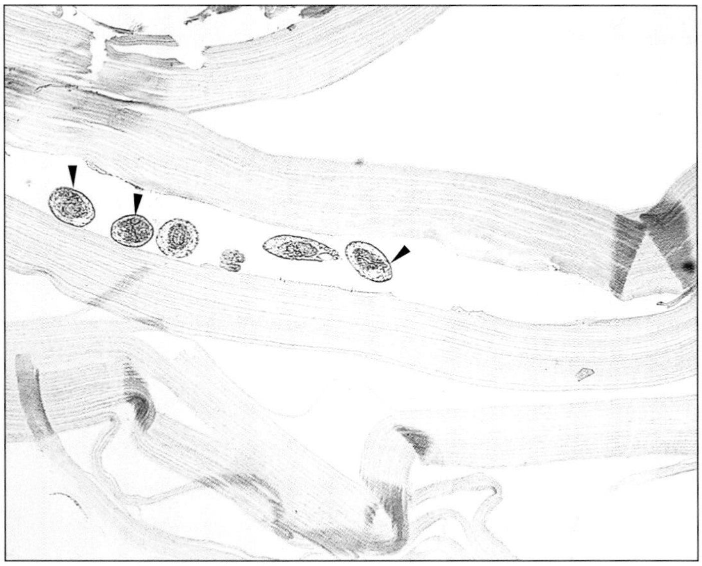
1

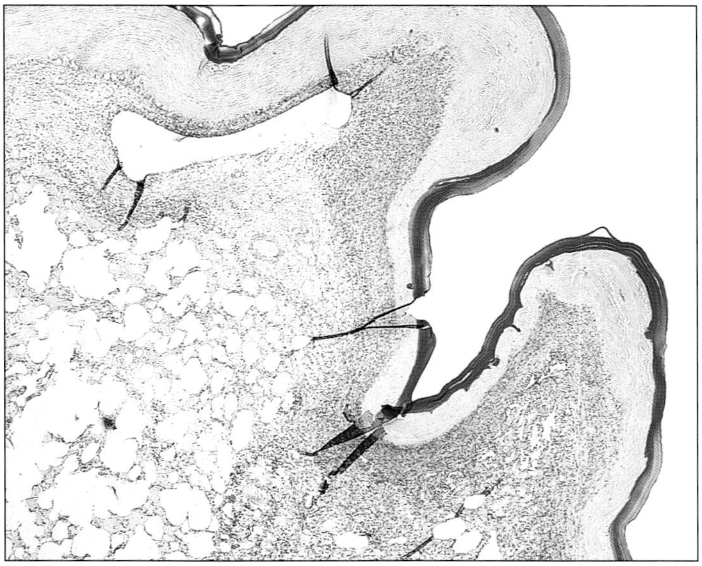
2

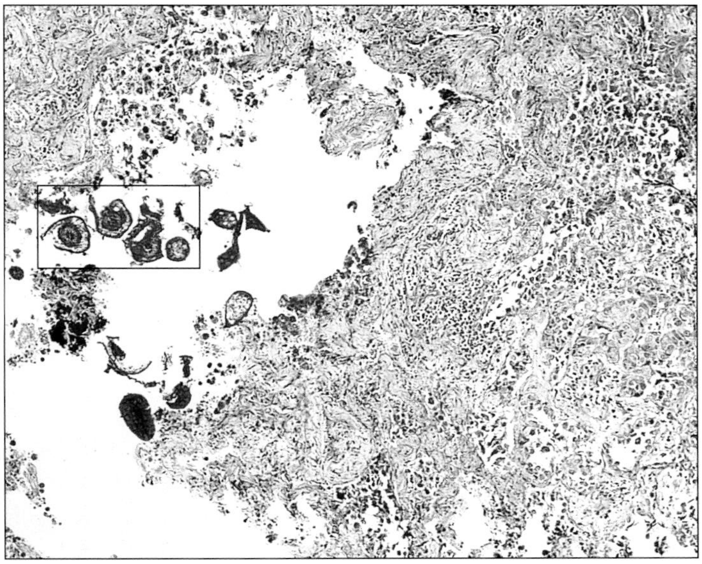
3

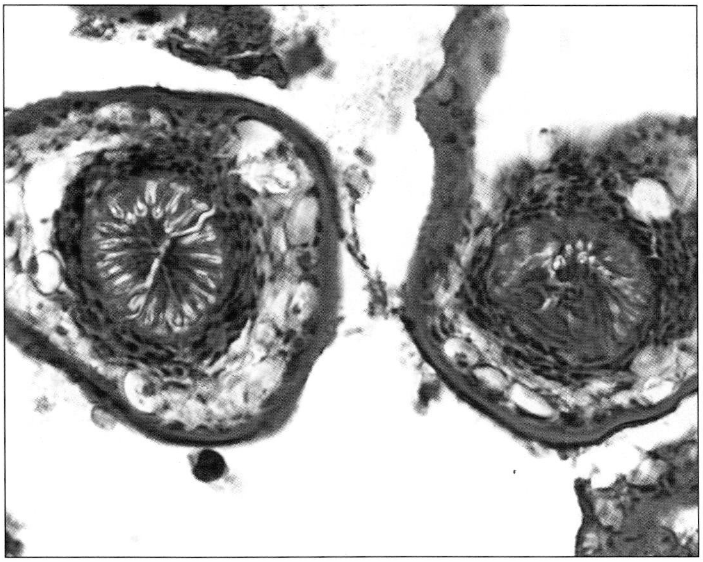
4

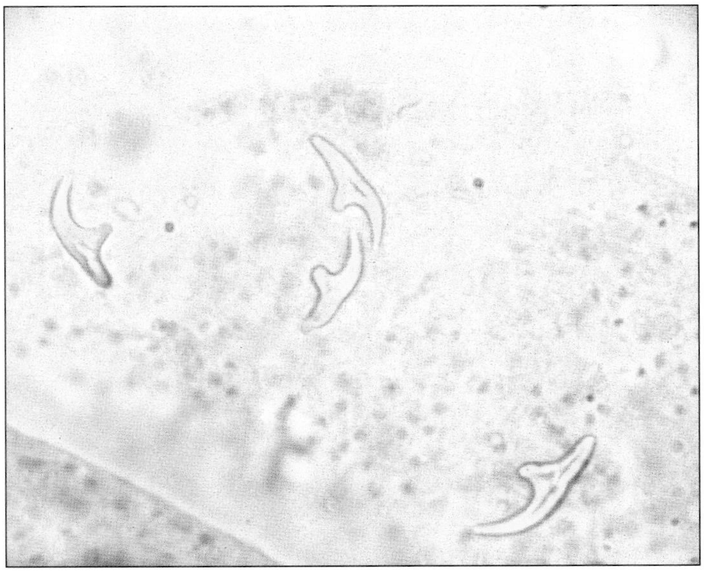
5

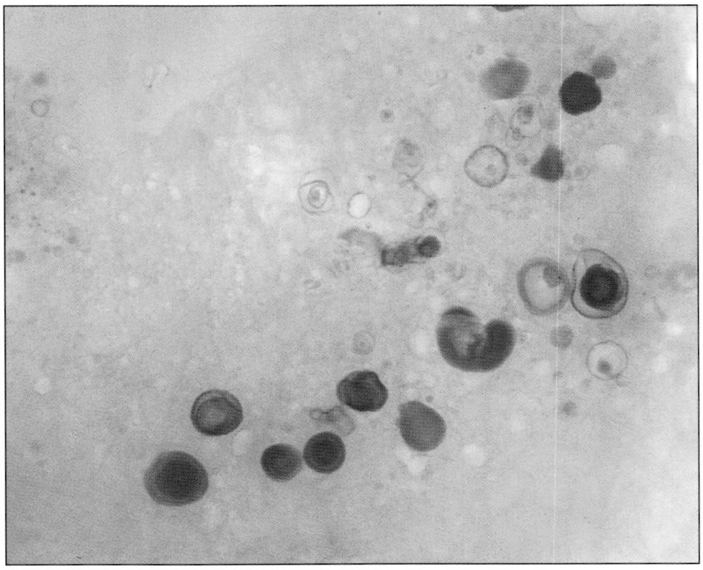
6

Echinococcus multilocularis and *E. vogeli*

Alveolar Hydatidosis

Although hydatidosis caused by *Echinococcus granulosus* is the most prevalent and important of the human hydatid infections, at least two other species of this genus also cause human disease. *Echinococcus multilocularis* causes alveolar hydatid disease, which is encountered primarily in arctic to temperate regions. In the Western Hemisphere, its distribution ranges from Alaska southward through Canada and into the upper Midwest of the United States. It is widely distributed in Europe, extending southward to Iran and Turkey, and occurs in northern parts of Japan, China, and India. *Echinococcus vogeli,* which has been found only in Central and South America, causes human polycystic hydatid disease.

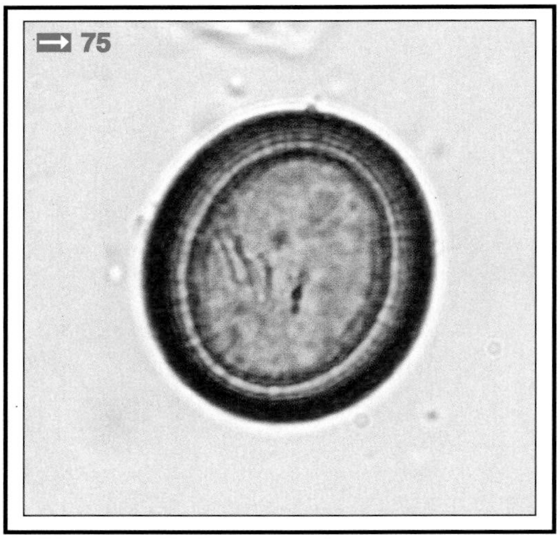

Biology and Life Cycle

Adult worms of *E. multilocularis* mature in the small intestine of various canid hosts, especially dogs and foxes. In some geographic areas the parasite has also been found to mature in domestic cats. Gravid proglottids shed typical taeniid-type eggs, which when passed in feces appear to be especially resistant to cold temperatures. Rodents, including field mice, voles, muskrats, ground squirrels, and others, are the intermediate hosts. The usual site of cystic development in these hosts is the liver. Exogenous budding of the germinal membrane makes this larval cestode highly invasive; it infiltrates the liver much like a malignancy does. Dissemination of protoscoleces from the cysts may result in the invasion of other organs and tissues, but the primary site of infection is the liver. In natural intermediate hosts, the cysts develop protoscoleces, which are infective to canid hosts, within only a few months. The cysts exhibit little growth once protoscoleces have been produced. The prepatent period in canids after ingestion of fertile cysts is approximately one month.

The natural cycle of *E. vogeli* involves bush dogs (*Speothos venaticus*), large rodents, and pacas (*Cuniculus paca*). The larval stage develops primarily in the liver. Numerous rodents and other mammals can be infected, either naturally or experimentally. Domestic dogs have been infected experimentally and are probably the main reservoir for human infections. The prepatent period for *E. vogeli* in dogs appears to be approximately 4 months.

Pathology and Clinical Manifestations

In humans, alveolar hydatid parasites typically mimic an invasive, slow-growing neoplasm of the liver. A correct diagnosis is difficult and is frequently made only at autopsy. Clinical presentation includes portal hypertension, bile duct obstruction, and ascites. Pathologically, the liver parenchyma is destroyed. The parasite is multivesicular, forming irregular spaces that consist of folded and collapsed hyaline membranes and germinal epithelium. A host-produced adventitial layer encapsulating the invasive mass is often lacking. Protoscoleces are produced in human infections only rarely, and calcareous corpuscles are also rare. The infiltration of the germinal membrane into blood vessels may result in metastases, principally to the lung and brain. The host response to the parasite typically involves chronic inflammatory cells, often with many eosinophils, and collagen deposition. Portions of the larval tissue may become calcified. The irregular, collapsed hyaline membranes do not stain well with H&E, though they stain more darkly with periodic acid–Schiff. In humans the polycystic hydatid form of *E. vogeli* produces clinical manifestations and disease similar to those produced by *E. multilocularis.* The liver is the primary organ affected, although metastases to the chest wall and cavity have been reported. As with alveolar hydatids, liver disease resembles that of hepatic carcinoma. Cysts may attain diameters of up to 8 cm or more. They contain aggregates of smaller cysts of various sizes, ranging from a few millimeters to a few centimeters in diameter. *Echinococcus vogeli* appears to be less pathogenic for humans than *E. multilocularis.*

Parasite Morphology

Adults of both species are similar to *E. granulosus* in that they have a scolex with an armed rostellum, a neck region, and three proglottids (immature, mature, and gravid). Adult worms of *E. multilocularis* are shorter than those of *E. granulosus*: they are only 1.2 to 3.7 mm long, whereas those of *E. vogeli* are similar in size. The eggs are of typical taeniid-type morphology and are indistinguishable from one another (75).

The larval stage of *E. multilocularis* in rodent intermediate hosts is a multivesicular, invasive structure that, unlike *E. granulosus* unilocular cysts, has no limiting host adventitial layer around it. As the larval mass expands, it assumes a multicompartmented appearance, with each compartment containing many protoscoleces and calcareous corpuscles (Plate 93:2 & 3). Unlike unilocular cysts, which contain fluid, the material in the alveolar cyst has a more gelatinous consistency. The alveolar hydatid proliferates both exogenously and endogenously through infiltration of cells from the germinal layer, resulting in cystlike or tubelike structures. In humans, the laminated and germinal layers are collapsed, folded, and scattered throughout the liver tissue (Plate 92:1, 2, 5, & 6). Protoscoleces are seen in human alveolar hydatid disease only rarely, and although there may be a few calcareous corpuscles, they are often absent (Plate 92:3 & 4). In *E. vogeli* infection of rodents, the polycystic hydatid demonstrates only endogenous proliferation, resulting in many brood capsules developing within the primary vesicle. The germinal membrane is thin, and calcareous corpuscles are scarce in both the primary vesicle and the brood capsules. Calcareous corpuscles are numerous in the protoscoleces, however. In humans, the polycystic hydatid may grow, contain fluid, proliferate both endogenously and exogenously, and produce brood capsules and protoscoleces (Plate 93:4–6). These features distinguish it from the alveolar hydatid.

In sections of human tissue, the typical alveolar hydatid shows infiltrating parasite tissue that is ductlike and often folded or convoluted. The parasite tissue lacks protoscoleces and calcareous corpuscles and has thin laminated and germinal layers surrounded by a thin layer of host fibrous tissue. Using standard H&E stain, the laminated layer is difficult to distinguish from surrounding host fibrous tissue. The use of PAS and Movat stains better distinguishes the laminated and germinal layers from host tissue response (Plate 92:5 & 6; Plate 93:1). In both rodents and humans, *E. vogeli* has vesiculate cysts containing protoscoleces and calcareous corpuscles.

The invasive nature of alveolar and polycystic hydatids requires that they be distinguished from malignant lesions. The presence of the characteristic laminated and germinal layers facilitates this distinction. Both the alveolar and polycystic hydatids differ from the typical unilocular hydatid with its three, clearly demarcated layers—host fibrous tissue, laminated layer, and germinal layer. Gomori methenamine silver stain nicely delineates the laminar layers of the laminated membrane, which aids in differentiating between the typical bladder wall of cysticerci and coenuri and the lipid pseudomembranes of membranous lipodystrophy.

References

D'Alessandro A, Rausch RL, Cuello C, et al. *Echinococcus vogeli* in man with a review on polycystic hydatid disease in Colombia and neighboring countries. *Am J Trop Med Hyg*. 1979;28:303-317.

Leducq R, Gabrion C. Developmental changes of *Echinococcus multilocularis* metacestodes revealed by tegumental ultrastructure and lectin-binding sites. *Parasitology*. 1992;104:129-141.

Marty AM, Hess SJ. Tegumental laminations in echinococci using Gomori's methenamine silver stain. *Lab Med*. 1991;22:419-420.

Ohbayashi M, Rausch RL, Fay FH. On the ecology and distribution of *Echinococcus* spp. (Cestoda: Taeniidae), and characteristics of their development in the intermediate host, II: comparative studies on the development of larval *E. multilocularis* Leuckart, 1863, in the intermediate host. *Jap J Vet Res*. 1971;19 (suppl 3):1-53.

Rausch R, D'Alessandro A, Rausch VR. Characteristics of the larval *Echinococcus vogeli* Rausch and Bernstein, 1972, in the natural intermediate host, the paca, *Cuniculus paca* L. (Rodentia: Dasyproctidae). *Am J Trop Med Hyg*. 1981;30:1043-1052.

Plate 92

Echinococcus multilocularis

Image 1

Section of human liver containing the alveolar hydatid of *E. multilocularis*. Collapsed, folded, thin laminated membranes are visible. A narrow band of host fibrous tissue surrounds this cystic larva (H&E, 62.5x).

Image 2

In this section, the collapsed laminated membrane is present within connective tissue surrounding a human lymph node. No protoscoleces are visible (H&E, 125x).

Image 3

In this section of human liver, several vesicles of an alveolar hydatid are visible. In the two largest cavities, dark-staining calcareous corpuscles are apparent (H&E, 125x).

Image 4

At higher magnification, a portion of the folded laminated membrane is visible. Sections through two protoscoleces are shown (arrows). Protoscolex formation is infrequent in human alveolar hydatid infection (H&E, 250x).

Image 5

Infection of human adrenal gland by *E. multilocularis*. In this section, the laminated layer, which is fragmented and convoluted, stains a more intense red than the surrounding tissue does with periodic acid–Schiff (PAS, 62x).

Image 6

In this section of human liver, the thickened and collapsed laminated membrane is enmeshed in host fibrous tissue and stains yellow with Movat (Movat, 250x).

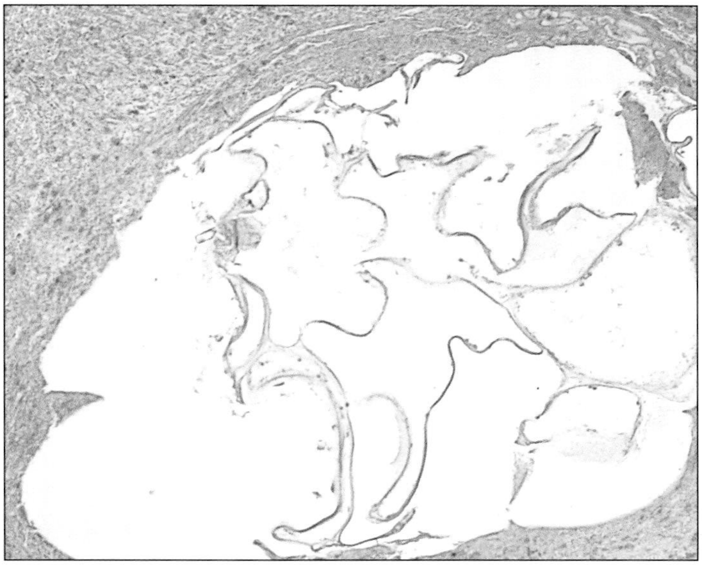
1

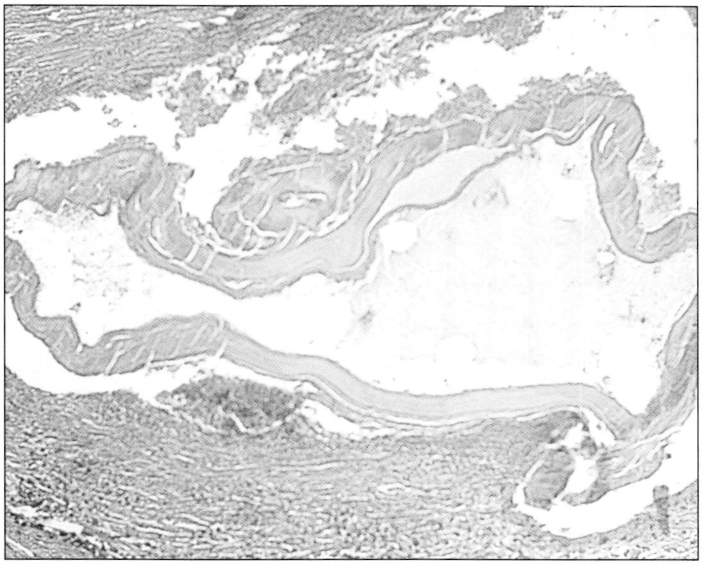
2

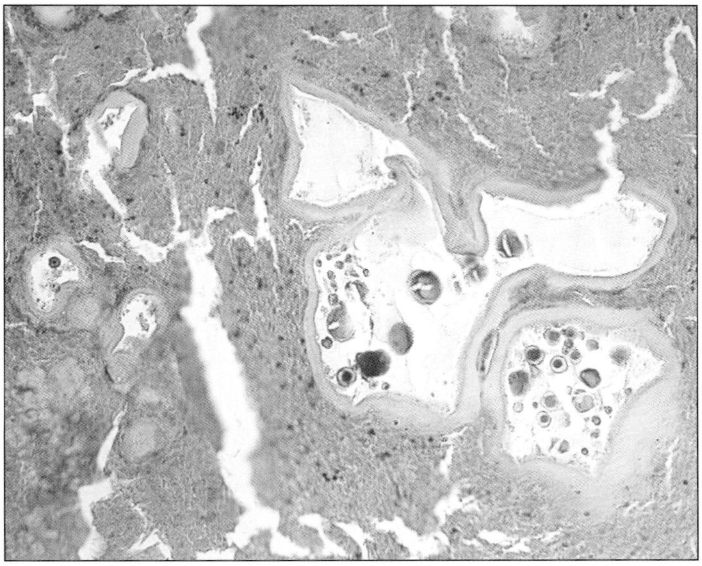
3

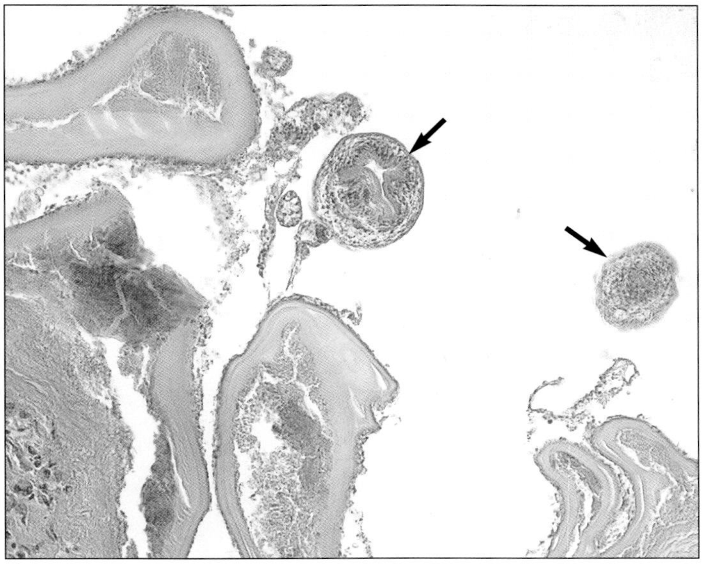
4

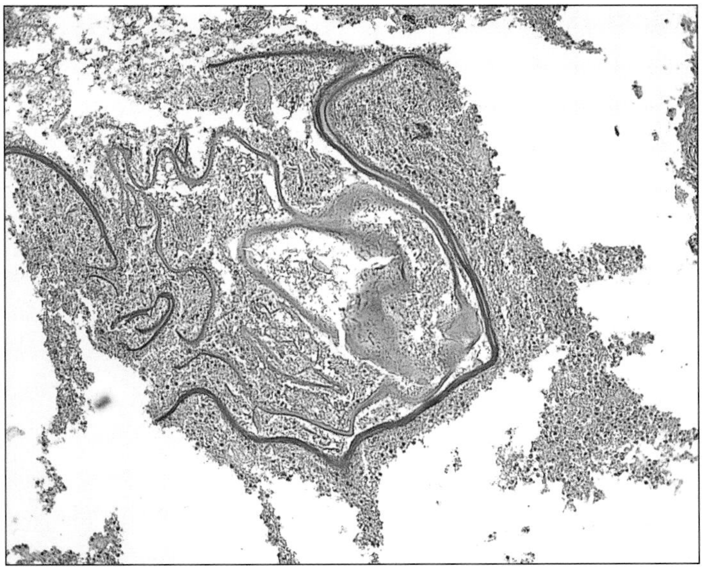
5

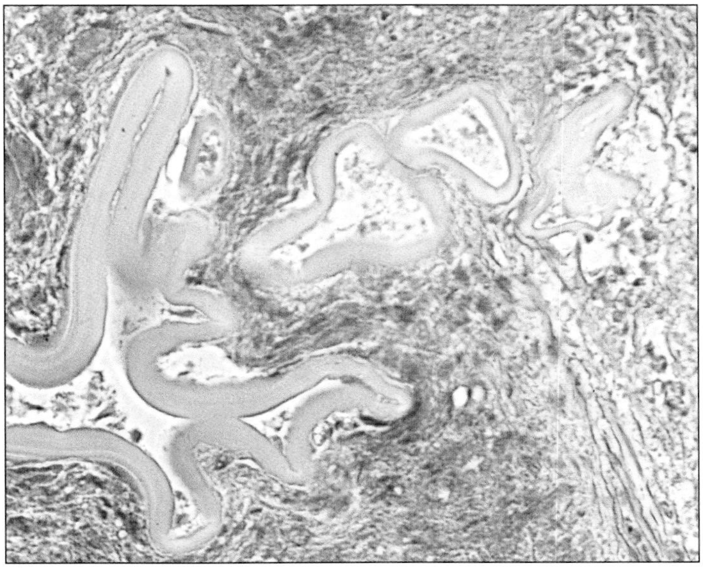
6

Echinococcus multilocularis and *E. vogeli*

Image 1

Multiple vesicles of an alveolar hydatid of *E. multilocularis* in a section of human liver stained with periodic acid–Schiff. The convoluted laminated membranes clearly stand out as dark-staining membranes (PAS, 125x).

Image 2

In this section of liver from a vole infected with *E. multilocularis*, many protoscoleces are seen within brood capsules. The vole and other rodents are the normal intermediate hosts of *E. multilocularis*. At this magnification, it is difficult to discern calcareous corpuscles (H&E, 62x).

Image 3

In the liver of a muskrat infected with *E. multilocularis,* protoscoleces and dark blue-staining, oval calcareous corpuscles are clearly seen. The laminated membrane (LM) and the germinal epithelium (keyline) are also visible (H&E, 125x).

Image 4

Section of human polycystic hydatid infection caused by *E. vogeli*. Note the thin, fragmented, convoluted laminated membrane (darts) (H&E, 62x).

Image 5

At higher magnification, portions of the laminated membrane (darts) are visible. With H&E stain, the laminated membrane is often difficult to distinguish from surrounding tissue (H&E, 125x).

Image 6

At even higher magnification, one can see hooklets (darts) that remain from protoscoleces that have undergone disintegration (H&E, 500x).

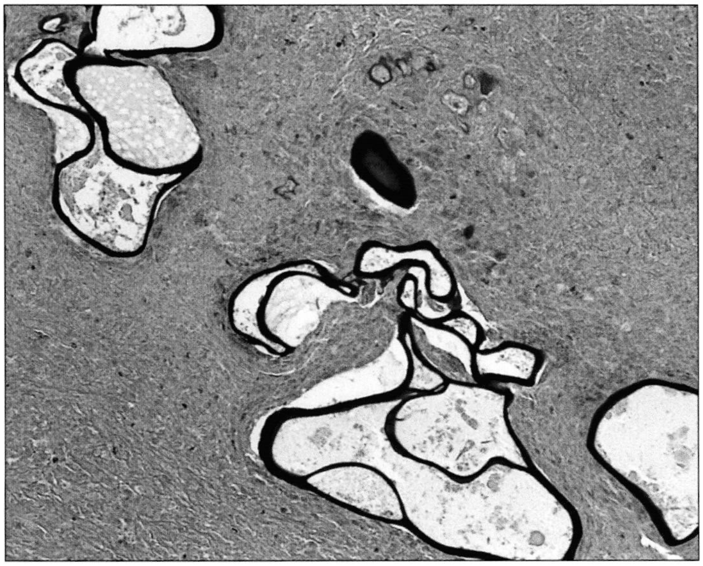

1

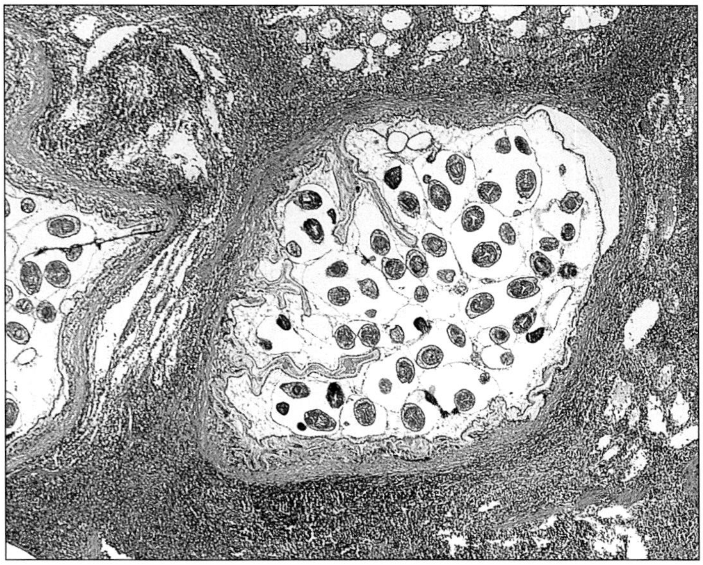

2

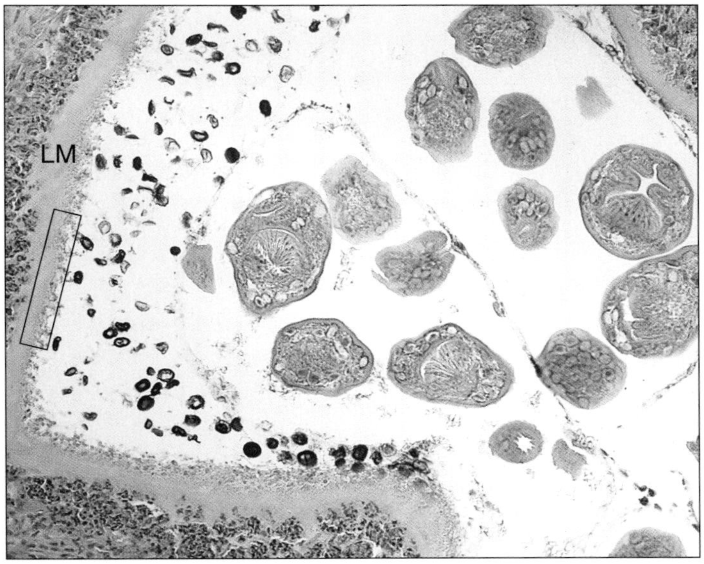

3

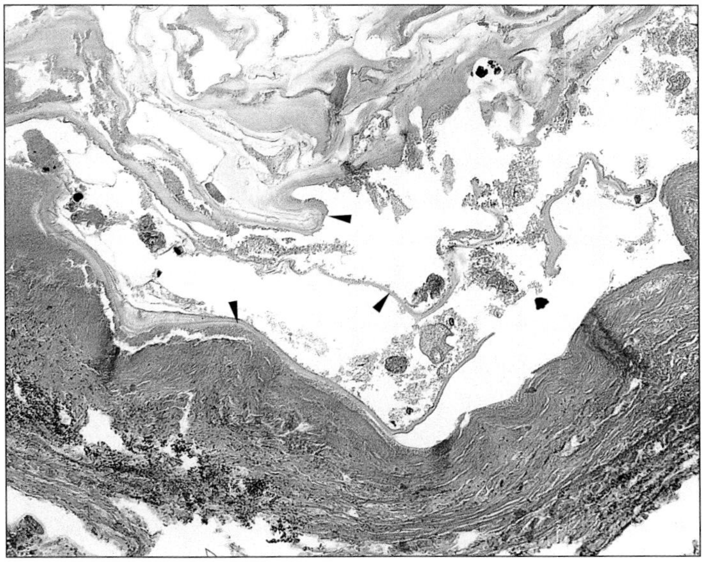

4

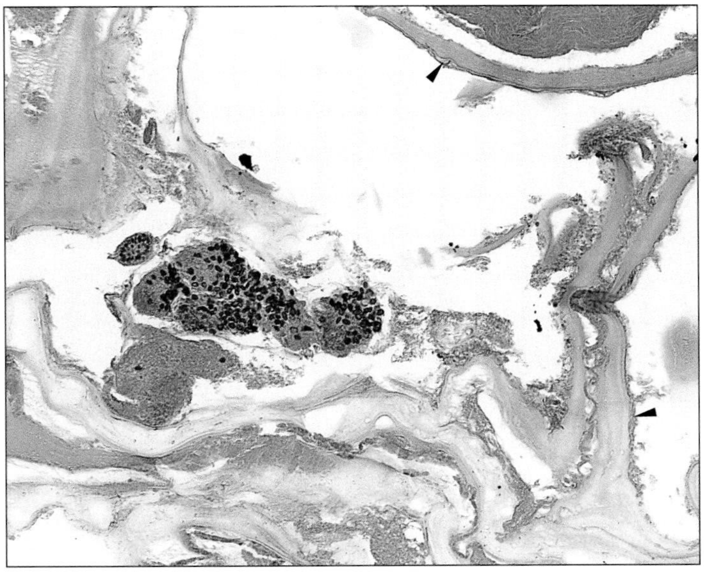

5

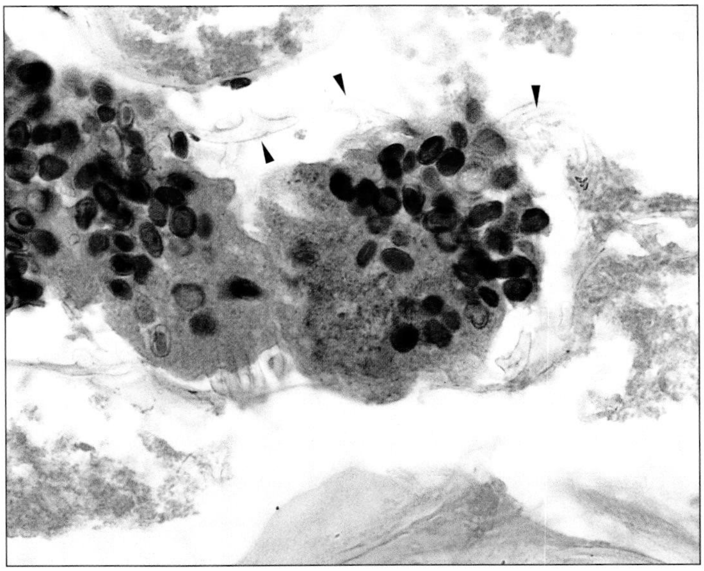

6

Acanthocephala

The acanthocephalans are commonly referred to as thorny-headed worms because they have a protrusible proboscis armed with spines at the anterior end of the body (⇨ 76). They belong to a phylum separate from the nematodes and the flatworms (trematodes and cestodes) and show few affinities to these and other phyla. Acanthocephalans are parasitic throughout their life and are found in the digestive tracts of various animals, especially fish, birds, and mammals in marine, freshwater, and terrestrial habitats. More than 600 species have been described. Human infections have been reported occasionally and from all parts of the world. *Macracanthorhynchus hirudinaceus*, a common parasite of pigs, is the most frequently reported agent of human infection. *Moniliformis moniliformis*, found in rats, ranks next. Other parasites identified at least once in humans include *Bolbosoma* species of marine animals, *Acanthocephalus bufonis* of Asian amphibians, *A. rauschi* of an unknown host, *Corynosoma* of seals, and *Macracanthorhynchus ingens* of the raccoon.

⇨ 76

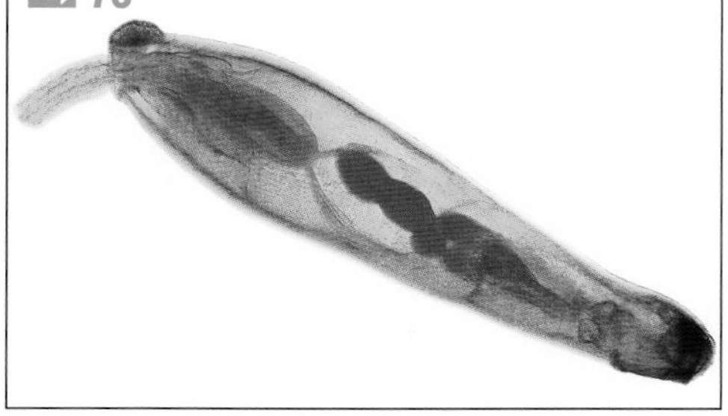

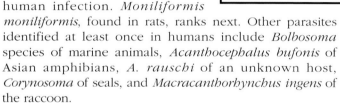

Biology and Life Cycle

The sexes of acanthocephalans are separate. They live in the digestive tract anchored to the gut wall by the spinous proboscis. Female worms discharge eggs, which contain a partially enveloped larva called an acanthor. When the eggs are ingested by an appropriate invertebrate (ie, an intermediate host such as an insect in the terrestrial environment or a crustacean in water), the acanthor hatches from the egg, enters the hemocoel, and develops into a more advanced larva called the acanthella, which over several weeks develops into a juvenile worm with rudiments of adult structures. The juvenile worm encysts in the tissues and is called a cystacanth. The infected insect or crustacean may be ingested by various animals other than the normal definitive host. These other animals (fish, amphibians, etc) serve as paratenic or transport hosts. The cystacanth maintains its infectivity until ingested. Definitive hosts are infected by ingesting the cystacanth in the insect or crustacean intermediate host or by eating the raw or inadequately cooked flesh of paratenic or transport hosts (fish) containing the same stage. The cystacanth is apparently able to mature in humans, because gravid adult worms are frequently recovered from human tissue.

Pathology and Clinical Manifestations

Infected individuals often present with acute abdominal pain that requires surgical intervention, while others experience no symptoms whatsoever. Worms often attach to the mucosa and produce ulceration and perforation. A report from China in 1983 revealed more than 200 surgical procedures to repair intestinal perforation caused by *M. hirudinaceus* in one province alone. The infections were typically in children with histories of eating raw or "cooked" beetles of various sorts, which were shown to naturally harbor cystacanth larvae.

Immature worms have also been found in the omentum and abdominal peritoneum of people at autopsy, but they did not contribute to death. A patent infection has been reported with *M. ingens,* and worms have been discharged in feces.

Parasite Morphology

The morphologic features of the acanthocephalans are so distinctive that the parasites are readily identified by gross features as well as their microanatomic structure. We will not identify the parasites at the generic or species level. Instead, we will simply indicate the morphologic features that permit identification of acanthocephalans in tissue sites.

Adult acanthocephalans are typically small, measuring about 2 cm long. However, species range in size from as small as 1.0 mm to larger than 1.0 m. Generally, the smaller species are found in fishes and the larger ones in birds and mammals. The body is usually cylindroid or somewhat flattened, with the proboscis and its hooks as the most conspicuous structure (Plate 94:1 & 2). The body wall differs in structure and appearance from the body wall in both the nematodes and the platyhelminthes (Plate 94:3 & 4). It consists of an outer tegument, a middle layer of circular muscles, and an inner layer of longitudinal muscles. The tegument is thick and divided into several layers, including an outer plasma membrane and three fibrous layers: a thin, outer layer; a thicker, feltlike middle layer; and a very thick, fibrous, inner layer, which includes channels that make up the lacunar system. The latter has a poorly defined structure and appears as holes in the feltlike syncytium of the inner layer (Plate 94:3 & 4). The lacunar system presumably contains nutritive fluid and serves as the food-distributing system of the organism. Beneath the three fibrous layers is a thin layer of tissue referred to as the dermis (Plate 94:4). The innermost lining of the body wall is the musculature and consists of outer circular and inner longitudinal fibers (Plate 94:4). Because acanthocephalans have no digestive tract, the reproductive system occupies the body cavity, or pseudocoelom. The sexes are separate. The reproductive organs are contained within or shrouded by a connective tissue sheath called the ligament sac, of which one or two may be present (Plate 94:6). The ligament sac is attached anteriorly to the body wall or the base of the proboscis sheath and posteriorly to other reproductive structures in the posterior extremity.

The female may have one or two ovaries, which typically break up into fragments called ovarian balls. When the ligament sac(s) ruptures as the female matures, the ovarian balls lie free in the pseudocoelom. The male usually has two testes enclosed in the ligament sac. The remainder of both systems is morphologically complex, but a description is not necessary here.

The anterior end of the parasite includes a pair of sacs called the lemnisci. These are generally long, slender structures that hang free in the pseudocoelom and apparently function as reservoirs for the fluid of the lacunar system.

Detailed knowledge of the structure of organ systems in the acanthocephalans is not necessary to identify them. Recognizing the unique structure of the body wall and the presence of structures such as the lemnisci, the proboscis, and the lacunar system is all that is needed to make an identification. More details about the lacunar system and the distribution of hooks on the proboscis and spines on the body surface, as well as other morphologic features, would be needed for further identification.

References

Beaver PC, Otsuji T, Otsuji A, Yoshimura H. Acanthocephalan, probably *Bolbosoma*, from the peritoneal cavity of man in Japan. *Am J Trop Med Hyg*. 1983;32:1016-1018.

Dingley D, Beaver PC. *Macracanthorhynchus ingens* from a child in Texas. *Am J Trop Med Hyg*. 1985;34:918-920.

Dunagan TT, Miller DM. Acanthocephala. In: Harrison FW, Ruppert EE, eds. *Microscopic Anatomy of Invertebrates, Vol IV: Aschelminthes*. New York, NY: Wiley-Liss, Inc; 1991.

Leng Y-J, Liang P-N. Human infection with *Macracanthorhynchus hirudinaceus* Travassos, 1916, in Guangdong Province with notes on its prevalence in China. *Ann Trop Med Parasitol*. 1983;77:107-109.

Plate 94

Acanthocephala

Image 1

Anterior end of Acanthocephalan embedded in the intestinal wall demonstrates the protrusible proboscis with its hooks (darts) and the anterior-most part of the body trunk (H&E, 40x).

Image 2

At high magnification, a transverse section through the proboscis shows the large hooks (darts) (H&E, 125x).

Image 3

Transverse section through the body of *Macracanthorhynchus ingens* in the intestine of a raccoon shows the typical structure of the body wall of the parasite. Note the dark-stained thin cuticle, thick epidermis (EP), both circular (arrow) and longitudinal muscles (keyline), and eggs (darts) (H&E, 40x).

Image 4

At high magnification, the major elements of the body wall are recognizable. Note the thin cuticle (arrows), the syncytial epidermis (EP) with its lacunae (LA), and the circular (dart) and longitudinal (keyline) muscles (H&E, 175x).

Image 5

Section through a granulomatous mass in the serosa of the ileum of a young Japanese man contains segments of an acanthocephalan parasite identified as a species of *Bolbosoma.* At this magnification, the structure of the parasite cannot be discerned (H&E, 6x).

Image 6

High magnification of a transverse section through the body of a worm. The body wall immediately identifies the parasite as an acanthocephalan. A portion of the reproductive system is visible within the pseudocoelom (H&E, 100x).

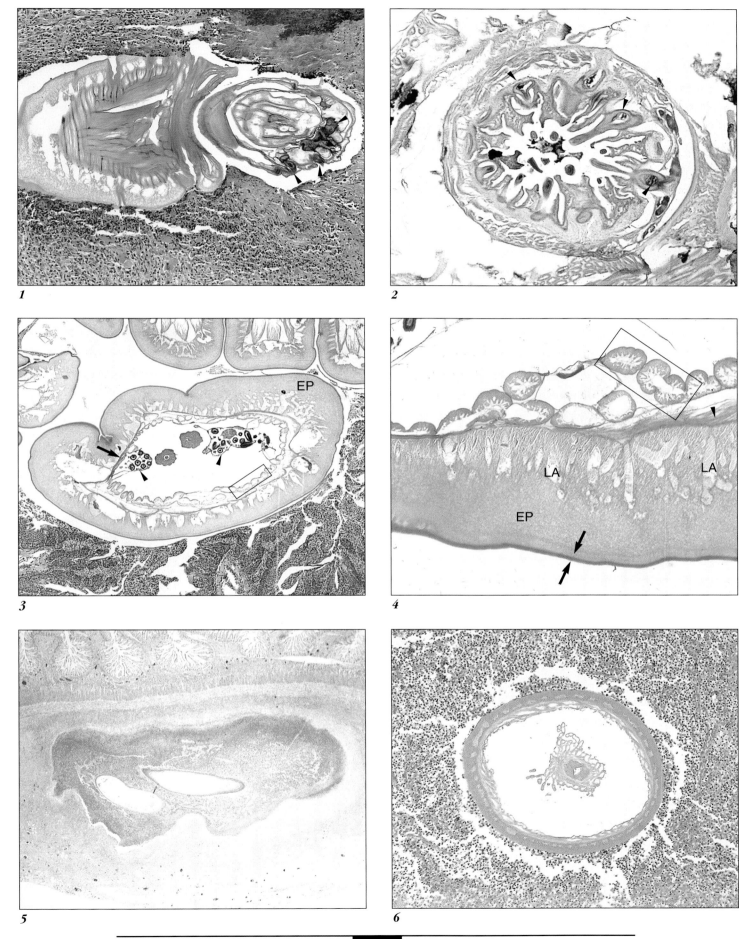

1

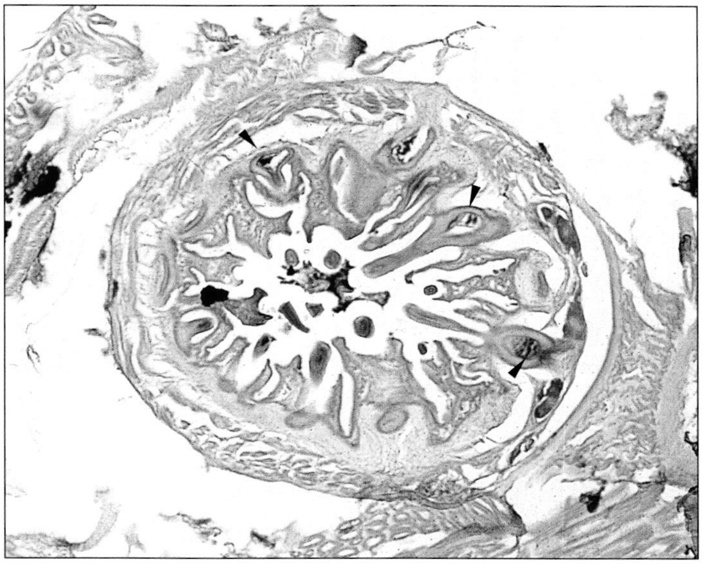

2

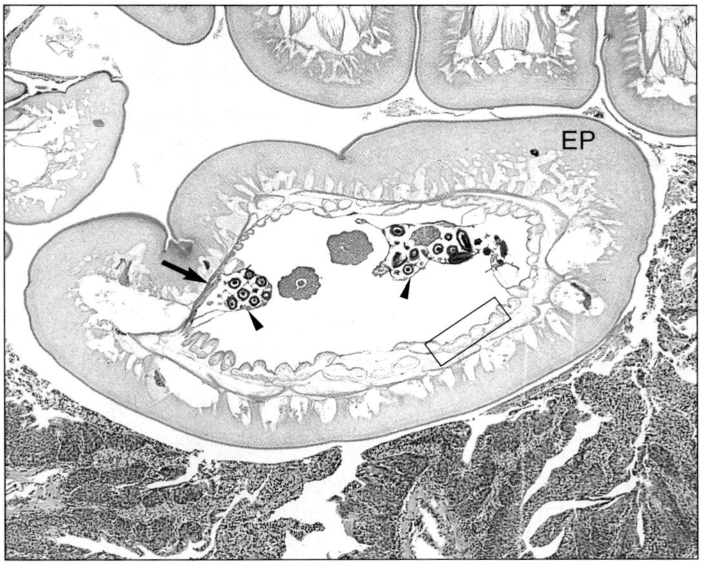

3

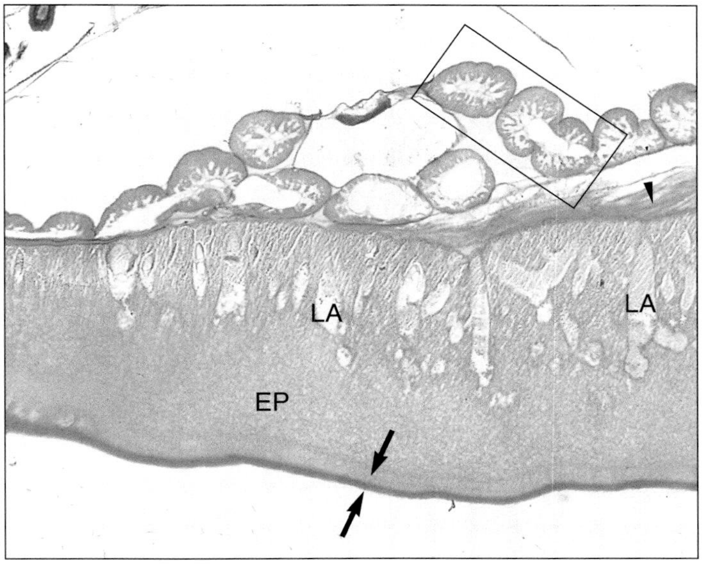

4

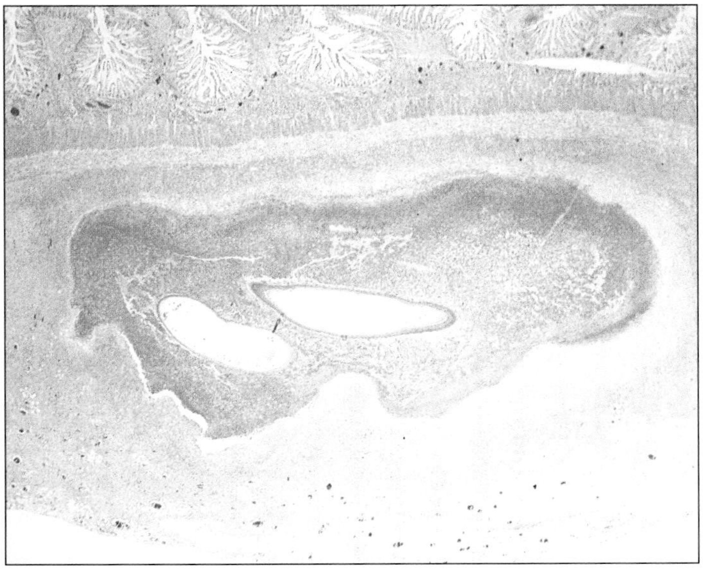

5

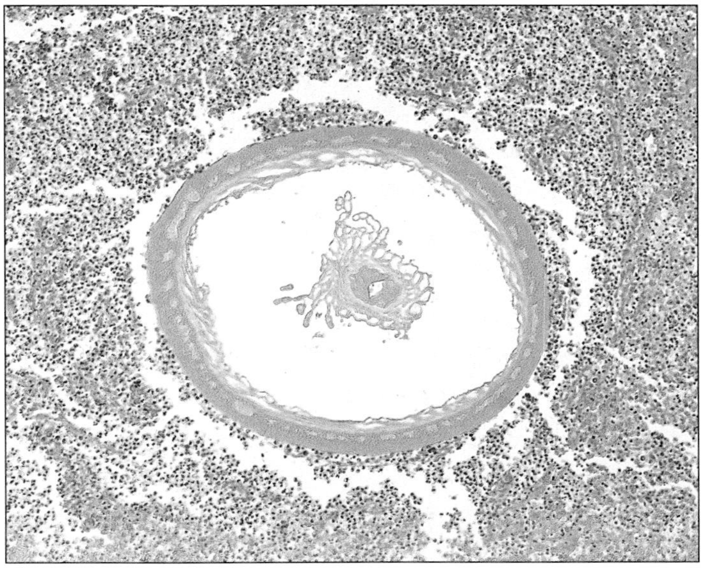

6

Pseudoparasites

Leeches, Planarians, Horsehair Worms

At times, objects allegedly found in fecal specimens (more accurately, they were found in, on, or associated with fecal specimens collected from grass, soil, toilet bowls, or dirty containers) are referred to the clinical laboratory for identification. When such objects are not immediately recognized, they are often submitted for histologic sectioning in hopes of obtaining diagnostic clues. Among the living objects one might encounter are earthworms, land planarians, mollusks, leeches, and horsehair worms. We describe typical histologic appearances of three of these creatures: the leech, the land planarian, and the horsehair worm.

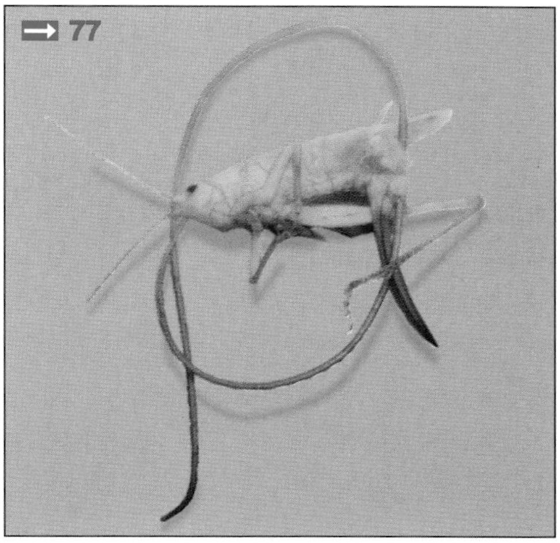

Leeches

Leeches belong to a small class (Hirudinea) of annelid worms. Most are found in inland waters or in damp terrestrial environments. Leeches range from small to large. They are coelomate animals and usually are hermaphroditic. The body is covered by a thin cuticle beneath which lies the epidermis. Conspicuous circular muscles and large bundles of longitudinal muscles eliminate the possibility of confusion with a trematode (Plate 95:1 & 2). The coelom is mostly filled with mesenchymatous tissue, within which lie the alimentary tract and reproductive, excretory, and nervous systems. Blood circulates within coelomic sinuses and not within blood vessels. Diagonal muscle fibers are seen within the body as well (Plate 95:1 & 2).

Planarians

Planarians are turbellarian flatworms, and like the trematodes and cestodes, they belong to the Phylum Platyhelminthes. Most planarians are free living, are dorsoventrally flattened (Plate 95:3) with rounded margins, and range from 5.0 mm to 5.0 cm in length. They are acoelomate. Planarians are most easily mistaken for trematodes. However, they are significantly different from trematodes: the body surface of the planarian is covered by a ciliated epithelium within which are usually rodlike structures called rhabdites. Often, ocelli, or eyes, are found along the margins of the body and on the dorsal surface (Plate 95:4). The parenchyma contains layers of circular and longitudinal muscle fibers as well as diagonal ones (Plate 95:3).

Horsehair Worms

The horsehair worms belong to the phylum Nematomorpha. Adult worms, which are free living, are long, slender, and filiform. Juvenile worms are parasitic in insects, crustaceans, and other arthropods (➡ 77). The sexes are separate. In histologic sections, the body wall is vaguely similar to the nematode body wall. The cortex of the thick cuticle may be heavily pigmented. The hypodermis (= epidermis) is thin and cellular. Nuclei are numerous in the submuscular area. A single large ventral chord is present, but no dorsal or lateral ones. The musculature is well developed and strong. Individual fibers are tall and slender, with the narrow, elongated cell nucleus toward the periphery rather than the base of the cell (Plate 95:5 & 6). The pseudocoelom is filled with mesenchyme. The intestine is more or less degenerate. The gonads or reproductive tubes are typically paired, cylindrical structures. Two genera, *Gordius* and *Paragordius,* have been reported from humans with the greatest frequency and are usually described as being passed in feces, urine, or vomitus.

References

Fernandez J, Tellez V, Olean N. Hirudinea. In: Harrison FW, Gardiner SL, eds. *Microscopic Anatomy of Invertebrates, Vol VII: Annelida.* New York, NY: Wiley-Liss Inc; 1992.

Bresciani J. Nematomorpha. In: Harrison FW, Ruppert EE, eds. *Microscopic Anatomy of Invertebrates, Vol IV: Aschelminthes.* New York, NY: Wiley-Liss Inc; 1991.

Plate 95

Pseudoparasites

Image1

Transverse section through a leech illustrates its typical anatomic features, including the band of circular muscle fibers (darts), bundles of longitudinal muscles (LM), and intestine (IN) (H&E, 75x).

Image 2

At higher magnification, the circular (CM) and longitudinal muscles (LM) are especially evident (H&E, 200x).

Image 3

Section through a land planarian allegedly vomited by a child. Note its morphologic similarity to a trematode (H&E, 150x).

Image 4

At higher magnification, the cellular epithelium and black-staining ocelli can be seen. The acoelomatous condition is clearly evident (H&E, 400x).

Image 5

Transverse section through a *Paragordius* species. The thick cuticle, cellular hypodermis, tall muscle layer, and ventral chord (dart) are clearly seen (H&E, 100x).

Image 6

At high magnification, note the thick cuticle (CU) with darkened cortical layer, the hypodermis (keyline), the muscles and their nuclei (MU), and the mesenchyme (ME) filling the pseudocoelom (H&E, 500x).

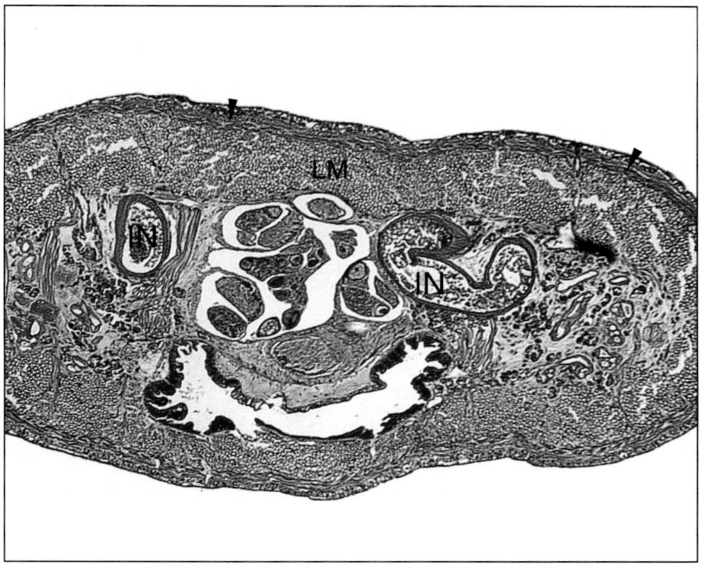

1

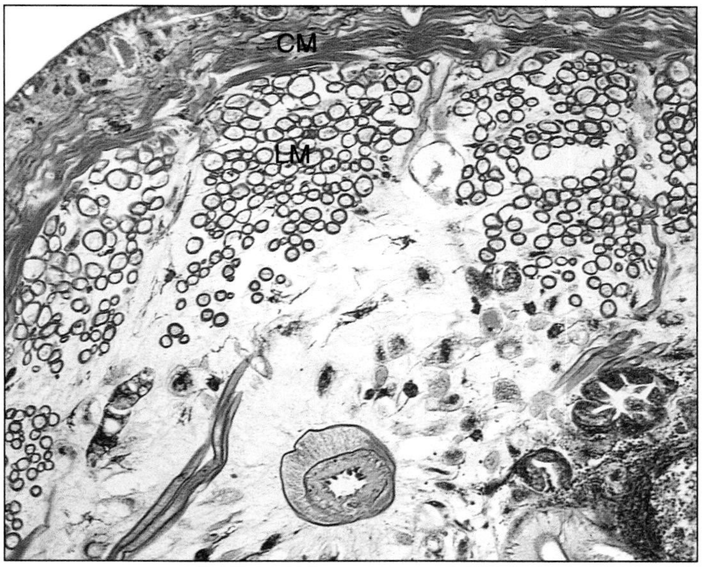

2

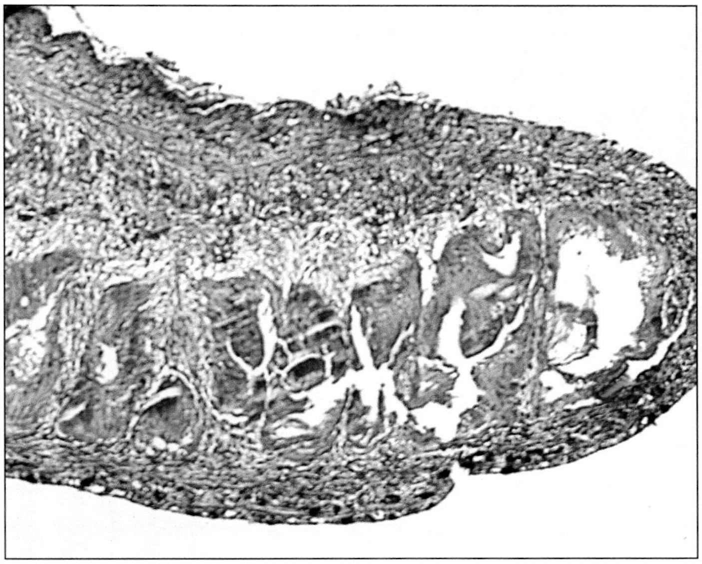
3

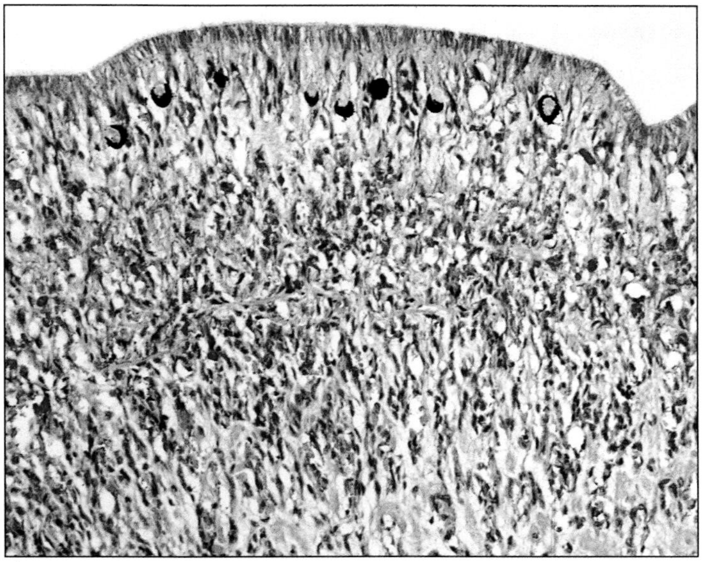
4

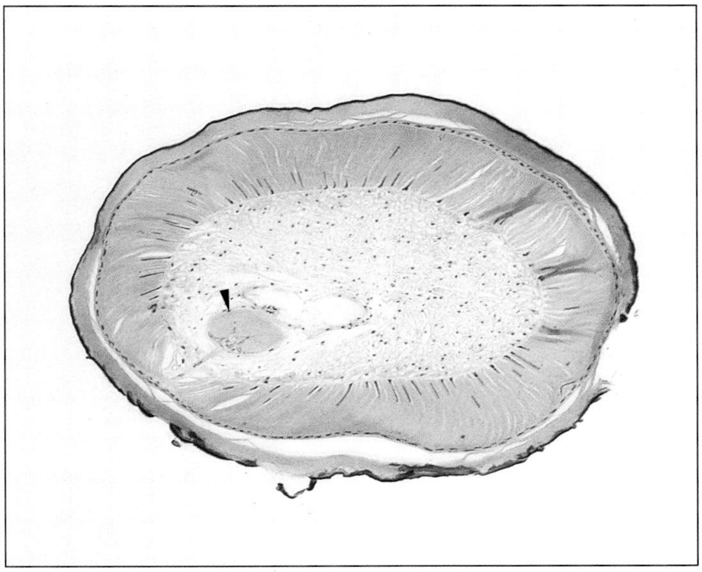
5

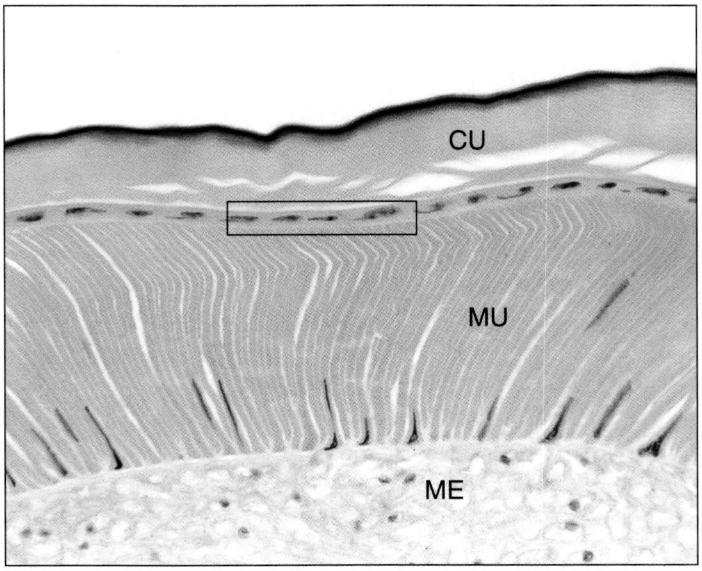

6

Pentastoma

Larval pentastomiasis is a zoonotic infection of humans that occurs principally in Asia, Africa, and the Middle East. Infections in North America are reported infrequently. The wormlike pentastomes are often referred to as tongue worms. Their zoologic classification has been controversial, because they have characteristics of both annelids and arthropods. Although they have been classified within the arthropods, more recent investigations suggest that they belong in a separate phylum, the Pentastomida. This phylum is divided into two orders, Cephalobaenida and Porocephalida, with the latter group containing two medically important families, the Linguatulidae and the Porocephalidae. The most important pentastome species causing human infections are *Armillifer armillatus* in the Porocephalidae and *Linguatula serrata* in the Linguatulidae.

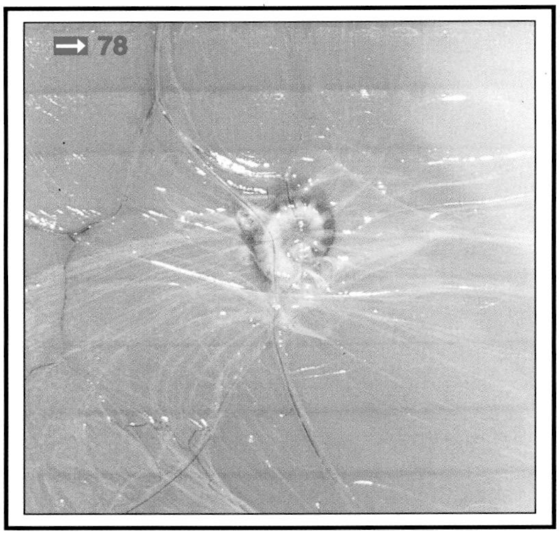

Biology and Life Cycle

Although most pentastomes, such as *Armillifer,* reach maturity in the respiratory tract of snakes, adults of *L. serrata* live in the nasopharynx of carnivores, especially dogs. In *Armillifer* infections, embryonated eggs containing first-stage larvae are excreted to the outside environment via respiratory secretions, saliva, or feces. In the normal life cycle, rodents ingest the eggs, and the larvae then migrate from the intestine to various organs and tissues. They undergo considerable growth and two molts to become third-stage larvae (which some authors refer to as nymphs). The larvae may encyst in the tissues. Infections are established in reptilian hosts by ingestion of these larvae. Humans usually acquire infection by accidentally ingesting embryonated eggs in contaminated food or water, and they may harbor both encysted and free larvae in various organs and tissues. Development of the parasite to the adult stage in humans has not been reported. In *L. serrata* infection, embryonated eggs are excreted to the outside environment via nasal secretions and feces. The eggs are ingested by various types of herbivorous animals such as sheep and goats. In herbivorous hosts the larvae migrate to various organs and tissues, including the liver and lymph nodes. In the normal life cycle, ingestion of infected tissues by carnivorous hosts results in the development of adult linguatulids in the nasopharyngeal region. Humans may be infected by accidentally ingesting infective eggs or by eating raw tissues of the herbivorous hosts.

Pathology and Clinical Manifestations

Humans appear to have a great tolerance for the larval stages of the pentastomes. The larvae are often incidental findings at surgery or autopsy. However, free larvae migrating through the tissues may grow considerably and invade vital organs and tissues. Encysted larvae are often found in mesenteries (➡ 78;Plate 96:4), the peritoneal cavity, or the lungs and liver (Plate 96:1). Larvae of *L. serrata* have occasionally been found in the anterior chamber of the eye in human cases from the southeastern United States. In the Middle East, *L. serrata* is responsible for the syndrome known variously as halzoun or marrara. The syndrome develops in individuals who have eaten local dishes made from the infected raw liver, lung, or stomach of various herbivorous animals. Infected individuals develop a self-limited nasopharyngitis within a few hours after eating and demonstrate coughing, hemoptysis, and vomiting along with pain, nasal discharges, and dyspnea. Third-stage larvae may be discharged during coughing and vomiting. In rare cases, *L. serrata* has reached maturity in humans.

Parasite Morphology

Adult pentastomids may reach up to 10 cm or more in length, with females larger than males. Linguatulids have a flattened body with transverse striations, whereas *Armillifer* adults are cylindrical with pronounced pseudoannulations. Early larval stages may measure less than 1 cm in length, with third-stage larvae up to several centimeters long. In *L. serrata,* the cuticle bears prominent spines, whereas in *Armillifer* the cuticle is smooth. The parasite has a simple gut. At the anterior end are two pairs of large hooks on either side of the mouth opening.

Larval stages in tissues are frequently coiled into a C shape and surrounded by a fibrous wall (Plate 96:1 & 5). The cuticle contains chitin, is 5 to 10 µm in thickness, and has sclerotized openings (Plate 96:4), which are diagnostic for pentastomids. In *Armillifer,* the pseudoannulations of the cuticle are readily seen (Plate 96:2 & 3). Beneath the cuticle lie subcuticular glands (Plate 96:3, 4, & 6) and striated muscle fibers (Plate 96:2 & 3). Sections through the anterior end of the larva demonstrate the hooks near the mouth opening (Plate 96:2). Prominent acidophilic glands can be seen in sections of larvae in tissues (Plate 96:2 & 3). The intestine is usually large and readily seen in section (Plate 96:2 & 5).

Pentastome larval stages in human tissues are usually found coiled on the surfaces of tissues or organs, including serosal surfaces, mesenteries, and the lung and liver. In histologic sections, the larval morphology is distinct from the roundworms and flatworms. The chitinous cuticle, the sclerotized openings, the striated muscle, and the acidophilic glands all contribute to the general identification of a pentastome. Identifying the genus may be difficult, however. Distinct cuticular pseudoannulations suggest *Armillifer,* whereas spines on the cuticle suggest *Linguatula.*

References

Baird JK, Kassebaum LJ, Ludwig GK. Hepatic granuloma in a man from North America caused by a nymph of *Linguatula serrata. Pathology.* 1988;20:198-199.

Drabick JJ. Pentastomiasis. *Rev Infect Dis.* 1987;9:1087-1094.

Esslinger JH. Development of *Porocephalus crotali* (Humboldt, 1808) (Pentastomida) in experimental intermediate hosts. *J Parasitol.* 1962;48:452-456.

Esslinger JH. Hepatic lesions in rats experimentally infected with *Porocephalus crotali* (Pentastomida). *J Parasitol.* 1962;48:631-638.

Murrell KD, Cross JH, Jones GS. *Armillifer* larvae in a ferret-badger (*Melogale personata*) from South Vietnam. *Bull Wildlife Dis.* 1969;5:144-145.

Pentastomes

Image 1

Sagittal section through a nymph of *Armillifer* species in the liver of a naturally infected monkey. The larva is flexed in a typical C shape. A host reaction to the presence of this encapsulated larva is lacking (H&E, 6x).

Image 2

Longitudinal section through a larva of *Armillifer* species coiled in a cyst from the mesentery of a ferret-badger (*Melogale personata*) from South Vietnam. The larvae present measured 9 to 12 mm in length and 1 to 2 mm in width. Partial sections of the four chitinized hooks (keyline) near the mouth opening are visible. The large, open tube is the gut, which is also represented just behind the hooks. The acidophilic glands (AG) are prominent. The pseudoannulations of the cuticle are evident (darts). Subcuticular glands and muscle are apparent, but detail is difficult to discern at this magnification (H&E, 25x).

Image 3

At higher magnification, the pseudoannulations of this species of *Armillifer* are well demonstrated (darts). Beneath the cuticle are the subcuticular glands and muscle. A small portion of the acidophilic glands (AG) can be seen (H&E, 250x).

Image 4

At even higher magnification, details of the tegument and underlying subcuticular glands and muscle are seen. One of the sclerotized openings (dart) in the cuticle is present (H&E, 500x).

Image 5

Section through the liver of a rat experimentally infected for four months with *Porocephalus crotali*, a pentastomid that matures in the lungs of cottonmouth water moccasins (*Agkistrodon piscivorus*). Two different sections of the same nymph are present within a well-developed fibrous capsule. The tubular structures in both sections are different levels of the gut. In the section to the right, acidophilic glands (keyline) are seen (H&E, 70x).

Image 6

At higher magnification, the dark-staining cuticle and the subcuticular glands are evident. Note the lack of pseudoannulations, as seen in *Armillifer* (H&E, 500x).

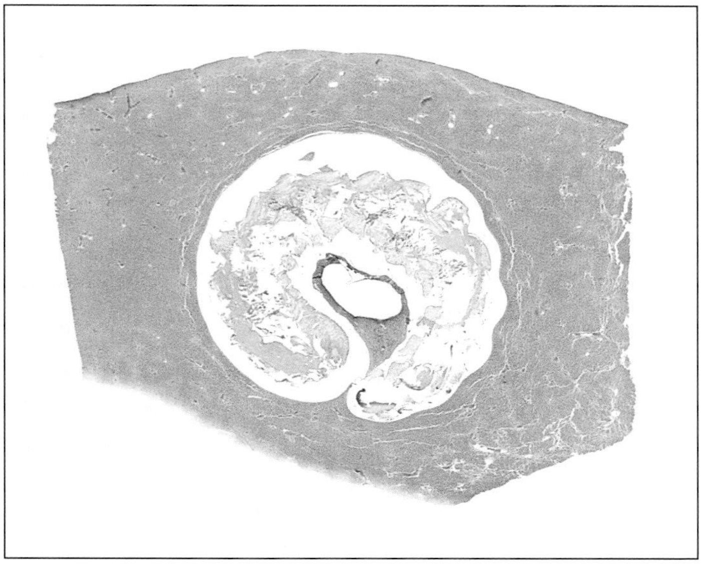

1

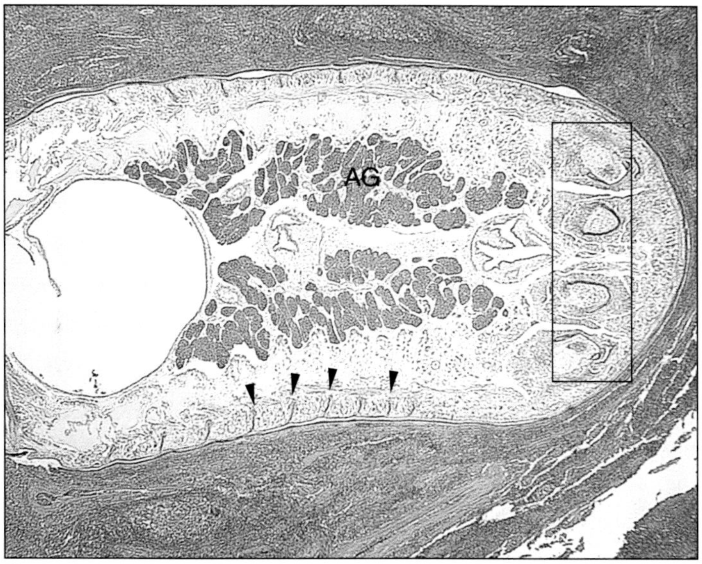

2

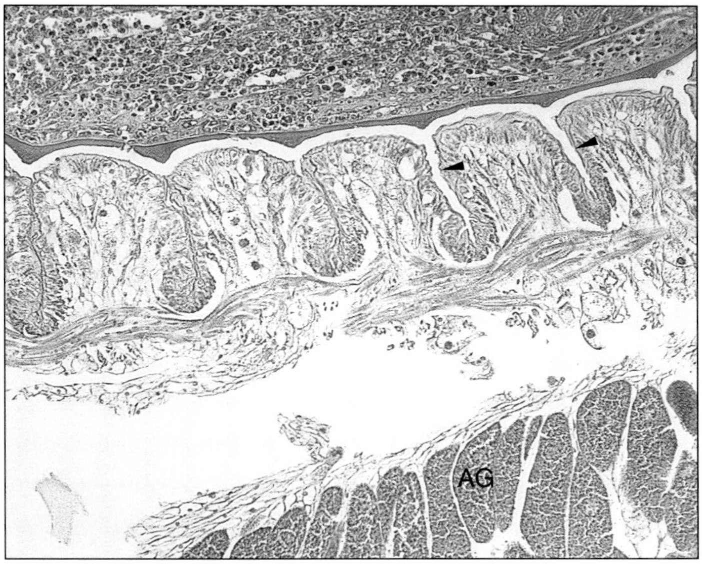

3

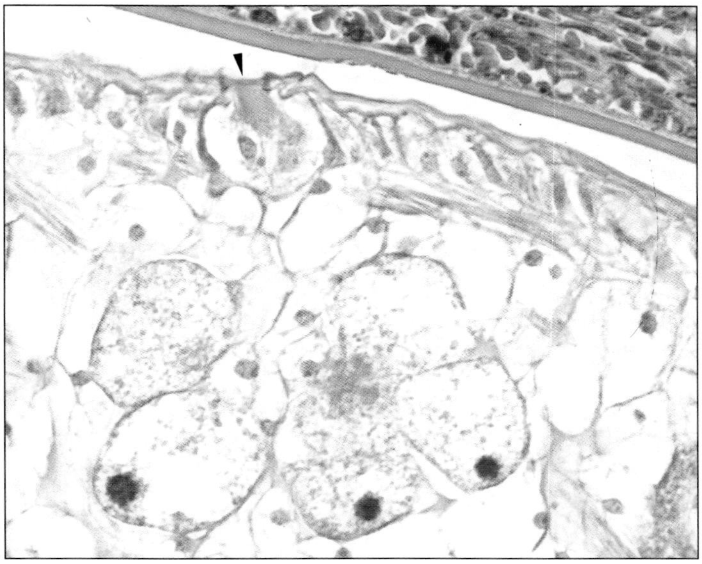

4

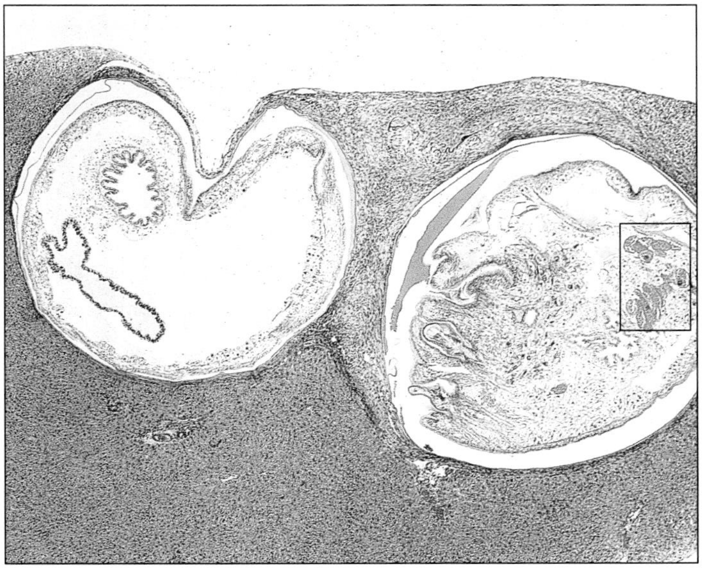

5

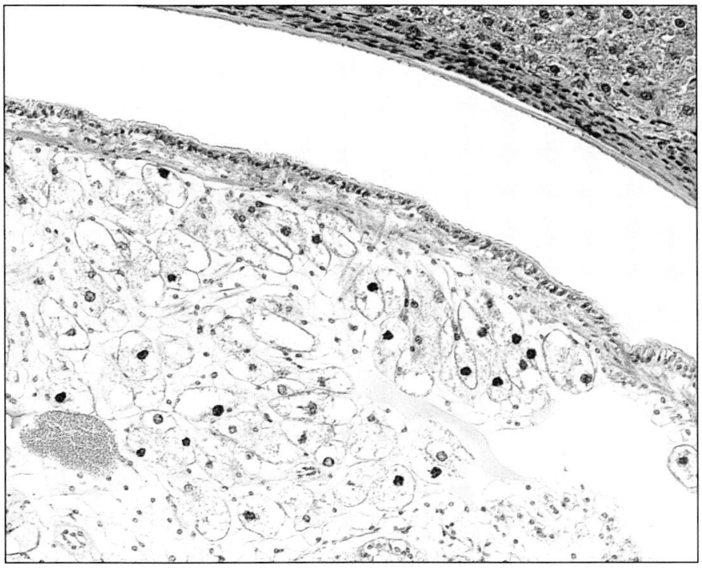

6

Arthropods

The arthropods comprise more than a million species of organisms, of which 70% to 80% are insects. They have in common a rigid, chitinized, or sclerotized exoskeleton; a segmented body; and three or more pairs of legs (appendages). Despite these basic morphologic similarities, the group has a tremendous morphologic and biologic diversity, which has led some to regard it as a polyphyletic group. Such extreme diversity precludes even a synoptic review of the major classes of the phylum here.

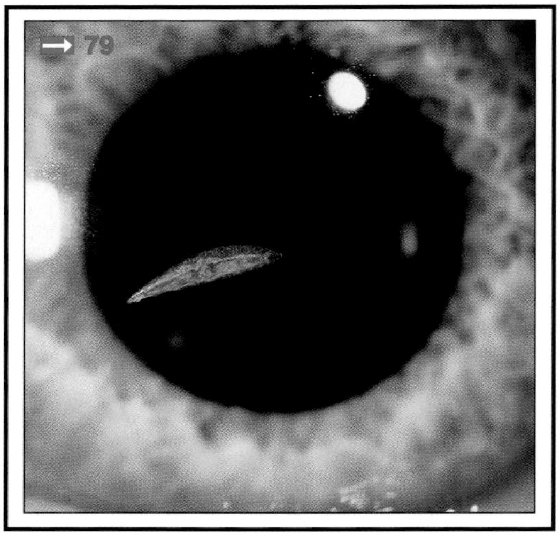

The arthropods develop from egg to adult by a process of metamorphosis, which may be incomplete or gradual (ie, egg, nymph, adult) or complete (ie, egg, larva, pupa, adult).

A large variety of arthropods are associated with human health and disease. Some, including mosquitoes, flies, and fleas, are biological or, less frequently, they are mechanical vectors of a wide spectrum of diseases caused by bacteria, viruses, and protozoan and metazoan parasites. Others, such as spiders, scorpions, wasps, and bees, are venomous and either bite or sting humans, causing mild to serious but usually transitory inflammatory or allergic responses. Still others, including the mange and follicle mites, flies, and fleas, are parasitic in human tissues during some stage of their life cycle.

We have restricted our coverage to the mites, *Sarcoptes* and *Demodex,* which parasitize the skin; the flies whose larvae invade the skin, flesh, and even the eye (➡ 79), causing myiasis; and *Tunga*, a flea that can penetrate the skin and produce a superficial cutaneous lesion.

Various body lice, mites, and fleas may infest the body surfaces, causing transitory dermatitis or allergic responses in some cases. However, because they do not actually occupy or parasitize the tissues, they are not included here.

Sarcoptes scabiei

This microscopic mite (➡ 80) is the agent of human scabies as well as a variant of the disease referred to as Norwegian scabies or Norwegian itch. It has cosmopolitan distribution and in the human population is especially common in overcrowded and poverty-stricken areas where personal hygiene may be neglected. Transmission is from human to human. Other species of *Sarcoptes* as well as varieties of *S. scabiei* parasitize the skin of various animals. These species and varieties can also infect humans, but such infections are typically transitory.

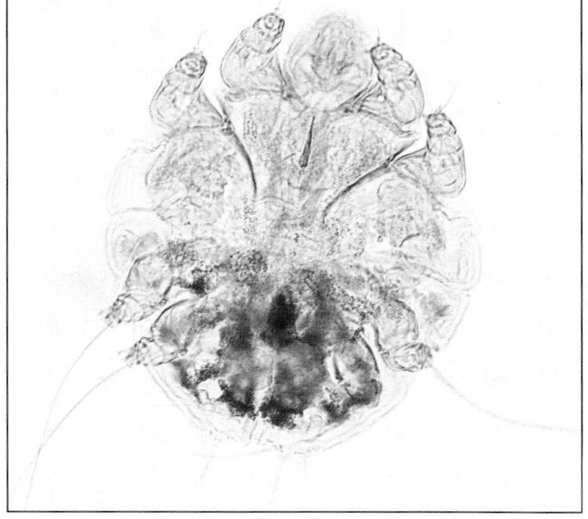

➡ 80

Biology and Life Cycle

The adult mites burrow in the superficial layers of the epidermis (Plate 97:1). The tunnels, although small and sinuous, are visible to the naked eye and may measure up to 3 or 4 cm in length, usually with a vesicle at one end. The mites burrow in the skin on any part of the body, but lesions are most frequently encountered on the hands and wrists, the interdigital, axillary, and inguinal folds, the buttocks, and the male genitalia. The female mite, which is typically positioned in the distal end of the tunnel, deposits a few eggs as well as fecal pellets in the burrows (Plate 97:2 & 3). The eggs hatch after a few days. The larvae molt three times and develop to the adult stage in two weeks or less. The adult female remains reproductive for about two months. Transmission results from direct contact between individuals or exposure to contaminated (infested) personal articles such as clothing.

Pathology and Clinical Manifestations

The mites prefer to burrow in the stratum corneum of the skin. The burrowing process and the secretions and excretions of the mite usually cause a dermatitis and intense itching. Scratching of affected areas facilitates dispersal of the organisms to other areas of the body. Manifestations include bleeding of the abraded areas, scab formation, and, frequently, secondary bacterial infection. Physicians rarely see uncomplicated scabies infections. The hyperkeratotic changes seen in the skin of patients with Norwegian scabies (Plate 97:1), along with the presence of many organisms and eggs, may be related to immunodeficiency in the host. The variable clinical presentations are probably related to host hypersensitivity.

Parasite Morphology

Mites may be obtained for diagnostic confirmation by scraping the affected skin or teasing the organisms out of their burrows and then examining the material under a microscope.

The living mite is tiny and opalescent in appearance. The female is dorsoventrally flattened, is oval to elongate, and measures up to 0.45 mm in length (➡ 80). Males are about half as large and have suckers on the hind legs. The mouthparts are conspicuously oriented in the midline of the anterior margins of the body. The first two pairs of legs are short and positioned close to the anterior margin, but the equally short third and fourth pairs are widely separated from the first two (➡ 80). On the dorsal surface of the body are parallel transverse ridges or striations with toothlike spines and hairs (Plate 97:4 & 5). A few hairs and bristles are found on the otherwise smooth ventral surface. The maximum dimension of the ovoidal egg with a visible developing larva is 100 to 150 µm (Plate 97:6).

Diagnosis depends on demonstrating the mites in skin scrapings. However, sections of tissue show the typical burrows in the cornified epithelium, with the mite's chitinized exoskeleton containing striations, spines, and hairs predominately on the dorsum of the body. Typical eggs containing developing larvae (Plate 97:6) are likely to be present as well. *Sarcoptes* is unlikely to be confused with the follicular mite, *Demodex,* because of differences in tissue habitats and body morphology.

References

Arlian LG. Biology, host relations, and epidemiology of *Sarcoptes scabiei*. *Ann Rev Entomol.* 1989;34:139-161.

Fernandez N, Torres A, Ackerman AB. Pathologic findings in human scabies. *Arch Dermatol.* 1977;113:320-324.

Glover R, Young L, Goltz RW. Norwegian scabies in acquired immunodeficiency syndrome: report of a case resulting in death from associated sepsis. *J Am Acad Dermatol.* 1987;16:396-399.

Head ES, MacDonald EM, Ewert A, Apisarnthanarax P. *Sarcoptes scabiei* in histopathologic sections of skin in human scabies. *Arch Dermatol.* 1990;126:1475-1477.

Plate 97

Sarcoptes scabiei

Image 1

Adults and eggs in burrows in skin (H&E, 30x).

Image 2

At higher magnification, sections through both adults (arrows) and eggs (darts) are visible (H&E, 120x).

Image 3

Yellow-brown fecal pellets deposited in the burrows by the mites (H&E, 120x).

Image 4

Section through an adult mite shows the thin exoskeleton, which bears spines (keyline), and portions of the legs (darts) (H&E, 120x).

Image 5

At high magnification, the semirigid exoskeleton, which bears large, toothlike spines as well as fine superficial ridges (keyline), is visible. Striated muscles (MU) are also evident (H&E, 500x).

Image 6

Section through an egg contains a developing hexapod larva (H&E, 410x).

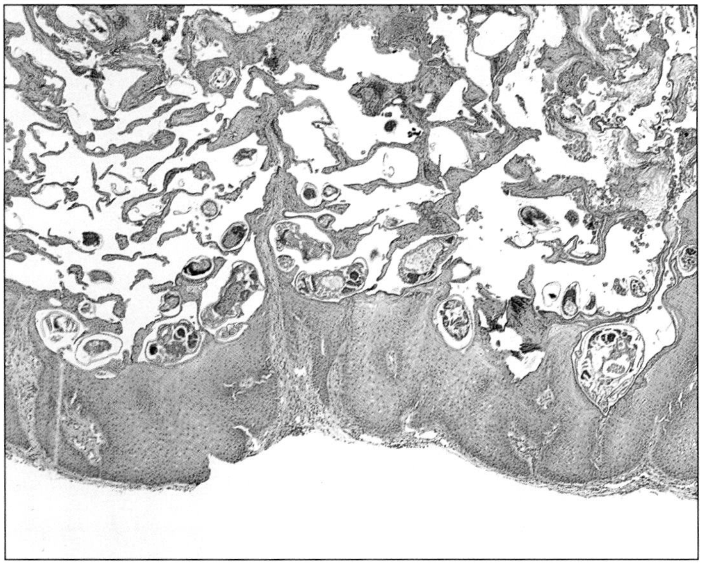

1

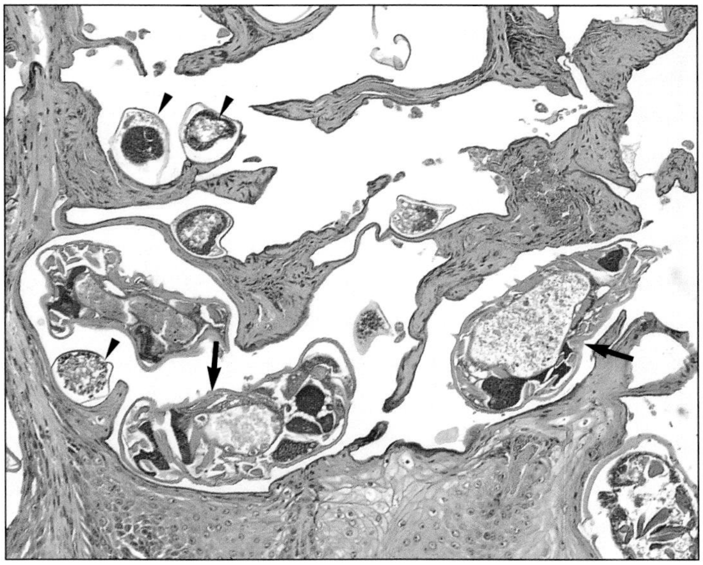

2

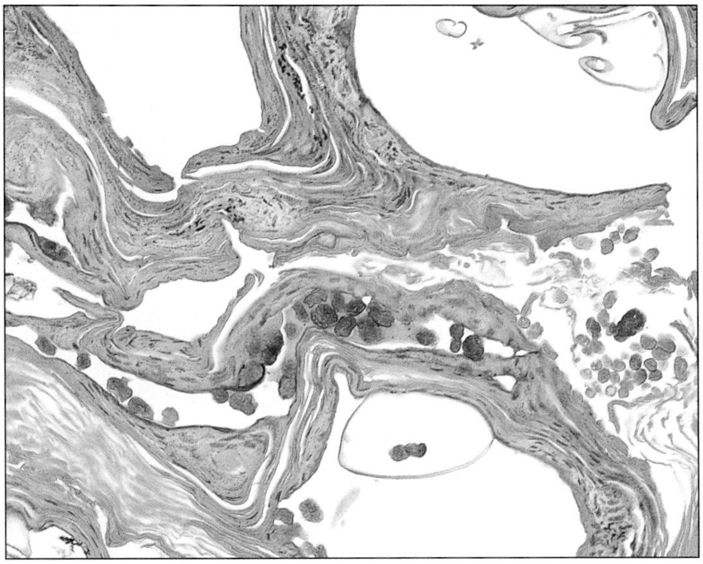

3

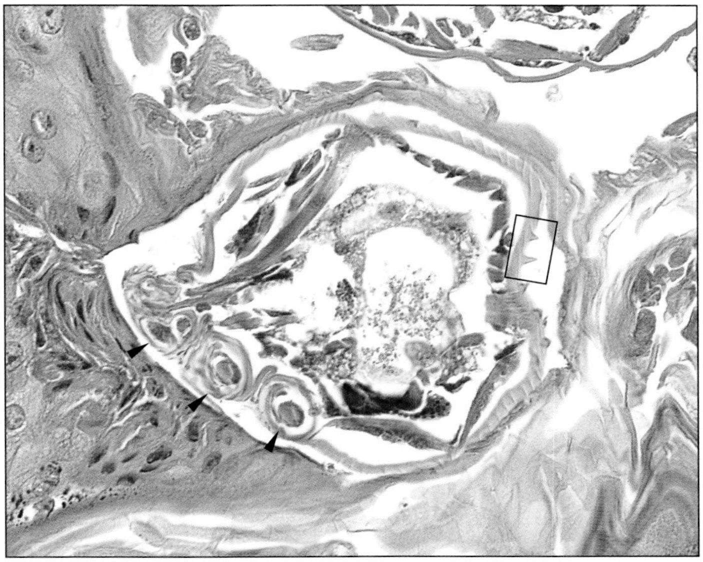

4

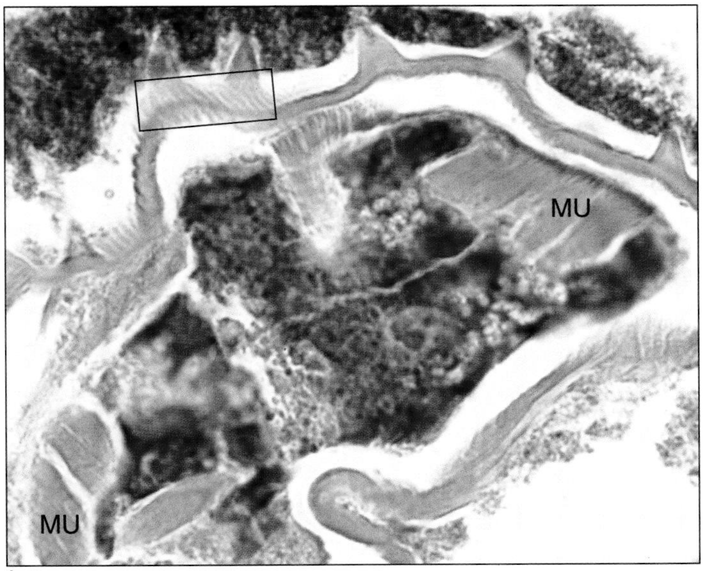

5

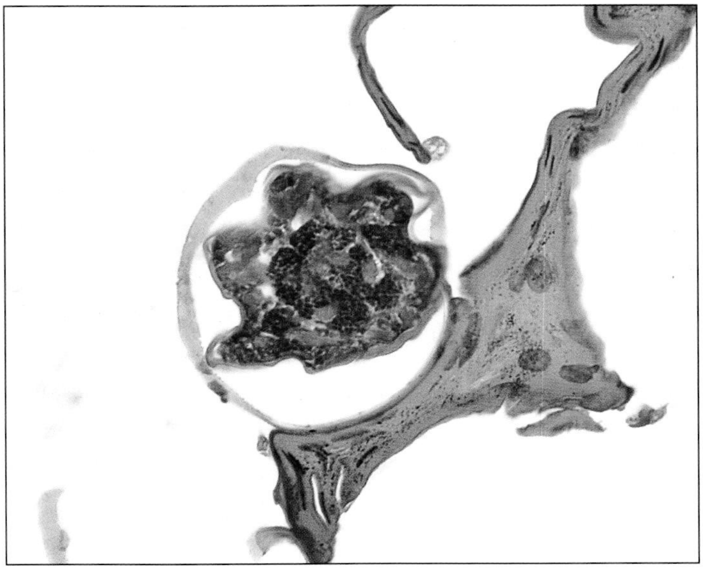

6

Demodex

Follice Mites

Almost everyone in the world is infected with the follicle mite, *Demodex*. These mites are obligate parasites of the pilosebaceous follicles on the face, particularly around the nose, forehead, and scalp. Two species are parasites of humans: *D. folliculorum* in the hair follicle itself and *D. brevis* in the associated sebaceous glands. These parasites are routinely and incidentally encountered in skin biopsy specimens. Although generally regarded as nonpathogenic, minor and occasionally major skin lesions of various sorts have been attributed to these organisms. Related species often cause severe diseases in animals such as dogs.

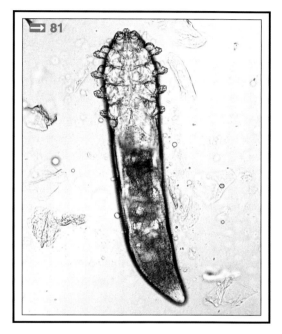

Biology and Life Cycle

Evidence suggests that *Demodex* never occurs in humans in tissues other than hair follicles and associated sebaceous glands. The parasite's entire life cycle, which includes several stages (ie, egg, larva, nymph, and adult), lasts about 14 days. The adult female survives for only about 5 days; males survive for an even shorter period. Females apparently produce only a few eggs during their brief life. Several mites, as many as 10 to 15, may occupy the same follicle, although the average seems closer to 6 or 8. *Demodex folliculorum* feeds on cells of the follicular epithelium. *Demodex brevis* appears to consume sebaceous gland cells.

Pathology and Clinical Manifestations

It has been suggested that *Demodex* plays a causal role in a wide variety of skin conditions, including blepharitis, pityriasis rosacea, and perioral dermatitis. The effects of the mites on the pilosebaceous system include follicular dilations, perifollicular inflammation, and the accrual of dense, homogeneous, eosinophilic material around a mite or groups of mites (Plate 98:2 & 5). On the whole, demodicosis produces no symptoms or grossly evident pathologic changes in the affected skin.

Parasite Morphology

The adults are minute and elongate (➡ 81). The female *D. folliculorum* has a mean length of about 300 μm and a diameter of 52 μm; males are only slightly smaller. Adult *D. brevis* are about 30% smaller than adult *D. folliculorum*. In both species the anterior one third of the body bears the mouthparts (gnathosoma) and the four pairs of short, stumpy legs (podosoma). The remainder of the body (opisthosoma) is transversely striated and rounded posteriorly (➡ 81). The eggs of *D. folliculorum* are spindle shaped and measure about 100 μm in length. Those of *D. brevis* are oval and smaller, measuring about 60 μm. In sections of skin, the anterior end of the body is most recognizable due to its more rigid structure (Plate 98:5 & 6). Several mites may be seen in one follicle (Plate 98:2 & 4).

The size, habitat, and characteristic morphologic features of these mites make it unlikely that they will be confused with any other arthropods in the skin.

References

Aylesworth R, Vance JC. *Demodex folliculorum* and *Demodex brevis* in cutaneous biopsies. *J Am Acad Dermatol*. 1982;7:583-589.

Burns DA. Follicle mites and their role in disease. *Clin Exp Dermatol*. 1992;17:152-155.

Nutting WB. Hair follicle mites (Acari: Demodicidae) of man. *Int J Dermatol*. 1976;15:79-98.

Plate 98

Demodex

Image 1

Living adult mite found in sebaceous material expressed from a hair follicle (Unstained, 200x).

Image 2

Section through hair follicle shows portions of several mites (H&E, 200x).

Image 3

Section through a mole excised from the skin shows mites in a follicle (dart) (H&E, 100x).

Image 4

At higher magnification, portions of at least three mites are visible (H&E, 180x).

Image 5

High magnification through the anterior portion of mite (H&E, 500x).

Image 6

At higher magnification, one sees the gnathosoma (keyline) and the podosoma, which bears the four pairs of legs (H&E, 1000x).

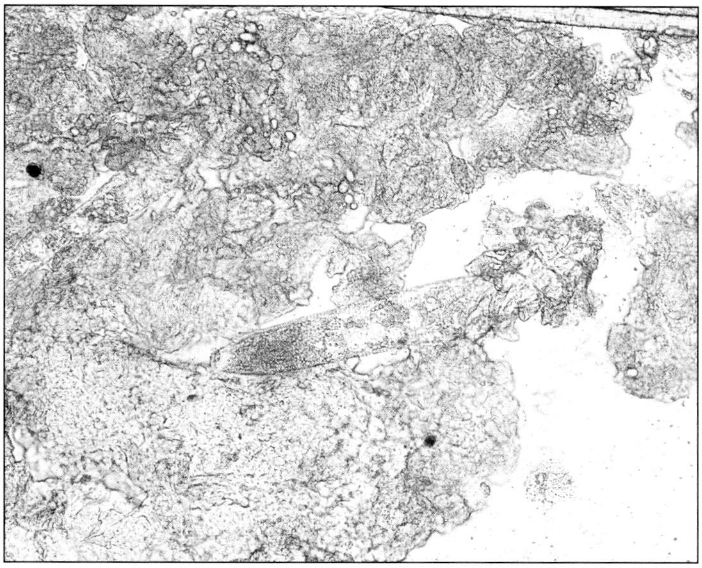
1

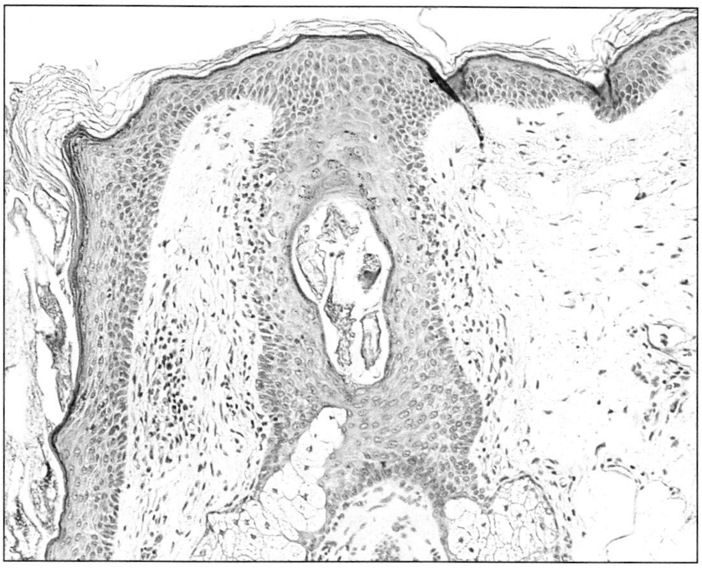
2

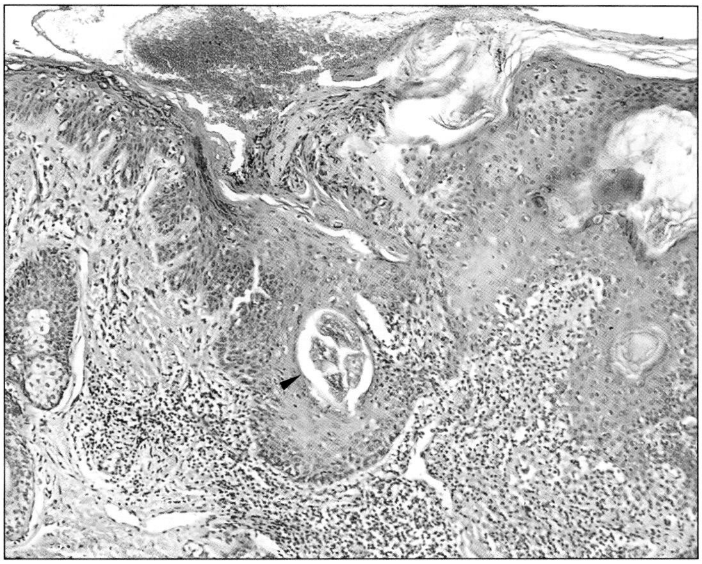
3

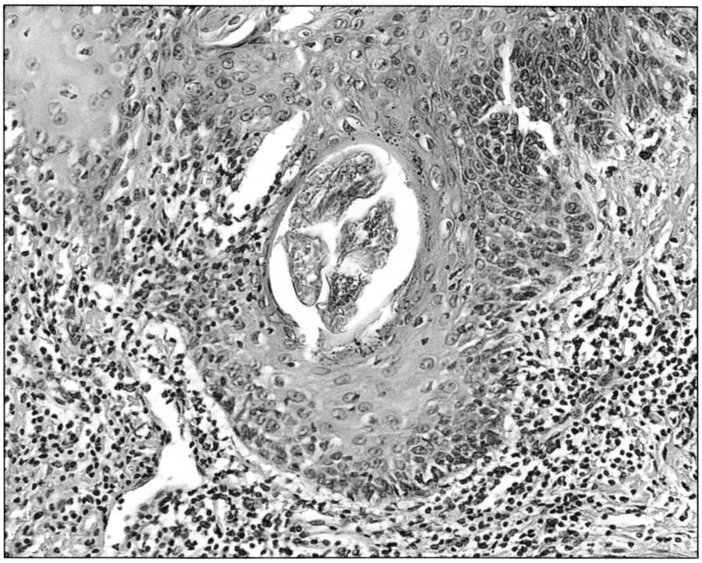
4

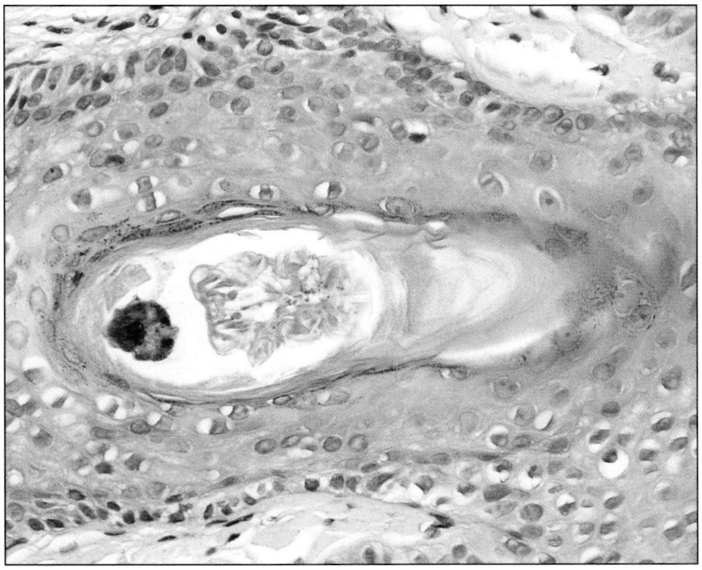
5

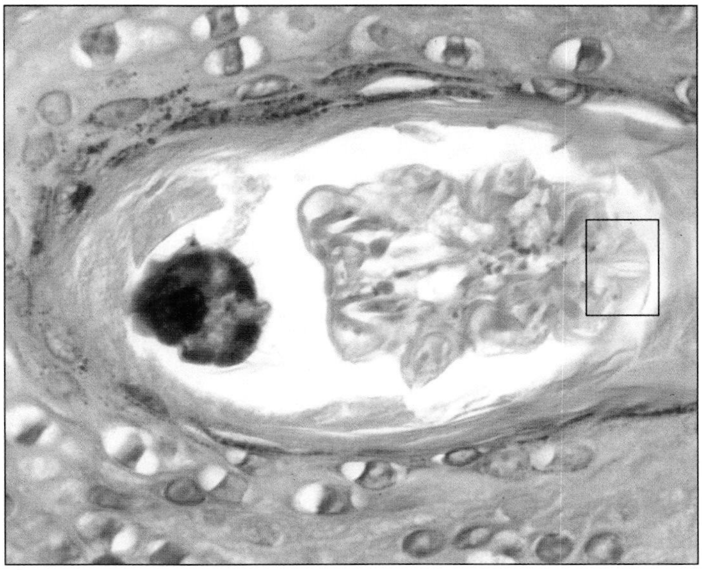
6

Myiasis

Several groups of flies have larvae that invade the tissues of vertebrate animals to feed on living or dead tissues, secretions, etc. Some are obligatory tissue parasites, such as the bot flies and screw worms, while others are semispecific, depositing their eggs or larvae in decaying flesh or diseased tissues (flesh flies). Occasionally, these flies invade human tissues. Human myiasis has cosmopolitan distribution and occurs in both tropical and temperate regions, including the United States and other parts of North America.

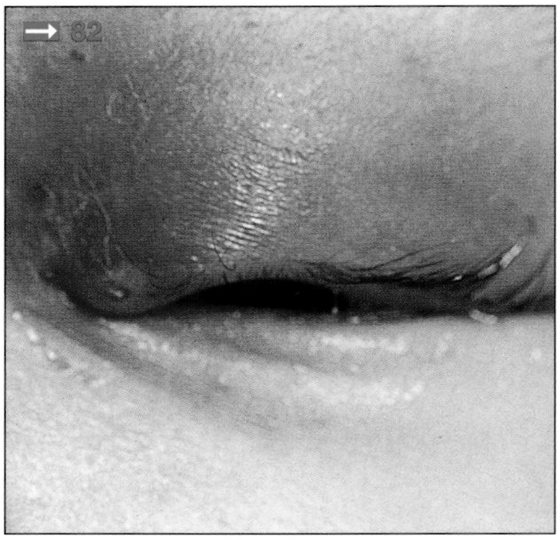

Biology and Life Cycle

In the course of their development, flies undergo a complete metamorphosis that involves the four basic stages of egg, larva, pupa, and adult. Eggs hatch quickly. The larvae, commonly referred to as maggots, are elongate, cone shaped, and without appendages. The larva develops through three instars and under normal circumstances then drops from the host and becomes a pupa, which ultimately transforms to an adult. The maggot is the stage most important in human myiasis and the only stage that occurs in humans. The entire life cycle may take weeks or months to complete.

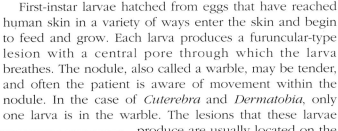

Cutaneous Myiasis

The skin and underlying dermis is the most common site for human myiasis. Many species of flies are responsible for these infections, but the most common agents are the bot flies, which include *Cuterebra*, *Gasterophilus*, *Dermatobia*, *Hypoderma*, and *Oestrus*, and the screw worms, which include *Cordylobia* and *Cochliomyia*.

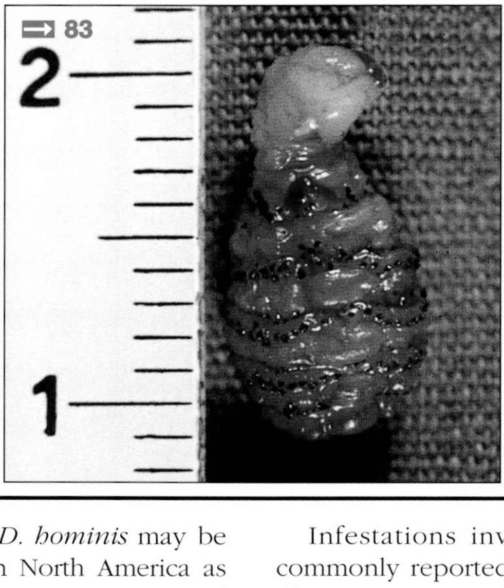

Baird et al (1989) reported that *Dermatobia hominis* is the most common agent of furuncular myiasis in the Western Hemisphere, with most cases occurring in Central and South America. Although *D. hominis* may be the cause of a majority of the cases in North America as well, *Cuterebra* species is the most common cause of infections among individuals who have not traveled abroad. Visitors to Africa occasionally become infected with the tumbu fly, *Cordylobia anthropophaga* or *Stasisia* (= *Cordylobia*) *rodhaini*.

First-instar larvae hatched from eggs that have reached human skin in a variety of ways enter the skin and begin to feed and grow. Each larva produces a furuncular-type lesion with a central pore through which the larva breathes. The nodule, also called a warble, may be tender, and often the patient is aware of movement within the nodule. In the case of *Cuterebra* and *Dermatobia*, only one larva is in the warble. The lesions that these larvae produce are usually located on the head, neck, and chest (*Cuterebra*), other areas of exposed skin, and the scalp (*Dermatobia*) (→ **82**). Infections with *Cordylobia* are usually found on any exposed areas of skin, and each warble may contain one to four larvae.

Gasterophilus (horse bot) larvae enter the skin and typically cause larva migrans. They then localize in a site but do not produce a warble. Occasionally, this larva migrates to deeper tissues and organs such as the lung (Plate 99:3 & 4).

Ophthalmomyiasis

Some of the same species of fly larvae found in the skin and subcutaneous tissues have been recovered from the eye and the orbit. The sheep bot, *Oestrus ovis*, is found wherever sheep are raised. It is a common cause of human ophthalmomyiasis and has been recovered from the human conjunctiva and adjacent tissues (Plate 100:1 & 2). In the United States, *Cuterebra* larvae have been found in the anterior and posterior chambers of the eye (→ **79**, p. 338) as well as in the eyelid. In Scandinavia the reindeer warble, *Hypoderma tarandi*, has been reported from the eye and eyelid of two children (Plate 100:4–6).

Other species of flies, including *Chrysomyia*, *Sarcophaga*, and *Wohlfahrtia*, have been identified as a cause of ophthalmomyiasis in different parts of the world.

Other Sites of Infection

Infestations involving many other tissue sites are commonly reported. Eggs of the Old World screw worm, *Chrysomyia*, are deposited on broken skin or mucous membranes such as the nares, nasal sinuses, gums, conjunctiva, and vagina. They hatch and burrow into the tissues, where they grow to the third-instar stage in a few days and then spontaneously leave the tissues between the 7th and 14th days. In the interim, they may produce foul-smelling, disfiguring lesions that can become secondarily infected.

Larvae of *Oestrus ovis* can infest the nasopharynx and nasal sinuses or the pharynx, causing considerable congestion, secretions, and pruritus. However, these symptoms disappear after a few days, when the larvae spontaneously exit from the tissues.

Gastrointestinal infections with fly larvae, particularly *Gasterophilus,* have been documented. However, intestinal and urogenital infections are difficult to confirm, perhaps because fecal and urine samples and vomitus, or the containers in which they were collected, were contaminated before or after the samples were obtained. Additionally, food may be contaminated with fly eggs prior to its consumption. Eggs may hatch in the intestine and the larvae may survive and even develop to some degree before they are expelled in feces.

Finally, fly maggots are frequently found in dead tissues (eg, bodies exposed to flies postmortem and prior to examination) or in diseased tissues or wounds in comatose individuals, even in hospitals. Infestations occur particularly in tropical environments and in circumstances where a wide variety of flies may alight on the tissues and deposit eggs or larvae. These represent accidental rather than obligatory myiasis.

Parasite Morphology

The fly larva (maggot) is the only stage of importance in myiasis. The typical larva is elongate and somewhat cone shaped and lacks appendages. The anterior end, which is usually narrower, bears mouthparts and anterior spiracles. The posterior end bears a pair of larger, conspicuous spiracles. The segmented body of the larva may bear rows of spines of different sizes and structure. The structure of the mouthparts and the detailed structure of the posterior spiracles are morphologic features important in identifying the species of larvae.

The larvae develop through three instars, resulting in considerable difference in size and gross appearance. Maggots range in size from less than a millimeter in the first-instar stage to almost 3.0 cm in the mature, third-instar stage (➡ 83). Larvae obtained from tissues are generally first- or second-instar stages. Mature larvae are obtained from tissues less commonly, because they are usually removed by the patient or an attending physician before they complete their maturation. Specific identification is typically straightforward and based on gross morphologic features (eg, mouthparts, spination, and spiracle morphology). Detailed descriptions of the important morphologic features of fly larvae are available in medical entomology or parasitology texts.

Identifying maggots in tissues is much more challenging than identifying the intact larva, and species identifications are often impossible. The patient's travel history as well as symptomatology and clinical presentation provide clues to diagnosis.

In tissue sections the morphologic features of these arthropods are different from those of all other parasites. The tegument may be sclerotized, with cuticularized spines and hooks (Plate 99:2 & 6; Plate 100:4 & 6). Striated muscle (Plate 99:2; Plate 100:2), tracheae (Plate 99:2, 4, & 5), and sometimes spiracles are evident. Portions of the chitinized mouthparts are often seen (Plate 100:2) as well.

A composite of morphologic features, the lesion, and patient history will lead to an adequate generic diagnosis.

References

Baird JK, Baird CR, Sabrosky W. North American cuterebrid myiasis: report of seventeen new infections of human beings and review of the disease. *J Am Acad Dermatol.* 1989;21:763-772.

De Kaminsky RG. Nosocomial myiasis by *Cochliomyia hominivorax* in Honduras. *Trans R Soc Trop Med Hyg.* 1993;87:199-200.

Kearney MS, Nilsson AC, Lyslo A, Syrdalen P, Dannevig L. Ophthalmomyiasis caused by the reindeer warble fly larva. *J Clin Pathol.* 1991;44:276-284.

Newman PE, Beaver PC, Kozarsky PE, Waring GO III. Fly larva adherent to corneal endothelium. *Am J Ophthalmol.* 1986;102:211-216.

Arosemena R, Booth SA, Su WPD. Cutaneous myiasis. *J Am Acad Dermatol.* 1993;28:254-256.

Plate 99

Cordylobia, Gasterophilus, and *Dermatobia*

Image 1

Longitudinal section through a maggot of *Cordylobia* excised with adjacent tissues from the scalp of an individual who had been in West Africa. Even at low power, the segmentation of the organism can be seen (H&E, 30x).

Image 2

At higher magnification, large yellow spines (darts) are seen on the surface of the tegument. Note also the extensive musculature (MU) and tracheal tubes (arrows). A portion of this parasite measured about 3 cm in length (H&E, 120x).

Images 3 and 4

Section through a coin lesion in the lung of a resident of West Virginia. A maggot estimated to be longer than 6.0 mm was identified. Large tracheal trunks (TT) are seen. Adjacent sections (not illustrated) showed sclerotized cuticular spines whose size, shape, spacing, and arrangement were consistent with those of a second-instar larva of the horse bot, *Gasterophilus*, probably *G. intestinalis* (H&E; 70x, 100x).

Image 5

Sections through a bot removed from the scalp of a woman who had been in Mexico before the onset of symptoms. The thickened tegument (TE), muscles (MU), and large tracheae (T) are visible (H&E, 15x).

Image 6

At higher magnification, some of the thick yellow spines on the tegument are seen. The morphologic features are those of *Dermatobia* (H&E, 90x).

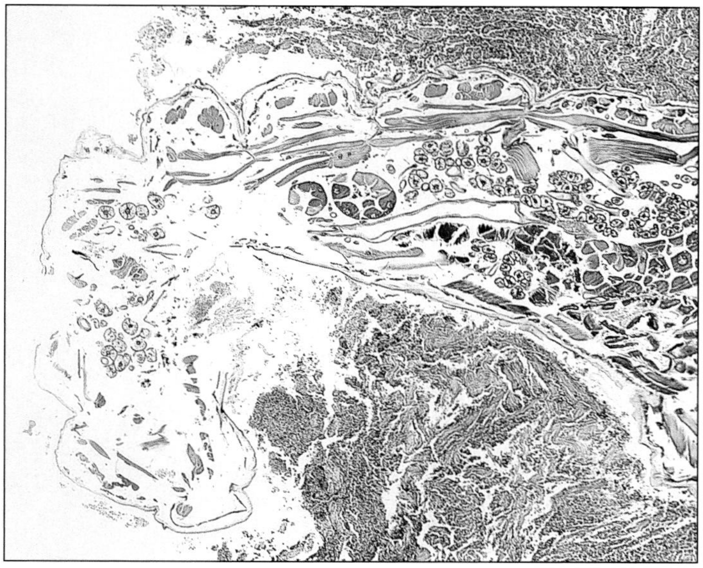

1

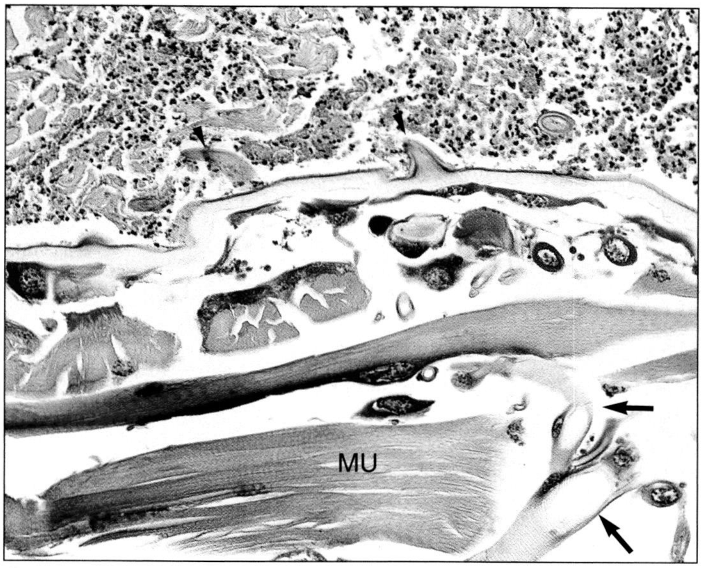

2

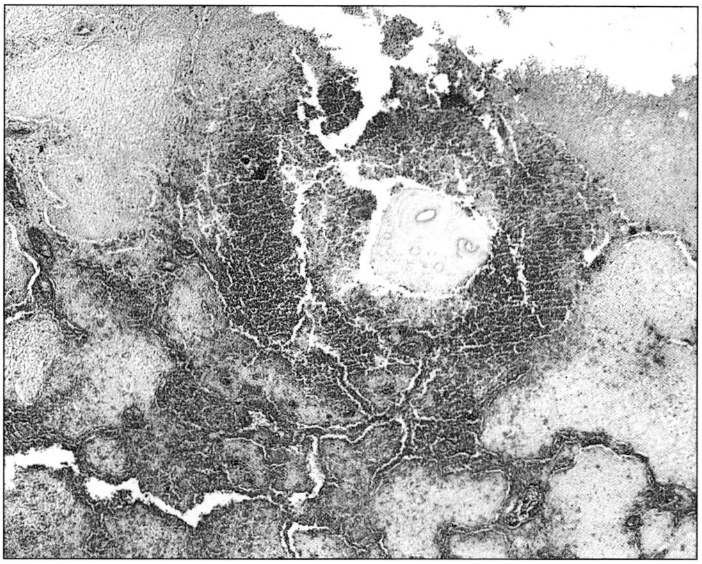

3

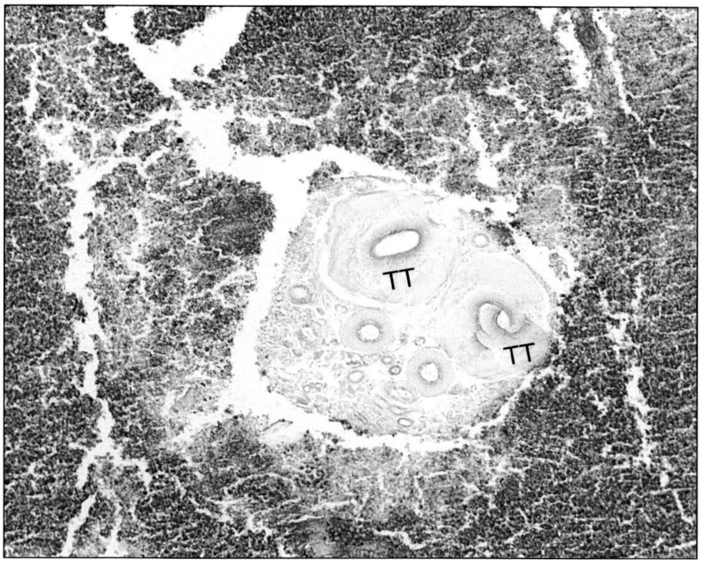

4

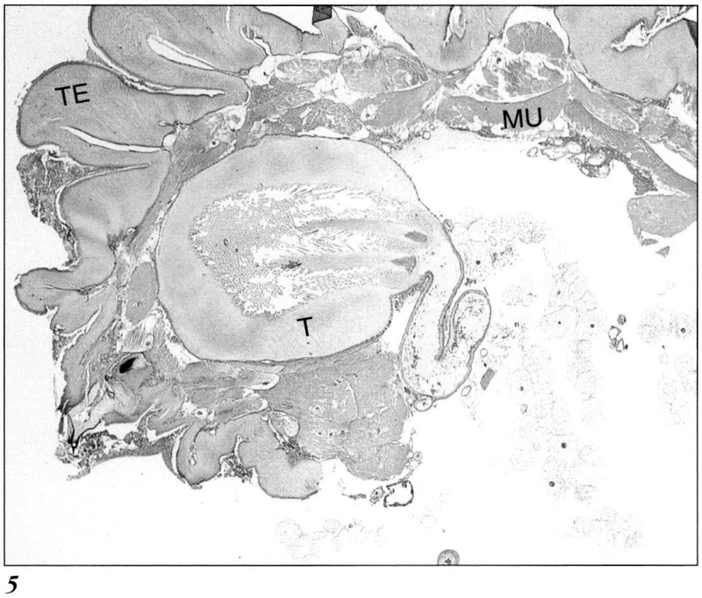

5

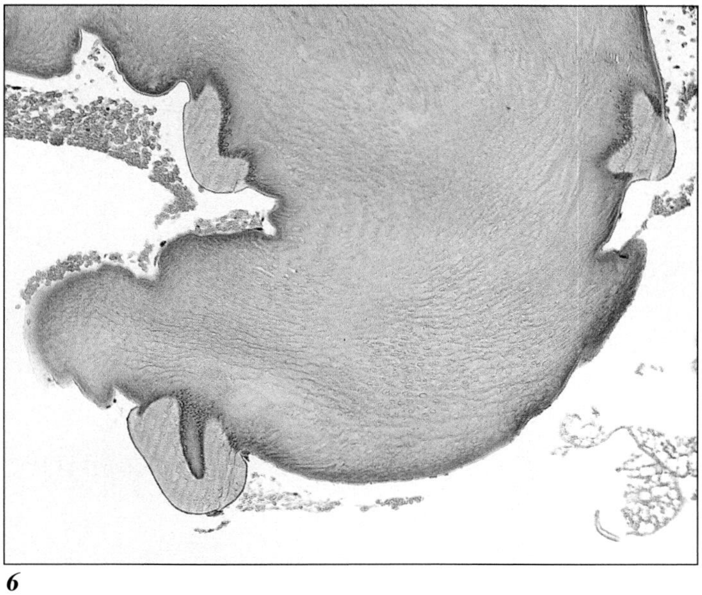

6

Plate 100

Oestrus ovis and *Hypoderma tarandi*

Images 1 and 2

Section through a bot identified as a first-instar larva of *Oestrus ovis* in the conjunctiva of a woman from Ohio. Typical morphologic features of a bot are visible: muscles (arrows), trachea (dart), and mouth parts (keyline). Note the inflammation surrounding the organism (H&E; 80x, 160x).

Image 3

Section through an excised portion of the eyelid of a Norwegian boy shows a maggot identified as *Hypoderma tarandi* within a warble. Even at this low magnification, segmentation is evident. The food channel (FC) is recognizable, but muscles and trachea, while present, are not individually identifiable at this magnification (H&E, 90x).

Image 4

At high magnification, spination (darts) in the tegument is evident (H&E, 800x). (Courtesy of M. Kearney.)

Image 5

At this magnification, the basic arthropod features, ie, trachea (dart) and muscles (arrow), are clear. Bits of the sclerotized mouth parts are present as well (keyline) (H&E, 400x).

Image 6

Degenerate portions of the body wall of the larva show a relatively well-preserved body spine (dart) (H&E, 750x).

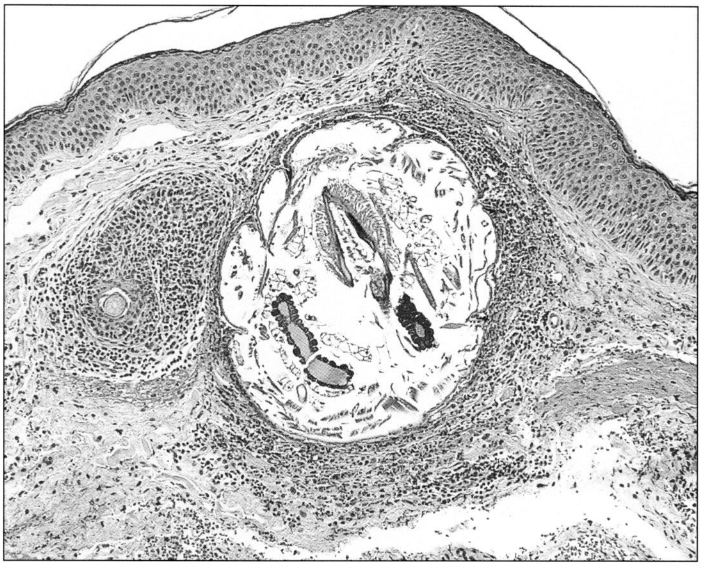

1

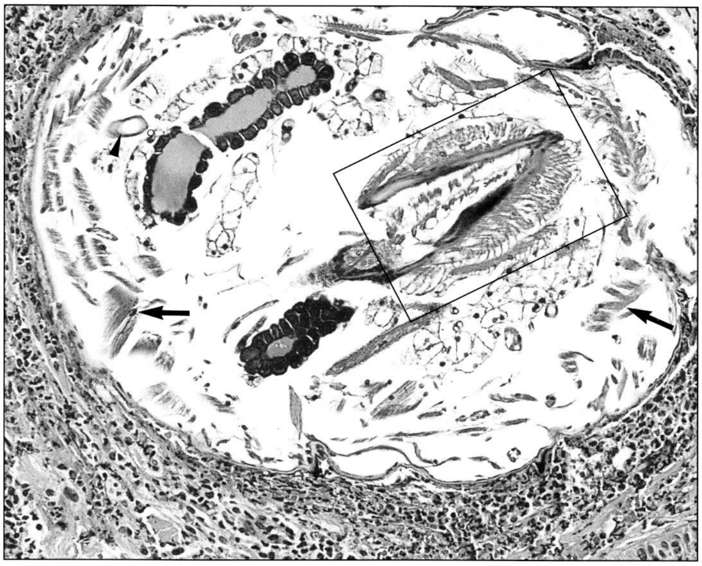

2

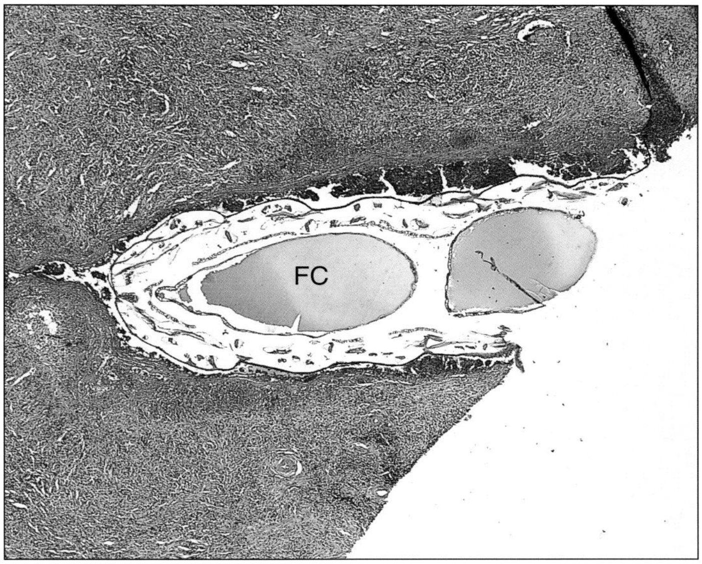

3

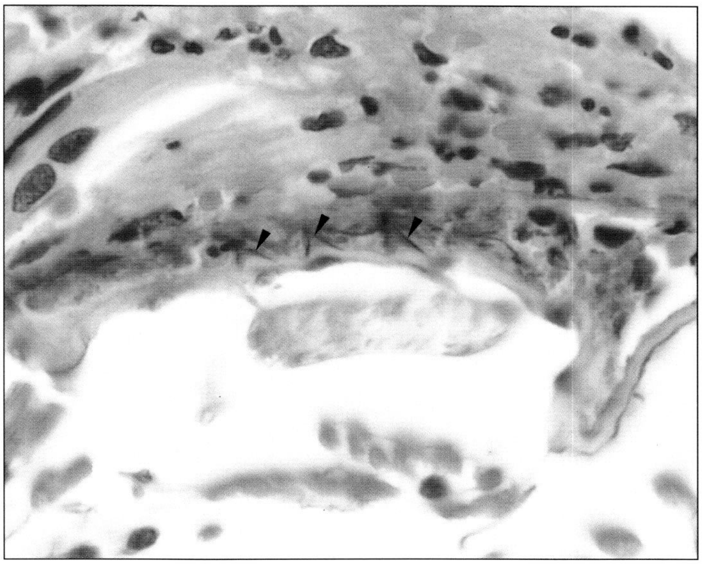

4

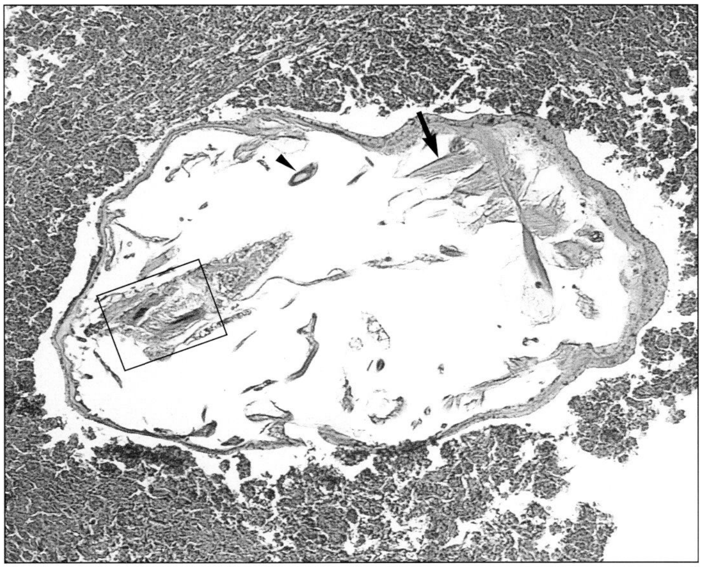

5

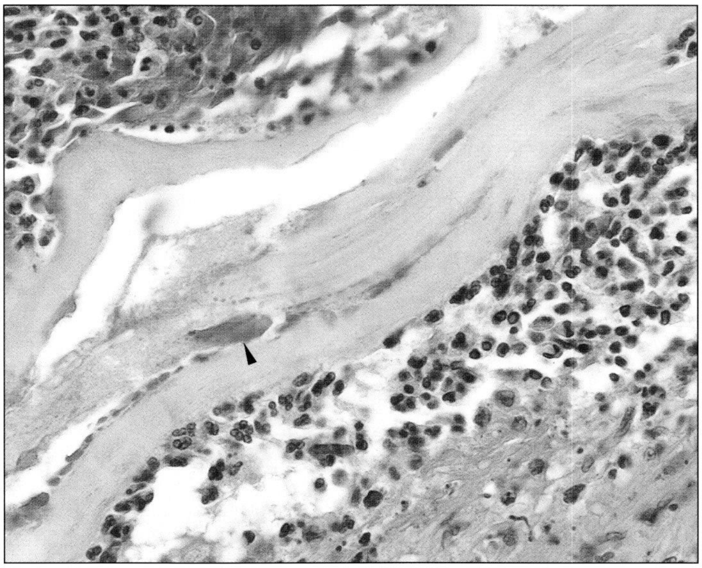

6

Other Arthropods

Tunga penetrans, the chigoe or sand flea (84), is the only flea that invades the human epidermis and produces nodular swellings that are painful and eventually ulcerate (85). Female fleas that have been fertilized in the external environment burrow into the skin and proceed to grow as they become engorged during their feeding process. The head end of the flea lacerates and takes blood from dermal blood vessels, while the posterior end remains exposed to the air through the small hole in the keratin. Eggs are extruded through this hole. After laying eggs, the female flea dies, and eventually the remnants of the flea and keratin will be sloughed. In areas where the sand flea is endemic (ie, tropical Africa, Central and South America, various Caribbean Islands, Pakistan, and the west coast of India), cutaneous lesions occur principally on the ankle, instep, between the toes, and under the nails. Infections are well known and readily diagnosed without histologic evaluation (85). If a lesion is excised and sectioned, it is not difficult to make the appropriate diagnosis (Plate 101:1 & 2).

84

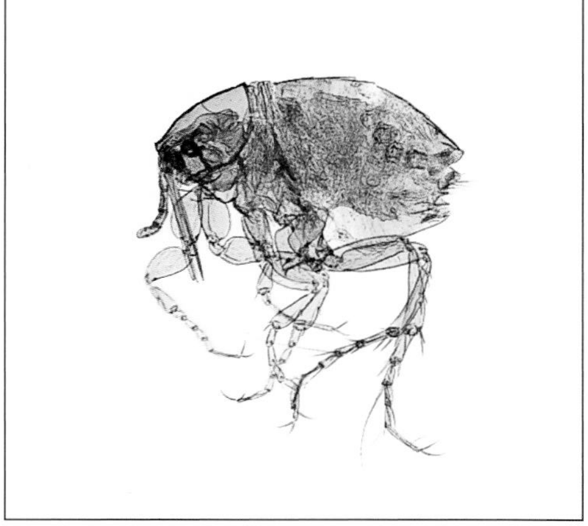

Maggots are frequently encountered in human tissues when corpses remain undiscovered and undergo decomposition. Forensically, the types of fly larvae present and the stages of their development are often useful in establishing the time of death. In most instances, however, the fly larva is identified from intact specimens. Maggots are more rarely encountered in sections of human tissues. The sections in Plate 101:3 & 4 were made from neck tissue of a Vietnamese man who had committed suicide by hanging. Because the corpse was not found for several days, the rope cut into the neck and eggs of an unknown species of fly were deposited on the lesion. The eggs hatched, liberating maggots. The dead man's country of origin suggested that these sections might represent a migrating immature lung fluke of the genus *Paragonimus*. However, it is apparent from the cuticle, the typical arthropod internal anatomy, and the dorsal spines that the section represents a maggot infestation and not a migrating trematode. The maggot's specific identification is not known, although it might be a species of *Lucilia* or a related group.

85

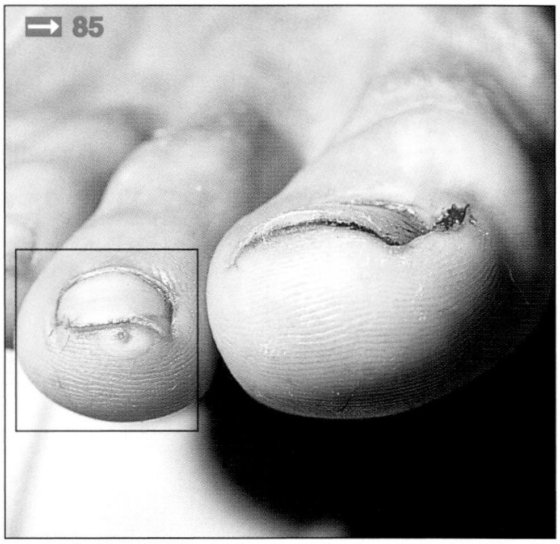

Ticks may provoke a tissue response from the host when they attach to the skin to take blood. Occasionally, attempts are made to remove the tick by traction. This often causes mouthparts of the organism to be left in the host tissues. Sometimes engorged ticks are discovered attached to the skin but are not recognized as such. The ticks may be removed and submitted to the pathology laboratory for diagnosis. Their characteristic arthropod morphology and occasionally the recognition of mouthparts make an accurate diagnosis possible (Plate 101:5 & 6).

References

Alexander JO. *Arthropods and Human Skin*. Berlin, Germany: Springer-Verlag; 1984.

James MT. The flies that cause myiasis in man. Miscellaneous Publication No. 631. Washington, DC: U.S. Department of Agriculture; 1947.

Lord WD, Catts EP, Scarboro A, et al. The green blow fly, *Lucilia illustris* (Meigen), as an indicator of human post-mortem interval: a case of homicide from Fort Lewis, Washington. *Bull Soc Vector Ecol*. 1986;11:271-275.

Smith KGV. *A Manual of Forensic Entomology*. New York, NY: Cornell University; 1986.

Zumpt F. *Myiasis in Man and Animals in the Old World*. London, England: Butterworths; 1965.

Arthropods

Image 1

Low-power image of a section through a nodular lesion in human skin contains a female *Tunga* (H&E, 30x).

Image 2

At higher magnification, the cuticularized body wall (dart), gut (G), tracheae (keyline), and developing eggs (arrows) are visible (H&E, 75x).

Image 3

Section of human tissue from the neck region includes sections through three or four maggots (H&E, 150x).

Image 4

At higher magnification, a section through a maggot illustrates the body wall. Small spines (darts) are visible on one portion, as well as the food channel (FC), Malpighian tubules, and respiratory tracheae (keyline) (H&E, 300x).

Image 5

A cystlike lesion removed from the umbilical area of a child and submitted for pathologic examination. Rather than human cutaneous and subcutaneous tissues, structures characteristic of arthropods are immediately recognizable. A structure outside the large mass (keyline) provides the clue for identification of the object (H&E, 90x).

Image 6

At high magnification, this structure is identifiable as the cuticularized mouth parts of a tick. Rather than a cyst, the tissues represent a portion of the body of a tick adhering to the skin of the child (H&E, 440x).

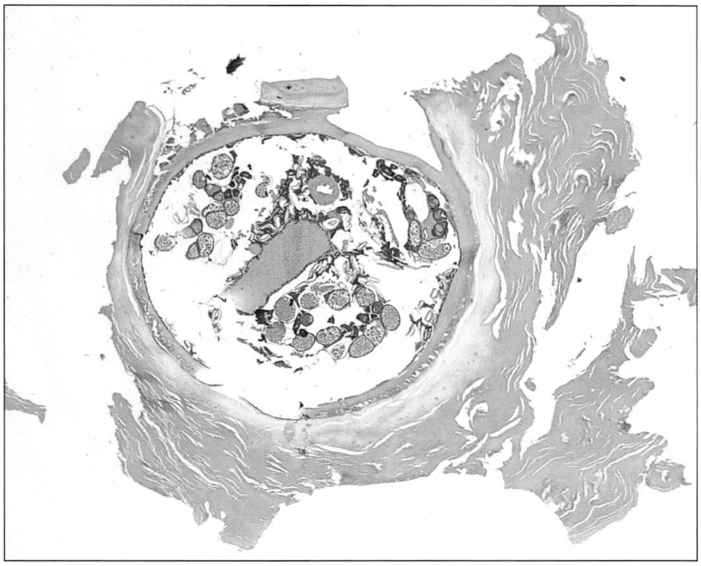

1

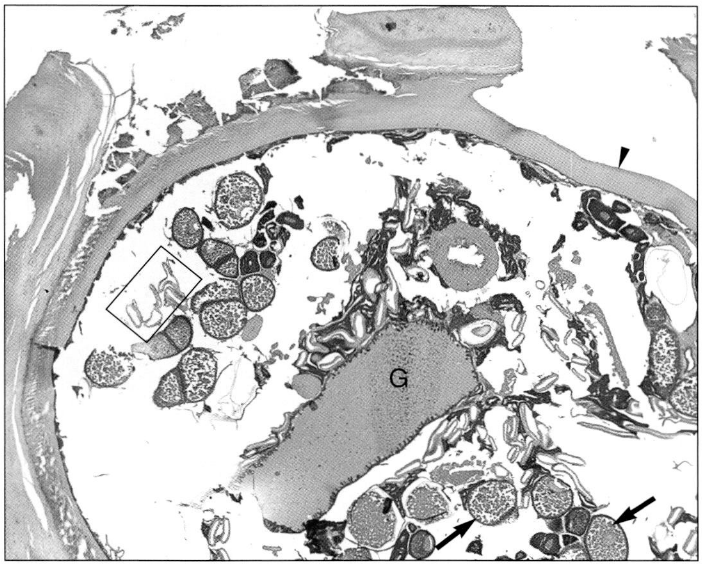

2

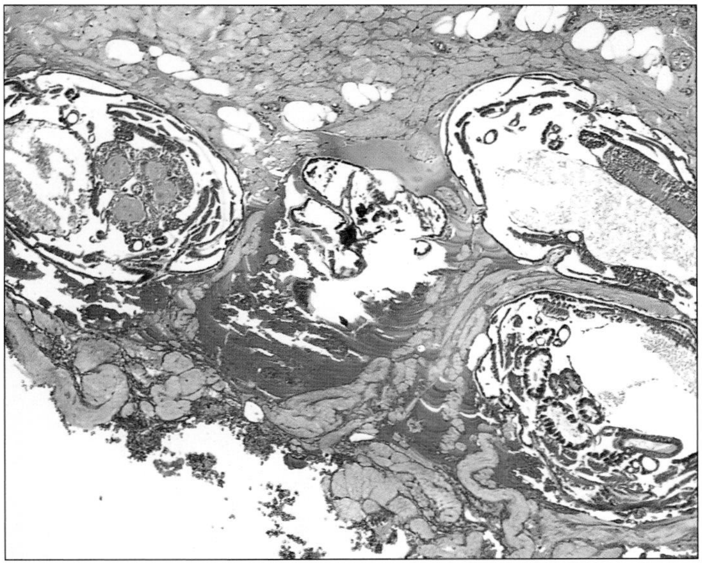

3

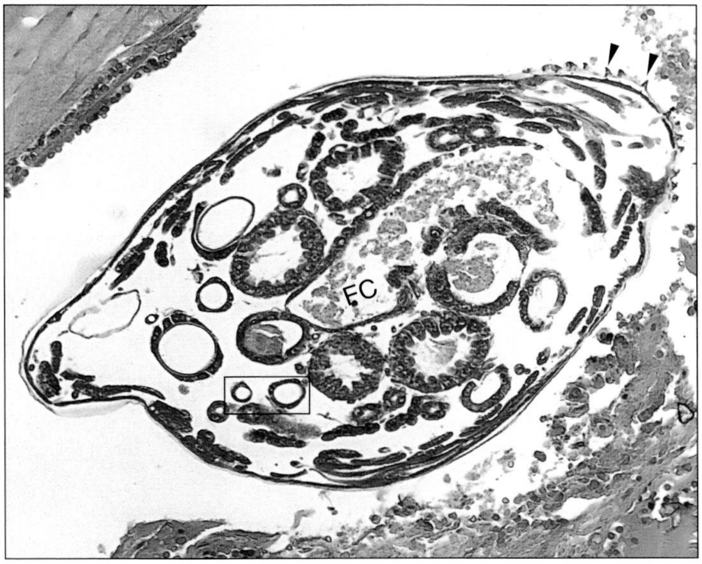

4

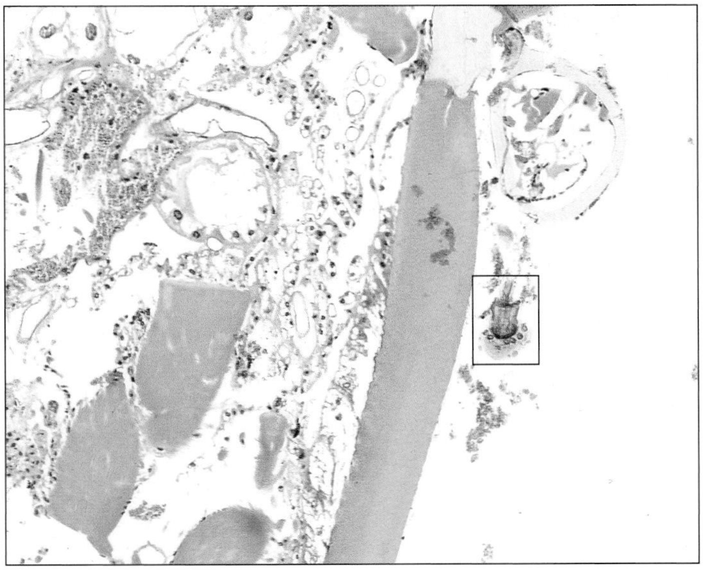

5

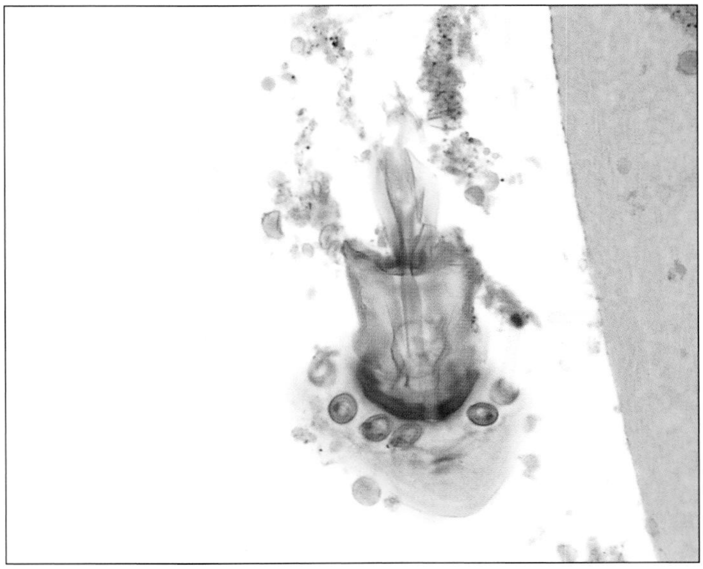

6

Artifacts

Nonparasitic Objects

From time to time, objects will be encountered in tissues that, because of their highly organized structure and vague or even strong resemblance to parasitic organisms or their eggs, are suspected of being some kind of parasite. With careful study and some knowledge of parasite anatomy and egg morphology, it is usually possible to determine whether the object is a parasite or not. Unfortunately, it is not always possible to identify what the nonparasite object is, because of the wide range of possibilities. Nevertheless, many objects or artifacts can be identified.

Many nonparasite elements are found in the intestine, particularly the appendix, which pathologists examine with possibly the greatest frequency. It is common to find seeds and other plant materials in appendices, and these often mimic parasites (Plate 102). Plant structures are not limited to the intestinal tract; for example, thorns may be found embedded in soft tissues (Plate 103:1 & 2). Although plant structures are readily identified grossly, in sections they pose a problem because of the general lack of knowledge of their microscopic structure. Seeds with prickly coats or burrs sometimes lodge in soft tissues of the throat. These are then removed and submitted for pathologic examination as a possible parasite or maggot (Plate 103:3 & 4). Plant debris, particularly starch granules, are encountered in a variety of sites, often in granulomas, and are frequently thought to be some kind of parasite egg (Plate 104:1–4). Other plant elements have been found in a range of unlikely sites (Plate 103:5 & 6; Plate 104:5 & 6).

In recent years, peculiar, ringlike, laminated structures have been detected in a variety of human tissues and aspirate material. These structures are called Liesegang rings after a German biochemist who first described them in the late 19th century. They are often found within cysts in tissues or in tissues that are inflamed, fibrotic, or undergoing necrosis. The kidney and closely associated tissues are important areas for their detection, but they have also been found in breast tissue, pericardium, synovium, conjunctiva and eyelid, and other tissues. The manner in which these structures form is not well understood, although it appears to be a complex physicochemical process. This complex process produces ringlike structures that are not always uniform in appearance and size, although they are basically similar in many other respects. The importance of Liesegang rings from a diagnostic perspective is that they have frequently been mistaken for parasites, both eggs and worms. Representative material from retroperitoneal masses near the kidney of two different human cases indicates the range in appearance of these interesting bodies (Plate 105).

Because of their size and structure, fungal spores and similar objects are often suspected of being various helminth eggs (Plate 106). Additionally, tissues and tissue fluids may be contaminated during histologic processing by foreign objects such as lint and dust mites (Plate 107).

References

Gupta RK, McHutchinson GR, Fauck R. Liesegang rings in a needle aspirate from a breast cyst. *Acta Cytol.* 1993;35:700-702.

Mahoney CA, Sherwood N, Yap EH, et al. Ciliated cell remnants in peritoneal dialysis fluid. *Arch Pathol Lab Med.* 1993;117:211-213.

Sun T, Turnbull A, Lieberman PH, et al. Giant kidney worm (*Dioctophyme renale*) infection mimicking retroperitoneal neoplasm. *Am J Surg Pathol.* 1986;10:508-512.

Tuur SM, Nelson AM, Gibson DW, et al. Liesegang rings in tissue: how to distinguish Liesegang rings from the giant kidney worm, *Dioctophyme renale*. *Am J Surg Pathol.* 1987;11:598-605.

Artifacts

Images 1 and 2

Sections of an appendix contain a structure that at low magnification appears to be a parasite. It was submitted with a tentative diagnosis of "parasite with chitinous parts." At higher magnification, it is evident that this is a seed with a thick, cellular outer coat (dart), a cellular inner layer that mimics muscle (arrows), and germ plasm (GP) that suggests an organ structure (H&E; 35x, 100x).

Images 3 and 4

Sections of an appendix show a transverse section of an adult pinworm (keyline) and a larger structure, a seed. This was interpreted as possibly a section through a tapeworm proglottid. At higher magnification of the "proglottid," the heavy cellular nature of the seed is apparent (see Plate 85:1 to compare this object with a tapeworm proglottid) (H&E; 35x, 90x).

Images 5 and 6

Sections through a pinfeather lodged in the appendix. Superficially, this resembles a parasite because of what appears to be a cuticle (pink stain) and an inner layer of muscle cells. At high magnification, the musclelike inner layer of the object is still striking. Note the cellular nature of the outer layer (Trichrome, 40x; 250x).

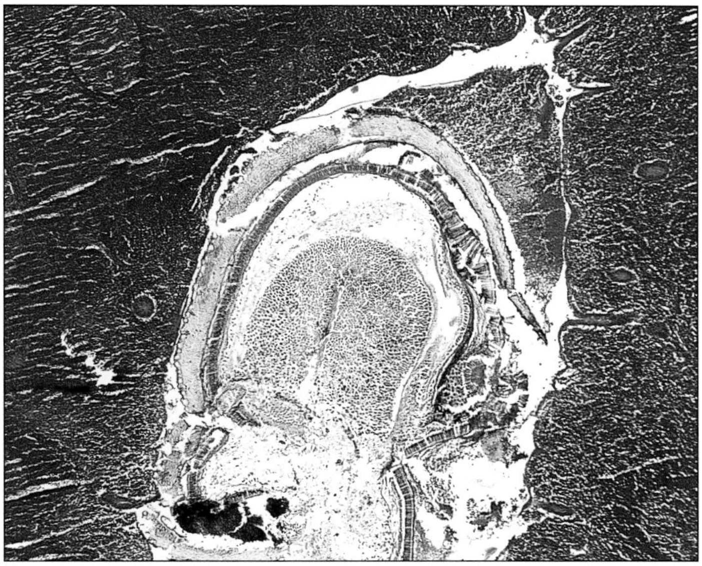

1

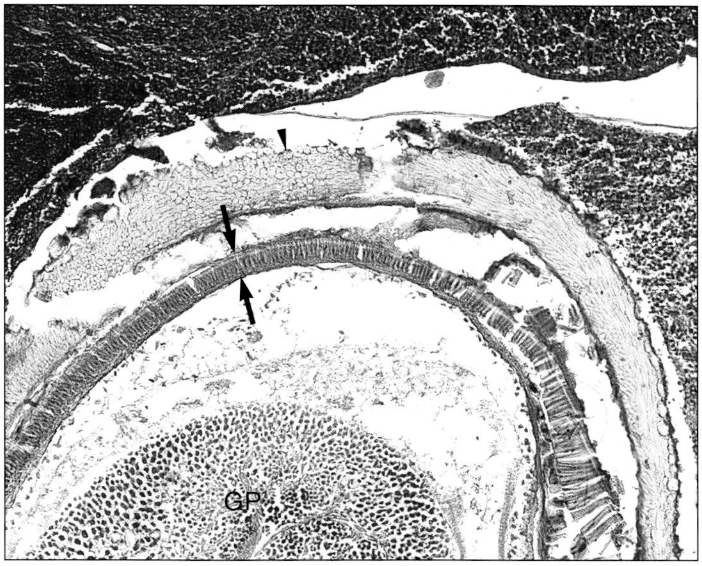

2

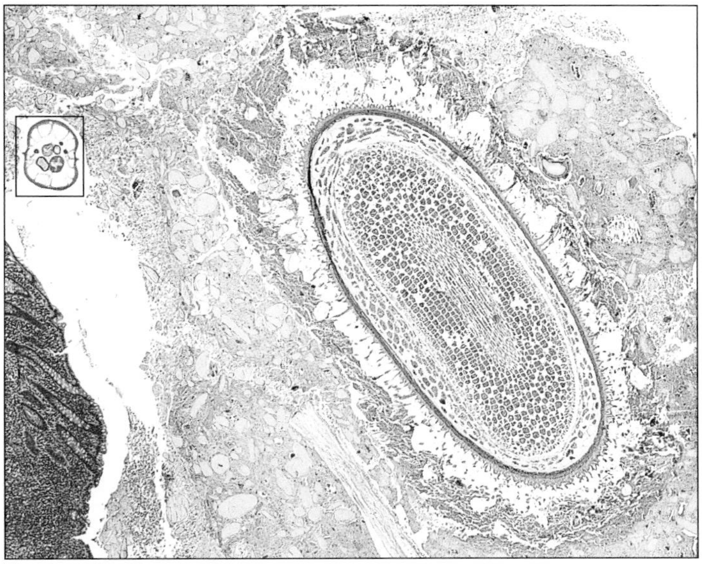

3

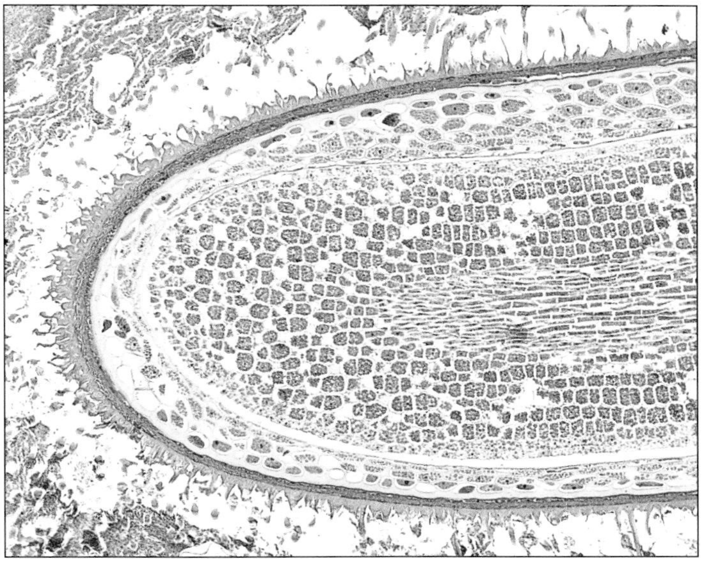

4

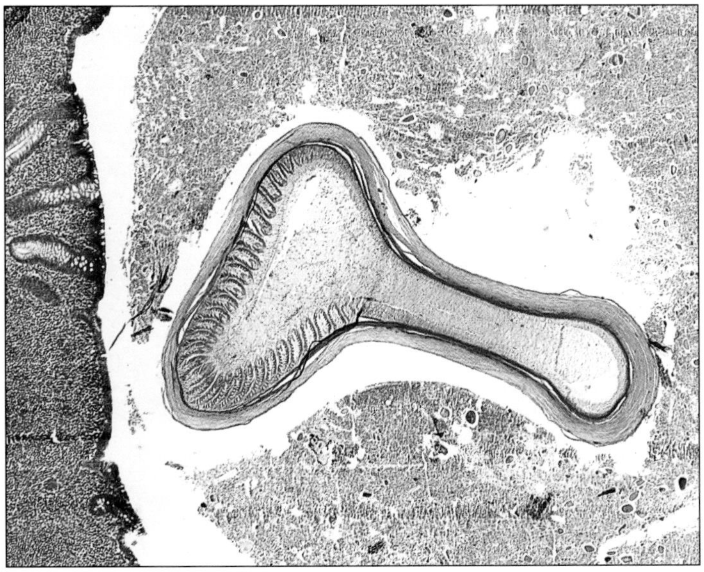

5

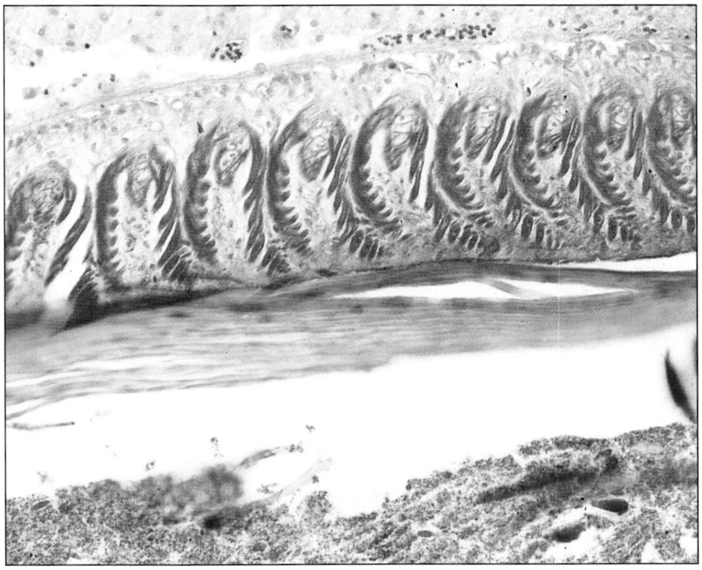

6

Artifacts

Images 1 and 2

Biopsy specimen of a mass palpated in an earlobe reveals the presence of what was believed to be a thorn. Its microscopic structure clearly ruled out parasitic material (H&E, 20x; 80x).

Images 3 and 4

Structure removed from the throat of an adult. The object measured 4.5 x 1.5 mm and was thought to be a parasite, possibly a pentastome. At high magnification, its structure is clearly that of a seed or burr. Note the similarity to the seed found in Plate 102:3 (H&E, 33x; 100x).

Images 5 and 6

Sections through a hematoma from a man who died of hemorrhage into the abdominal cavity. The yellow-staining objects, which are especially evident at higher magnification, are plant material from the intestine (stain unknown, 30x; 200x).

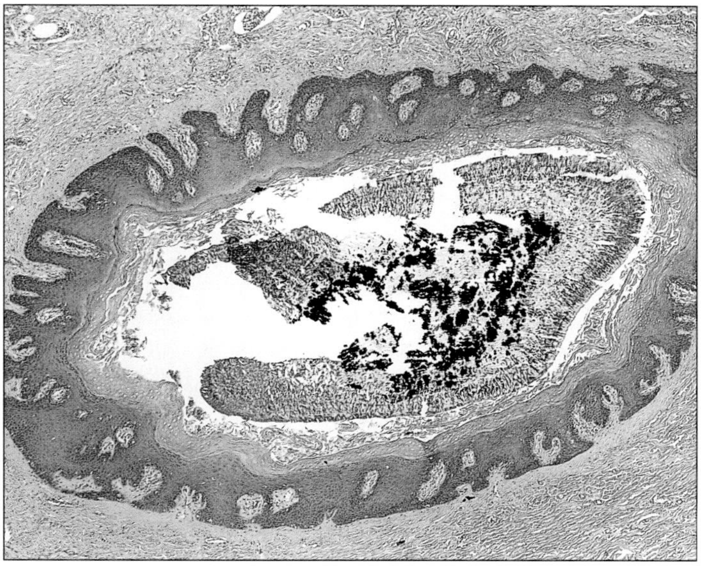

1

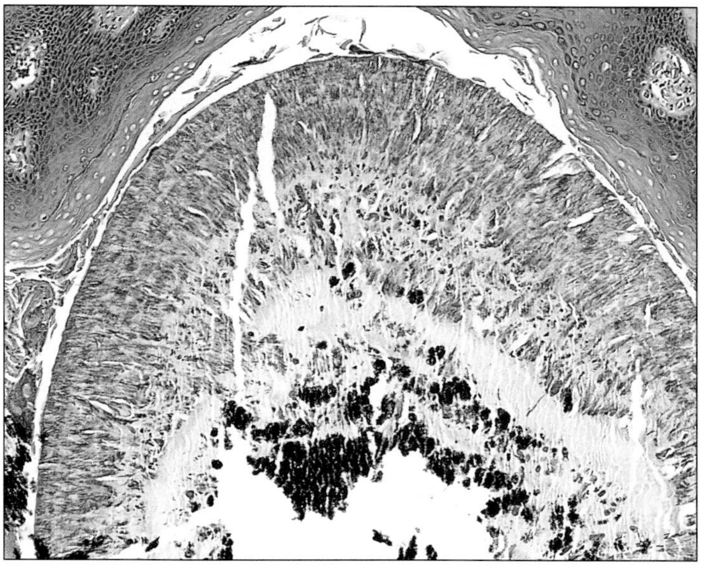

2

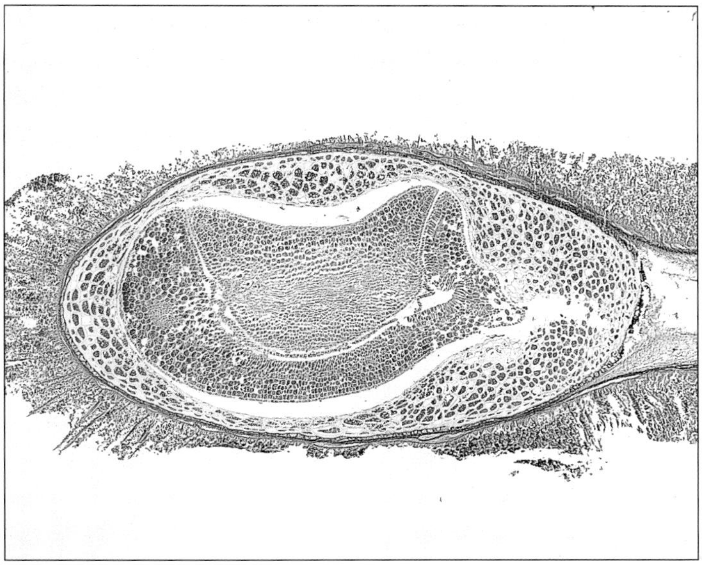

3

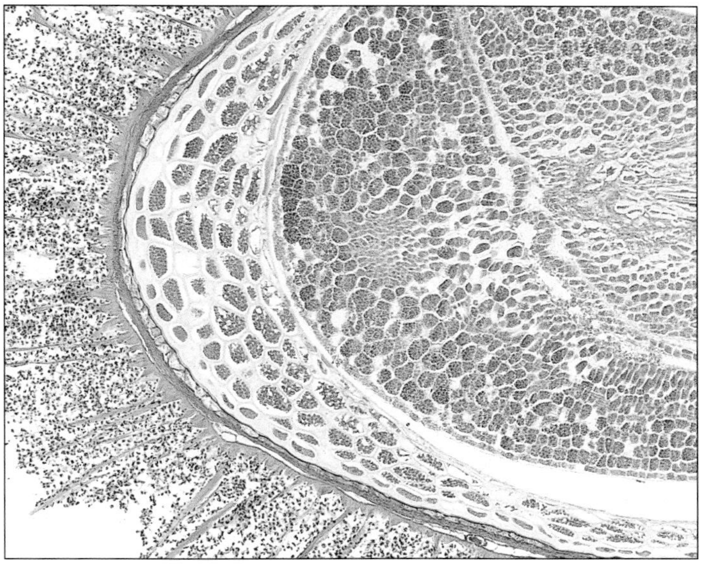

4

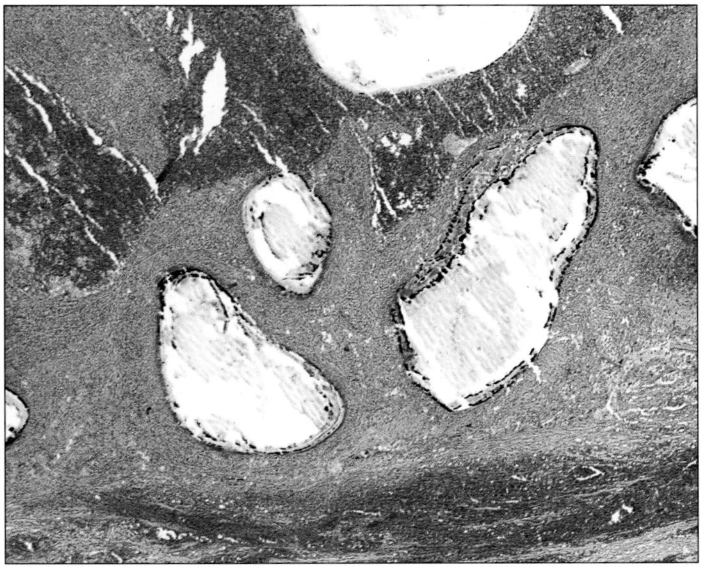

5

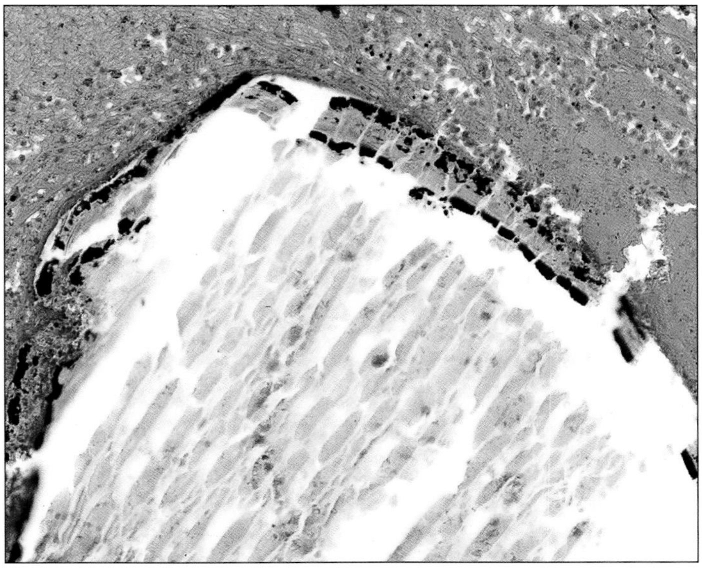

6

Plate 104

Artifacts

Images 1 and 2

Section of lung examined during routine autopsy of an individual who died of a stroke. The object within the inflammatory lesion is a starch grain, which has a characteristic appearance at high magnification. Starch grains are often suspected of being parasite eggs or parasites. These were probably aspirated into the lung (H&E; 300x, 500x).

Images 3 and 4

Starch grains (keyline) in the base of a peptic ulcer. The typical starch grains are apparent at higher magnification. These were originally interpreted as "remnants of a nematode" (H&E; 30x, 100x).

Images 5 and 6

A granuloma removed from a woman contains what was suspected to be a maggot. The tentative diagnosis was based on the presence of so-called "tracheoles," which are found in insects. At higher magnification, the "tracheoles" were found to be plant spiral fibers (GMS, 35x; 400x).

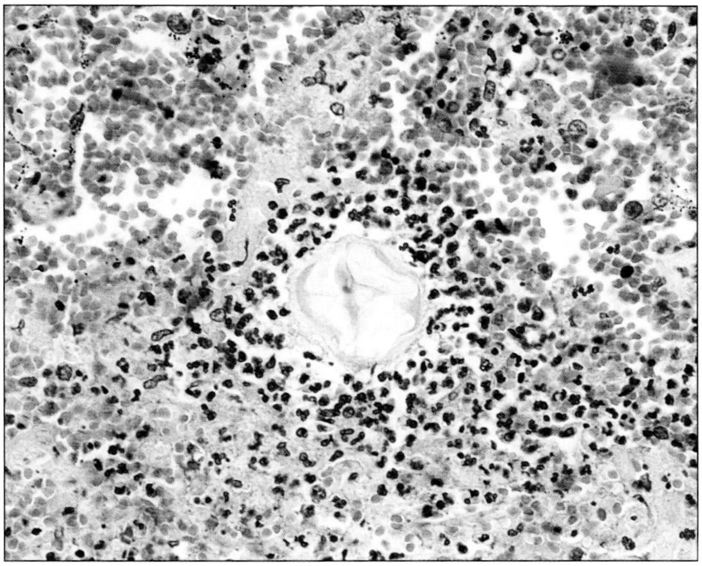
1

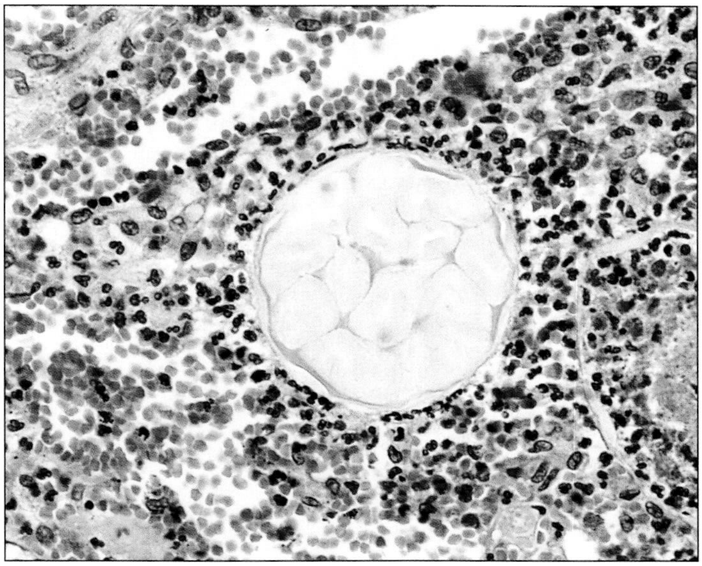
2

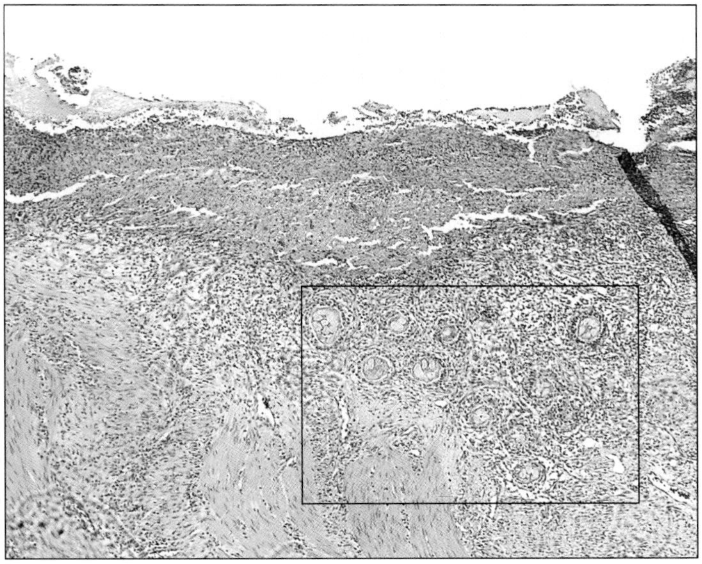
3

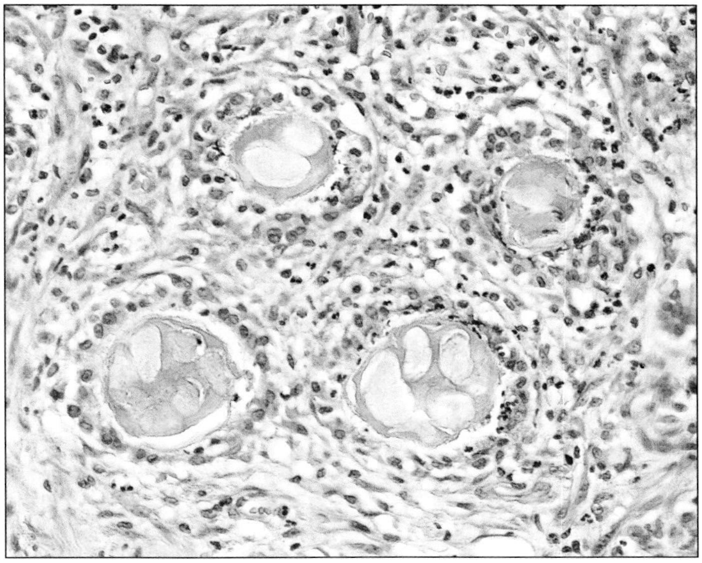
4

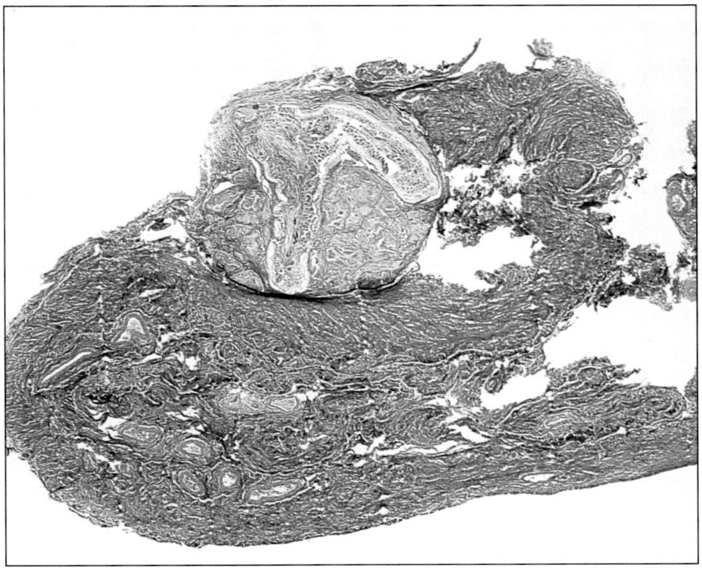
5

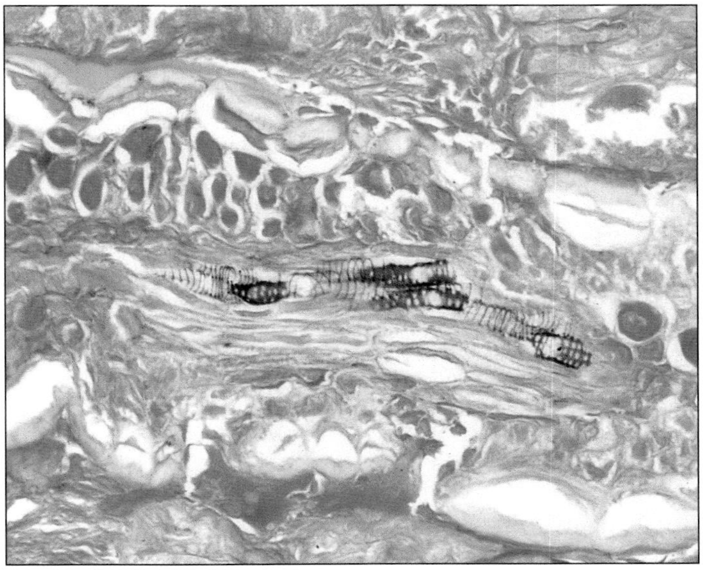
6

Plate 105

Artifacts

Image 1

Several objects of different sizes identified as Liesegang rings or Liesegang bodies. To the inexperienced, these do bear a superficial resemblance to parasite eggs. The striated walls vaguely suggest *Taenia* eggs. Others suggest that they look like *Dioctophyme* eggs (H&E, 1000x).

Image 2

In this section from the same case, a relatively large Liesegang body is present along with several smaller ones. The large one is different in appearance from those seen in the previous figure within the same field (H&E, 500x).

Image 3

Section from a human case in which Liesegang bodies were initially and incorrectly identified as eggs and adults of the nematode parasite *Dioctophyme renale*, the giant kidney worm. The numerous ringlike structures measure 25 to 35 µm in diameter and have a relatively thick wall (H&E, 500x).

Image 4

At slightly higher magnification, several rings can be seen. Their variability in shape and appearance should suggest objects other than parasite eggs. They have no features suggesting nematode structures, and therefore should not be confused with sections of worms (H&E, 700x).

Image 5

In another field, the structures are much larger, measuring up to 60 µm in length, and are different in appearance from those in Image 1. The differences in size and shape from one field to another suggest artifactual changes rather than organisms (H&E, 500x).

Image 6

At higher magnification, a large, elongated Liesegang body is seen. These bodies may attain lengths of 75 to 100 µm, and they have been interpreted as remnants of an adult parasitic worm (H&E, 1000x).

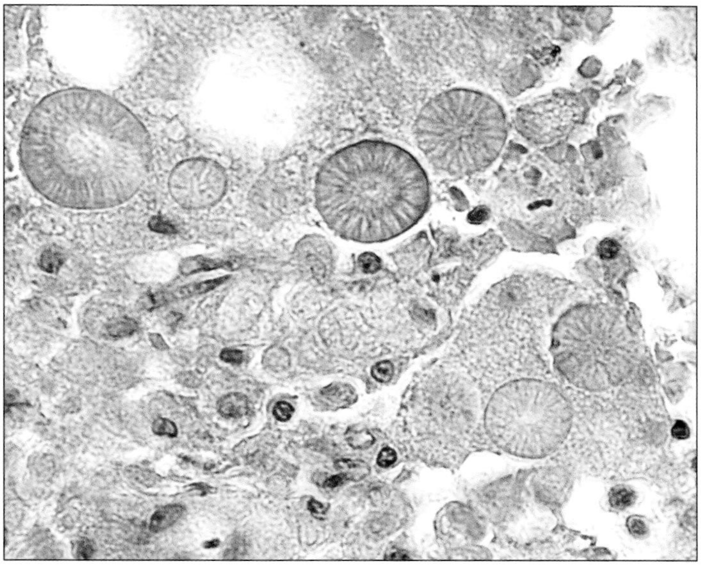

1

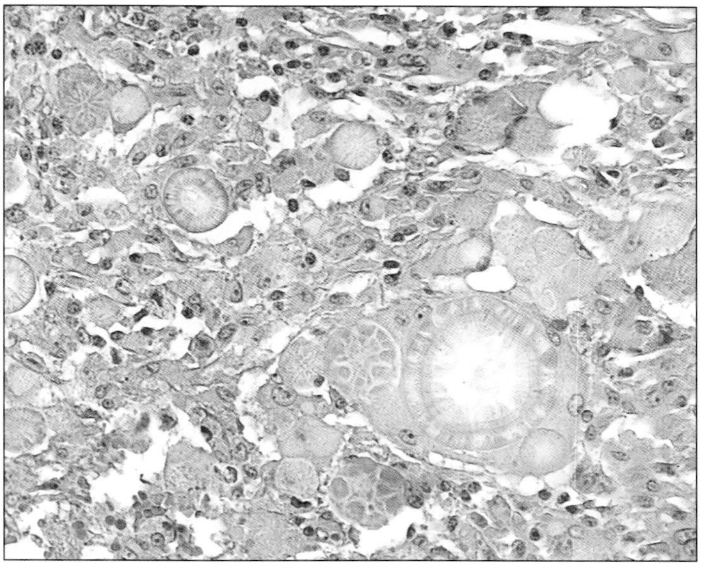

2

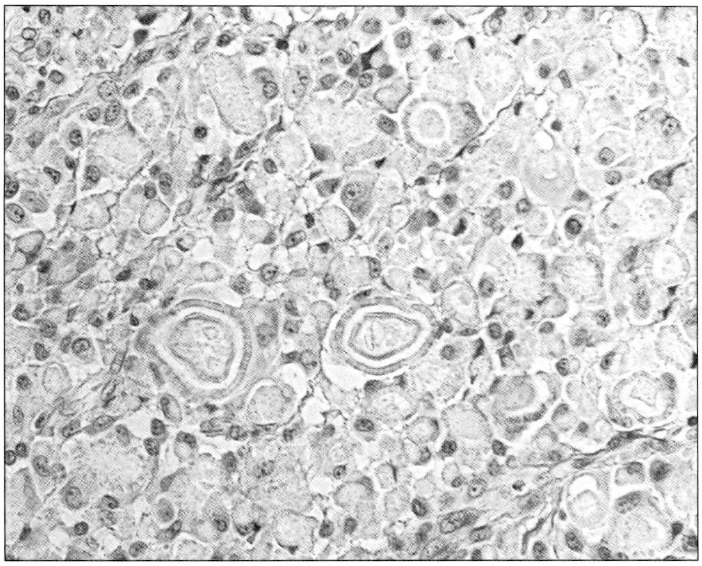

3

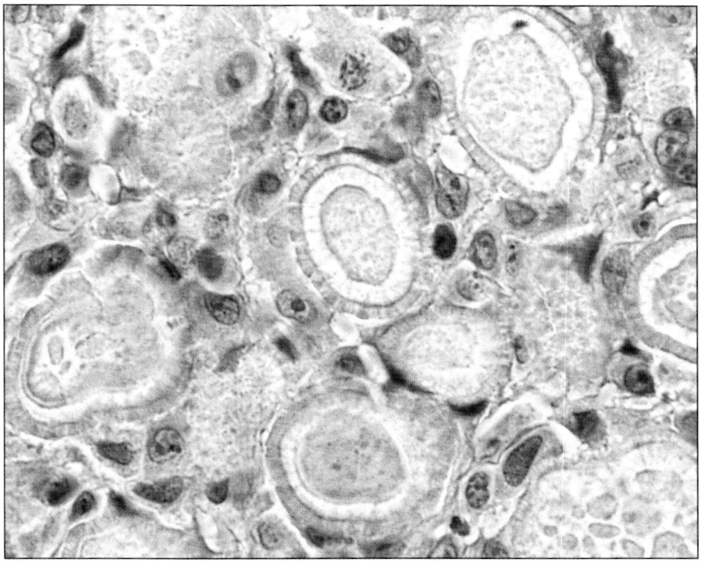

4

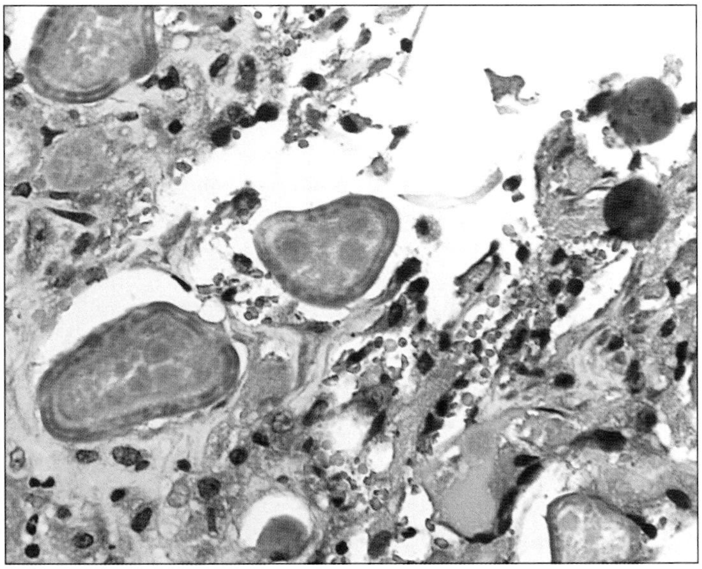

5

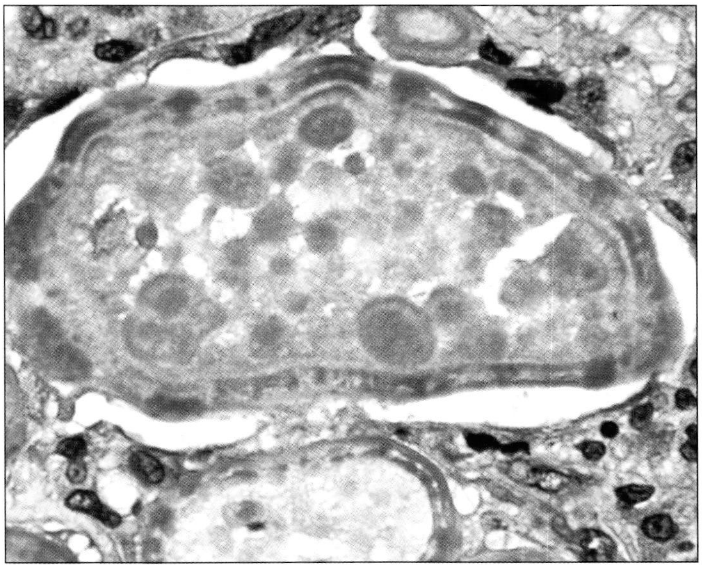

6

Plate 106

Artifacts

Image 1

Unidentified spores (arrows) found in material collected by fine-needle aspiration from a "pseudotumoral, paraaortic mass." These objects, which were identified as fragments of the nematode *Dirofilaria repens*, measured 20 to 35 µm in diameter. They appear to have a thick wall with an amorphous content (700x).

Image 2

At higher magnification, a thick, golden wall with an internal amorphous mass lacks any structure suggestive of a nematode parasite or a nematode egg. These objects appear to be contaminants of the aspirated material that was sectioned for study (H&E, 1200x).

Image 3

Object seen in an intestinal biopsy specimen and initially identified as the ciliate *Balantidium coli*. The objects seen in various sections measured about 35 to 45 µm in diameter (H&E, 1000x).

Image 4

A different object, found in the same specimen as that shown in Image 3, displays a striated outer membrane. Although not inconsistent with *B. coli* from the standpoint of size, the external limiting membrane and the internal contents suggest a spore of some kind. The dark-staining mass in the "cytoplasm" of the object suggested to the initial viewer the macronucleus of *B. coli*. This object is probably a spore (H&E, 1000x).

Images 5 and 6

Section of lung from a resident of Honduras in which small, egglike objects (keyline) can be seen. They were suspected to be eggs of *Paragonimus*, although they are really a hyphomycete, *Emmonsia*. At higher magnification, none of the features suggest a diagnosis of *Paragonimus* (H&E; 50x, 100x).

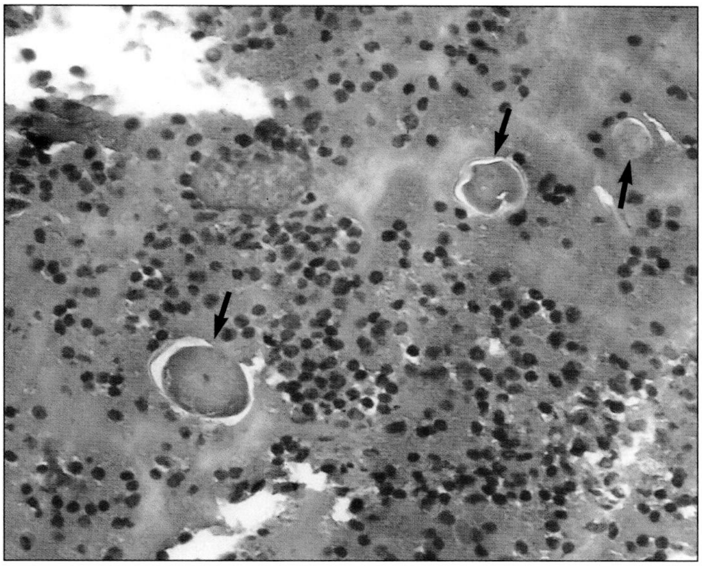
1

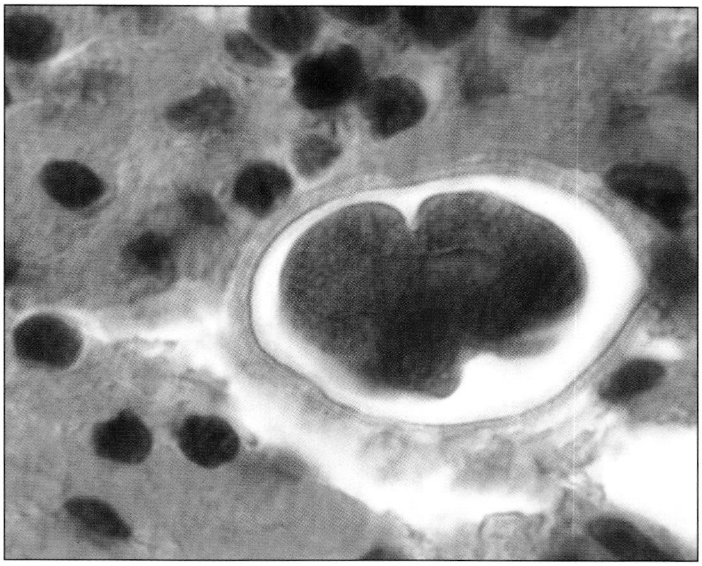
2

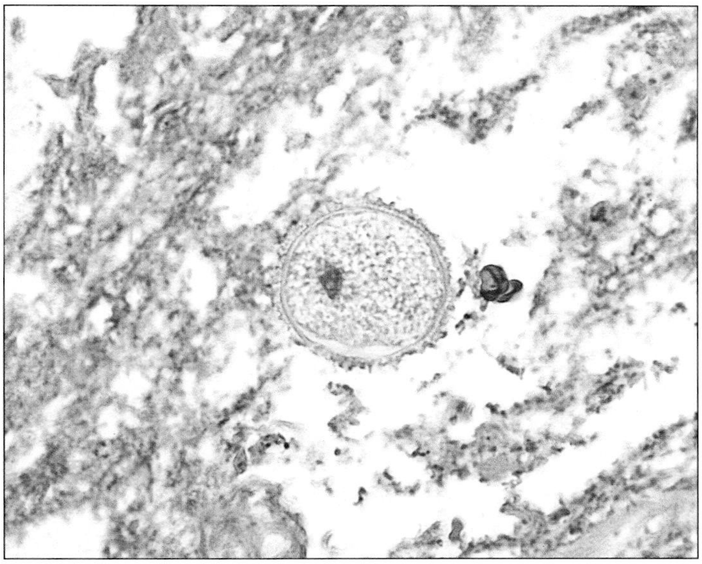
3

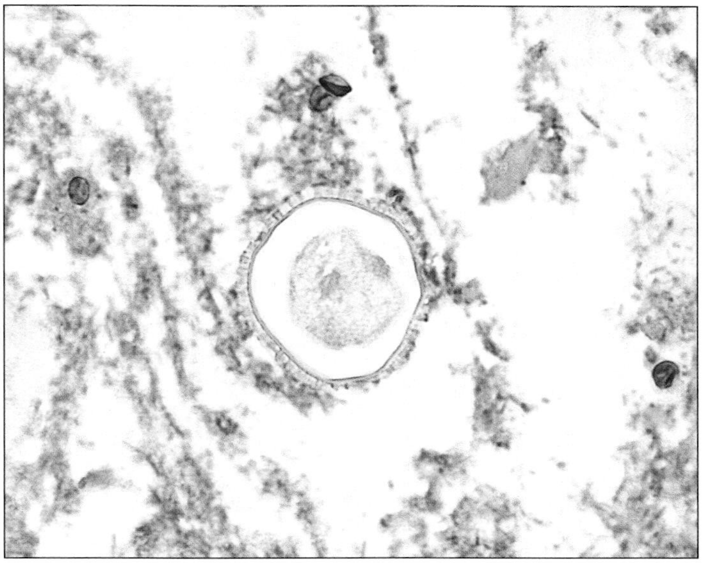
4

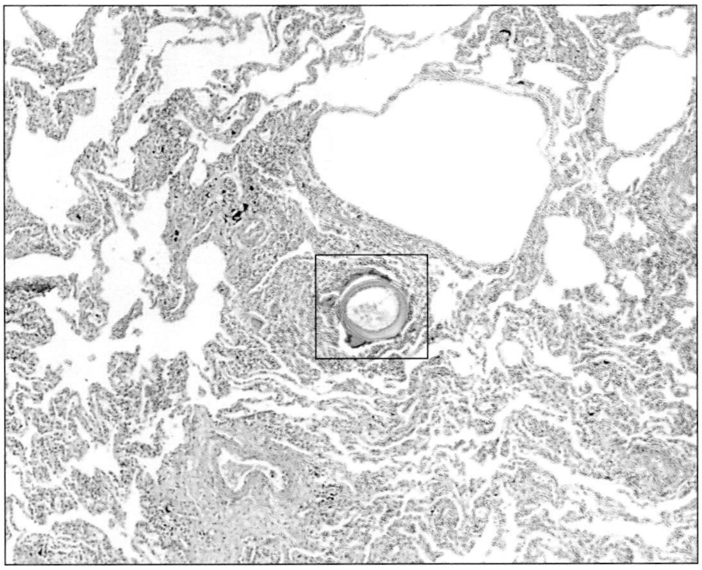
5

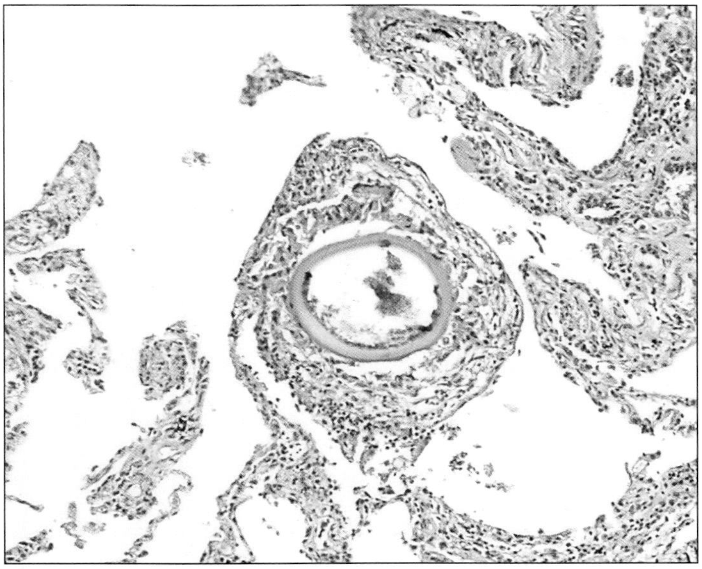
6

Plate 107

Artifacts

Images 1 and 2

Section of bone marrow containing "things" (darts). The individual submitting the sample noted, "We see [them] frequently and have not been able to figure out exactly what they are." These are cotton fibers that have contaminated the tissue sample, probably in the collection process. The fibers are approximately 30 µm in diameter and are hollow (H&E, 100x; 200x).

Images 3 and 4

Dust mites contaminating another bone marrow sample. In Image 3, a portion of the body and some of the legs and spines of the mite are visible (keyline). In Image 4, a mite cut in longitudinal section shows the major portion of the body as well as a leg, mouth parts, and an antenna (H&E; 200x, 400x).

Image 5

In this vaginal smear, a detached ciliary tuft of columnar epithelial cells is present. These may be seen in a variety of tissue fluids, secretions, and the like (Papanicolaou, 1200x).

Image 6

A fiber lodged on a Nuclepore® filter. Blood had been passed through the filter in a search for microfilariae. When examined at high magnification, this structure did not show any structural features of a microfilaria (Hematoxylin, 300x).

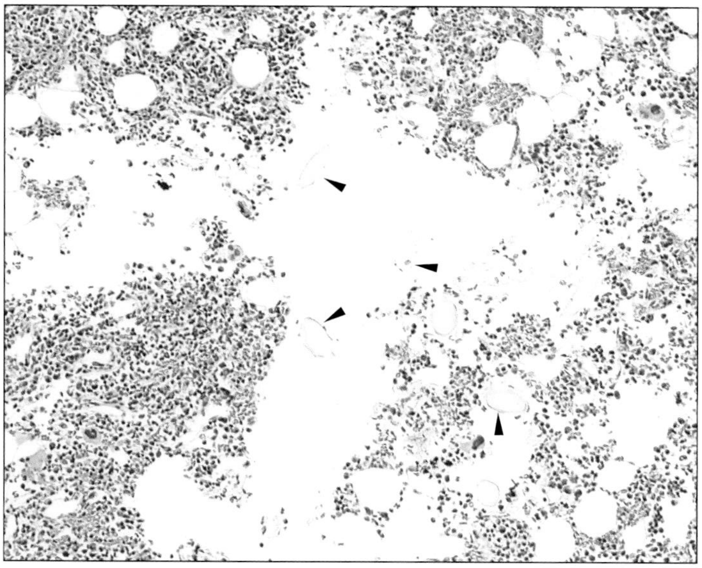
1

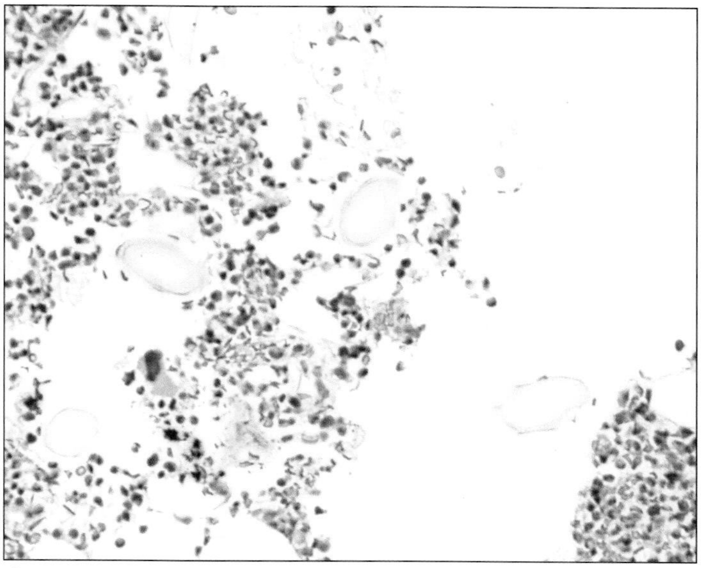
2

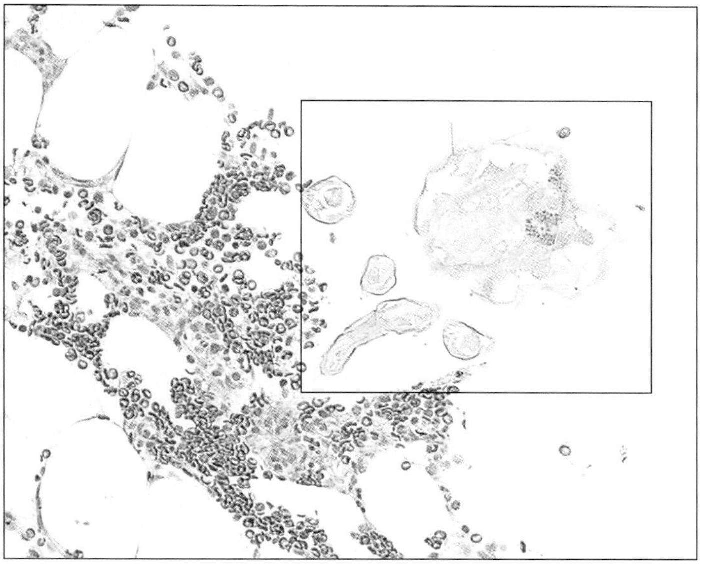
3

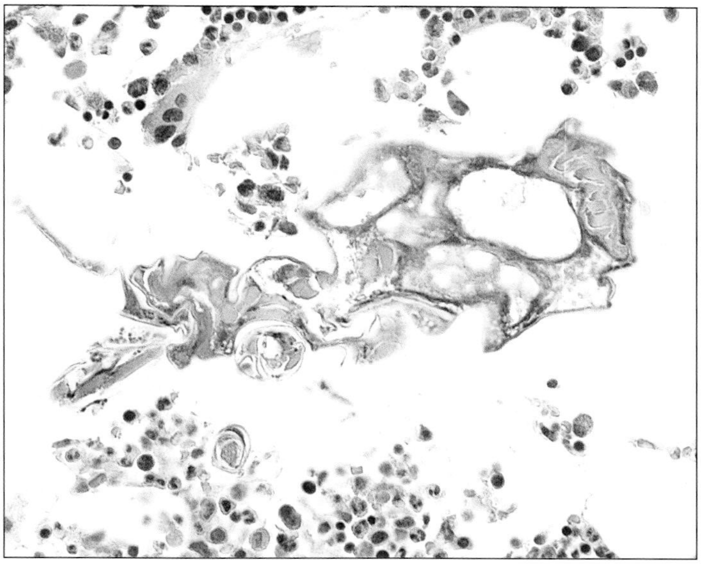
4

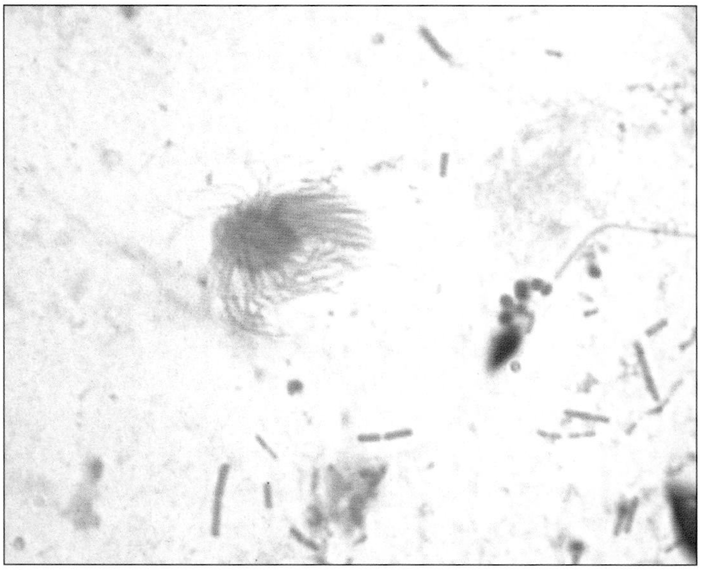
5

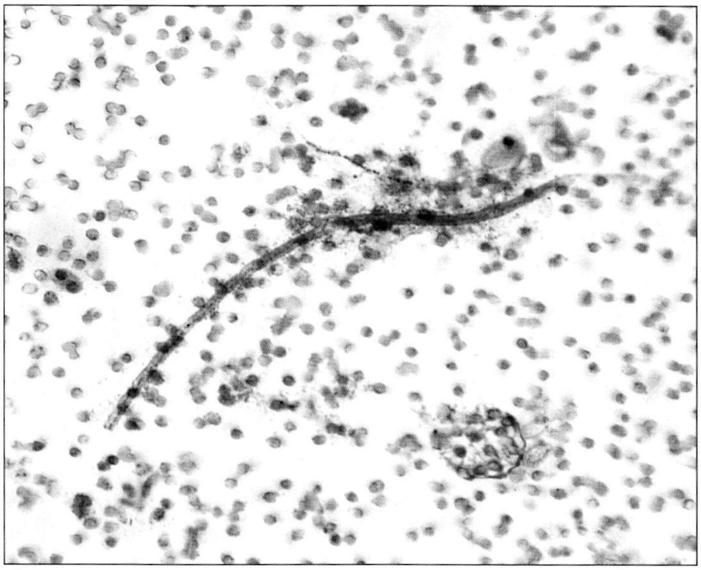
6

Glossary

Acanthella. Larva of an acanthocephalan that develops from the acanthor.

Acanthor. Larval stage of an acanthocephalan that hatches from an egg.

Acetabulum. Another name for the ventral sucker of a trematode. This term also applies to the suckers on the scolex of a tapeworm.

AIDS. Acquired immune deficiency syndrome.

Alae. Longitudinal thickenings or projections of the cuticle of nematodes, usually situated in lateral or sublateral regions of the body. These are especially prominent in larval stages.

Amastigote. Small, rounded, intracellular morphologic stage found in species of *Leishmania* and in *Trypanosoma cruzi*. Amastigotes lack an external flagellum. Also called Leishman-Donovan body or leishmanial stage.

Ameboma. Chronic granulomatous lesion caused by *Entamoeba histolytica* that may develop in the cecal or rectosigmoid region of colon.

Amphidelphic. Condition of reproductive system in nematodes in which the paired uteri are opposed and proceed separately in anteriad and posteriad directions from the opening of the vagina.

Anisakid. Nematodes belonging to the Family Anisakidae. Adult worms principally live in sea mammals. Larval stages develop in fish and when eaten by humans cause anisakiasis.

Axoneme. The core of a cilium or flagellum that is made up of microtubules in a "9 + 2" arrangement.

Axostyle. Rodlike supporting organelle extending from apical to posterior end of certain flagellate protozoa. The axostyle may project from the posterior end in some species.

Bacillary band. Structure present in trichinelloid nematodes; composed of hypodermal gland cells that communicate with the surface through cuticular pores.

Ballonets. Four inflatable areas of the head bulb of *Gnathostoma* species, each of which is connected to a cervical sac lying adjacent to the esophagus.

Basal body. Structure from which the axoneme arises in flagellates; also called a blepharoplast, kinetosome, or centriole.

Bilharziasis. Disease caused by *Schistosoma* species; synonymous with schistosomiasis.

Blepharoplast. *See* basal body.

Bosses. Blisterlike inflations or plaques on the surface of the cuticle of some nematodes (eg, *Gongylonema*).

Bot fly. Flies of the Family Gasterophilidae. Bot-fly maggots parasitize the stomach and other tissues of equids and other mammals.

Bothrium. Shallow dorsal or ventral groove on the scolex of some pseudophyllidean tapeworms (eg, *Diphyllobothrium*).

Bradyzoite. A type of merozoite that develops slowly within tissue cysts in chronic infections of some of the intestinal coccidia (eg, *Toxoplasma, Sarcocystis*).

Bulb. Posterior expanded portion of muscular esophagus in some nematodes (eg, *Enterobius*).

Bursa. Expanded, umbrellalike modification of posterior end of strongylid male nematodes. Used in copulation, the bursa is supported by fingerlike, muscular rays and is useful for taxonomy (eg, hookworms, trichostrongyles, metastrongyles).

Calabar swellings. Transient swellings of joints and subcutaneous tissues associated with infection with *Loa loa*; also known as "fugitive" swellings.

Calcareous corpuscles. Small round or oval bodies enclosed in a cell membrane. These occur in platyhelminthes and are seen most prominently in the parenchyma of cestodes. Calcareous corpuscles have an organic matrix organized into concentric layers that chemically contain calcium, magnesium, phosphorus, and carbonate. They are especially prominent in larval cestodes.

Cercaria. Tailed, free-swimming larval stage of trematodes, which is produced by asexual reproduction in the molluscan intermediate host. Cercaria may infect definitive hosts directly (eg, schistosomes) or undergo encystation to the metacercarial stage in other intermediate hosts.

Chagas' disease. Human infection with *Trypanosoma cruzi*.

Chagoma. An erythematous, indurated area that develops at the site of initial infection with metacyclic trypomastigotes of *Trypanosoma cruzi*.

Charcot-Leyden crystals. Crystals of varying size formed from breakdown products of eosinophils. These crystals are slender and shaped like a double pyramid with pointed ends. They are found in the sputum, feces, or tissues of patients with allergic conditions and often indicate tissue invasion by helminth parasites.

Chigoe flea. Common name for *Tunga penetrans*.

Chitin. Nitrogenous polysaccharide that occurs in the cuticle of arthropods.

Chords. The bulging of the hypodermis into the pseudocoelom of nematodes, typically in the dorsal, ventral, and lateral positions. The lateral chords vary in size and morphology among nematode groups and are an extremely useful morphologic characteristic when identifying nematodes in tissue sections.

Cilium. Essentially the same as a flagellum, except that a flagellum is usually much longer. These hairlike or whiplike organelles arise from a basal body and project from the body surface of the organism. With electron microscopy, the internal axoneme is composed of microtubules in a "9 + 2" arrangement.

Circomyarian. Type of muscle cell in nematodes in which the cytoplasmic portion of cell is entirely surrounded by contractile fibers.

Cirrus. Muscular male copulatory organ found in trematodes and cestodes.

Coelomocytes. Cells of mesenchymatous origin present in the pseudocoelom of nematodes and other invertebrates.

Coelomyarian. Muscle cell type in which contractile fibrils are perpendicular to the hypodermis and also extend up the lateral margins of the cytoplasmic portion of the cell in various nematodes.

Coenurus. Larval tapeworm (metacestode) of some species of the Family Taeniidae (*Taenia,* formerly placed in genus *Multiceps).* The coenurus is characterized by its multiple scoleces, which invaginate into a fluid-filled bladder.

Conoid. When visualized by electron microscopy, this hollow, electron-dense structure is found within the polar ring at the anterior end of merozoites, tachyzoites, bradyzoites, and some other stages of apicomplexan protozoans. It is composed of spirally coiled microtubules (eg, *Toxoplasma, Sarcocystis*).

Copepod. Aquatic, invertebrate, intermediate host of numerous helminth parasites (eg, *Diphyllobothrium, Spirometra, Dracunculus, Gnathostoma*).

Coracidium. A ciliated, six-hooked embryo present in eggs of pseudophyllidean tapeworms (eg, *Spirometra, Diphyllobothrium*).

Corpus. The narrow anterior portion of the muscular esophagus of certain nematodes (eg, *Enterobius*).

Creeping eruption. Synonymous with cutaneous larva migrans and "ground itch," creeping eruption is caused by skin-penetrating nematodes, which migrate through skin and subcutaneous tissues (eg, dog and cat hookworm larvae, *Ancylostoma* species).

Cryptosporidiosis. Intestinal infection with the coccidian *Cryptosporidium* species.

Cysticercosis. Tissue infection with the larval stage of *Taenia* species. The infection is caused by a metacestode with a single scolex invaginated into a fluid-filled bladder (eg, *T. solium*).

Cysticercus. The larval stage of many tapeworms belonging to the genus *Taenia.* A single scolex is invaginated into a fluid-filled bladder (eg, *T. solium, T. saginata*).

Cuticle. The nonliving, noncellular layer secreted by the underlying hypodermis in nematodes.

Cytophaneres. Thickly set projections or villi on the tissue cyst wall of numerous coccidian species of the genus *Sarcocystis*.

Definitive host. The host in which the adult stage of a parasite develops. Frequently, but not always, the host in which sexual reproduction of the parasite occurs.

Demodicidosis. Infestation of the skin with *Demodex* species.

Didelphic. Female nematodes with paired reproductive tubes.

Dioecious. Having separate sexes.

Distome. Fluke with an oral and a ventral sucker.

Diurnal periodicity. Microfilariae found in the peripheral blood only during the day (eg, *Loa loa*).

Ectopic. Infection that occurs in a location other than the normal or expected site.

Ectoplasm. Outer layer of cytoplasm that typically is clear and nongranular in amebic trophozoites (eg, *Entamoeba histolytica*).

Endodyogeny. Formation of two individual daughter cells, each surrounded by its own membrane, while still in mother cell (eg, *Toxoplasma, Sarcocystis*).

Endoplasm. Inner, granular layer of cytoplasm in amebic trophozoites (eg, *Entamoeba histolytica*).

Eosinophilic meningoencephalitis. Although this may occur in a number of helminthic infections, it usually describes human infection with *Angiostrongylus cantonensis.*

Epimastigote. Morphologic stage of trypanosomes and leishmanias. The flagellum arises anteriad to the centrally located nucleus and emerges laterally, forming a short undulating membrane as it runs along the remainder of the body and emerges as a free flagellum at the anterior end.

Espundia. Disfiguring tissue destruction of the nose and mouth caused by leishmanial organisms in mucocutaneous leishmaniasis (eg, *Leishmania braziliensis*).

Filariform larva. Infective-stage larva of various nematodes in which the esophagus is long, slender, and lacks a bulb (eg, *Strongyloides,* hookworms).

Flagellum. *See* cilium. Many types of flagella on parasitic organisms are characterized by their number, their position, and whether they are associated with an undulating membrane.

Fluke. A common name for a trematode.

Gametocyte. Sexual cell (macrogametocyte in the female; microgametocyte in the male) that produces gametes in apicomplexan protozoans. Also called a gamont.

Genital atrium. Cavity in the body wall of trematodes and cestodes into which the male and female genital ducts open.

Genital primordium. Small group of cells that give rise to the adult reproductive system.

Gnathosoma. The region bearing mouthparts in arthropods.

Gubernaculum. Sclerotized accessory reproductive structure in some nematodes that usually forms a troughlike structure in the posterior part of body in which the spicules may slide. The gubernaculum may be simple or complex in morphology and is often useful for taxonomic purposes.

Gynecophoral canal. A ventral folding of the lateral margins of the male schistosome; within this troughlike structure the female worm is held in permanent or semipermanent copula.

Halzoun. Congestion of the nasopharyngeal mucosa resulting in respiratory difficulties; caused by larval pentastomes (eg, *Linguatula* species).

Helminth. Term used for nematodes (nemathelminthes) and trematodes and cestodes (platyhelminthes).

Hemozoin. Metabolic waste product of malarial parasites that is composed of hematin and excess protein. Hemozoin appears as brown pigment granules in organisms and macrophages and is often referred to as malarial pigment.

Hermaphroditism. Presence of male and female reproductive systems in the same individual (eg, cestodes and most trematodes).

Hexacanth embryo. *See* oncosphere.

Hydatid cyst. Larval (metacestode) stage of *Echinococcus* species that may be unilocular (*E. granulosus*), multilocular (*E. multilocularis*), or polycystic (*E. vogeli*).

Hydatid sand. Sediment found in a hydatid cyst that consists of free, degenerating protoscoleces, hooks, and calcareous corpuscles.

Hypnozoite. Dormant exoerythrocytic stage of sporozoites of *Plasmodium vivax* and *P. ovale* occurring in the liver parenchymal cells of a mammalian host. Hypnozoites are regarded as the source of relapses of malarial infection in these species.

Hypodermis. Structure that secretes an overlaying cuticle. The bulging of the hypodermis into the pseudocoelom occurs in nematodes to form typically dorsal, ventral, and lateral chords. Also called epidermis.

Intermediate host. A host in the life cycle of some parasites in which required larval development occurs. Following this development, the larva will be infective to the definitive host or, less frequently, a second intermediate host.

Kala-azar. Disease caused by *Leishmania donovani, L. chagasi,* or *L. infantum.* Another name for visceral leishmaniasis.

Karyosome. Single, sometimes fragmented body of densely packed, DNA-rich, nuclear chromatin within the nucleus of protozoa. Karyosomes are Feulgen positive. Their position and morphology are especially useful for identification of amebae.

Kinetosome. *See* basal body.

Lacunar system. System of canals within the body wall of acanthocephalans that function as a circulatory system.

Larva migrans. Migration of larval stages of parasites in human tissues (eg, *Toxocara canis, Gnathostoma* species). *See* creeping eruption.

Leishman-Donovan body. The amastigote stage of some hemoflagellates (eg, *Leishmania* species).

Liesegang bodies. Ringlike, laminated structures found in various human tissues and aspirates. Liesegang bodies develop by a complex process of supersaturated solutions precipitating in colloidal systems.

Loeffler's syndrome. Pneumonitis caused by migrating larvae of *Ascaris lumbricoides.* Clinical picture includes transient, migratory lung infiltrates on x-rays, cough, and marked peripheral eosinophilia.

Macrogametocyte. Cell that becomes a female gamete.

Macronucleus. Large, kidney-bean–shaped nucleus seen in *Balantidium coli.*

Megacolon. Pathologic condition seen in chronic Chagas' disease in which the colon is much enlarged, flabby, and contains large amounts of liquid feces.

Megaesophagus. Distention of the esophagus in chronic Chagas' disease, resulting in dysphagia.

Meromyarian. Presence of only a few (two to five) muscle cells in each quadrant between the chords in the body wall of nematodes.

Merozoite. Daughter cells resulting from schizogony (eg, malaria).

Mesenchyme. Nonspecialized connective tissue occurring in trematodes and cestodes.

Mesocercaria. A larval stage of the trematode genus *Alaria.* This nonencysted form can migrate in both human and animal tissues.

Metacercaria. A stage in most trematode life cycles between the cercaria and adult worm. It encysts in tissues or on vegetation and is the infective stage for the definitive host.

Metacestode. A larval cestode.

Metrocyte. Large, round cell occurring in tissue cysts of certain coccidians. This cell undergoes division by endodyogeny to form new metrocytes that mature to become bradyzoites (eg, *Sarcocystis* species).

Microfilaremia. The presence in the bloodstream of microfilariae, which are produced by adult filarial worms.

Microfilariae. Embryos produced by filarial worms. Microfilariae are released into the bloodstream or tissues and are infective to the arthropod vector.

Microgametocyte. Cell that produces male gametes.

Microtriches. Minute projections from the tegument of cestodes that increase the absorptive area of tegument.

Miracidium. Ciliated embryo that develops in trematode eggs. This stage is infective for the snail intermediate host.

Monodelphic. Having only a single set of reproductive organs. Typical for some nematodes.

Myiasis. Infestation of the tissues by fly larvae (maggots).

Nocturnal periodicity. Microfilariae found in the peripheral blood only during nighttime hours (eg, *Wuchereria bancrofti*).

Onchocercoma. Subcutaneous nodule containing adult worms of *Onchocerca volvulus*.

Oncosphere. Six-hooked larva in cestode eggs. Synonymous with hexacanth embryo.

Oocyst. Cyst form in apicomplexan protozoans that results from sporogony. It may (eg, *Toxoplasma, Cryptosporidium*) or may not (*Plasmodium* species) have a hard, resistant membrane.

Ookinete. Motile zygote of malaria parasite. The ookinete occurs in the stomach of the mosquito intermediate host and is produced from the fusion of male and female gametes.

Operculum. Specialized lidlike structure on parasite eggs (eg, trematodes and pseudophyllidean tapeworms) through which the larval stage escapes.

Parasitophorous vacuole. A fluid-filled vacuole within a host cell that surrounds developing intracellular apicomplexan protozoans. The membrane of the vacuole is derived from the host cell.

Paratenic host. A host that is not required in the life cycle of a parasite but when utilized by larval stages enhances their opportunity to be ultimately ingested by a definitive host. Little or no necessary growth of the larval stage occurs in this host. Same as a transport host (eg, *Anisakis, Diphyllobothrium*).

Parthenogenesis. Type of reproduction in which the organism undergoes development without fertilization by a male gamete (eg, *Strongyloides stercoralis*).

Pentastomiasis. Disease caused by species of the Phylum Pentastomida (eg, *Armillifer, Linguatula*).

Platymyarian. Muscle cell type in nematodes in which the contractile portion of the cell is wide, shallow, and perpendicular to the hypodermis.

Plerocercoid. A ribbonlike larval cestode that follows the procercoid stage. This is the infective stage for the definitive host, and it may make extensive use of paratenic hosts (eg, *Diphyllobothrium* species, *Spirometra* species). Synonymous with sparganum.

Polar tube. Extrusible organelle of microsporidians that is spirally coiled within the spore. Sporoplasm from the spore is ejected into the host cell via this tube.

Prepatent period. The biologic incubation period from entry of an infective parasite stage into the body until the parasites or their products can be demonstrated in feces, blood, or other excreta by diagnostic procedures.

Procercoid. Larval cestode that develops within a copepod intermediate host after it is infected by a coracidium. Typical in some pseudophyllidean cestodes (eg, *Spirometra* species).

Prodelphic. In nematodes, uteri are parallel and directed anteriorly from the point of origin at the vagina.

Proglottid. A single segment of an adult tapeworm that contains a set of both male and female reproductive organs and can be divided into immature, mature, and gravid forms.

Protoscolex. Juvenile scolex found within a coenurus or a hydatid cyst.

Pseudocoelom. Body cavity of nematodes that is not completely lined with epithelium of mesodermal origin. Also referred to as the pseudocoel.

Pseudocyst. Cystlike stage containing numerous cells of a protozoan parasite in which the surrounding wall or membrane is of host origin (eg, *Toxoplasma gondii*).

Rhabditiform larva. A nematode larva in which the esophagus consists of the anterior corpus, a narrowed isthmus, and an expanded bulb (eg, hookworm and *Strongyloides*).

Rhoptries. Elongate, electron-dense, tubular or club-shaped organelles that occur within the polar ring of the apical complex of apicomplexan protozoans.

Romaña's sign. Conjunctivitis and unilateral edema of the upper and lower eyelids (often involving the cheek) that occurs in individuals recently infected with *Trypanosoma cruzi*.

Rostellum. Cone-shaped or cylindrical projection at the anterior end of the scolex of some tapeworms. It may or may not be retractable and may have hooklets (*Taenia solium*) or lack hooklets (*T. saginata*).

Schizogony. Asexual multiplication by multiple fission in malarial parasites in which merozoites are formed. Exoerythrocytic schizogony occurs in parenchymal cells of liver, and erythrocytic schizogony occurs in red blood cells.

Sclerotized. Hardened or thickened areas of the cuticle and other structures in nematodes as well as the exoskeleton in arthropods.

Scolex. The head end or holdfast organ of tapeworms; may have bothria or suckers.

Sheath. Cuticle of larval nematodes that is retained around the body by some species after a molt (eg, hookworm filariform larvae). Also refers to vitelline membrane that has been retained around the body of some microfilariae (eg, *Wuchereria bancrofti, Brugia malayi, Loa loa*).

Sparganum. *See* plerocercoid. When humans are infected, the disease is referred to as sparganosis.

Spicules. Rod-shaped, sclerotized accessory reproductive structures, usually paired, at the posterior end of male nematodes. The spicules aid in copulation, are simple to complex in morphology, and are often useful for nematode classification.

Sporoblast. Cell mass that differentiates into a sporocyst within the oocyst of certain coccidians (eg, *Isospora belli*, *Sarcocystis* species).

Sporocyst. A cyst stage within some of the intestinal coccidians that contains sporozoites (infective stages).

Sporogony. Asexual process of multiplication by repeated division of a zygote, which results in the formation of sporocysts (if present in the life cycle) and sporozoites. Typical in coccidians and other sporozoans.

Sporozoite. Slender, spindle-shaped, motile infective stages in coccidian life cycles; the result of sporogony.

Stichosome. Column of stichocytes (esophageal gland cells) that surround and are a source of secretion into the thin capillary esophagus of nematodes belonging to the Trichinelloidea (eg, *Trichuris, Trichinella*).

Stoma. Mouth cavity of nematodes that lies between the oral opening and the beginning of the esophagus.

Striae. Transverse markings of the cuticle of nematodes that vary in width and depth. The striae may also be longitudinal and give a blocklike appearance to the cuticle.

Strobila. Structure that encompasses the entire chain of proglottids of a tapeworm, excluding the scolex and neck.

Tachyzoites. Fast-developing merozoites that divide in host cells by endodyogeny during the acute stage of infection (eg, *Toxoplasma gondii*).

Tetrathyridium. Large, solid-bodied, cysticercoid-type cestode larval stage that occurs in the genus *Mesocestoides*.

Tracheae. Small, cuticular-lined tubes that are part of the respiratory system in many arthropods.

Transport host. *See* paratenic host.

Trophozoite. Active, vegetative, feeding stage of a protozoan.

Trypomastigote. Morphologic form of trypanosomatid flagellates in which the flagellum arises near the posterior end of the body, posterior to the nucleus. The flagellum emerges laterally to form a long, undulating membrane as it runs along the length of the body before emerging as a free flagellum at the anterior end. This occurs in the bloodstream and is often referred to as trypanosome (eg, *Trypanosoma cruzi*).

Vector. Living carrier or transporter, usually an arthropod or mollusk, that transmits parasites from one host to another.

Ventriculus. Glandular modification of the posterior portion of the esophagus in some nematodes; may have a cecum arising from it (eg, *Anisakis, Pseudoterranova*).

Visceral larva migrans. This expression originally referred to the specific migration of larval ascarids (*Toxocara canis* and *T. cati*) in the human body; however, it may be used to describe the larval migration of all helminths in the deeper parts of the body.

Vitellaria. Yolk glands of trematodes and cestodes.

Zoonosis. Disease of animals that is transmissible to humans.

Recommended References

Atlases, Texts, and General References

Acha PN, Szyfres B. *Zoonoses and Communicable Diseases Common to Man and Animals.* 2nd ed. Washington, DC: Pan American Health Organization; 1987. Scientific Publication No. 503.

Ash JE, Spitz S. *Pathology of Tropical Diseases: An Atlas.* Philadelphia, Pa: WB Saunders Co; 1945.

Ash LR, Orihel TC. *Atlas of Human Parasitology.* 3rd ed. Chicago, Ill: ASCP Press; 1990.

Beaver PC, Jung RC, Cupp EW. *Clinical Parasitology.* 9th ed. Philadelphia, Pa: Lea & Febiger; 1984.

Binford CH, Connor DH. *Pathology of Tropical and Extraordinary Diseases: An Atlas.* Vols. 1 & 2. Washington, DC: Armed Forces Institute of Pathology; 1976.

Brown WJ, Voge M. *Neuropathology of Parasitic Infections.* Oxford, England: Oxford University Press; 1982.

Chitwood BG, Chitwood MB. *An Introduction to Nematology.* Baltimore, Md: Monumental Printing Co; 1950.

Chitwood MB, Lichtenfels JR. Identification of parasitic metazoa in tissue sections. *Exp Parasitol.* 1972;32:407–519.

Coombs I, Crompton DWT. *A Guide to Human Helminths.* London, England: Taylor & Francis; 1990.

Gutierrez Y. *Diagnostic Pathology of Parasitic Infections With Clinical Correlation.* Philadelphia, Pa: Lea & Febiger; 1990.

Harrison FW, Corliss JO. *Microscopic Anatomy of Invertebrates: Platyhelminthes and Nemertina.* New York, NY: Wiley-Liss Inc; 1991.

Harrison FW, Gardiner SL, eds. *Microscopic Anatomy of Invertebrates; Annelida.* New York, NY: Wiley-Liss Inc; 1992.

Hyman LH. *The Invertebrates: Platyhelminthes and Rhynchocoela.* New York, NY: McGraw-Hill Book Co Inc; 1951.

Hyman LH. *The Invertebrate: Acanthocephala, Aschelminthes, and Entoprocta.* New York, NY: McGraw-Hill Book Co Inc; 1951.

Kean BH, Sun T, Ellsworth RM. *Color Atlas/Text of Ophthalmic Parasitology.* New York, NY: Igaku-Shoin; 1991.

Marcial-Rojas RA, ed. *Pathology of Protozoal and Helminthic Diseases With Clinical Correlation.* Baltimore, Md: Williams & Wilkins Co; 1971.

Margulis L, Schwartz KV. *Five Kingdoms. An Illustrated Guide to the Phyla of Life on Earth.* San Francisco, Calif: WH Freeman Co; 1982.

Mehlhorn H, ed. *Parasitology in Focus: Facts and Trends.* Berlin, Germany: Springer-Verlag; 1988.

Miyazaki I. *An Illustrated Book of Helminthic Zoonoses.* Tokyo, Japan: International Medical Foundation of Japan; 1991.

Neafie RC, Marty AM. Unusual infections in humans. *Clin Microbiol Rev.* 1993;6:34-56.

Peters W, Gilles HM. *A Colour Atlas of Tropical Medicine and Parasitology.* 3rd ed. Boca Raton, Fla: CRC Press; 1989.

Reeder MM, Palmer PES. *The Radiology of Tropical Diseases With Epidemiological, Pathological and Clinical Correlation.* Baltimore, Md: Williams & Wilkins Co; 1981.

Salfelder K, Liscano TR, Sauerteig E. *Atlas of Parasitic Pathology.* Dordrecht, The Netherlands: Kluwer Academic Publishers; 1992.

Shaw AC, Lazell SK, Foster GN. *Photomicrographs of Invertebrates.* London, England: Longman Group Ltd; 1974.

Protozoa

Aikawa M, Sterling CR. *Intracellular Parasitic Protozoa.* New York, NY: Academic Press; 1974.

Anderson OR. *Comparative Protozoology. Ecology, Physiology, Life History.* Berlin, Germany: Springer-Verlag, 1988.

Canning EU, Lom J. *The Microsporidia of Vertebrates.* London, England: Academic Press; 1986.

Dubey JP, Beattie CP. *Toxoplasmosis of Animals and Man.* Boca Raton, Fla: CRC Press;1988.

Dubey JP, Speer CA, Fayer R. *Sarcocystosis of Animals and Man.* Boca Raton, Fla: CRC Press; 1988.

Gardiner CH, Fayer R, Dubey JP. *An Atlas of Protozoan Parasites in Animal Tissues.* Washington, DC: U.S. Department of Agriculture; 1988. Agriculture Handbook No. 651.

Harrison FW, Corliss JO. *Microscopic Anatomy of Invertebrates: Protozoa.* New York, NY: Wiley-Liss Inc; 1991.

Hughes WT. *Pneumocystis carinii Pneumonitis.* Boca Raton, Fla: CRC Press; 1987.

Lee JJ, Hutner SH, Bovee EC, eds. *An Illustrated Guide to the Protozoa.* Lawrence, Kan: Society of Protozoologists; 1985.

Martinez AJ. *Free-Living Amebas: Natural History, Prevention, Diagnosis, Pathology, and Treatment of Disease.* Boca Raton, Fla: CRC Press; 1985.

Meyer EA, ed. *Giardiasis.* Amsterdam, The Netherlands: Elsevier; 1990.

Molyneux DH, Ashford RW. *The Biology of Trypanosoma and Leishmania Parasites of Man and Domestic Animals.* London, England: Taylor & Francis; 1983.

Peters W, Killick-Kendrick R, eds. *The Leishmaniases in Biology and Medicine.* London, England: Academic Press; 1987.

Ravdin JI, ed. *Amebiasis: Human Infection by Entamoeba histolytica.* New York, NY: John Wiley & Sons; 1988.

Rondanelli EG, Scaglia M, eds. *Atlas of Human Protozoa.* Milan, Italy: Masson; 1993.

Tizard I, ed. *Immunology and Pathogenesis of Trypanosomiasis.* Boca Raton, Fla: CRC Press; 1985.

Wernsdorfer WH, McGregor I, eds. *Malaria: Principles and Practice of Malariology.* Edinburgh, Scotland: Churchill Livingstone; 1988.

Nematodes

Anderson RC. *Nematode Parasites of Vertebrates: Their Development and Transmission.* Wallingford, England: CAB International; 1992.

Bird AF, Bird J. *The Structure of Nematodes.* 2nd ed. San Diego, Calif: Academic Press Inc; 1991.

Boreham PFL, Atwell RB, eds. *Dirofilariasis.* Boca Raton, Fla: CRC Press; 1988.

Campbell WC, ed. *Trichinella and Trichinosis.* New York, NY: Plenum Press; 1983.

Gibbons LM. *SEM Guide to the Morphology of Nematode Parasites of Vertebrates.* Farnham Royal, United Kingdom: CAB International; 1986.

Gilles HM, Ball PAJ. *Hookworm Infections.* Amsterdam, The Netherlands: Elsevier; 1991.

Grove DI, ed. *Strongyloidiasis: A Major Roundworm Infection of Man.* London, England: Taylor & Francis; 1989.

Harrison FW, Ruppert EE, eds. *Microscopic Anatomy of Invertebrates: Aschelminthes.* New York, NY: Wiley-Liss Inc; 1991.

Ishikura H, Kikuchi K, eds. *Intestinal Anisakiasis in Japan.* Tokyo, Japan: Springer-Verlag; 1990.

Ishikura H, Namiki M, eds. *Gastric Anisakiasis in Japan: Epidemiology, Diagnosis, Treatment.* Tokyo, Japan: Springer-Verlag; 1989.

Levine ND. *Nematode Parasites of Domestic Animals and of Man*. 2nd ed. Minneapolis, Minn: Burgess Publishing Co; 1980.

Sasa M. *Human Filariasis*. Baltimore, Md: University Park Press; 1976.

Trematodes

Malek EA. *Snail-Transmitted Parasitic Diseases*. Boca Raton, Fla: CRC Press; 1980.

Rollinson D, Simpson AJG. *The Biology of Schistosomes: From Genes to Latrines*. London, England: Academic Press; 1987.

Smyth JD, Halton DW. *The Physiology of Trematodes*. 2nd ed. Cambridge, Mass: Cambridge University Press; 1983.

Cestodes

Arme C, Pappas PW, eds. *Biology of the Eucestoda*. London, England: Academic Press; 1983.

Flisser AKW, Willms K, Laclette JP, et al, eds. *Cysticercosis: Present State of Knowledge and Perspectives*. New York, NY: Academic Press; 1982.

Schmidt GD. *Handbook of Tapeworm Identification*. Boca Raton, Fla: CRC Press; 1986.

Slais J. *The Morphology and Pathogenicity of the Bladder Worms: Cysticercus cellulosae and Cysticercus bovis*. Prague, Czechoslovakia: Academia Publishing House of the Czechoslovak Academy of Sciences; 1970.

Smyth JD, McManus DP. *The Physiology and Biochemistry of Cestodes*. Cambridge, Mass: Cambridge University Press; 1989.

Thompson RCA, ed. *The Biology of Echinococcus and Hydatid Disease*. London, England: George Allen & Unwin; 1986.

Arthropods

Alexander JO. *Arthropods and Human Skin*. Berlin, Germany: Springer-Verlag; 1984.

Burgess NRH, Cowan GO. *A Colour Atlas of Medical Entomology*. London, England: Chapman & Hall Medical; 1993.

Goddard J. *Physician's Guide to Arthropods of Medical Importance*. Boca Raton, Fla: CRC Press; 1993.

Harwood RF, James MT. *Entomology in Human and Animal Health*. 7th ed. New York, NY: Macmillan Publishing Co Inc; 1979.

James MT. *The Flies That Cause Myiasis in Man*. Washington, DC: U.S. Department of Agriculture; 1947. Miscellaneous Publication No. 631.

Lane RP, Crosskey RW. *Medical Insects and Arachnids*. London, England: Chapman & Hall Medical; 1993.

Peters W. *A Colour Atlas of Arthropods in Clinical Medicine*. London, England: Wolfe Publishing Ltd; 1992.

Rothschild M, Schlein Y, Ito S. *A Colour Atlas of Insect Tissues via the Flea*. Weert, The Netherlands: Wolfe Publishing Ltd; 1986.

Zumpt F. *Myiasis in Man and Animals in the Old World*. London, England: Butterworths; 1965.

Veterinary Parasitology and Parasites of Laboratory Animals

Dunn AM. *Veterinary Helminthology*. 2nd ed. London, England: William Heinemann Medical Books Ltd; 1981.

Flynn RJ. *Parasites of Laboratory Animals*. Ames, Iowa: Iowa State University Press; 1973.

Georgi JR. *Parasitology for Veterinarians*. 2nd ed. Philadelphia, Pa: WB Saunders Co; 1974.

Levine ND. *Veterinary Protozoology*. Ames, Iowa: Iowa State University Press; 1985.

Soulsby EJL. *Helminths, Arthropods and Protozoa of Domesticated Animals*. 7th ed. Philadelphia, Pa: Lea & Febiger; 1982.

Index

Page numbers in boldface indicate clinical images and color plates. See the quick reference tables (pp.xiv–xxi) and the glossary (p.371) for additional references to the subjects indexed below.

C

O

P